D1563319

# MEDICINE MEETS VIRTUAL REALITY 13

# Studies in Health Technology and Informatics

This book series was started in 1990 to promote research conducted under the auspices of the EC programmes Advanced Informatics in Medicine (AIM) and Biomedical and Health Research (BHR), bioengineering branch. A driving aspect of international health informatics is that telecommunication technology, rehabilitative technology, intelligent home technology and many other components are moving together and form one integrated world of information and communication media.

The complete series has been accepted in Medline. In the future, the SHTI series will be available online.

Series Editors:
Dr. J.P. Christensen, Prof. G. de Moor, Prof. A. Hasman, Prof. L. Hunter,
Dr. I. Iakovidis, Dr. Z. Kolitsi, Dr. Olivier Le Dour, Dr. Andreas Lymberis, Dr. Peter
Niederer, Prof. A. Pedotti, Prof. O. Rienhoff, Prof. F.H. Roger France, Dr. N. Rossing,
Prof. N. Saranummi, Dr. E.R. Siegel and Dr. Petra Wilson

## Volume 111

*Recently published in this series*

ISSN 0926-9630

# Medicine Meets Virtual Reality 13

*The Magical Next Becomes the Medical Now*

Edited by

James D. Westwood

Randy S. Haluck MD FACS

Helene M. Hoffman PhD

Greg T. Mogel MD

Roger Phillips PhD CEng MBCS

Richard A. Robb PhD

Kirby G. Vosburgh PhD

IOS
*Press*

Amsterdam • Berlin • Oxford • Tokyo • Washington, DC

ISBN 1 58603 498 7
Library of Congress Control Number: 2004117290


*Publisher*
IOS Press
Nieuwe Hemweg 6B
1013 BG Amsterdam
The Netherlands
fax: +31 20 620 3419
e-mail: order@iospress.nl


*Distributor in the UK and Ireland*
IOS Press/Lavis Marketing
73 Lime Walk
Headington
Oxford OX3 7AD
England
fax: +44 1865 750079

*Distributor in the USA and Canada*
IOS Press, Inc.
4502 Rachael Manor Drive
Fairfax, VA 22032
USA
fax: +1 703 323 3668
e-mail: iosbooks@iospress.com

PRINTED IN THE NETHERLANDS

*Medicine Meets Virtual Reality 13*
*James D. Westwood et al. (Eds.)*
*IOS Press, 2005*

v

# Preface
# The Magical Next Becomes
# the Medical Now

James D. WESTWOOD and Karen S. MORGAN
*Aligned Management Associates, Inc.*

*Magical* describes conditions that are outside our understanding of cause and effect. What cannot be attributed to human or natural forces is explained as magic: super-human, super-natural will. Even in modern societies, magic-based explanations are powerful because, given the complexity of the universe, there are so many opportunities to use them.

The history of medicine is defined by progress in understanding the human body – from magical explanations to measurable results. Metaphysics was abandoned when evidence-based models provided better results in the alleviation of physical suffering. The pioneers of medicine demonstrated that when we relinquish magic, we gain more reliable control over ourselves.

In the 16th century, religious prohibitions against dissection were overturned, allowing surgeons to explore the interior of the human body first-hand and learn by direct observation and experimentation. No one can deny that, in the years since, surgical outcomes have improved tremendously.

However, change is marked by conflict: medical politicking, prohibitions, and punishments continue unabated. Certain new technologies are highly controversial, including somatic cell nuclear transfer (therapeutic cloning) and embryonic stem cell research. Lawmakers are deliberating how to control them. The conflict between science and religion still affects the practice of medicine and how reliably we will alleviate human suffering.

To continue medical progress, physicians and scientists must openly question traditional models. Valid inquiry demands a willingness to consider all possible solutions without prejudice. Medical politics should not perpetuate unproven assumptions nor curtail reasoned experimentation, unbiased measurement, and well-informed analysis.

\* \* \* \* \*

For thirteen years, MMVR has been an incubator for technologies that create new medical understanding via the simulation, visualization, and extension of reality. Researchers create imaginary patients because they offer a more reliable and controllable experience to the novice surgeon. With imaging tools, reality is purposefully distorted to reveal to the clinician what the eye alone cannot see. Robotics and intelligence networks allow the healer's sight, hearing, touch, and judgment to be extended across distance, as if by magic.

At MMVR, research progress is sometimes incremental. This can be frustrating: one would like progress to be easy, steady, and predictable. Wouldn't it be miraculous if revolutions happened right on schedule?

But this is the real magic: the "Eureka!" moments when scientific truth is suddenly revealed after lengthy observation, experimentation, and measurement. These moments are not miraculous, however. They are human ingenuity in progress and they are documented here in this book.

MMVR researchers can be proud of the progress of thirteen years – transforming the medical *next* into the medical *now*. They should take satisfaction in accomplishments made as individuals and as a community. It is an honor for us, the conference organizers, to perpetuate MMVR as a forum where researchers share their eureka moments with their colleagues and the world.

Thank you for your magic.

*Medicine Meets Virtual Reality 13*
*James D. Westwood et al. (Eds.)*
*IOS Press, 2005*

## MMVR13 Proceedings Editors

James D. Westwood
MMVR Program Coordinator
Aligned Management Associates, Inc.

Randy S. Haluck MD FACS
Director of Minimally Invasive Surgery
Director of Surgical Simulation
Associate Professor of Surgery
Penn State, Hershey Medical Center

Helene M. Hoffman PhD
Assistant Dean, Educational Computing
Adjunct Professor of Medicine
Division of Medical Education
School of Medicine
University of California, San Diego

Greg T. Mogel MD
Assistant Professor of Radiology and Biomedical Engineering
University of Southern California;
Director, TATRC-W
U.S. Army Medical Research & Materiel Command

Roger Phillips PhD CEng MBCS
Research Professor, Simulation & Visualization Group
Director, Hull Immersive Visualization Environment (HIVE)
Department of Computer Science
University of Hull (UK)

Richard A. Robb PhD
Scheller Professor in Medical Research
Professor of Biophysics & Computer Science
Director, Mayo Biomedical Imaging Resource
Mayo Clinic College of Medicine

Kirby G. Vosburgh PhD
Associate Director, Center for Integration of Medicine and
Innovative Technology (CIMIT)
Massachusetts General Hospital
Harvard Medical School

## MMVR13 Organizing Committee

Michael J. Ackerman PhD
High Performance Computing & Communications,
National Library of Medicine

Ian Alger MD
New York Presbyterian Hospital;
Weill Medical College of Cornell University

David C. Balch MA
DCB Consulting LLC

Steve Charles MD
MicroDexterity Systems;
University of Tennessee

Patrick C. Cregan FRACS
Nepean Hospital,
Wentworth Area Health Service

Henry Fuchs PhD
Dept of Computer Science,
University of North Carolina

Walter J. Greenleaf PhD
Greenleaf Medical Systems

Randy S. Haluck MD FACS
Dept of Surgery,
Penn State College of Medicine

David M. Hananel
Surgical Programs,
Medical Education Technologies Inc.

Wm. LeRoy Heinrichs MD PhD
Medical Media & Information Technologies/ Gynecology & Obstetrics,
Stanford University School of Medicine

Helene M. Hoffman PhD
School of Medicine,
University of California, San Diego

Heinz U. Lemke PhD
Institute for Technical Informatics,
Technical University Berlin

Alan Liu PhD
National Capital Area Medical Simulation Center,
Uniformed Services University

Greg T. Mogel MD
University of Southern California;
TATRC/USAMRMC

Kevin N. Montgomery PhD
National Biocomputation Center,
Stanford University

Makoto Nonaka MD PhD
Foundation for International Scientific Advancement

Roger Phillips PhD CEng MBCS
Dept of Computer Science,
University of Hull (UK)

Richard A. Robb PhD
Mayo Biomedical Imaging Resource,
Mayo Clinic College of Medicine

Jannick P. Rolland PhD
ODA Lab, School of Optics / CREOL,
University of Central Florida

Ajit K. Sachdeva MD FRCSC FACS
Division of Education,
American College of Surgeons

Richard M. Satava MD FACS
Dept of Surgery, University of Washington;
DARPA; TATRC/USAMRMC

Rainer M.M. Seibel MD
Diagnostic & Interventional Radiology,
University of Witten/Herdecke

Steven Senger PhD
Dept of Computer Science,
University of Wisconsin - La Crosse

Ramin Shahidi PhD
Image Guidance Laboratories,
Stanford University School of Medicine

Faina Shtern MD
Beth Israel Deaconess; Children's Medical Center;
Harvard Medical School

Don Stredney
Interface Laboratory,
OSC

Julie A. Swain MD
Cardiovascular and Respiratory Devices,
U.S. Food and Drug Administration

Kirby G. Vosburgh PhD
CIMIT; Massachusetts General Hospital;
Harvard Medical School

Dave Warner MD PhD
MindTel LLC;
Institute for Interventional Informatics

Suzanne J. Weghorst MA MS
Human Interface Technology Lab,
University of Washington

Mark D. Wiederhold MD PhD FACP
The Virtual Reality Medical Center

Medicine Meets Virtual Reality 13
James D. Westwood et al. (Eds.)
IOS Press, 2005

# Contents

*Medicine Meets Virtual Reality 13*
*James D. Westwood et al. (Eds.)*
*IOS Press, 2005*

# Dynamic Generation of Surgery Specific Simulators – A Feasibility Study

Eric ACOSTA and Bharti TEMKIN PhD.

*Department of Computer Science, Texas Tech University*
*Department of Surgery, Texas Tech University Health Science Center*
*PO Box 2100, Lubbock 79409*
*e-mail: Bharti.Temkin@coe.ttu.edu*

**Abstract.** Most of the current surgical simulators rely on preset anatomical virtual environments (VE). The functionality of a simulator is typically fixed to anatomy-based specific tasks. This rigid design principle makes it difficult to reuse an existing simulator for different surgeries. It also makes it difficult to simulate procedures for specific patients, since their anatomical features or anomalies cannot be easily replaced in the VE.

In this paper, we demonstrate the reusability of a modular skill-based simulator, LapSkills, which allows dynamic generation of surgery-specific simulations. Task and instrument modules are easily reused from LapSkills and the three-dimensional VE can be replaced with other anatomical models. We build a nephrectomy simulation by reusing the simulated vessels and the clipping and cutting task modules from LapSkills. The VE of the kidney is generated with our anatomical model generation tools and then inserted into the simulation (while preserving the established tasks and evaluation metrics). An important benefit for the created surgery and patient-specific simulations is that reused components remain validated. We plan to use this faster development process to generate a simulation library containing a wide variety of laparoscopic surgical simulations. Incorporating the simulations into surgical training programs will help collect data for validating them.

## 1. Introduction

Virtual Reality based surgical simulators have the potential to provide training for a wide range of surgeries with a large set of pathologies relevant for surgical training [1,2]. However, in order to fully leverage the capabilities of surgical simulators it is necessary to overcome some of the bottlenecks imposed by the complexity of developing and validating them.

The generalized modular architecture of LapSkills [3] makes it possible to dynamically generate or modify surgery and patient-specific simulations with minimum programming. The construction process involves 1) importing or generating VE(s) with the associated physical properties for the anatomical structures, 2) selecting tasks and instruments with the associated evaluation metrics, 3) integrating the models and tasks into the simulation, and 4) integrating the new simulation into LapSkills. This allows LapSkills to be used as a general platform to run new simulations and collect performance data for validating the newly built simulation.

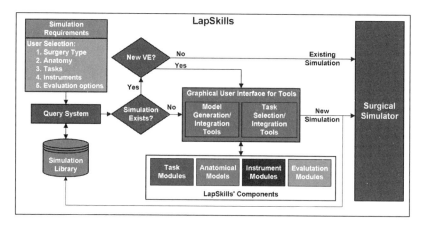

**Figure 1.** User selection based simulation generation.

To show the feasibility of generating new simulations from LapSkills, a nephrectomy simulation has been developed. The VE for the kidney, including vessels such as renal artery and vein, was generated with our anatomical model generation tools and then inserted into the simulation while preserving the established clipping and cutting tasks and evaluation metrics. Furthermore, the VE has been interchanged with other patient specific VEs from other modalities, such as the Visible Human dataset and other patient-specific datasets.

## 2. Dynamic simulation generation

Extending the capabilities of LapSkills, to also function as a simulation generator, provides the ability to rapidly create new customized and partially validated surgery and patient-specific simulations. Various possibilities offered by this system, illustrated in Figure 1, cover a large set of pathologies relevant for the training needs of surgeons. Based on the desired requirements, such as surgery type, anatomy, tasks included, selection of instruments, and evaluation options, LapSkills queries its library of existing simulations to determine if the required simulation already exists. If a match is found, the existing simulation can be used for training. However, if the needed simulation does not exist then a new user specified simulation is generated and seamlessly integrated into the simulation library to become an integral part of LapSkills. Interfacing several tools (described in sections 2.2 and 2.3) to LapSkills makes it possible to reuse the components of its architecture in order to create or modify simulations.

### 2.1. LapSkills architecture

The architecture consists of several reusable modules shown in Figure 2. Task modules consist of basic subtasks that can be used to define a skill, listed in Table 1. The instrument module contains the simulated virtual instruments. Each task and instrument module has built-in evaluation metrics that are used to acquire performance data. Thus, reusing these modules automatically incorporates the associated evaluation metrics. The evaluation modules contain different evaluation models. An evaluation model determines

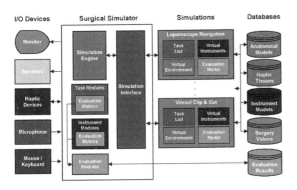

**Figure 2.** Architecture of LapSkills.

**Table 1.** Sample reusable subtasks contained within task modules.

| Task List |
|---|
| Clip \<object\> |
| Cut \<object\> |
| Extract \<object\> |
| Grasp \<object\> |
| Locate \<object\> |
| Move \<object\> |
| Touch \<object\> |
| Insert \<instrument\> |
| Withdraw \<instrument\> |

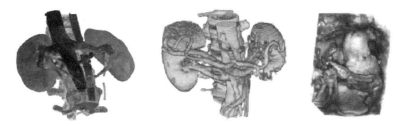

**Figure 3.** Volumetric anatomical models generated from (left) the Visible Human in 75 seconds, (middle) CT dataset in 10 seconds, and (right) 3D Ultrasound in 1 second.

how to interpret the data collected by the task and instrument metrics to evaluate the user's performance.

A simulation specification file represents the task list, virtual instruments, and evaluation model, and describes the VE for each skill. The task list consists of a sequence(s) of subtasks that are used to simulate the skill. The instrument and evaluation components specify which virtual instruments and evaluation modules are used. The VE describes which anatomical models (contained in the database) are to be used and specifies their properties such as orientation, haptic tissue properties, etc. The information stored in the specification file is used by the simulation interface in order to dynamically build and perform the skill at run-time.

A simulation engine allows the simulator to step through the sequence of tasks that are defined for a skill. It incorporates a state machine (which is constructed when a simulation file is loaded) that transitions through the list of subtasks as the user performs them.

Several databases are utilized by LapSkills including anatomical and instrument models, haptic tissue properties that define the feel of the structures, surgery videos, and evaluation results.

## 2.2. Anatomical model generation and integration tools

The anatomical models, or Virtual Body Structures (VBS), are generated from the Visible Human (vh-VBS) and patient-specific (ps-VBS) datasets, with some examples illustrated in Figure 3. The model generation times are based on a Pentium 4 1.8 GHz with

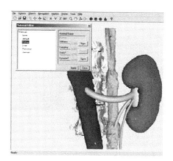

**Figure 4.** Model and task integration tool.

1 GB RAM. Using an existing segmentation of the Visible Human data makes it easy to add, remove, and isolate structures to assemble the desired VE. Structures of interest are selected using a navigational system and then generated for real-time exploration [4–6].

Tissue densities from medical datasets such as CT, MRI, and Ultrasound are used to generate ps-VBS [4]. Manipulation capabilities are included to explore the ps-VBS. A range of densities can be adjusted in order to target specific densities associated with structures of interest. Density-based controlled segmentation is used to isolate ps-VBS. Presets make it possible to return to the current state when the dataset is reloaded and help locate anatomical structures from different datasets of the same modality. Adjustable slicing planes are also provided to clip the volume to remove unwanted portions of the data and to view the structures internally.

Once structures of interest are isolated from a dataset, models are generated and exported for simulator use. Three types of VBS models can be created: surface-based, volumetric, or finite element. A surface-based model is a 3D geometric model that uses polygons to define the exterior of an anatomical structure. Volumetric models use voxels to completely define all internal sub-structures and external structures. FEM models are created using surface-based models and a commercially available FEM package. The package makes it possible to specify the elements of the model, assign material properties, and to export deformable models with pre-computed force and displacement information. Conversion from a volumetric model to a surface model is also possible using our tools.

The model integrator incorporates components for adding, removing, replacing, and orienting VBS in the VE, as shown in Figure 4. VBS can be manipulated and placed in any location within the VE. Scene manipulations such as pan, zoom, rotate, setting the field of view, and changing the background image are also possible. A material editor is available to change or assign haptic tissue properties to surface-based VBS, making them touchable [7,8]. Several tissue properties such as stiffness, damping, and static/dynamic friction are used to define the feel of VBS. An expert in the field of anatomy or surgery can interactively tweak the values for each structure and save the properties into a library of modeled heuristic tissues [8]. Existing modeled tissue properties in the library can be directly applied to the structures of the VE.

### 2.3. Task integration tool

The task integrator allows the task and instrument modules of LapSkills to be incorporated in a simulation, Figure 4. The task integrator also allows for specification of all

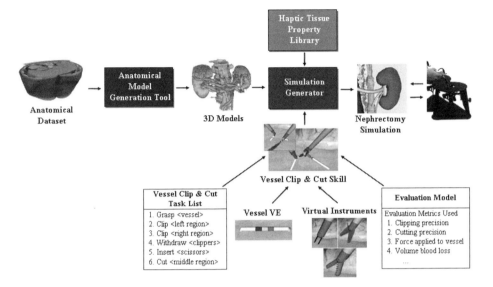

**Figure 5.** Generating the nephrectomy simulation based on LapSkills.

the necessary information needed to carry out a task, including the order of the subtasks. Instructions are provided for each task to guide the user while training with a simulation. User evaluation metrics associated with the tasks and instruments are automatically incorporated as default. However, they can be modified based on the evaluation model that is specified by the user.

## 3. Laparoscopic nephrectomy simulation

The laparoscopic live donor nephrectomy procedure is method of kidney removal that reduces post-operative complications from open surgery [9]. In this procedure, the tissues surrounding the kidney are dissected to access its connected blood vessels and the ureter. The blood vessels and the ureter are clamped and cut to free the kidney. The kidney is then placed into a bag and removed.

Figure 5 shows the process used to build the nephrectomy simulation via LapSkills. The patient-specific VE, consisting of the kidneys and selected structures of interest, was generated and then integrated into the nephrectomy simulation. These structures can also be interchanged with other vh-VBS and ps-VBS via the model integration tool. The vessel clipping and cutting subtasks, instruments, and evaluation model were imported from the existing skill of LapSkills.

The nephrectomy simulation focuses on simulating a left-sided approach. It currently allows the surgeon to locate the kidney and free it by clipping and cutting the renal artery, renal vein, and the ureter. Instrument interactions with a vessel, as it is grasped or stretched, are felt with the haptic device. Force feedback is computed based on a mass-spring system used to model the vessel. Clip application is simulated using a ratchet component on the device handle. The simulator settings and evaluation metrics for this simulation are similar to the existing clipping and cutting skills [3].

## 4. Discussion and future work

In general, many issues remain to be solved for tissue modeling and virtual environment generation. These include 1) segmentation and registration, 2) real-time model generation and rendering for desired model types (e.g. surface, volume, or FEM), 3) changes in model resolution and accuracy while switching from one model type to another for real-time computation, 4) tissue property generation and assignment, and 5) limitations of the haptic hardware, such as haptic resolution. Many software development problems still remain for tool tissue interactions such as model deformation and collision detection.

Generating tissue properties and simulating palpation of different tissue types is a major hurdle. While basic research in quantitative analysis of biomechanics of living tissue has made tremendous progress, integration of all the facets of the field has yet to become a reality. It is a great challenge to produce reliable data on a large number of tissue types and utilize the in-vivo data to model deformable tissues in simulators.

Replacing models in a simulation requires automatic transfer of the tissue properties for anatomical structures. For surface-based models, the current model integration tools allow automatic transfer of the physical parameters for the sense of touch. For instance, when a haptic surface-based visible human model is exchanged with a surface-based patient specific model, the new patient specific model is automatically touchable with the same tissue properties. However, while exchanging model geometries, seamless transfer of haptic properties between model types (e.g. surface to volumetric) remains to be implemented.

Once the structures are segmented, we are able to generate models of different types. Currently, LapSkills works only with surface-based models and FEM models derived from surface-based models. Haptic rendering methods for non-deformable VBS and simple deformable soft bodies [10] have been utilized, but the general problem of rendering dynamic tissue manipulations remains unsolved.

Building a library of simulations can help collect the performance data needed to validate the use of simulations in surgical training. After statistically significant performance data is collected for different categories of surgeons, including expert and novice surgeons, the evaluation metrics and models used in LapSkills can be used to create a performance scale for measuring laparoscopic skills [3].

## 5. Conclusion

We build a nephrectomy simulation reusing LapSkills' modules to demonstrate that its modular architecture, along with tools interfaced to LapSkills, simplifies the software development process for dynamically building new simulations. This makes it possible to provide a library of surgery and patient specific simulations with a large set of pathologies relevant for surgical training.

## Acknowledgements

We would like to thank Colleen Berg for making it possible to create FEM models. The 3D ultrasound data used in Figure 3 is courtesy of Novint Technologies, Inc.

# References

[1]  Satava R. *Cybersurgery: Advanced Technologies for Surgical Practice*. New York, NY: John Wiley & Sons, Inc, 1998.

[2]  Dawson S. L. "A Critical Approach to Medical Simulation." *Bulletin of the American College of Surgeons*, 87(11):12–18, 2002.

[3]  Acosta E., Temkin B. "Haptic Laparoscopic Skills Trainer with Practical User Evaluation Metrics." To appear in *Medicine Meets Virtual Reality 13*, 2005.

[4]  Acosta E., Temkin B. "Build-and-Insert: Anatomical Structure Generation for Surgical Simulators." *International Symposium on Medical Simulation (ISMS)*, pp 230-239, 2004.

[5]  Temkin B., Acosta E., et al. "Web-based Three-dimensional Virtual Body Structures." *Journal of the American Medical Informatics Association*, Vol. 9 No. 5 pp 425-436, Sept/Oct 2002.

[6]  Hatfield P., Acosta E., Temkin B. "PC-Based Visible Human Volumizer." *The Fourth Visible Human Project Conference*, 2002.

[7]  Acosta E., Temkin B., et al. "G2H – Graphics-to-Haptic Virtual Environment Development Tool for PC's." *Medicine Meets Virtual Reality 8*, pp 1-3, 2000.

[8]  Acosta E., Temkin B., et al. "Heuristic Haptic Texture for Surgical Simulations." *Medicine Meets Virtual Reality 02/10: Digital Upgrades: Applying Moore's Law to Health*, pp 14-16, 2002.

[9]  Fabrizio M. D., Ratner L. E., Montgomery R. A., and Kavoussi L. R. "Laparoscopic Live Donor Nephrectomy." *Johns Hopkins Medical Institutions, Department of Urology*, http://urology.jhu.edu/surgical_techniques/nephrectomy/.

[10] Burgin J., Stephens B., Vahora F., Temkin B., Marcy W., Gorman P., Krummel T., "Haptic Rendering of Volumetric Soft-Bodies Objects", *The third PHANToM User Workshop (PUG)*, 1998.

*Medicine Meets Virtual Reality 13*
*James D. Westwood et al. (Eds.)*
*IOS Press, 2005*

# Haptic Laparoscopic Skills Trainer with Practical User Evaluation Metrics

Eric ACOSTA and Bharti TEMKIN PhD.
*Department of Computer Science, Texas Tech University*
*Department of Surgery, Texas Tech University Health Science Center*
*PO Box 2100, Lubbock 79409*
*e-mail: Bharti.Temkin@coe.ttu.edu*

**Abstract.** Limited sense of touch and vision are some of the difficulties encountered in performing laparoscopic procedures. Haptic simulators can help minimize these difficulties; however, the simulators must be validated prior to actual use. Their effectiveness as a training tool needs to be measured in terms of improvement in surgical skills. LapSkills, a haptic skill-based laparoscopic simulator, that aims to provide a quantitative measure of the surgeon's skill level and to help improve their efficiency and precision, has been developed. Explicitly defined performance metrics for several surgical skills are presented in this paper. These metrics allow performance data to be collected to quantify improvement within the same skill over time. After statistically significant performance data is collected for expert and novice surgeons, these metrics can be used not only to validate LapSkills, but to also generate a *performance scale* to measure laparoscopic skills.

## 1. Haptic Laparoscopic Skills Trainer - LapSkills

Efforts have been made to establish performance metrics to validate the effectiveness of surgical simulators [1–6]. This requires collecting user performance data. If the preset level of difficulty and the skill of the user are mismatched, the task of collecting data becomes difficult. Real-time feedback modeled using explicitly defined metrics for task performance would allow surgeons to quickly establish their current skill level. It would then be possible to adjust the level of difficulty as the user becomes more proficient and to measure the performance progress. These features have been incorporated into our adaptable and quantifiable haptic skill-based simulator, LapSkills. The simulator settings, such as the surgical task, virtual instruments, and the level of task difficulty, can be easily changed with voice commands. Real-time customization of voice commands with a microphone makes LapSkills user friendly and responsive to the needs of the surgeon. Surgeons can switch activities with voice commands without interruptions associated with mouse and keyboard interfaces.

LapSkills allows a surgeon to master several fundamental skills such as laparoscope navigation and exploration, hand-eye coordination, grasping, applying clips, and cutting, Figure 1. Laparoscope navigation requires the user to travel through a tube in order to locate objects. Lateral movement of the laparoscope is confined to the inside of the tube using force feedback. Laparoscope exploration teaches how to navigate the laparoscope

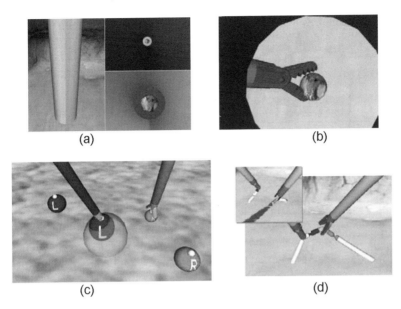

**Figure 1.** Skills simulated in LapSkills: (a) Laparoscope navigation, (b) Laparoscope exploration, (c) Hand-eye coordination, and (d) Vessel clipping and cutting.

around obstacles to locate randomly placed objects and remove them with graspers. A tube is placed around the laparoscope to control the field of view of the camera.

In hand-eye-coordination, surgeons collect randomly placed objects (by a marked spot) and place them into a collection bin. The objects are labeled with "L" or "R" to signify which hand must be used to grab them. Each object has a life that indicates how long it is displayed before it disappears. The location of the collection bin also changes after a timeout period expires.

To exercise vessel clipping and cutting, the user clips and cuts a vessel within high-lighted regions. Failure to apply the clip to the entire width of the vessel results in blood loss when cut. If the vessel is stretched too far, it will rupture and begin to bleed.

## 2. Practical User Evaluation Metrics

The embedded, explicitly defined metrics for each skill, listed in Table 1, allow three categories of performance data to be collected to quantify improvement within the same skill over time and to generate an overall performance scale to measure laparoscopic skills.

## 3. Conclusion

We have developed an adaptable and quantifiable haptic skill-based simulator that is responsive to surgeons needs. With LapSkills we have addressed two issues of existing laparoscopic simulators: 1) making the simulator dynamic for the user and 2) offering real-time evaluation feedback without interruption while training. The explicitly defined

**Table 1. Evaluation metric categories.** The task difficulty and performance metrics evaluate the user for specific tasks. Task difficulty metrics are used to change the levels of task difficulties at any time while training with LapSkills. General performance metrics are task independent and apply to all skills.

| Task | Task Difficulty | Task Performance |
|---|---|---|
| Lap. Nav. in Tube | • Tube length and radius<br>• Object distance from tube bottom center | • Number of times tube is touched<br>• Force applied to tube<br>• Camera steadiness |
| Lap. Explore | • Camera obstruction<br>• Object size and placement | • Time between locating objects<br>• Number of times obstacles are touched<br>• Camera steadiness |
| Hand-eye Coord. | • Number of objects per hand<br>• Object size and life<br>• Grasping marker size<br>• Area size where objects appear<br>• Timeout before bin moves | • Manual dexterity-fraction objects collected per hand<br>• Accuracy- (In)correct collected objects<br>• Precision-proximity to marker where object is grasped<br>• Depth perception-deviation from minimal path between object and collection bin |
| Vessel Clip/Cut | • Clipping region size<br>• Cutting region size<br>• Vessel thickness<br>• Vessel rupture strength | • Clipping/cutting precision-proximity to regions<br>• Clipping efficiency-fraction correctly placed clips<br>• Number clips dropped and picked up<br>• Amount of force applied to vessel<br>• Volume blood loss |

**General performance metrics:**

- Task completion time–total time taken to complete the task.
- Path length–distance taken by the instrument tip is given by
  $\sum_{i=1}^{N-1} \sqrt{(x_{i+1} - x_i)^2 + (y_{i+1} - y_i)^2 + (z_{i+1} - z_i)^2}$, where $x_i$, $y_i$, and $z_i$ are the instrument tip coordinates taken from the $i^{th}$ sample point.
- Motion smoothness–measures abrupt changes in acceleration given by $\frac{1}{N-1} \sum_{i=1}^{N-1} \sqrt{(a_{i+1} - a_i)^2}$, where $a_i$ represent the acceleration of the instrument tip computed from the $i^{th}$ sample point.
- Rotational orientation–measures placement of the tool direction for tasks involving grasping, clipping, and cutting, given by $\frac{1}{N-1} \sum_{i=1}^{N-1} \sqrt{(\theta_{i+1} - \theta_i)^2}$, where the angle $\theta_i$, in polar coordinates, is computed from the $i^{th}$ sample point.

performance metrics are used to model the real-time feedback provided for the essential surgical skills, and to quantify the improvement resulting from the use of the tool. A performance scale can be defined for each specific skill or procedure and then used for the validation of LapSkills. The simulator can also be configured to the requirements of different procedures and skill levels, and can be converted into a surgery specific simulator [7].

# References

[1] Metrics for objective assessment of surgical skills workshop. Scottsdale Arizona (2001). Final Report available at http://www.tatrc.org/website_metrics/metrics_final/finalreport.html.
[2] Satava R.M., Cuschieri A, et al. "Metrics for objective assessment." *Surgical Endoscopy*, 17:220-226, 2003.
[3] Payandeh S., Lomax A., et al. "On Defining Metrics for Assessing Laparoscopic Surgical Skills in Virtual Training Environment." *Medicine Meets Virtual Reality 02/10*, pp. 334-340, 2002.

[4] Cotin S., Stylopoulos N., Ottensmeyer M., et al. "Metrics for Laparoscopic Skills Trainers: The Weakest Link!" *Proceedings of MICCAI 2002, Lecture Notes in Computer Science* 2488, 35-43, 2002.

[5] Liu A., Tendick F., et al. "A Survey of Surgical Simulation: Applications, Technology, and Education." *Presence: Teleoperators and Virtual Environments*, 12(6):599-614, 2003.

[6] Moody L., Baber C., et al. "Objective metrics for the evaluation of simple surgical skills in real and virtual domains." *Presence: Teleoperators and Virtual Environments*, 12(2):207-221, 2003.

[7] Acosta E., Temkin B. "Dynamic Generation of Surgery Specific Simulators – A Feasibility Study." To appear in *Medicine Meets Virtual Reality 13*, 2005.

*Medicine Meets Virtual Reality 13*
*James D. Westwood et al. (Eds.)*
*IOS Press, 2005*

# Desktop and Conference Room VR for Physicians

Zhuming AI and Mary RASMUSSEN

*VRMedLab, Department of Biomedical and Health Information Sciences,*
*University of Illinois at Chicago*
*e-mail: zai@uic.edu*

**Abstract.** Virtual environments such as the CAVE™and the ImmersaDesk™, which are based on graphics supercomputers or workstations, are large and expensive. Most physicians have no access to such systems. The recent development of small Linux personal computers and high-performance graphics cards has afforded opportunities to implement applications formerly run on graphics supercomputers. Using PC hardware and other affordable devices, a VR system has been developed which can sit on a physician's desktop or be installed in a conference room.

Affordable PC-based VR systems are comparable in performance with expensive VR systems formerly based on graphics supercomputers. Such VR systems can now be accessible to most physicians. The lower cost and smaller size of this system greatly expands the range of uses of VR technology in medicine.

## 1. Introduction

Virtual environments such as the CAVE™and the ImmersaDesk™, which are based on graphics supercomputers or workstations, are large and expensive. Most physicians have no access to such systems. The recent development of small Linux personal computers (PC) and high-performance graphics cards has afforded opportunities to implement applications formerly run on graphics supercomputers. Using PC hardware and other affordable devices, a VR system has been developed which can sit on physician's desktop or be installed in a conference room.

## 2. Method

### 2.1. Hardware Configuration

Because of the parallel processing of VR applications, a dual-processor hyper-threading Pentium IV PC is used in this VR system. The Linux operating system is used so that it is easy to port most current VR applications from Unix platforms. Linux is very stable and free, and many software development tools are also free. We have tested different combinations of graphics card/driver/stereo glasses for the VR system. The StereoEyes stereo glasses and emitter from StereoGraphics works well. For graphics card drivers there are three options that we have investigated. Software from Xig supports many different graphics cards, but it is not free. NVIDIA's driver supports stereo display for their Quadro-based graphics cards, and FireGL from ATI also supports stereo. NVIDIA Quadro4 based graphics cards perform very well with our application software. High quality CRT monitors are needed to generate stereo vision for the desktop configuration. By adding two projectors, polarizing filters, and a screen the VR system can be used in a conference room. A variety of tracking devices have been interfaced with this system to provide viewer centered perspective and 3-dimensional control. A Linux kernel module has been developed to allow the use of an inexpensive wireless remote control.

## 2.2. Software Development Tools

Many software development tools used in a SGI environment are available for Linux. These include CaveLib, QUANTA, Performer, Inventor (Coin3D), and Volumizer. Performer for Linux can be used for surface rendering. Open Inventor and its clones, such as Cone, can also be used. SGI Volumizer can be used to develop volume rendering applications. VTK is also a very useful development tool. Networking software QUANTA is used for collaboration.

## 2.3. Applications

CAVE and ImmersaDesk applications have been ported to the PC-based VR system. A networked volume data manipulation program is under development. A component to support collaboration among medical professionals has been developed. This is based on the Quality of Service Adaptive Networking Toolkit (QUANTA) [1] developed at EVL, UIC. A collaborative VR server has been designed. It has a database to store the shared data such as CT or MR data. Collaborators' information is also stored in the database. Client applications can connect to the server to join existing collaborative sessions or open new sessions. Real-time audio communication is implemented among collaborators. This is implemented using the multicasting feature in QUANTA so that it can deliver real-time audio to a large number of collaborators without a $n^2$ growth in bandwidth. A standard protocol will be set up so that all our applications will be able to connect to the server and share information. Physicians can use the application to study volume data collaboratively in a virtual environment from their desktops or conference rooms.

A direct volume rendering algorithm for Linux PCs has been developed. Three-dimensional texture mapping features in NVIDIA graphics cards are used. The algorithm has built-in adaptive level-of-detail support. It can interactively render a gray-scale volume up to the size of $512 \times 512 \times 256$ or a full color volume of $256 \times 256 \times 256$ on an NVIDIA Quadro FX3000 card. If texture compression is used, the algorithm can interactively render a gray-scale or full color volume up to the size of $512 \times 512 \times 512$ on the graphics card. The volume can be shown in stereo. We are also working on a cluster-based solution to handle even bigger datasets.

## 3. Results

A Linux based VR system for the physician's desktop and conference room has been developed. We have ported the Virtual Pelvic Floor [2] and Virtual Nasal Anatomy (Figure 1) applications to the system. A new application for eye disease simulation has been

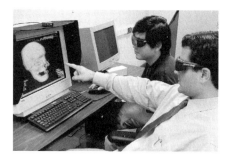

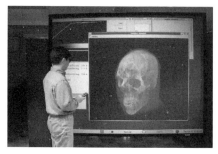

**Figure 1.** The Virtual Nasal Anatomy application on the desktop VR system.

**Figure 2.** The volume rendering application on the conference room VR system.

developed for this new system. A networked volume rendering application has been developed (Figure 2). The Virtual Pelvic Floor application runs faster on the PC-based VR system then on the ImmersaDesk powered by a SGI Onyx2.

## 4. Conclusion and Discussion

Affordable PC-based VR systems are comparable in performance with expensive VR systems formerly based on graphics supercomputers. Such VR systems can now be accessible to most physicians. The lower cost and smaller size of this system greatly expands the range of uses of VR technology in medicine.

Most tele-immersive VR features are kept on the PC-based VR system. Video camera based tracking systems are being developed by our collaborators and may provide a more natural interface for the physicians [3].

## Acknowledgments

This project has been funded in part with federal funds from the National Library of Medicine/ National Institutes of Health, under contract No. N01-LM-3-3507.

## References

[1]  J. Leigh, O. Yu, D. Schonfeld, R. Ansari, et al. Adaptive networking for tele-immersion. In *Proc. Immersive Projection Technology/Eurographics Virtual EnvironmentsWorkshop (IPT/EGVE)*, Stuttgart, Germany, May 2001.
[2]  Zhuming Ai, Fred Dech, Jonathan Silverstein, and Mary Rasmussen. Tele-immersive medical educational environment. *Studies in Health Technology and Informatics*, 85:24–30, 2002.
[3]  J. Girado, D. Sandin, T. DeFanti, and L. Wolf. Real-time camera-based face detection using a modified lamstar neural network system. In *Proceedings of IS&T/SPIE's 15th Annual Symposium Electronic Imaging 2003, Applications of Artificial Neural Networks in Image Processing VIII*, pages 20–24, San Jose, California, January 2003.

*Medicine Meets Virtual Reality 13*
*James D. Westwood et al. (Eds.)*
*IOS Press, 2005*

# A Biologically Derived Approach to Tissue Modeling

Tim ANDERSEN, Tim OTTER, Cap PETSCHULAT, Ullysses EOFF, Tom MENTEN,
Robert DAVIS and Bill CROWLEY

*Crowley Davis Research, 280 South Academy Ave, Eagle, ID 83616*

**Abstract.** Our approach to tissue modeling incorporates biologically derived primitives into a computational engine (CellSim® coupled with a genetic search algorithm. By expanding an evolved synthetic genome CellSim® is capable of developing a virtual tissue with higher order properties. Using primitives based on cell
signaling, gene networks, cell division, growth, and death, we have encoded a 64-
cell cube-shaped tissue with emergent capacity to repair itself when up to 60%
of its cells are destroyed. Other tissue shapes such as sheets of cells also repair
themselves. Capacity for self-repair is an emergent property derived from, but not
specified by, the rule sets used to generate these virtual tissues.

## 1. Introduction

Most models of biological tissues are based on principles of systems engineering [1]. For
example, tissue structure and elasticity can be modeled as dampened springs, electrically
excitable tissues can be modeled as core conductors, and tissues such as blood can be
modeled according to principles of fluid mechanics. As different as these models are,
they share a number of general features: they are constructed from the perspective of an
external observer and designer of the system; they are grounded in laws (Hook, Kirchoff,
Ohm, Bernoulli, etc.) that describe predictable behavior of the physical world in a manner
that can be verified empirically, by measurement; they incorporate feedback controls to
optimize system performance by tuning of adjustable elements; their complexity requires
some kind of computational approach.

Although models based on a systems engineering approach contain a number of features that mimic the way that natural living systems are built and how they function,
such models differ from natural systems in important ways (Table 1). Notably, living
organisms have been designed by evolutionary processes characterized by descent with
modification from ancestral forms, not by a single-minded, purposeful, intelligent architect. This means that natural designs are constrained by evolutionary legacies that may
be suboptimal but unavoidable consequences, for example, of the process of development in a given species. Even so, living systems incorporate a number of remarkable
features that human-designed systems lack, such as self-construction via development,
self-repair, plasticity, and adaptability – the ability to monitor and respond to complex,
unpredictable environments.[1]

In an attempt to devise tissue models that conform more closely to the living systems they emulate, we have begun to incorporate biologically-derived primitives into a

**Table 1.** General features of natural and human-designed systems.

|  | **Natural Systems** | **Human-engineered Systems** |
|---|---|---|
| Design | Selection by evolutionary process | Optimization by architect |
| Construction | Self-constructs by development; continuous turnover of components | Built by a separate process and apparatus prior to operation |
| Control | Feedback, homeostasis, self-repair, regeneration | Automated feedback |
| Tuning/ Operation | Contingent, adaptable and plastic; monitors complex, unpredictable environment | Task-specific; monitors only a few parameters |

**Table 2.** Biological Primitives and Their Representation in CellSim®.

| **Biological Primitive** | **Representation in CellSim®** |
|---|---|
| Compartments | Cells, each with genome containing gene-like elements |
| Self-replication & Repair | Cell division and growth; replacement of dead cells |
| Adaptation | GA search engine with genetic operators and defined fitness function |
| Selective Communication | Signals to/from environment and neighboring cells; gene regulatory networks |
| Energy Requirement | Growth substance $\geq$ threshold value |

computational framework [3,4]. Relevant features include: 1) a developmental engine (CellSim®) that expands a synthetic genome to develop a virtual tissue composed of cells; 2) an evolutionary selection process based on genetic algorithms; 3) rule-based architecture using cellular processes such as growth, division, and signaling; and 4) higher order (emergent) properties such as self-repair. In summary, such an automated modeling process minimizes human intervention, reduces human error, and yields robust, versatile rule-based systems of encoding.

## 2. Computational Platform

### 2.1. Biological Primitives

Our computational platform is designed to incorporate principles of biology, particularly those primitive features of living systems that are fundamental to their construction and operation and that distinguish them from non-living. Living organisms share five basic features (Table 2): 1) compartmental organization (a form of anatomical modularity); 2) self-replication and repair; 3) adaptation (sensitivity to environment and ability to evolve); 4) selective communication among components; 5) requirement for energy (dissipative, non-equilibrium).

Each of the above features is intertwined with at least one of the others. For example, despite their sometimes static appearance, living organisms are in a continual state of repair and renewal. This requires energy to build, replicate, disassemble, monitor and repair components. In addition, regulatory capacities such as homeostasis derive from the processes of cell signaling, compartmental organization, and selective feedback communication among components.

The most fundamental compartment of living systems is the cell, the smallest unit capable of self-replication. Each cell contains a genome, and it has a boundary that both delimits the cell and its contents and mediates exchange and communication between the cell and its surroundings. Accordingly, we have chosen to focus our simulations on a cellular level of granularity: processes such as division, differentiation, growth, and death are encoded in gene-like data structures, without reference to their complex biochemical basis *in vivo*. However, signaling and control of gene expression are treated computationally as molecular processes.

## 2.2. Basic Operation of CellSim®

The computational engine CellSim® models tissue phenotype (appearance, traits, properties) as the result of a developmental process, starting from a single cell and its genome. Properties such as tissue morphology and self-repair arise from the interaction of gene-like elements as the multicellular virtual tissue develops.

CellSim® defines and controls all of the environmental parameters necessary for development, including placement of nutrients, defining space for cells to grow, sequencing of actions, and rules that govern the physics of the environment. To make CellSim® more flexible, all of the environmental parameters (e.g., rules governing the calculation of molecular affinity and the placement and concentration of nutrients or other molecules) are configurable at run-time. If no value is specified for a parameter, default settings apply.

After the parameters of the CellSim® environment are configured, development is initiated by placing a single cell into that environment. The cell's genome then interacts with any molecules in the environment as well as any molecules that are produced internally by the cell. Depending upon these interactions, each gene within the cell may be turned on (or off). When a gene is turned on, the transcription apparatus of the cell produces the molecules defined by the gene's structural region. These newly produced molecules may in turn interact with the cell's genome, affecting rates of transcription at the next time step. Development is thus governed by inputs from the external environment, and also by internal feedback mechanisms.

In addition to transcription, two primary actions – cell death (apoptosis) and cell growth/division – are available to each cell in the current version of CellSim®. The genome of a cell may include genes that encode death molecules (and/or growth molecules) and as the genes that encode either growth or death molecules are transcribed, the concentration of these molecules in the cell's cytoplasm increases. Growth or death is then a function of the concentration of these two types of molecules. When a cell dies, it is removed from the CellSim® environment. Alternately, if a cell grows and divides, a new cell is placed in a location adjacent to the existing (mother) cell. If all adjacent positions are already occupied, that cell may not divide even if the concentration of growth substance exceeds the threshold for growth.

## 2.3. Cell Signaling

In addition to environmental factors and internally produced molecules, a cell may also receive information from neighboring cells. The simplest neighborhood of a cell consists of those cells that are spatially adjacent to (touching) the cell of interest. However,

CellSim® allows a cell's neighborhood to be configured as any arbitrary group of cells. For example, a neighborhood (the cells to/ from which it will send/ receive signals) could include cells that are not adjacent, as occurs *in vivo* with cells that are able to signal nonlocal cells via hormones.

Cellular signaling is based on a handshake approach that requires both the sender and the receiver to create specific molecules in order for a signal to be transmitted. To send a signal, a cell must create molecules of type 'signal'. At each time step, each cell determines which cells are in its neighborhood and presents the signal(s) it has produced to its neighbors. For a cell to receive a signal that is being presented to it, the cell must build receiver molecules that are tuned to the signal. This completes the handshake portion of the cell signaling process – i.e. in order for a signal to be passed between two cells, the sender cell's signal must be compatible with the receiver molecules built by the receiver cell. Finally, when a receiver senses a signal for which it is designed it generates an internal signal that is defined by the receiver molecule (which is ultimately defined and produced by the cell's genome), but is independent of the particular signal a receiver molecule is designed to detect. This third component has been decoupled from the receiver and signal to allow different cells to produce entirely different internal signals from the same external stimulus. The strength of the internal signal is a configurable function of the concentration of signal molecules produced by the sender and the concentration of receiver molecules that the receiver has produced.

## 2.4. GA-Based Search

To automate the process of tissue modeling, genetic algorithms (GAs) are used to search for a genome with proper encoding to render the desired (target) tissue shape and function [3,4]. Typically a seed population of cells, each with a different genome, develop to yield a population of individuals, each a multicellular tissue with different properties. An individual is defined by both its genome and the CellSim® configuration that develops it; during evolution this permits modification of the genome (using genetic operators) or alteration of the context for development, or both.

Three basic steps are required to process each individual in the population. First, a CellSim® environment is instantiated using the configuration specified by the individual, and a single cell with a defined genome is placed in that environment. Then the CellSim® engine is allowed to run until a stable configuration is reached (or a maximum number of time steps is reached). If the configuration stabilizes, the fitness of the resulting individual is evaluated.

Currently, we have chosen to focus on the relatively simple problem of producing a multicellular tissue with a particular shape. Accordingly, the fitness of an individual is a function of how closely the stable configuration of cells matches the target shape. As we begin to produce more complex tissues, other target properties such as elasticity, connectivity, reactivity, contraction, and cellular state of differentiation will be incorporated into more complex fitness functions. After each individual in a population has been evaluated and scored according to a fitness function, the GA selects a subpopulation, usually those individuals with the highest fitness, as the starting set for the next generation. Genetic operators (mutation, duplication, deletion, or cross-over) increase the genetic variation of the seed population for another round of development by CellSim®, and the cycle repeats.

## 3. Simple Virtual Tissues

### 3.1. Initial Conditions

To test the capabilities of our computational platform and search algorithms we chose a cube as one of the first target tissue shapes. A cube is a relatively simple shape, but it is not necessarily easy to encode using CellSim®, because CellSim® naturally lends itself to developing shapes with curved surfaces and smooth edges (e.g., ellipses or spheroids), but shapes with large, flat surfaces and sharp edges pose a greater challenge.

The target shape for the GA search was a $4 \times 4 \times 4$ cell cube, and the developmental engine was initialized with a population of 50 individuals, each defined by its genome and by its CellSim® configuration. Each individual's starting genome was a single gene with two control regions, one promoter and one repressor, linked to a single structural region coding for cell growth factor. In addition, the GA search algorithm was configured with 13 different types of mutation operators, most of which alter the control and structural regions of the cell's genome, modifying parameters that dictate the type of molecule a particular control region interacts with, the effect of this interaction on transcription, and the type(s) of molecule(s) encoded by the structural region. The other mutation operators modify the CellSim® configuration, in particular the placement and concentration of molecules in the environment. The mutation rate varied between 10 and 20 percent, depending upon the type of mutation operator.

### 3.2. Evolving a Cube-Shaped Tissue

The best individual in the starting population had a fitness of 0.37 (fitness = 1.0 indicates a perfect match). Fitness remained constant until the 19th generation, when an individual of fitness 0.64 was produced. At this point, the best individual's genome and the CellSim® starting configuration had been modified extensively by mutation, with relatively large changes in the parameters governing interaction of the gene control regions, and addition of 4 point sources of growth molecules to the CellSim® environment. Over the next 31 generations the GA produced incremental improvements to the average fitness of the population, until at the 50th generation the GA converged to a perfect solution, and the search terminated (Fig. 1A).

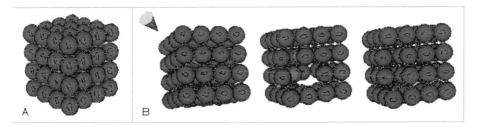

**Figure 1.** Evolved cube-shaped tissues. (A) Best individual (fitness 1.0) produced by a GA-based search. (B) Self-repair of the tissue cube after being damaged by a projectile (conical shape, panel B, upper left). The projectile approaches the cube from the upper left, passing downward, through, and exiting near the midpoint of the lower back edge, leaving a visible hole (B, middle image). As lost cells are replaced (B, right image), the damage is eventually repaired completely.

## 3.3. Self-Repair

The GA-based search is able to find an individual that matches the target shape but furthermore, this individual is capable of sustaining a relatively large amount of damage to its structure during development without compromising its ability to produce a stable cube. Indeed, even after the individual produces a stable cube shape, if the cube sustains damage (loss of up to 60% of its structure) the individual detects the damage and repairs it. Although the undisturbed cube appears static, injury reveals that the capacity for self repair remains latent.

Using other starting genomes and CellSim® configurations we have been able to evolve tissues with different shapes, such as single- or multi-layered sheets of cells. While not all of the tissue shapes that have been produced in our experiments can repair damage during all phases of the development process, all of the shapes produced to date do have some ability to repair damage, depending upon when the damage is introduced. For example, using a more complicated development process that involves cell signaling to cause death of cells that grow in undesired positions and to terminate cell growth at the appropriate time, we have evolved an individual that produces a stable $5 \times 5$ single-layer sheet of cells. In this case, incoming signals from neighboring cells cause other cells to adopt a state that stabilizes the sheet, but also inhibits the ability to repair damage to the sheet. Consequently, this individual is not as resilient to damage as the cube. Nevertheless, while the sheet individual is in the growth/development phase, it can sustain moderate damage yet it still produces the desired target shape.

## 4. Discussion and Conclusions

This paper presents an automated, bottom-up approach to tissue modeling, the goal of which is to derive higher-level properties of biological systems –self-directed development, self-repair, feedback, resilience to perturbation, and adaptability– from low-level biological primitives, allowing the system to assemble these primitives to achieve a desired target. This differs significantly from standard, top-down tissue modeling, where any higher-level biological properties must be explicitly designed and encoded into the system.

The ability to repair damage or injury is an emergent property of tissues evolved by the GA/ CellSim® system. Tissue phenotype results from interaction of genetically encoded elements with the environment defined by CellSim® , and improvements in phenotype arise through an iterative evolutionary process guided by a GA-based search strategy. Capability for self-repair was not specifically encoded in any gene, nor was this capability a factor in calculating the fitness during the GA-based search, but rather, capacity for self-repair arises from the biological primitives incorporated in CellSim® (e.g., molecular interaction, gene networks, feedback mechanisms, etc.). None of these biological primitives *explicitly* encodes the ability to repair damage, but when taken together they tend to make the process of construction robust to relatively large disruptions.

We are currently exploring ways to generate more complex self-repairing shapes and to incorporate biological primitives that support other tissue properties such as mechanical deformability.

## Acknowledgement

This work was supported by contract # DAMD17-02-2-0049 (TATRC) and W81XWH-04-2-0014 (DARPA).

## Note

1. As an extreme example of versatility, among certain reef fishes the largest female in a harem changes sex and becomes the dominant, functional male if the original dominant male dies or is removed [2]. Thus, changing the social environment triggers a complete reorganization of the (former) female body plan. By analogy, this could be seen as the equivalent of a house spontaneously reorganizing its floor plan and plumbing to accommodate an increased number of party guests as the holiday season approaches.

## References

[1] Sun, W. and P. Lal (2002) Computer Methods and Programs in Biomedicine 67: 85-103.
[2] Robertson, D.R. (1972) Science 177:1007-1009.
[3] Forbes, N. (2004) *Imitation of Life: How Biology Is Inspiring Computing*. MIT Press, Cambridge, MA, pp. 13-50.
[4] Langton, C.G. (1989) In *Artificial Life*, vol. VI, C.G. Langton, ed., Addison-Wesley, NY, pp.1-47.

*Medicine Meets Virtual Reality 13*
*James D. Westwood et al. (Eds.)*
*IOS Press, 2005*

# Grid Enabled Remote Visualization of Medical Datasets

Nick J. AVIS, Ian J. GRIMSTEAD and David W. WALKER
*Cardiff School of Computer Science, Cardiff University, Queen's Buildings,*
*5 The Parade, Roath, Cardiff CF24 3AA, United Kingdom*

**Abstract.** We present an architecture for remote visualization of datasets over the Grid. This permits an implementation-agnostic approach, where different systems can be discovered, reserved and orchestrated without being concerned about specific hardware configurations. We illustrate the utility of our approach to deliver high-quality interactive visualizations of medical datasets (circa 1 million triangles) to physically remote users, whose local physical resources would be otherwise overwhelmed. Our architecture extends to a full collaborative, resource-aware environment, whilst our presentation details our first proof-of-concept implementation.

## 1. Introduction

3D medical datasets (point based, polygonal or volumetric) and their rendering and visualization are important elements of a growing number of medical diagnosis, treatment planning, training and education activities. Traditionally to process these large datasets would require direct access to specialist graphics supercomputers, often tightly coupled to local display systems (ranging from the standard desktop to large scale immersive facilities such as CAVEs [1]). Dataset size continues to grow faster than Moore's Law [2], so whilst local processing capacities are increasing, such datasets can quickly overwhelm standard local computational infrastructures especially when users demand interactive data visualization and navigation.

Increases in network speed and connectivity are simultaneously allowing more cooperation between geographically remote teams and resources. Such developments break some of previous dependencies on the availability of local resources and afford new ways of working. Grid computing, based on service-oriented architectures such as OGSA [3], permits users to remotely access heterogeneous resources without considering their underlying implementations. This simplifies access for users and promotes the sharing of specialised equipment (such as rendering hardware). The motivation for this work arises from the desire to both investigate how interactive services can be supported within a Grid infrastructure and to remove the constraint on physical co-location of the end user with the high capability visualization engines.

We briefly review current Grid-based visualization systems and introduce our Resource-Aware Visualization Environment (RAVE). We present an overview of its architecture, and show initial test results of remote visualization using a PDA to observe remotely-rendered complex polygonal objects. We conclude this paper with a discussion of our findings and future work.

## 2. Previous Work

Remote access to rendering hardware enables expensive, specialist hardware to be used without having to move from the user's current place of work to a specific site. This is especially important when the user cannot move to the machine (for instance, a surgeon performing an operation) - the machine must come to the user.

OpenGL VizServer 3.1 [4] enables X11 and OpenGL applications to be shared remotely, with machines that do not have specialist high-performance graphics hardware. VizServer renders the OpenGL remotely, and transmits the rendered frame buffer to the collaborator. This has been used in a collaboration between the Manchester Royal Infirmary and the Manchester Visualization Centre [5,6], where MRI data is processed remotely by VizServer. The three-dimensional output is projected in the operating theatre, for the surgeon to refer to during the operation. This is in contrast to the two-dimensional image slice films that are usually viewed on a standard lightbox.

COVISE [7] is a modular visualization package, where one user is the master with control over the entire environment, whilst other users are slaves that can only observe. COVISE takes advantage of local processing on the slaves by only transmitting changes in data. For instance, the master sends changes in viewpoint, and the slaves then render the new view using a local copy of the data. COVISE also supports running slaves without a GUI – these machines become remote compute servers, enabling the Master to distribute processes over multiple machines.

For a fuller review of remote visualization applications refer to [8] and [9].

## 3. RAVE Architecture

We propose a visualization system that will respond to available resources, provide a collaborative environment, and be persistent (enabling users to collaborate asynchronously with previously recorded sessions). The system must not only react to changes in resources, but also make best use of them by sharing resources between users. To implement our visualization system, we have three components: a data service, a render service and a thin client. The architecture is presented in Figure 1.

The data service imports data from either a static file/web resource or a live feed from an external program. The data service forms a persistent, central distribution point for the data to be visualized. Multiple sessions may be managed by the same data service, sharing resources between users. The data are intermittently streamed to disk, recording any changes in the form of an audit trail. A recorded session may be played back at a later date; this enables users to append to a recorded session, collaborating asynchronously with previous users who may then later continue to work with the amended session.

A client with local rendering capability (referred to as an "active client") may connect to the data service and request a copy of the data. A user can interact with the shared data through the client by modifying their viewpoint or the actual scene itself. This permits large immersive displays such as an Immersadesk R2 to be used, along with commodity hardware. The client informs the data service of any changes, which are then reflected to all other clients, to ensure all clients have an up-to-date copy of the dataset. Multiple clients simultaneously visualize the same data, forming a collaborative environment where each client is represented in the dataset by a simple avatar.

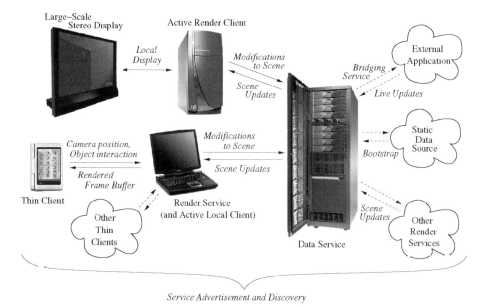

**Figure 1.** Diagram of RAVE architecture.

Whereas the active client is a render-capable client for the data service, a thin client (such as a PDA) represents a client that has no local rendering resource. The thin client must make use of remote rendering, so it connects to a render service and requests rendered copies of the data. Render services connect to the data service, and request a copy of the latest data in an identical manner to an active client, except that the render service can render off-screen for remote users, utilizing available rendering resources. Multiple render sessions are supported by each render service, so multiple users may share available rendering resources. If multiple users view the same session, then a single copy of the data is stored in the render service to save resources. The thin client can still manipulate the camera and the underlying data, but the actual data processing is carried out remotely whilst the thin client only deals with information presentation (such as displaying the remotely rendered dataset).

Once Grid/Web resources (with a known API) are exposed as services, they can be inter-connected without knowledge of the contents of the modules. To open our system to any resource, we chose to implement Grid/Web services and advertise our resources through Web Service Definition Language (WSDL) documents. WSDL can be registered with a UDDI server [10], enabling remote users to find our publicly available resources and connect automatically (no configuration is required by the client, although resources may need to have access permissions modified to permit new users).

## 4. Initial Test Results

We used three machines in this test; a laptop running Linux as the render service, an SGI Onyx as the data service, and a Sharp Zaurus PDA as the thin client. Files are supplied remotely to the data service via HTTP or FTP connections. The use of Grid middleware permits these resources to be substituted transparently, with the user being isolated from these implementation details.

The actual demands on the PDA are for a network connection, enough memory to import and process a frame buffer (120kB for a 200x200 pixel image with 24 bits per pixel, 480kB for a 400x400 image) and a simple GUI. We are platform and operating system agnostic, so any PDA could be selected or other devices running Microsoft Windows or Sun Solaris.

### 4.1. Test Models

Two test models (a skeletal hand and a skull) were obtained from the Large Geometric Models Archive at Georgia Institute of Technology [11]. The models were in PLY format, converted to Wavefront OBJ and then imported into our data service. The skeletal hand is from the Stereolithography Archive at Clemson University, with a view presented from the PDA in Figure 2. The skull is a section of the Visible Man project (from the National Library of Medicine), where the skeleton was processed by marching cubes and a polygon decimation algorithm. Two sample datafiles provided with VTK [12] were also imported; the frog skeleton and the scan of a human head (both isosurfaces). The VTK files are presented in Figure 2, as displayed on the active RAVE client (running on a laptop).

### 4.2. Web Services, UDDI and RAVE

The GUIs presented in Figure 2 shows an identical menu structure, but the PDA client operates through Web Services, whilst the active client can modify local geometry directly. With the PDA, the render service is interrogated for available interactions, whilst the active client can directly contact the scene graph. The interactions are then used to populate the menu, and are activated either via a standard Web Service call or a standard

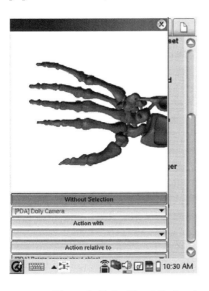
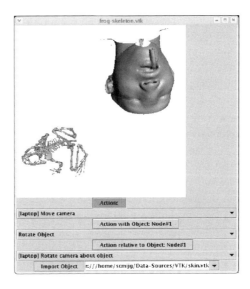

**Figure 2.** Skeletal hand displayed on PDA (C++), and VTK files on active client (Java).

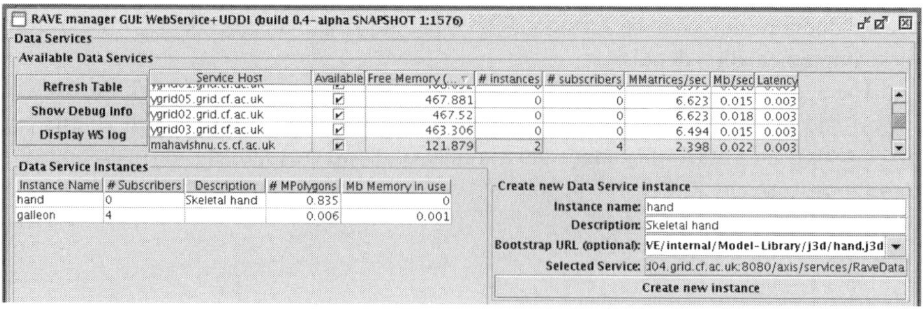

RAVE manager GUI: WebService+UDDI (build 0.4-alpha SNAPSHOT 1:1576)

**Data Services**

**Available Data Services**

| | Service Host | Available | Free Memory ( | # instances | # subscribers | MMatrices/sec | Mb/sec | Latency |
|---|---|---|---|---|---|---|---|---|
| Refresh Table | ygrid01.grid.cf.ac.uk | ✓ | | | | | | |
| | ygrid05.grid.cf.ac.uk | ✓ | 467.881 | 0 | 0 | 6.623 | 0.015 | 0.003 |
| Show Debug Info | ygrid02.grid.cf.ac.uk | ✓ | 467.52 | 0 | 0 | 6.623 | 0.018 | 0.003 |
| Display WS log | ygrid03.grid.cf.ac.uk | ✓ | 463.306 | 0 | 0 | 6.494 | 0.015 | 0.003 |
| | mahavishnu.cs.cf.ac.uk | ✓ | 121.879 | 2 | 4 | 2.398 | 0.022 | 0.003 |

**Data Service Instances**

| Instance Name | # Subscribers | Description | # MPolygons | Mb Memory in use |
|---|---|---|---|---|
| hand | 0 | Skeletal hand | 0.835 | 0 |
| galleon | 4 | | 0.006 | 0.001 |

**Create new Data Service instance**

Instance name: hand
Description: Skeletal hand
Bootstrap URL (optional): VE/internal/Model-Library/j3d/hand.j3d
Selected Service: j04.grid.cf.ac.uk:8080/axis/services/RaveData

Create new instance

**Figure 3.** RAVE UDDI manager.

Java interface. All interactions take the form of a mouse/pen drag, with an optional previously selected object. This enables us to use a standard API common to all interfaces (such as a pen based thin client PDA or mouse-based active client).

To discover what RAVE sessions are in progress, and what resources are available, we publish our services to a UDDI server, which we can then interrogate via our RAVE manager GUI, as presented in Figure 3. The services can be sorted by resource: available memory (as in Figure 3), number of session instances, million matrices processed per second, network bandwidth or latency. Only the data service section is shown here; the render service section is similar, except with an additional field, "polygons per second" for rendering performance. The user can now create a new session (providing a URL to a data source if required, otherwise an empty session can be started, ready for clients to remotely insert datasets into the session). Active or thin client sessions may also be launched from this GUI.

### 4.3. Timings

An 802.11b wireless card was used on the PDA, which contacted the render service on the laptop via a wireless access point. This implementation of the RAVE architecture uses a simple run-length encoding scheme for images, so we are limited by network bandwidth. A 400x400 true colour (24 bits per pixel) image was transmitted, with timings presented in Table 1. The on-screen render speed is shown for an active client as a contrast against that for the thin client. The time taken to render the image at the render server is shown as "Render Time", and the time to transmit/receive the image as "Image Transmission". Note that images are continuously streamed to the PDA, forming an interactive environment, rather than a batch-processing model.

It can be seen that the render time is dominated by the image transmission (between 60% and 95%). The peak laptop rendering throughput was around 4.5 million triangles/sec, but the laptop was running at around 10% load. Further investigation showed that Java3D off-screen rendering was significantly slower than that of on-screen rendering (varying between 10 to 30%, depending on the number of triangles in the model being rendered). However, other clients can use the unused resources; the render server is then limited to available network bandwidth to support multiple clients.

The image receipt times indicate a logical network bandwidth of between 2.6Mb/s and 0.6Mb/s. A direct socket test between the Zaurus and the main network returns an available bandwidth of 0.6Mb/s, so although our image compression is working, our

**Table 1.** Benchmarking timings for 400x400 pixel image.

| Model Name | Number Triangles | Active Client FPS | Thin Client FPS | Image Transmission | Render Time |
|---|---|---|---|---|---|
| Skeletal Hand | 834,884 | 5.4 | 3.2 | 0.172s | 0.134s |
| Frog Skeleton | 663,926 | 6.3 | 3.6 | 0.111s | 0.162s |
| Visible Man Skull | 473,281 | 10.1 | 1.3 | 0.625s | 0.108s |
| Human Head | 72,701 | 45.1 | 2.7 | 0.342s | 0.025s |

system is still limited by the available network bandwidth. We need to investigate more efficient encoding schemes for image streaming, as run-length encoding produces little benefit with highly varying images (such as the visible man skull dataset).

Various issues were encountered when using the mobile edition of Java (J2ME, available on the Zaurus), so we were forced to use C++ to implement the PDA client. For further detail refer to [8].

## 5. Discussion

The current OGSA model [3] of Grid services is changing rapidly, converging with the WS-Resource Framework [13]. This means that service implementations must not become tied to any particular infrastructure, as this is subject to change. We wrap our serving technology inside OGSA, Web Services or a test environment, so our service "engine" is unaffected by changes in infrastructure, only the wrapper needs to be modified.

Our initial framework is a proof of concept; we now have to react to available resources (e.g. network bandwidth, overloaded machines). This includes alternative transmission schemes to cope with lower bandwidth, and automatically switching from an overloaded or faulty service (providing a degree of fail safe operation). We will investigate volume rendering and "bridging" libraries, where we can plug existing applications into RAVE, effectively adapting a single-user application into a collaborative, remote environment.

Many medical imaging applications combine the requirements for high capability computing and data storage with the need for human-in-the-loop supervision. The value of the latest generation of tomographic scanners and digital imaging systems cannot be realised unless appropriate processing and dissemination of the images take place. As such there is a need to move many of the existing batch-oriented services of present Grids to interactive or responsive service provision.

We maintain that the above prototype system represents present state-of-the-art in terms of Grid-enabled remote visualization and provides a platform for further development and refinement for applications such as intraoperative imaging.

## References

[1] C. Cruz-Neira, D.J.Sandin and T.A. DeFanta. Surround-Screen Projection-Based Virtual Reality: The Design and Implementation of the CAVE. In *ACM Computer Graphics*, Vol. 27, Number 2, pages 135-142, July 1993.

[2] Gordon E. Moore. Cramming more components onto integrated circuits. In *Electronics*, Volume 38, Number 8, April 1965.

[3]   Ian Foster, Carl Kesselman, Keffrey M. Nick, and Steven Tuecke. The Physiology of the Grid: An Open Grid Services Architecture for Distributed Systems Integration. Technical report, Globus, February 2002.

[4]   SGI. SGI OpenGL VizServer 3.1. Data sheet, SGI, March 2003.

[5]   N. W. John. High Performance Visualization in a Hospital Operating Theatre. In *Proceedings of the Theory and Practice of Computer Graphics (TPCG03)*, pages 170-175. IEEE Computer Society, June 2003.

[6]   R. F. McCloy and N. W. John. *Computer Assisted Radiology and Surgery (CARS)*, chapter Remote Visualization of Patient Data in the Operating Theatre During Helpato-Pancreatic Surgery, pages 53-58. Elsevier, 2003.

[7]   High Performance Computing Centre Stuttgart. COVISE Features. http://www.hlrs.de/organization/vis/covise/features/, HLRS, September 2000.

[8]   Ian J. Grimstead, Nick J. Avis and David W. Walker. Automatic Distribution of Rendering Workloads in a Grid Enabled Collaborative Visualization Environment. In *Proceedings of SuperComputing 2004 (SC2004)*, November 2004.

[9]   K. Brodlie, J. Brooke, M.Chen, D. Chisnall, A. Fewings, C. Hughes, N. W. John, M. W. Jones, M. Riding and N. Roard. *Visual Supercomputing – Technologies, Applications and Challenges*. STAR – State of the Art Report, Eurographics, 2004.

[10]  Organization for the Advancement of Structured Information Standards (OASIS), Universal Description, Discovery and Integration (UDDI) – Version 2 Specification, http://www.oasis-open.org/committees/uddi-spec/doc/tcspecs.htm, July 2002.

[11]  The Large Geometric Models Archive. http://www.cc.gatech.edu/projects/large_models/, Georgia Institute of Technology.

[12]  Visualization ToolKit (VTK), downloadable from http://www.vtk.org/

[13]  Grid and Web Services Standards to Converge. Press release at http://www.marketwire.com/mw/release_html_b1?release_id=61977, GLOBUSWORLD.

Medicine Meets Virtual Reality 13
James D. Westwood et al. (Eds.)
IOS Press, 2005

# Surface Scanning Soft Tissues

Nick J. AVIS, John McCLURE and Frederic KLEINERMANN

*Cardiff School of Computer Science, Cardiff University, Queen's Buildings,*
*5 The Parade, Roath, Cardiff CF24 3AA, United Kingdom*
*Directorate of Laboratory Medicine, Manchester Royal Infirmary, Oxford Road,*
*Manchester, M13 9WL, United Kingdom*
*Research Group WISE, Department of Computer Science, VrijeUniversiteit Brussel,*
*Pleinlaan 2, B-1050 Brussel, Belgium*

**Abstract.** We investigate and report a method of 3D virtual organ creation based on
the RGB color laser surface scanning of preserved biological specimens. The surface attributes of these specimens result in signal degradation and increased scanning time. Despite these problems we are able to reproduce 3D virtual organs with
both accurate topology and colour consistency capable of reproducing pathological
lesions.

## 1. Introduction

3D computer based training tools and surgical simulators are emerging as useful teaching tools in a variety of different situations [1]. The construction of these simulators in
challenging in many areas. Whilst there has been considerable interest and developments
recently regarding the physically based modelling of soft tissues to allow real time deformation due to surgical interaction [2], the visual representation of both normal and diseased tissues and organs has been a relatively neglected area. Existing 3D virtual organ
models are often "hand crafted" using conventional 3D content creation tools employing
standard polygonal modeling and texture mapping techniques. As such it is difficult and
time consuming to create a library of 3D virtual organs to expose the trainee to a range of
virtual organs that represent biological variability and disease pathology. Furthermore,
such virtual organs must be both topologically correct and also exhibit color consistency
to support the identification of pathological lesions.

We investigated a new method of virtual organ creation based on a commercially
available RGB color laser surface scanning technology and point based rendering techniques applied in the first case to a number of preserved biological specimens. These
specimens represent the "gold standard" anatomical teaching resources presently available within teaching hospitals.

## 2. Surface Scanning

The test objects included: a plastic facimile of a human skull, a rubber model of a human
liver, untreated porcine and ovine material obtained from a local high street butcher, a

plastinated human heart and preserved porcine and human specimens. Specific permissions from the relevant authorities were sought and obtained to allow the use of human materials of these purposes. Prior to scanning the preserved specimens were removed from their jar, washed and excess water removed via light application of an absorent lint-free cloth. The specimens were scanned using the Arius3D system (www.arius3d.com). This system employs a scanning laser and the triangulation technique to determine the distance of each measured point. The laser head is mounted on a coordinate measuring machine (CMM). Unlike most laser scanning systems the Arius3D scanner records color information as well as distance at each measured point by combining the signals from three color lasers (red, green and blue) and constructs a "texture" image which is aligned and at the same spatial resolution as the reconstructed surface [3]. Since the pitch between measured point is small (of the order of 100 to 200 micros) a visual representation of the object can be presented using point based rendering techniques without the need to generate a polygonal surface representation [4]. Conversion to a surface representation can be performed as a post data acquisition and merging operation using a number of commercially available third party tools.

## 3. Results

Unlike the plastic and rubber specimens all the biological specimens exhibited highly reflective surfaces. In addition the objects themselves were not self supporting and were highly deformable.

In many scan passes the system was unable to detect a signal and effect a reconstruction of the scanned area. This was due to the reflective nature of the surface being scanned. Similar problems had previously been encountered when attempting to use photogrammetry and other laser based surface scanning technologies on similar specimens [5]. The need for multiple scans at slighly different angles to obtain sufficient data to effect a reconstruction proved problematical both in terms of increased scan time and dataset size, but also regarding issues surrounding the movement of the specimen. Figure 1 show the test specimens and the reconstructed "virtual organ" using the Arius3D scanner data and point based rendering techniques.

## 4. Discussion

The utility of virtual organs showing pathological lesons depends on color consistency in the representation of the lesions. The Arius3D system is unique, as far as we are aware, in that it recovers both toplogy and color from the scanned object. The physics associated with surface and sub-surface reflections and how these affect the scanner require further investigation. Nevertheless of the test objects scanned we were able to effect a 3D reconstruction albeit with considerably more scan time and post processing effort that originally anticipated.

## 5. Conclusion

The surface scanning of biological soft tissues promises a quick and easy means to construct virtual organs for use within surgical simulators and other computer based medical

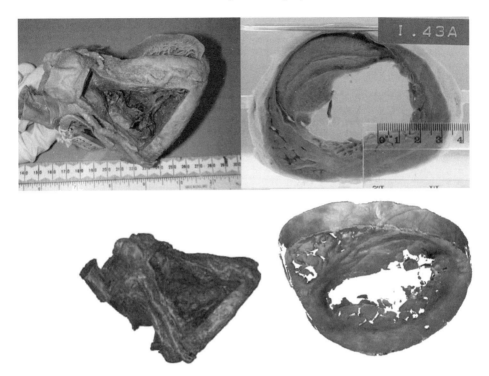

**Figure 1.** Test objects and virtual organ representations. The virtual organs contain 13,385,767 and 585,508 data points respectively. The images show models using point based rendering techniques and have not been converted to a polygonal mesh. Color consistency within and between models is important to support pathological lesion identification.

education packages. However, as outlined here, the surface and subsurface reflections associated with the tissues of many organs, present additional challenges to scanning systems and result in data drop-out. This combined with the deformable nature of much of this material and the challenge of a simple and effective means of capturing the surface topology and texture of deformable biological specimens in-vivo or ex-vivo remains.

## Acknowledgements

This study was in part supported by grants from the Pathological Society of Great Britain and Ireland and from the North Western Deanery for Postgraduate Medicine and Dentistry.

## References

[1]  N J Avis. Virtual Environment Technologies. Journal of Minimally Invasive Therapy and Allied Technologies, Vol 9(5) pp333- 340, 2000.
[2]  A Nava, E Mazza, F Kleinermann, N J Avis and J McClure. Determination of the mechanical properties of soft human tissues through aspiration experiments. In MICCAI 2003, R E Ellis and T M Peters (Eds.) LNCS (2878), pp 222-229, Springer-Verlag, 2003.

[3]  Rejean Baribeau. Optimized Spectral Estimation Methods for Improved Colorimetry with Laser Scanning Systems. Proc. 1st International Symposium on 3D Data Processing Visualization and Transmission (3DPVT'02), 2002.

[4]  M Zwicker, H Pfister, J van Baar and M Gross. Surface Splatting, SIGGRAPH 2001, Proc. 28th Annual Conference on Computer Graphics and Interactive Techniques, pp 371-378, 2001.

[5]  Nick J Avis, Frederik Kleinermann and John McClure. Soft Tissue Surface Scanning – A comparison of commercial 3D object scanners for surgical simulation content creation and medical education application. In International Symposium Medical Simulation (ISMS 2004), S Cotin and D Metaxas (Eds.) LNCS 3078, pp 211-220, Springer-Verlag, 2004.

*Medicine Meets Virtual Reality 13*
*James D. Westwood et al. (Eds.)*
*IOS Press, 2005*

# Validation of a Bovine Rectal Palpation Simulator for Training Veterinary Students

Sarah BAILLIE [a,c], Andrew CROSSAN [a], Stephen BREWSTER [a],
Dominic MELLOR [b] and Stuart REID [b]

[a] *Glasgow Interactive Systems Group, Department of Computing Science*
[b] *Faculty of Veterinary Medicine, University of Glasgow, UK*
[c] *Clyde Veterinary Group, Lanark, UK*
*e-mail: {sarah, stephen}@dcs.gla.ac.uk*

**Abstract.** Bovine rectal palpation is a necessary skill for a veterinary student to learn. However, lack of resources and welfare issues currently restrict the amount of training available to students in this procedure. Here we present a virtual reality based teaching tool - the Bovine Rectal Palpation Simulator - that has been developed as a supplement to existing training methods. When using the simulator, the student palpates virtual objects representing the bovine reproductive tract, receiving feedback from a PHANToM haptic device (inside a fibreglass model of a cow), while the teacher follows the student's actions on the monitor and gives instruction. We present a validation experiment that compares the performance of a group of traditionally trained students with a group whose training was supplemented with a simulator training session. The subsequent performance in the real task, when examining cows for the first time, was assessed with the results showing a significantly better performance for the simulator group.

## 1. Introduction

Bovine rectal palpation is performed by veterinarians for pregnancy diagnosis, fertility assessment and as part of a clinical examination. The procedure is difficult to learn and requires a great deal of practice to identify structures palpated. In the United Kingdom the number of veterinary undergraduates has increased in recent years and the opportunities to gain sufficient farm animal experience to develop the required skills are becoming limited [1]. Welfare guidelines limit the number of examinations allowed per cow and this further reduces the opportunities to practice.

A Bovine Rectal Palpation Simulator has been developed at the University of Glasgow as a teaching tool to supplement existing training methods [2]. An iterative design process was used to create a virtual environment with simulations of the bovine reproductive tract, including models of the cervix, uterus and ovaries positioned within the pelvis and abdomen. Nine veterinarians were involved in the development and evaluation of the simulations and this resulted in the creation of a range of realistic models. During simulator training, the student palpates the virtual objects while interacting with

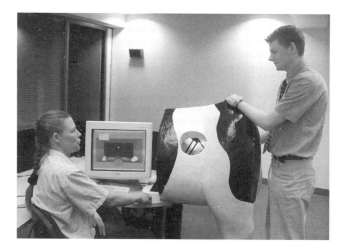

**Figure 1.** Simulator training. The teacher provides instruction while the student palpates virtual models of the bovine reproductive tract inside the fibreglass cow using a PHANToM.

a PHANToM haptic device (from SensAble Technologies), which is positioned inside a model of a fibreglass rear-half of a cow (Figure 1). The teacher follows the student's action inside the virtual cow on the monitor and provides instruction. A teaching protocol has been developed where the student learns initially to locate the uterus in different positions, mastering this fundamental skill before progressing on to performing fertility examinations and diagnosing pregnancy.

Validation is a key factor if simulators are to become widely adopted in medical and veterinary training. Without it, the benefits that simulators provide are uncertain; trainees may develop a false sense of confidence or learn techniques that actually degrade their performance in the real task. There have been previous attempts to validate virtual reality based palpation simulators, a human prostate simulator [3] and a horse ovary palpation simulator (HOPS) [4]. Both measured the performance of groups representing different skill levels but failed to differentiate between the groups during simulator tests. A comparison of students trained on HOPS with those receiving only traditional training demonstrated equal performance levels for both groups in a post-training test [5]. Additionally, assessments were made using either the simulated environment [3,4] or when examining *in vitro* specimens [5], which are both approximations for the real task.

A preliminary evaluation of the bovine simulator has been conducted and students considered their subsequent performance examining cows had improved [2]. However, this evaluation depended on students assessing their own technique and therefore, an independent, objective assessment of performance was needed to validate the teaching tool.

## 2. Methods

Sixteen undergraduate veterinary students from the University of Glasgow with no prior experience of performing bovine rectal palpation were randomly selected and allocated to two groups, A and B. The students were in the third year of the veterinary course, the stage at which they were about to embark on their first placement training examin-

**Table 1.** Uterus identification rates per 4 cows examined for the eight pairs of students.

| Group                 Pair: | 1 | 2 | 3 | 4 | 5 | 6 | 7 | 8 | Group total |
|---|---|---|---|---|---|---|---|---|---|
| Group A: Simulator trained | 1 | 3 | 2 | 3 | 2 | 3 | 2 | 2 | 18 / 32 |
| Group B: Traditional training only | 0 | 0 | 0 | 0 | 0 | 1 | 0 | 0 | 1 / 32 |

ing cows on farms with veterinarians. All of the students had undergone the traditional training provided in the preclinical course, consisting of anatomy lectures and laboratory practical sessions. Group A was trained with the simulator whereas Group B received only the traditional training. The students were divided into pairs, one from each group, and each pair examined four non-pregnant cows on-farm. The task was to find and identify the uterus during a five minute examination and correct identification was verified using video-recorded images from an ultrasound probe taped to the palm of the student's hand.

## 3. Results

All students in Group A located the uterus in one or more of the four cows examined, compared with only one student in Group B (Table 1). There were 18 successful identifications for Group A from a maximum of 32 (8 students ×4 cows per group), verified by ultrasound, and only one for Group B. These results indicated that Group A was significantly better at finding the uterus than Group B (p-value < 0.001).

## 4. Conclusion

The Bovine Rectal Palpation Simulator provided more effective training than the traditional method alone and the poor performance of Group B underlines the difficulties currently experienced by novices. The simulator-trained students had learned skills that enabled them to locate the uterus when examining cows, demonstrating the validity of the simulator as a teaching tool for one of the key components of bovine rectal palpation.

## 5. Discussion

There is a need to find ways of supplementing existing methods for training veterinary students to perform bovine rectal palpation and a simulator has been developed as a potential solution. The validation of the simulator was undertaken to demonstrate that students were acquiring skills that transferred to the real task and not, for example, just learning to use the simulator. As part of the preparation for clinical placement training, equipping students with basic skills using the simulator will enable them to make more effective use of animals as a learning resource. This is important when the opportunities to practice on farms are increasingly limited. Additionally, training novices for an invasive procedure in a virtual environment prior to the first real examination has benefits for animal welfare. During the simulator sessions, the teacher has the advantage of being able to see the student's actions, which is not possible in the real cow. Therefore, the teacher is able to provide more effective training, guiding movements, identifying structures palpated and providing feedback on performance.

The bovine simulator provides a complement to existing training methods. Additional models have been developed including a wide range of fertility cases and some examples of pathology and the training sessions can be customised to individual student's learning needs. The simulator also has potential to provide training for clinical scenarios in other species and further developments are planned.

## References

[1] C. D. Penny, "Education – A University View," Cattle Practice, vol. 10, no. 4, pp. 255-256, 2002.
[2] S. Baillie, A. Crossan, S. Reid, and S. Brewster, "Preliminary Development and Evaluation of a Bovine Rectal Palpation Simulator for Training Veterinary Students," Cattle Practice, vol. 11, no. 2, pp. 101-106, 2003.
[3] G. Burdea, G. Patounakis, V. Popescu, and R. E. Weiss, "Virtual Reality-Based Training for the Diagnosis of Prostate Cancer," IEEE Transactions on Biomedical Engineering, vol. 46, no. 10, pp. 1253-1260, 1999.
[4] A. Crossan, S. Brewster, S. Reid, and D. Mellor, "Comparison of Simulated Ovary Training over Different Skill Levels", In Proc. EuroHaptics, 2001, pp. 17-21.
[5] A. Crossan, S. Brewster, D. Mellor, and S. Reid, "Evaluating Training Effects of HOPS", In Proc. Euro-Haptics, 2003, pp. 430-434.

Medicine Meets Virtual Reality 13
James D. Westwood et al. (Eds.)
IOS Press, 2005

# Predictive Biosimulation and Virtual Patients in Pharmaceutical R&D

Alex BANGS

*Entelos, Inc., 110 Marsh Dr., Foster City, CA 94404*

**Abstract.** In the automotive, telecommunication, and aerospace industries, modeling and simulation are used to understand the behavior and outcomes of a new design well before production begins, thereby avoiding costly failures. In the pharmaceutical industry, failures are not typically identified until a compound reaches the clinic. This fact has created a productivity crisis due to the high failure rate of compounds late in the development process. Modeling and simulation are now being adopted by the pharmaceutical industry to understand the complexity of human physiology and predict human response to therapies. Additionally, virtual patients are being used to understand the impact of patient variability on these predictions. Several case studies are provided to illustrate the technology's application to pharmaceutical R&D and healthcare.

## 1. Introduction

The pharmaceutical industry is facing a productivity crisis. Many current blockbuster drugs are coming off patent and new drugs are not being introduced at a fast enough pace to meet investor expectations [1]. It currently costs over $800M and takes an average of 14 years to develop a new drug [2]. The Food and Drug Administration recently announced the Critical Path Initiative, which attempts to address the issues of cost and time in the drug development process, and outlined the need for the industry to adopt technologies that may help [3].

A key challenge for the pharmaceutical industry is the high failure rate of drugs, particularly those in late in late phase development. In the automotive, aerospace, and telecommunication industry, modeling and simulation are used to design and test new products well before they are commercially produced. For example, the Boeing 777 flew many times in a computer before it was constructed [4]. Modeling and simulation have been used in some aspects of drug development, notably for molecular modeling and drug pharmacokinetics, but have not been widely applied in industry to modeling biological systems and in particular human physiology. The technology and methods now exist to build large-scale biosimulation models for pharmaceutical R&D. In fact, such models have already been built and applied, resulting in saving in terms of time and money, and lowered risk of drug failures.

## 2. Predictive Biosimulation Models

A number of approaches are being taken to understand complex biological systems [5]. Many of these approaches focus on analyzing data from high throughput technologies, such as gene expression arrays. These approaches seek possible correlations to behaviors that may indicate relationships not previously identified or understood. Other approaches are focused on automatically or manually constructing relationship models based on information in the scientific literature. In most of these cases, the result is a static model of biological relationships. Missing from these approaches is the ability to understand the dynamics of the system (*e.g.,* what the quantities and signals are at any point in time, the relative effects of those quantities and signals, how feedback affects the system) and how they translate into therapeutic efficacy. In order to achieve this capability, a more quantitative approach is required.

A biosimulation model quantitatively captures biological elements (*e.g.,* proteins, cytokines, cell populations) and their relationships. The relationships between elements are represented using differential equations, allowing simulation techniques to predict the behavior of the system and the quantities of the biological elements over time. The model may be configured with parameter changes to predict new outcomes for different scenarios, *e.g.,* for new drug targets or new clinical trial protocols.

Constructing such models requires a significant amount of data about the biological elements, their states, and their relationships. Historically, much of the biosimulation work has been accomplished using "bottom-up" techniques, *i.e.,* building models of biochemical pathways or subcellular systems based on the data gathered on these systems. Another technique focuses on a "top down" approach to modeling biological systems [6].

The goal of the top-down approach is to build a model that can simulate a pathology or behavior in the context of a particular disease. This approach starts by defining a model scope, which is based on the disease characteristics and their related physiological systems, as well as the anticipated uses of the model. For example, a model of obesity may need to include the gastrointestinal tract, organ systems for processing and storing macronutrients (*e.g.,* the liver and adipose tissue), and brain regulation of appetite. Given the disease focus, the model does not need to include details of bone structure or lung tissue function. The underlying philosophy of the top-down approach is Einstein's maxim that things should be made "as simple as possible, but no simpler."

If the model is to be used for evaluating drug targets, the physiological systems where those targets play a role must be included in sufficient detail so that the target effects can be modeled. This does not require that every subcellular biochemical pathway in the body be included. Instead, many of these systems are modeled with the functional effects of the underlying biological pathways aggregated and represented at a higher level of detail. For example, rather than include all the dynamics of a cell type's intracellular pathways, it may be sufficient to include enough dynamics of intercellular behavior that, under specific conditions, the cell produces cytokines at specified rates. Where necessary, the models include a deeper representation of the biological pathways to capture dynamics of interest at a lower level (*e.g.,* around a protein target of interest).

These models are constructed using a wide range of data. For example, data from laboratory studies is used to confirm the existence of biological relationships, and where possible, determine their dynamics. At the top level, clinical data is used to validate the model, ensuring that the full system behaves as a patient would under the same clinical protocol. The result is a model that simulates a patient with the disease of interest.

## 3. Virtual Patients

The diseases being studied in pharmaceutical research today are highly complex. It is typical to hear a scientist refer to a disease such as asthma as being not one but rather many different diseases clustered together. Complex diseases do not result from a single gene defect, but rather, an interaction of multiple genetic and environmental factors. Therefore, a model needs to represent not just "the disease," but also the range of patients that may present with the disease, as well as the unique set of genetic and environmental variations they incorporate.

In addition, while building a model, there will be knowledge gaps. These may include a lack of specific information about the rate of a particular biological process, or the quantities of various biological elements at specific times. In some cases, these may be reverse engineered, which may be time consuming or even impossible given technical limitations. The first question in attempting to bridge any knowledge gap is therefore "Is this unknown significant?"– will the predictions of the model change based on changes in this unknown? Therefore, a system to explicitly represent these gaps, and the possible variations of their solutions, can help us identify the key knowledge gaps. With this information, experiments can be defined to resolve them.

The concept of a *virtual patient* was developed to encompass the variations required to study the broad range of patients and the underlying uncertainties about patient biology [7]. The modeling platform supports the representation of virtual patients, along with the tests required to validate them as being "real" in terms of their physiological readouts. Once virtual patients are constructed, "what if" experiments are performed to validate, for example, whether manipulating a particular drug target has the desired effect in a diverse set of potential patients.

## 4. Case Studies

Entelos has developed a modeling approach and technology platform to construct large-scale physiological models of human disease. These platforms, called PhysioLab® systems, facilitate pharmaceutical R&D in a number of immune/inflammatory diseases, including asthma and rheumatoid arthritis, and in diseases related to metabolism, including obesity and diabetes. These models have been applied to a wide variety of R&D problems (Figure 1). To illustrate their use, a selection of case studies is included below.

### 4.1. Drug Target Validation

Entelos collaborated with Pfizer to evaluate phosphodiesterase 4 (PDE4) as a drug target in asthma [8]. The process started with defining all of the known functions of PDE4 based on the scientific literature. Additional hypothesized functions were added where PDE4 was thought to have an effect, but for which it had not been explicitly measured. These functions and hypotheses were then represented in the model, allowing the mathematical effect of inhibiting PDE4 to be simulated. In addition, a set of moderate asthmatic virtual patients were constructed with different mediator expression profiles.

The PDE4 inhibitory effect was then simulated against the set of virtual asthma patients. First, all the functions were inhibited simultaneously to evaluate the potential

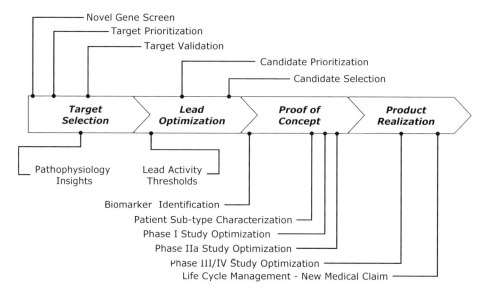

**Figure 1.** Applications of PhysioLab technology in pharmaceutical R&D.

efficacy of target inhibition. Under these conditions, the model predicted the target would have a significant clinical effect on all the patients, improving their ability to breathe as measured through forced expiratory volume in one section ($FEV_1$) scores. Second, each of the functions was inhibited individually. This analysis showed that of the 50+ pathways where PDE4 was thought to play a role, only four had a significant effect on the clinical outcome. Based on this information, Entelos provided recommendations for wet lab confirmation of the simulation results, including advice on the development of predictive, *in vitro* assays. Following this initial target validation analysis, a set of PDE4 inhibitor compounds were simulated to show the effects of different dosing strategies on the efficacy of PDE4 inhibition.

This approach provides unique value in target validation, providing new information on drug target effects, reducing the time for target validation and predicting human results well before a drug enters clinical trials. Additionally, the positive prediction of PDE4 efficacy increased the company's confidence in moving the target forward in the research pipeline.

## 4.2. Clinical Trial Design

Entelos collaborated with Johnson & Johnson Pharmaceutical Research and Development (J&JPRD) on designing a Phase 1 clinical trial for a new diabetes drug [10]. With new glucose-lowering drugs, there is a concern about patients becoming hypoglycemic. To ensure that this would not be an issue with the new drug, J&JPRD had planned to run a trial in healthy patients with escalating doses to see if there was any risk of hypoglycemia. Entelos simulated the trial using healthy virtual patients, and predicted that the hypoglycemic effects between the different doses would not be easily observable, and that there did not appear to be any adverse effects at the highest dose.

The trial was run with a smaller patient population and only the highest dose *versus* placebo was examined. The simulation results were confirmed by the trial results.

Overall the process resulted in cost and time savings. J&JPRD was able to run a shorter trial with fewer dosing arms, reducing patient recruitment. The result was a 40% reduction in time and 66% reduction in patients for the Phase 1 trial. Further simulations were performed in a population of virtual patients to provide additional information, including biomarkers and the optimization of a backup compound.

### 4.3. Biomarker/Diagnostic Identification

With the complex, chronic diseases being studied today, it is important to be able to characterize patients and understand what therapeutic regimen would best fit each patient. To achieve this, biomarkers (*e.g.*, patient measurements, diagnostic tests), are needed to differentiate and diagnose patients. Biomarkers are also used during clinical trials to identify which patients best respond to a drug or to identify whether the drug is having a desired effect.

Entelos collaborated with Roche Diagnostics to identify a new biomarker for insulin sensitivity [9]. A signal in a patient's progression to diabetes is their increased insensitivity to insulin. Early identification of this condition could have a significant impact on patient care, but existing markers were not very predictive. The goal was to identify a new, more predictive marker that would be based on simple tests using measurements from a single blood sample.

To perform this analysis, Entelos evaluated potential markers in 62 virtual patients with diverse phenotypes and pathophysiologies. In addition, a novel prevalence weighting methodology was developed that allowed the results from the virtual patients to be compared to a typical clinical population. The markers were further evaluated against a number of patient scenarios, including different diets.

The result was a new, more predictive biomarker of insulin sensitivity. The marker was defined faster and more easily than would be possible with regular patients. In the future, this technology may be used not only to create new diagnostics, but applied directly to patient care, helping to characterize patients and identify the best treatment regimen for an individual patient.

## 5. Conclusion

The pharmaceutical industry is starting to benefit from biological modeling and simulation – learning early which products will work in the marketplace and how best to bring them to market. The result will be cost and time savings, and ultimately, more effective products being brought to market. The technology can also be extended into the healthcare arena, identifying new tests to improve patient care, and eventually, applying it directly to individual patient care.

## References

[1]  Arlington S., Barnett S., Hughes S., *Pharma 2010: The Threshold of Innovation*, IBM Business Consulting Services (2002).
[2]  DeMasi J., Hansen R., Grabowski, H., "The price of innovation: new estimates of drug development costs," *Journal of Health Economics*, Vol.22; 325-30 (2003).

[3]   *Innovation or Stagnation? Challenge and Opportunity on the Critical Path to New Medical Products,* Food and Drug Administration (2004).

[4]   Norris, G., "Boeing's seventh wonder," *Spectrum IEEE,* Vol.32(10); 20-23 (1995).

[5]   Butcher, E., Berg, E., Kunkel, E., "Systems biology in drug discovery," *Nature Biotechnology,* Vol.22(10); 1253-1259 (2004).

[6]   Paterson, T., "Applying simulation technology to the life sciences," in *Frontiers of Engineering* (Washington D.C: National Academy Press, 2002) 87-90.

[7]   Michelson, S., Okino, M., "The virtual patient: capturing patient variability using biosimulation," *Preclinica,* Vol.2(1); 33-37 (2004).

[8]   "Best practices awards: discovery and development participants," *BioIT World,* 15 July 2003.

[9]   Uehling, M., "I, virtual patient," *BioIT World,* 18 August 2004, 50.

[10]  Trimmer, J., McKenna, C., Sudbeck, B., Ho, R. "Use of systems biology in clinical development: design and prediction of a type 2 diabetes clinical," in *PAREXEL's Pharmaceutical R&D Sourcebook 2004/2005* (Waltham, MA: PAREXEL Internat'l Corp., 2004) 131.

Medicine Meets Virtual Reality 13
James D. Westwood et al. (Eds.)
IOS Press, 2005

# Simulating Surgical Incisions without Polygon Subdivision

Yogendra BHASIN, Alan LIU and Mark BOWYER

*National Capital Area Medical Simulation Center*
*e-mail: ybhasin@simcen.usuhs.mil; url: http://simcenusuhs.mil*

**Abstract.** Modeling cuts, bleeding and the insertion of surgical instruments are essential in surgical simulation. Both visual and haptic cues are important. Current methods to simulate cuts change the topology of the model, invalidating pre-processing schemes or increasing the model's complexity. Bleeding is frequently modeled by particle systems or computational fluid dynamics. Both can be computationally expensive. Surgical instrument insertion, such as intubation, can require complex haptic models. In this paper, we describe methods for simulating surgical incisions that do not require such computational complexity, yet preserve the visual and tactile appearance necessary for realistic simulation.

## 1. Introduction

Simulation is increasingly used for surgery training. Surgical simulators allow users to improve their skills prior to operating on a patient. These systems can assist surgical training by providing different training scenarios and quantifying user performance. Making surgical incisions is a fundamental task of most procedures. Simulating incisions require the portrayal of visual and tactile effects like cutting, bleeding and instrument insertion. These cues provide important feedback. Cuts change the visual appearance of the tissue. The incision's length, depth, and orientation vary by procedure. Blood can obscure the surgeon's view, and make surgery difficult. Tissue consistency and resilience affects the amount of pressure to apply on the scalpel. Due to its importance, cutting, bleeding and instrument insertion are frequently simulated surgical effects. A number of methods have been proposed to address them. In this section, we review current research.

Many methods simulate cuts by modifying the topology of the model. Some simulators simply remove model elements from the object along the cut path [1]. This creates an uneven appearance and unrealistic gaps in the model. Subdivision methods implement cuts by splitting the polygons along its boundaries or path of incision in real-time. [2] proposed cutting surface-based meshes while re-meshing the cut to achieve the required level of smoothness. [3] used volumetric models in the form of tetrahedral mesh for cutting. While such methods can produce visually pleasing cuts, they increase the size of the mesh, resulting in increased computational burden. In addition, some methods for real-time deformation modeling rely on pre-processing the model's geometry. Cuts change the model's topology and can invalidate these schemes [4].

Bleeding is commonly modeled using mathematical representations of fluid flow or particle systems. Computational fluid dynamics methods based on Navier-Stokes equations provide accurate fluid flow models. Although some simplified forms of these equations [5] have been developed, they can be difficult to implement in real-time simulations. [6] introduced particle systems as a technique for a class of fuzzy objects. Both particle-based Lagrangian approach [5] and grid-based Eulerian approach [7] have been used to simulate fluids. Although easy to animate, these require many particles for realism and impose high computational overhead. [8] developed a particle based texture animation method to simulate arterial bleeding. Other methods include temporal texture synthesis [9], or video capture [10]. Such schemes can be inefficient, or provide limited realism.

Modeling instrument insertion is difficult because of interactions with complex anatomical models. Many simulators focus on specific aspects of the surgical task and assume that the instruments are already inserted in the operation site [8,11]. Some simulators rely on mannequins for the actual instrument insertion [12]. The actual process of inserting the instruments hasn't received much attention, yet this task is crucial in some procedures, such as diagnostic peritoneal lavage [13].

Many surgical procedures such as cricothyroidotomy, chest tube insertion, and diagnostic peritoneal lavage, require only small incisions be made. The cuts are small, and often do not bleed profusely. When surgical instruments such as tubes or needles are inserted, resistance is felt due to anatomical structures beneath the skin however these structures cannot be seen. In these cases, it is possible to provide realistic visual and haptic feedback without the computationally intensive methods outlined above.

## 2. Method

We propose an alternative way to model some surgical incisions. Rather than using polygon subdivision, we use animated texture maps and local haptic models. The underlying patient model is untouched. We have implemented this approach on a prototype cricothyroidotomy simulator currently under development [14]. Cricothyroidotomy is an emergency procedure that is performed when the patient's airway is blocked, and less invasive attempts to clear it have failed. The simulator enables medical students to practice making the incision on the throat, then inserting surgical instruments to widen and maintain the airway. In this section, we describe our method for modeling the visual and tactile effects of small surgical incisions.

### 2.1. Visual Feedback During Cutting

Animated and dynamic textures can allow interactive applications with little impact on the rendering performance [15]. Textures provide visually acceptable details of small scale structures. Our method is similar to [16], but has been extended to include the simulation of blood trails and oozing wounds. In our method, dynamic updates of the skin texture are implemented using the OpenGL's function glTexSubImage2D(). This function allows us to overwrite selective portion of a texture map by specifying the location of the rectangular sub-region to be replaced. Two types of textures are used, one for the wound, another for bleeding. The wound texture consists of a red spot in the center of a $5 \times 5$ image [Fig 1.1]. The texture is radially blurred using Adobe Photoshop so that the intensity of adjacent textures is identical at the edges. A cut is modeled by placing

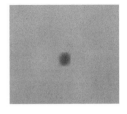

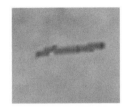

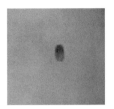

**Figure 1.1.** Single wound texture.    **Figure 1.2.** A Cut modeled using successive wound textures.    **Figure 1.3.** A blood droplet

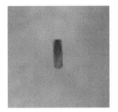

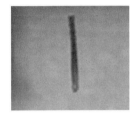

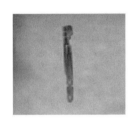

**Figure 1.4.** Expanded droplet.    **Figure 1.5.** A blood drop with trail    **Figure 1.6.** Overlapping drops with transparent regions.

successive wound textures at the point of contact of the scalpel. This gives an appearance of a continuous cut [Fig 1.2].

Bleeding is modeled in two parts: the leading droplet, and the trail. Figure 1.3 shows a single blood droplet overwritten on skin. The droplet is expanded by successively replacing it with a longer drop texture [Fig 1.4]. As these drops flow down the skin, they leave behind a blood trail, giving an oozing effect. The region of the drop that joins the trail is Gaussian blurred so that the intensity of the two textures is consistent with each other and they blend together nicely [Fig 1.5].

Blood drops and trails do not occupy the entire region of a rectangular image and have transparent regions. In the OpenGL implementation, subtextures do not blend with existing blood trace on the main texture but overwrites them. This produces undesirable effects as shown in figure 1.6. So blood textures cannot be implemented using subtextures alone. To fix this problem, we model the droplets and the trails as RGBA images. The transparent regions of the images are identified using the alpha channel. These transparent regions are then tracked and manually rasterized using glDrawPixels() function so that the original texture is maintained on the main image [Fig. 3.1].

## 2.2. Haptic Feedback During Cutting

For small incisions a simplified haptic model can provide tactile fidelity comparable to more complex techniques. Unlike models that require change in the model's topology, our method uses a local model based on reaction forces as the blade is pressed into skin, and constrained motion in a plane. The haptic feedback during cutting is primarily governed by two effects. Reaction forces correspond to the tissue resistance felt as the scalpel is pressed deeper into the cut. The second effect corresponds to the blade's motion constrained by the surrounding tissue to move in the cut direction. In this section we describe how we implement these effects in our simulator.

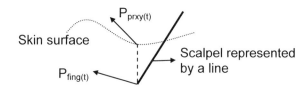

**Figure 2.1.** Reachin's haptic interaction model when a scalpel is penetrated inside the skin surface.

We use the haptic interaction model provided by Reachin API [17]. Define the haptic device position as $P_{fing(t)}$ where time $t$ is the instance after the first contact. $P_{fing(t)}$ moves freely in the space and can penetrate object surfaces. In our simulator, $P_{fing(t)}$ corresponds to the scalpel's tip. When $P_{fing(t)}$ penetrates the model, the ReachIn API defines an additional point, $P_{prxy(t)}$. As shown in figure 2.1, this is the nearest point on the surface of the object to $P_{fing(t)}$. $P_{fing(0)}$ and $P_{prxy(0)}$ are correspondingly defined at the instance of the first contact.

Let, $S_{x(t)}$ and $S_{y(t)}$ be the unit vectors at time $t$ along the scalpel's local $x$ and $y$ axis respectively. Let $K_x$, $K_n$, $K_y$, $K_{xz}$ and $K_d$ be constants set according to the desired tissue properties.

**Implementing the reaction effect.** Reaction forces model the resistance of the cut tissue. The user feels greater resistance as the scalpel is penetrated deeper into the skin. This force is proportional to the depth of penetration of the scalpel along the unit vector from $P_{fing(t)}$ to $P_{prxy(t)}$ denoted by $S_{n(t)}$. Thus,

$$F_{n(t)} = -K_n \cdot \left[ (P_{fing(t)} - P_{fing(0)}) \cdot S_{n(t)} \right] \cdot S_{n(t)},$$

where

$$S_{n(t)} = (P_{prxy(t)} - P_{fing(t)})/|P_{prxy(t)} - P_{fing(t)}|$$

**Implementing the constrained motion effect.** Once the scalpel is within the incision, the blade cannot move easily in a direction perpendicular to the cut. We implement this effect by constraining the motion of the blade in a plane containing the cut. A correction force is applied whenever the scalpel drifts from the plane. This force $F_{x(t)}$ acts in the direction perpendicular to the blade (along scalpel's $x$-axis) at time $t$. It is proportional to the distance of the scalpel from the cut-plane and is computed by projecting this distance onto the $x$-axis. Figure 2.2 illustrates. Thus,

$$F_{x(t)} = -K_x \cdot [(P_{fing(t)} - P_{fing(0)}) \cdot S\_x(0)] \cdot S_{x(0)}.$$

**Stability.** The ReachIn API employs an event-driven paradigm to update system variables. For efficiency reasons, updates may not occur immediately after an event occurs. This occasionally results in inconsistent values for $P_{fing(t)}$ and $P_{prxy(t)}$ and in turn $S_{n(t)}$. Instead of a smooth reaction force, the user may feel occasional jerkiness. To reduce this effect, $S_{n(t)}$ is averaged over the past $n$ iterations as,

$$S_{navg(t)} = \sum_{i=t-n}^{t} S_{ni} \left/ \left| \sum_{i=t-n}^{t} S_{ni} \right| \right.$$

Occasionally the user might feel certain vibrations in the system because of lower update rates. This is overcome by applying a damping force $F_{d(t)}$ proportional to the velocity $V_{(t)}$ of $P_{fing(t)}$ and is computed as, $F_{d(t)} = K_d \cdot V_{(t)}$.

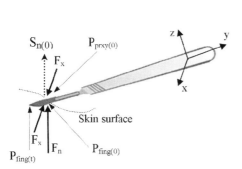
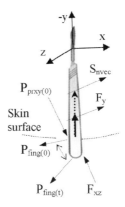

**Figure 2.2.** Reflected forces on the scalpel handle during incision enlargement.

**Figure 2.3.** Reflected forces on the scalpel's during cutting.

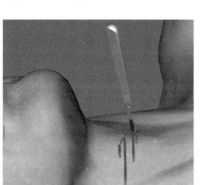
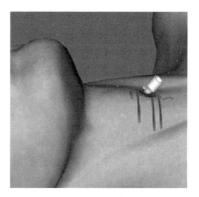

**Figure 3.1.** Cricothyroidotomy simulator showing bleeding due to an incision.

**Figure 3.2.** Endotracheal tube inserted inside the trachea.

## 2.3. Haptic Feedback During Instrument Insertion

In cricothyroidotomy, once an incision is made, the handle of the scalpel is used to enlarge the incision so that the tube can be inserted in the trachea. As shown in figure 2.3, the tactile feedback during instrument insertion is similarly modeled using reaction and constraining forces. We describe them in more detail.

**Implementing the reaction effect.** The reaction force $F_{y(t)}$ is proportional to the depth of penetration of the instrument along $S_{n(t)}$. $F_{ort(t)}$ is used to model the resistance of the instrument depending on the orientation of the handle. The instrument can be easily inserted inside the incision if it is orientated along the cut direction. However, the user feels more resistance if it is inserted in other directions. It is computed as the normalized scalar product of the handle's orientation and the cut direction. The reaction force is given by,

$$F_{y(t)} = -K_y \cdot [(P_{fing(t)} - P_{fing(0)}) \cdot S_{navg(t)}] \cdot S_{navg(t)} \cdot F_{ort(t)}$$

**Implementing the constrained motion effect.** The instruments inserted inside the incision site cannot cut the skin surface. However they can expand the soft tissue to a limited extent when penetrated deeper. This behavior is modeled using a constraining force that is proportional to the distance of the instrument from its initial contact position and is computed as,

$$F_{xz(t)} = K_{xz} \cdot \left\{ \left[ (P_{prxy(t)} - P_{fing(t)}) - (P_{prxy(0)} - P_{fing(0)}) \right] \right.$$
$$\left. \cdot (P_{prxy(t)} - P_{fing(t)}) \right\} \cdot (P_{prxy(0)} - P_{fing(0)})$$

## 3. Results

We have implemented the techniques on a cricothyroidotomy simulator. In our simulator, incisions can be made at arbitrary locations. The incisions open and can bleed freely, with blood trails developing and flowing down the neck in a convincing fashion [Fig. 3.1]. The enlargement of the incision can be done using the handle of the scalpel. If an incision is made at the correct location, the insertion of a breathing tube can be performed [Fig. 3.2]. The user experiences the same tactile feedback as in the actual procedure. Our method makes no changes to the underlying model's topography. Bleeding is modeled by dynamically updating the skin with wound and blood sub-textures. Tactile feedback during incisions is modeled using reaction and constraining forces. As an initial test of validity, surgeons familiar with the procedure were invited to test the system. Many have responded favorably to the tactile and visual realism of the simulation.

## 4. Discussion and Conclusion

For many surgical procedures, accurate physical modeling of cutting and instrument insertion may be unnecessary. We have developed techniques that do not require computationally intensive algorithms, yet achieve similar visual and tactile effects. Initial feedback from surgeons familiar with the procedure suggests that our techniques are a viable approach. Further studies are necessary to quantify the degree of acceptance. While our method works well for small, straight-line incisions, it may not work as well for more complex procedures.

## Acknowledgements

This work is supported by the USAMRMC under contract no. DAMD17-03-C-0102. The views, opinions and/or findings contained in this report are those of the author(s) and should not be construed as an official Department of the Army position, policy or decision unless so designated by other documentation.

## References

[1] M. Bro-Nielsen, "Finite element modeling in medical VR", Journal of the IEEE, Vol. 86, No. 3, pp. 490-503, 1998.
[2] F. Ganovelli, C. O'Sullivan, "Animating cuts with on-the-fly re-meshing", Eurographics, pp. 243–247, 2001.

[3]  A. B. Mor, T. Kanade, "Modifying soft tissue models: Progressive cutting with minimal new element creation", MICCAI, pp. 598-607, 2000.

[4]  G. Song, N. Reddy, "Tissue cutting in virtual environments," Interactive Technology and the New Paradigm for Healthcare, Studies in Health Technology and Informatics, IOP Press, pp. 359-364, 1995.

[5]  M. Kass, G. Miller, "Rapid, stable fluid dynamics for computer graphics", Computer Graphics, Vol. 24, No. 4, pp. 49-57, 1990.

[6]  W. T. Reeves, "Particle systems - A technique for modeling a class of fuzzy objects", Computer Graphics, Vol. 17, No. 3, pp. 359-376, 1983.

[7]  J. Stam, "Stable fluids", ACM SIGGRAPH, pp. 121-128, 1999.

[8]  U. Kühnapfel, H. K. Çakmak, H. Maass, "Endoscopic surgery training using virtual reality and deformable tissue simulation", Computers and Graphics, pp. 671-682, 2000.

[9]  G. Doretto, S. Soatto, "Editable dynamic textures", ACM SIGGRAPH Sketches and Applications, 2002.

[10]  P. Oppenheimer, A. Gupta, S. Weghorst, R. Sweet, J. Porter, "The representation of blood flow in endourologic surgical simulations", Medicine Meets Virtual Reality, pp. 365-371, 2001.

[11]  LapSim, Surgical Science, www.surgical-science.com.

[12]  AccuTouch Endoscopy Simulator, Immersion Medical, www.immersion.com.

[13]  A. Liu, C. Kaufmann, T. Ritchie, "A computer-based simulator for diagnostic peritoneal lavage", Medicine Meets Virtual Reality, 2001.

[14]  A. Liu, Y. Bhasin, M. Bowyer, "A Haptic-enabled Simulator for Cricothyroidotomy", To appear in Medicine Meets Virtual Reality, 2005.

[15]  S. Soatto, G. Doretto, and Y. Wu, "Dynamic textures", International Journal of Computer Vision, Vol. 51, No. 2, pp. 91-109, 2003.

[16]  F. Neyret, R. Heiss, F. Sénégas, "Realistic rendering of an organ surface in real-time for laparoscopic surgery simulation", The Visual Computer, Vol. 18, No. 3, pp. 135-149, 2002.

[17]  Reachin Technologies AB, www.reachin.se.

*Medicine Meets Virtual Reality 13*
*James D. Westwood et al. (Eds.)*
*IOS Press, 2005*

# 3D Real-time FEM Based Guide Wire Simulator with Force Feedback

Suraj BHAT, Chandresh MEHTA, Clive D'SOUZA and T. KESAVADAS
*Virtual Reality Laboratory, Department of Mechanical Engineering,*
*State University of New York at Buffalo*
*e-mail: {sbhat,crmehta,crdsouza,kesh}@eng.buffalo.edu*

**Abstract.** Minimally invasive surgical techniques using catheter is now used in many procedures. Development of surgical training of such procedures requires real-time simulation of tool-organ interaction. In such processes, each subsequent step of interaction would be based on the current configuration of the surgical tool (guidewire in this case), leading to development of techniques to solve and visualize the configuration of tool at every time step. This paper presents a Finite Element (FEM) based approach to simulate the tool-organ interaction.

## 1. Introduction

Much minimally invasive treatment involves a catheter-based approach where the goal is to access a weak vessel, for example an aneurysm, and place an angioplasty balloon and stent at the location. To simulate such process, in this paper we have developed a guidewire vessel contact simulation where the current deformed configuration of the vessel and compliant surgical tool (guidewire) dictates the subsequent surgical procedure to be adopted. To improve the safety and efficacy of surgery simulation, interventionalist should be presented with a very accurate estimate of the contact mechanics such as force and orientation of the guide wire at every moment of the procedure. To achieve this, one could either prepare a database of 3D images to cover most likely resultant scenarios or numerically find out, using FEM or any other method, the deformed shape of the guidewire/catheter and artery vessel.

Alderliesten et al [1], have incorporated a quasi-static mechanics approach to simulate the propagation of the guide wire within a vascular system. Their work, however, treats the entire process analytically rather than using FEM to solve the problem.

Our work presents a FEM based approach to simulating guidewire – organ interaction (figure 1).

## 2. Methodology

### 2.1. Schematic

The movement of the guide-wire in vessel is considered as the sum of rigid body displacement and deformation [2]. The system schematic for our simulator is shown below (figure 2).

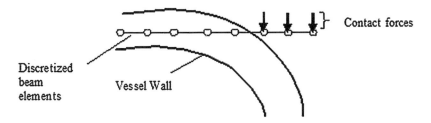

**Figure 1.** Contact force Computation & application on discretized beam elements.

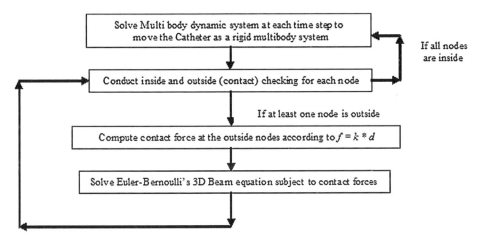

**Figure 2.** System Schematic.

Newton's second law of motion determines the rigid-body displacements of the guide-wire. On obtaining the equilibrium configuration from the rigid body displacement analysis, we carry out a simple 'inside' 'outside' check for each of the nodes. Vasculature is considered as a rigid tube for simplifying the computation. For each node that lies outside the tube, a force is determined which acts as a point load on that node. FEM is then used to find the deformed configuration of the 3D beam elements.

## 2.2. FEM

The guidewire is modeled as a series of 'N' 3D beam elements. Each beam is further divided into $n$ sub-elements. Since this choice involves nodal values and slopes, we use the Hermite shape functions as they satisfy the nodal values and slope continuity requirements.

From elementary beam theory for small deformations $\bar{u}_i$, we have the equilibrium equation for the $i$th beam:

$$\nabla^2\left(EI\left(\nabla^2\bar{u}_i\right)\right) - \bar{f}_i = 0 \tag{1}$$

Where $E$ is the Young's Modulus of the material; $I$ is the moment of inertia of the section about the neutral axis and $f$ is the distributed load per unit length.

In our case the $E$ and $I$ are assumed to be constant throughout the length of the guidewire. Hence the strong form equation for the beam can be expressed as follows:

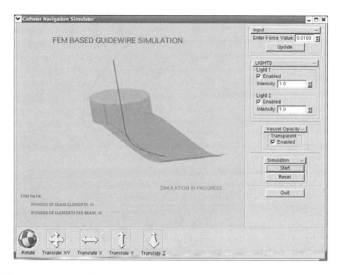

**Figure 3.** User Interface depicting the guide wire deformation during simulation.

$$EI\nabla^4 \bar{u}_i = \bar{f}_i \tag{2}$$

Essential boundary conditions are:

$$\bar{u}_i(0) = 0 \quad \text{for } i = 1,$$
$$= \bar{u}_{i-1}(L) \quad \text{for } i = 2 \text{ to } N$$
$$\bar{u}'_i(0) = 0 \quad \text{for } i = 1$$
$$= \bar{u}'_{i-1}(L) \quad \text{for } i = 2 \text{ to } N$$

And Normal boundary conditions are:

$$\bar{u}''_i(0) = 0 \quad \text{for } i = 1 \text{ to } N$$
$$EI\bar{u}'''_i(0) = 0 \quad \text{for } i = 1 \text{ to } N$$

The strong form of the equation is simplified into matrix form for $e^{\text{th}}$ sub-element of each beam as:

$$\sum_{b=1}^{4} K^e_{ab} u_b = F^e_a, \quad a = 1, 2, 3, 4 \tag{3}$$

After assembling all the sub-elemental matrix equations (Eq. 3) for each beam we solve the resultant global matrix to obtain nodal displacements and slopes.

## 3. Results

The user interface for visualizing guide-wire navigation inside a vasculature was created using GLUI. The rendering is done using OpenGL and GLUT. The code for our project is written using C++ in Linux.

The force input at the proximal end can be input by the user and can be varied by the user at each step of the guide-wire navigation. A simulation option, allows the user to view the entire wire navigation at a constant force input. The system is found to be generic and easily extensible.

## 4. Future Work

Currently we are working on interfacing our system with a force-feedback device. Simultaneously, we are in the process of using clinical data sets for generating patient specific vessel geometry for testing the guidewire simulation.

## References

[1] Alderliesten T,Konings MK, Niessen WJ,*" Simulation of GuideWire Propogation for Minimally Invasive Vascular Interventions", MICCAI* 2002, pp245-252,2002.
[2] Wang YP, Chui CK, Lim H, Cai YY, Mak K, *"Topology Supported Finite Element Method Analysis of Catheter/Guidewire Navigation in Reconstructed Coronary Arteries"*, Computers in Cardiology , 1997, Vol 24, pp 529-532.
[3] Subramanian N, Kesavadas T, Hoffmann KR *"A Prototype Virtual Reality System for Pre-Operative Planning of Neuro-Endovascular Interventions"*. In Proceedings of Medicine Meets Virtual Reality 12, 2004, pp 376-381.

*Medicine Meets Virtual Reality 13*
*James D. Westwood et al. (Eds.)*
*IOS Press, 2005*

# Determining the Efficacy of an Immersive Trainer for Arthroscopy Skills

James P. BLISS, Hope S. HANNER-BAILEY and Mark W. SCERBO

*Old Dominion University*

**Abstract.** The present study examined the effectiveness of an immersive arthroscopic simulator for training naïve participants to identify major anatomical structures and manipulate the arthroscope and probe. Ten psychology graduate students engaged in five consecutive days of practice sessions with the arthroscopic trainer. Following each session, participants were tested to see how quickly and accurately they could identify 10 anatomical landmarks and manipulate the arthroscope and probe. The results demonstrated steady learning on both tasks. For the anatomy task, participants correctly identified an average of 7.7 out of 10 structures correctly in the first session and 9.5 in the last. During the manipulation task, participants collided 53.5 times with simulated tissues in the first session and 13.2 times during the final session. Participants (n=9) also demonstrated minimal performance degradation when tested 4 weeks later. These data suggest that the immersive arthroscopic trainer might be useful as an initial screening or training tool for beginning medical students.

## 1. Background

The knee has been characterized as the most complex and frequently injured joint in the human body [1]. Knee arthroscopy has been performed for many years, since Kenji Takagi of Tokyo University performed the procedure first in 1918. The Virtual Reality in Medicine and Biology Group at the University of Sheffield has developed a VE-based simulator to represent arthroscopy [2], as has the Fraunhofer Institute for Computer Graphics [3]. Some simulators have been designed with force feedback to allow trainees to interact more realistically with anatomical structures of the knee. The increasing popularity and sophistication of arthroscopic simulation has prompted some medical personnel to call for the routine use of VE-based simulation in arthroscopic training [4]. Such training, it is claimed, allows trainees to practice without relying on animal models, cadavers, or actual patients. The current experiment is part of a larger program to investigate the effectiveness of an immersive arthroscopic trainer. Our plan was to determine whether naïve participants could use the simulator to learn fundamental anatomy and probe manipulation and navigation. Based on prior data from other medical simulators, we expected that participants would quickly and successfully demonstrate learning and would retain the acquired knowledge across a four-week period.

## 2. Methodology

### 2.1. Participants

Ten psychology graduate students from Old Dominion University participated. It was impractical to use medical students or residents because the present study required participants to practice with the simulator for five consecutive days and to be tested four weeks later. Participants included four males and six females, and participants did not have prior medical experience. They ranged in age from 21 to 55 years ($M = 27.5, SD = 10.0$). The participants were paid \$150 for their participation.

### 2.2. Apparatus and Procedure

The simulator used for this experiment was the Procedicus™ Virtual Arthroscopy (VA) trainer, manufactured by Mentice Corporation. Though the simulator includes modules for training complex skills such as loose body removal and subacromial decompression, we concentrated on only two basic skills: identifying anatomical landmarks and manipulating the arthroscope and probe. Participants were personally contacted to determine their interest in the project. Twenty-four hours before the experiment, participants studied a short information sheet that described ten anatomical landmarks within the knee and several anatomical terms. After arriving at the hospital laboratory, participants completed an informed consent form and were given ten minutes to review the background study material. They then spent 15 minutes manipulating the arthroscope to review knee landmarks. They were then tested to determine their ability to recognize the landmarks. After a brief break, participants spent 15 minutes practicing arthroscope and probe manipulation by locating and intersecting blue balls randomly placed within the simulated knee. After the practice session, participants were tested to see how quickly and accurately they could intersect 11 balls. They then completed an opinion questionnaire and were dismissed until the next day. Participants repeated the experimental procedure for five consecutive days. They were then brought back into the hospital laboratory four weeks later, at which time they repeated the test procedures.

## 3. Results

Participants demonstrated steady learning on both tasks, correctly identifying an average of 7.7 out of 10.0 anatomy structures in the first session, 8.2 in the second, 8.9 in the third, 9.2 in the fourth, and 9.5 in the last. Manipulation score averages (out of 100) were 2.9, 28.5, 49.1, 54.8, and 56.2 for sessions 1-5, respectively. Mean times to complete manipulation were 495.73, 322.45, 185.33, 167.95, and 161.47 seconds for sessions 1-5 respectively. During the manipulation task, participants collided with simulated tissue 53.5, 25.5, 7.4, 7.7, and 13.2 times, respectively. During the retention session, participants correctly identified an average of 8.4 anatomy structures. Furthermore, the mean manipulation time to complete the manipulation task was 167.31 seconds and the mean number of tissue collisions was 9.0.

In addition to mean differences across time, several significant correlations were observed. Although sex was not found to significantly correlate with any variable, older participants had more video game experience ($r = .85, p < .01$), and longer retention manipulation times ($r = .83$, $p < .01$). Furthermore, participants who reported difficulty with the simulator tended to have lower manipulation scores ($r = -.84$, $p < .01$) and more frequent collisions ($r = .81$, $p < .01$). Manipulation time was also negatively related to perceived helpfulness of visual aids ($r = -.84$, $p < .01$). Questionnaire data indicated that participants believed that the simulator was an effective tool for learning anatomy and manipulation basics.

## 4. Discussion

The data reported here illustrate learning rates for naïve participants. Throughout the five days of training, participants performed better and experienced less frustration on the anatomy exercise than they did the manipulation task. The anatomy task required the manipulation of only the scope, while the manipulation exercise required simultaneous use of the scope and probe. Thus, the manipulation task necessitated greater psychomotor ability. Equally important, however, was the level of retention demonstrated. Although there was a slight drop in the number of anatomical structures correctly identified after the four-week period, participants actually made fewer collisions with tissues during retention than they did at Day 5. The time to complete the manipulation task during retention was only marginally longer (5.84 seconds) than it was during the final day of training. Interestingly, there was minimal degradation of performance for both the anatomy and manipulation tasks. The anatomy task may have been slightly more difficult for participants during retention given that it is a more cognitively demanding exercise.

The major drawback of the present study was the small sample size. In the future, researchers should examine the learning curve of the Procedicus VA simulator with a larger sample and across a longer time period. Despite these limitations, it was encouraging that the tasks were not too difficult for naïve trainees to master. This suggests that the arthroscopic trainer might be useful as an initial screening or training tool for beginning medical students.

## 5. Conclusions

These data show that naïve participants can use the Procedicus VA trainer to learn basic anatomy and tool manipulation skills. Of the two tasks, manipulation seems to be more difficult, and may require extended practice for participants to master it.

## References

[1] McCarthy, A. D., & Hollands, R. J. (1997). Human factors related to a virtual reality surgical simulator: The Sheffield Knee Arthroscopic Training System. *Proceedings of the 4th Virtual Reality Special Interest Group Conference*. Leicester, England.
[2] Hollands, R. J., Trowbridge, E. A., Bickerstaff, D., Edwards, J. B., & Mort, N. (1995). The particular problem of arthroscopic surgical simulation: A preliminary report. In R. A. Earnshaw & J. A. Vince (Eds.) Computer *Graphics: Development in Virtual Environments*. London: Academic Press.
[3] Ziegler, R., Brandt, C., Kunstmann, C., Mueller, W., & Werkhaeuser, H. (1997). Haptic displays for the VR arthroscopy simulator. *Proceedings of the SPIE Conference*.
[4] Hardy, P. (2001). Arthroscopic surgery and virtual reality : Development of a virtual arthroscopic trainer. Newsletter of the International Society of Arthroscopy, Knee Surgery, and O Paper presented at the Advanced Technology Applications for Combat Casualty Care Annual Meeting, St. Pete Beach, FL.

Medicine Meets Virtual Reality 13
James D. Westwood et al. (Eds.)
IOS Press, 2005

# Teaching Intravenous Cannulation to Medical Students: Comparative Analysis of Two Simulators and Two Traditional Educational Approaches

Mark W. BOWYER [a], Elisabeth A. PIMENTEL [a], Jennifer B. FELLOWS [a],
Ryan L. SCOFIELD [a], Vincent L. ACKERMAN [a], Patrick E. HORNE [a], Alan V. LIU [a],
Gerald R. SCHWARTZ [a] and Mark W. SCERBO [b]

[a] *National Capital Area Medical Simulation Center of the Uniformed Services,
University of the Health Sciences, 4301 Jones Bridge Road, Bethesda, MD, 20814
url: http://simcen.usuhs.mil/*
[b] *Old Dominion University, Norfolk, VA*

**Abstract.** This study examines the effectiveness of two virtual reality simulators when compared with traditional methods of teaching intravenous (IV) cannulation to third year medical students. Thirty-four third year medical students were divided into four groups and then trained to perform an IV cannulation using either CathSim[TM], Virtual I.V.[TM], a plastic simulated arm or by practicing IV placement on each other. All subjects watched a five minute training video and completed a cannulation pretest and posttest on the simulated arm. The results showed significant improvement from pretest to posttest in each of the four groups. Students trained on the Virtual I.V.[TM] showed significantly greater improvement over baseline when compared with the simulated arm group (p < .026). Both simulators provided at least equal training to traditional methods of teaching, a finding with implications for future training of this procedure to novices.

## 1. Background

Health care providers must be taught basic clinical skills prior to performing these skills on patients. One of the most basic (and critical) skills taught to healthcare providers is obtaining venous access via intravenous (IV) cannulation. This type of clinical skills education is typically not part of a standardized curriculum, relying mostly on the initiative of faculty to teach medical students these basic skills [1]. Traditionally, teaching methods for IV cannulation have ranged from students being taught using an orange as a model or practicing on a plastic arm, to practicing the procedure on each other and actual patients. These methods may get the job done but they offer inconsistent educational opportunities, a limited variability of case content for the simulated arm, require the willingness of one's fellow student to be repetitively stuck with a needle, require a high faculty-to-student ratio, and are ultimately cost-ineffective [1,2]. Additionally, once IV cannulation skills have been obtained, the opportunities to become proficient and keep these skills current has become increasingly difficult due to the decreasing opportunities to practice on patients and the reality that many of these basic skills are delegated to ancillary personnel in the clinical setting [2].

Virtual reality (VR) simulators have been an integral part of aerospace and military training for decades and are starting to have increased utilization in the medical community. Simulators offer a variety of potential benefits to medical education and here, specifically, to teaching IV cannulation. Simulators offer a fail-safe environment in which to learn. The student may practice limitless times and is free to fail without the anxiety of causing pain or injury to an actual patient. Both the student's anxiety and the patient's anxiety are removed from the training environment. These devices typically require minimal faculty involvement beyond an initial orientation to operating the product. Thus, the simulator may be more cost effective without even considering the costs associated with the necessary IV supplies and disposal requirements. Additionally, many different levels of health care providers can be trained on a single machine, possibly reducing the cost further. It also may be possible for those training to insert IV catheters to move farther up the learning curve prior to real patient interaction [2]. As simulators become a technology increasingly available to medical educators, it has become important to validate these different systems to ensure tomorrow's health care providers are being properly trained.

There are at least two specific VR systems for teaching IV cannulation available today. CathSim™ (Immersion Medical, Gaithersburg, MD) has been available for 5 years. To date, limited attempts to validate this system have failed to show an advantage over traditional methods of education [2,3]. An additional VR system for teaching IV cannulation, the Virtual I.V.™ (Laerdal Medical, Gatesville, TX) has recently become available and has yet to undergo extensive testing.

The purpose of this study is to examine the effectiveness of these two VR simulators when compared to the traditional modes of using a plastic arm and students practicing on each other for training 3$^{rd}$ year medical students (MS-III) how to perform IV cannulation.

## 2. Methodology

### 2.1. Materials

#### 2.1.1. Plastic Simulated Arm

A Laerdal Multi-Venous IV Training Arm was used for the pretest, the posttest and as a training modality. The simulated arm has a layer of plastic skin covering a network of latex veins. In the simulated arm, venipuncture is possible in the antecubital fossa and dorsum of the hand and the accessible veins include the median, basilic and cephalic veins. Artificial blood is connected to the arm. Gravity draws the artificial blood into the venous system of the simulated arm, allowing for flashback when the IV catheter is properly inserted. Additional materials used with both the simulated arm and with the group of students who practiced on each other include latex gloves, tourniquets, alcohol swabs, gauze pads, 20-gauge IV catheter needles, 3-mililiter sterile syringes for flushing the catheter, sterile saline, tape and a biohazard sharps container for proper disposal.

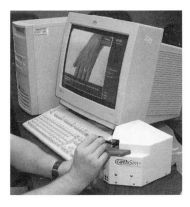

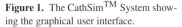

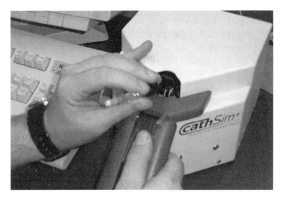

**Figure 1.** The CathSim™ System showing the graphical user interface.

**Figure 2.** CathSim™ AccuTouch® Tactile Feedback device allows for tactile (haptic) interaction with the patient on the screen.

## 2.1.2. CathSim™

The CathSim™ system is available from Immersion Medical, Inc. The CathSim™ system (Figure 1) is a microcomputer-based simulator originally developed by HT Medical Systems, Inc., in collaboration with the Department of Nursing, Food and Nutrition of Plattsburgh State University of New York [4,5]. The CathSim™ system provides training on IV catheterization. The physical system consists of an IBM-compatible computer accompanied by an AccuTouch® Tactile Feedback device, a six-degree-of-freedom haptic feedback device, which simulates the catheter needle/hub assembly and a section of the skin for traction. The AccuTouch® Tactile Feedback device (Figure 2) is designed to allow students to experience the tactile responses associated with inserting a needle into the skin and vein. The student also receives audio feedback in the form of patient vocalization that ranges from a crying baby as the IV is inserted to an adult patient saying "ouch!" [3,6].

CathSim™ has a variety of cases for teaching IV catheterization. The patients in each case have different levels of difficulty. For instance, there is an adult male with no complications, and pediatric and geriatric cases with varying complications. A student first selects a patient using the computer mouse. Upon choosing a case, the student must then choose an appropriate site for insertion. The selected insertion site appears on the screen and the student uses a computer's mouse to apply a tourniquet, palpate the vein and cleanse the site by pointing and clicking and dragging objects from a menu of IV catheterization supplies on the screen. Then the student selects the appropriate gauge needle and using the mouse and the AccuTouch® Tactile Feedback device positions the needle and applies the skin traction. Skin traction is simulated by pulling down in the rubber stripping portion of the device with the thumb (Figure 2). Next, the needle is inserted by first fully retracting the simulated catheter and needle of the AccuTouch® Tactile Feedback device and then inserting it as an IV catheter should be inserted. The student is simultaneously looking at the computer monitor to ensure vein access and confirmation of blood backflow. The student then withdraws the needle to complete the procedure. The system automatically ends the simulation once the needle has been withdrawn from the catheter. CathSim™ records many different performance metrics [5,6].

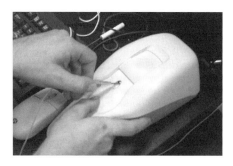

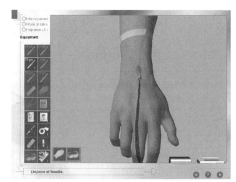

**Figure 3.** Virtual I.V.™ haptic interface. The lower portion allows for stretching the skin and inserting the needle, and the upper for palpating the vein and applying pressure.

**Figure 4.** Virtual I.V.™. This screen capture depicts the IV catheter in the vein with bleeding that has resulted from failure to remove the tourniquet and apply pressure.

## 2.1.3. Virtual I.V.

The Virtual I.V.™ system is available from Laerdal Medical. It is a VR simulator designed to train students on IV cannulation. The physical system is an IBM-compatible computer accompanied by a haptic interface that simulates the catheter needle/hub assembly and two sections of skin to allow for palpation and application of pressure (to stop bleeding) as well as skin traction. The haptic interface (Figure 3) is designed to support palpation, skin stretch and needle insertion with forces dependent on the scenario. The students also receive feedback in the form of bleeding, bruising, swelling, as well as other patho-physiological reactions [7].

The Virtual I.V.™ provides greater case depth than the CathSim$^{TM}$ with over 150 distinct case scenarios. The student can choose from four disciplines: nurses, doctors, EMTs and military care providers. Each patient case is customized to be specifically relevant to one of these disciplines. Then within each discipline are cases with increasing levels of difficulty [7].

A student first selects a discipline and then a level of difficulty within the discipline. A brief history of the patient and why he or she needs an IV is presented. The student must then select the appropriate supplies and the appropriate quantities of these supplies from a menu that contains over a dozen virtual supplies to include biohazard containers and the correct needle gauge for the patient case. The student is then presented with the limb in which the IV catheter will be placed. The student must select the appropriate site on the limb and palpate using the uppermost area of skin on the haptic interface. Then the site must be prepared using the supplies he or she gathered earlier. The student "uses" these supplies by using the computer mouse to click and drag supplies to the appropriate locations. The student then must use the haptic interface to retract the skin using the lowermost skin area and then insert the catheter (Figure 3). Once inserted and the needle is removed, if pressure is not applied to the upper skin area on the haptic interface the patient will bleed (Figure 4). The Virtual I.V.™ system records and evaluates a student's performance using varied performance metrics [7].

## 2.2. Participants

The participants in this study were thirty-four 3$^{rd}$ year medical students at the Uniformed Services University (USU) selected on the basis of prior IV experience. The students participated as part of their introduction to the third-year clinical surgical clerkship. They ranged in age from 23 to 39 years old (Average =26). The study was approved as an exempt protocol by the Investigational Review Board at USU.

All participants were novices, meaning they had never started an IV. A few students had significant experience with other types of simulators, e.g. flight, driving. None of the students had previous experience with other medical simulators and all students were regular computer users.

## 2.3. Procedure

All thirty-four third-year medical students viewed a 5-minute training video as a part of their normal curriculum on IV catheterization. All students were asked to fill out a background questionnaire. The students then completed a cannulation pretest on the simulated arm. Performance on the pretest was assessed using a modified version of a standard instrument used to certify this procedure. The instrument is based on a task analysis of the procedure and is scored from 0 to a maximum of 82 points. The students were then randomly divided into four groups. The first group (Each other or **EO**) consisted of 13 students who practiced IV cannulation on each other for a period of one hour with one faculty member helping and instructing each pair of students. The second group (Virtual I.V.™ or **V**) of 6 students had up to one hour to practice on the Virtual I.V.™. The third group (CathSim™ or **CS**) of 7 students had up to one hour to practice on the CathSim™. The final group (Simulated Arm or **A**) of 8 students practiced for an hour on the IV arm. Upon completion of training, all 34 students performed a post-test on the IV arm within 72 hours of completion of training. Their performance was assessed with the same instrument used for the pretest. The differences in performance between the groups were evaluated using ANOVA and paired t-tests with $\alpha$ set at $p < 0.05$.

## 3. Results

The results of the pre- and posttest and the change in score (delta) from pre- to posttest is shown in Table 2. There was significant improvement from pretest to posttest overall ($p < .00001$) and in each of the four groups (Table 1).

Comparison of each group with all others revealed no significant difference in pre- or posttest scores between the groups (by ANOVA). However, comparison of the delta or improvement from pre- to posttest revealed that the students practicing on the Virtual I.V.™ had significantly greater improvement than the traditional IV arm group ($p < .026$) and though not significant trending towards it for the EO group ($p < .079$) and the CS group ($p < .058$) (Table 2).

There were no significant differences in performance found based on the gender or age of the participating students. Additionally, there was no correlation between the performance of the four groups based on any previous exposure to non-medical simulators or computer usage.

**Table 1.** Mean Assessment Scores on pre- and posttest overall (all) and for each of the groups. EO=each other; V= Virtual I.V.™; CS= CathSim$^{TM}$; A=Simulated Arm. All Values are listed as the mean + or – one standard deviation.

| Group | n | Pretest % | Posttest % | p value | Delta |
|-------|---|-----------|------------|---------|-------|
| EO | 13 | 60.5 (9.7) | 73.8 (6.6) | **< .0003** | 13.2(11) |
| V | 6 | 55.0(12.1) | 75.7(3.7) | **< .0003** | 20.7(7.8) |
| CS | 7 | 66.6(11.8) | 78.4(5.2) | **< .02** | 11.9(12) |
| A | 8 | 65.3 (6.0) | 74.9(8.1) | **< .009** | 9.6(10.3) |
| All | 35 | 63.7(10.1) | 76.4(4.6) | **< .00001** | |

**Table 2.** Comparison of the delta or improvement from pre- to posttest among groups. Values reflect p value with significance at p < .05.

| | EO | V | CS | A |
|---|----|----|-----|----|
| EO | | p < .079 | p < .41 | p < .24 |
| V | | | p < .058 | **p < .026** |
| CS | | | | p < .36 |

## 4. Discussion/Conclusions

A review of the limited previous literature of Virtual Reality (VR) simulators has shown that simulators in general are inferior to the traditional methods (the plastic simulated arm) of teaching IV cannulation [1,2,8]. Additionally, no study was found to have compared VR simulators with the method of students practicing on each other to gain experience in IV placement. The results of this study indicate that all four methods of teaching IV cannulation were effective in teaching 3$^{rd}$ year medical students by virtue of improvement over the baseline assessment. Of note is the significantly greater improvement over baseline the students using the Virtual I.V.™ had when compared with those students who learned by practicing on the plastic simulated arm. This finding needs to be confirmed with additional subject accrual. However, this is of particular importance considering that previous studies comparing the CathSim$^{TM}$ to a plastic simulated arm found the students were better trained using the simulated arm. Additionally, one might expect that the students practicing on the simulated arm to have an advantage over the Virtual I.V.™ group as the assessments were performed on the same type of plastic simulated arms. Despite this possible advantage, the Virtual I.V.™ trained students had significantly greater improvement over baseline than those students trained on the plastic simulated arms.

When comparing the other training modes used to teach students to perform IV cannulation, there was no statistically significant difference found. This in and of itself is an important finding as it indicates that both simulators provided at least *equal* training to the more costly and faculty dependent traditional modes of teaching IV cannulation. This means that environments where faculty involvement is constrained have an additional option when considering how to best to maximize their educational resources.

While the results of this study suggest that VR simulators are useful tools in training health care providers, the underlying question is whether the significant improvement all students had over the baseline assessment regardless of training method will translate into improved performance on actual patients. This remains to be seen and is the focus of future study. Additional areas of focus for future study should include measures of skill degradation over time with interval testing in the four training groups. One of the limitations of this study is that the students were not trained to proficiency. This was due to the limited time these students had available before beginning the third year Surgery Clerkship; however, this deserves emphasis in future studies. Another limitation is the small number of participants. Clearly further study and subject accrual is required to delineate the role of these potentially valuable tools for training.

## References

[1] Prystowsky JB, Regehr G, Rogers DA, Loan JP, Hiemenz LL, Smith KM. A virtual reality module for intravenous catheter placement. The American Journal of Surgery 1999; 177:171-5.
[2] Engum SA, Jeffries P, Fisher, L. Intravenous catheter training system: Computer-based education versus traditional learning methods. The American Journal of Surgery 2003; 186:67-74.
[3] Scerbo MW, Bliss JP, Schmidt EA, Thompson SN, Cox TD, Polan HJ. A comparison of the CathSim™ system and simulated limbs for teaching intravenous cannulation. In J.D. Westwood et al. (Eds.), *Medicine meets virtual reality* 2004; 340-6. Amsterdam: IOS Press.
[4] Barker VL. CathSim™. In J.D. Westwood et al. (Eds.), *Medicine meets virtual reality* 1999; 36-37. Amsterdam: IOS Press.
[5] Ursino M, Tasto JL, Nguyen BH, Cunningham R, Merril GL. CathSim™: An intravascular catheterization simulator on a PC. *In J.D. Westwood et al. (Eds.), Medicine meets virtual reality* 1999; 360-6. Amsterdam: IOS Press.
[6] http://www.immersion.com/medical/products/vascular_access/.
[7] http://www.laerdal.com/document.asp?subnodeid=6473945.
[8] Chang KK, Chung JW, Wong TK. Learning intravenous cannulation: A comparison of the conventional method and the CathSim™ intravenous training system. Journal of Clinical Nursing 2002; 11: 73-78.

*Medicine Meets Virtual Reality 13*
*James D. Westwood et al. (Eds.)*
*IOS Press, 2005*

# Validation of *SimPL* – A Simulator for Diagnostic Peritoneal Lavage Training

Colonel Mark W. BOWYER M.D., Alan V. LIU Ph.D. and James P. BONAR M.D.

*National Capital Area Medical Simulation Center of the Uniformed Services*
*University of the Health Science, 4301 Jones Bridge Road, Bethesda, MD, 20814*
*url: http://simcen.usuhs.mil/*

**Abstract.** This study describes a comparison between an animal model and a haptic enabled, needle based, graphical user interface simulator (*SimPL*), for teaching Diagnostic Peritoneal Lavage (DPL). Forty novice medical students were divided into two groups and then trained to perform a DPL on either a pig or the *SimPL*. All subjects completed a pre and post test of basic knowledge and were tested by performing a DPL on a *TraumaMan*™ mannequin and evaluated by two trauma surgeons blinded to group. The results showed significant improvement over baseline knowledge in both groups but more so in the *SimPL* group. The simulator group performed better on site selection (p<0.001) and technique (p<0.002) than those who trained on a pig. The finding that a simulator is superior to an animal model for teaching an important skill to medical students has profound implications on future training and deserves further study.

## 1. Background

Diagnostic Peritoneal Lavage (DPL) is one of the core skills taught in the Advanced Trauma Life Support (ATLS®) given to more than 20,000 students per year. DPL is performed to diagnose the presence of blood in the abdomen in traumatically injured patients [1]. This skill has traditionally been taught using an animal model with the inherent expense and ethical concerns. Most providers once trained have very few occasions to practice this skill and therefore predictable skill degradation occurs. In response to the continued need to train this important skill we have developed a DPL simulator (*SimPL*) and a program for validating its usefulness [2].

### 1.1. The Technique of Diagnostic Peritoneal Lavage

The classic "closed" or Seldinger DPL technique involves placing a needle into the abdominal cavity below the umbilicus through the skin, the anterior abdominal fascia and the peritoneum. After entering the abdomen a guide wire is passed through the needle into the abdomen, the needle removed and a catheter then advanced into the abdomen over the wire. The wire is removed and a syringe is placed on the catheter and aspirated. If blood is aspirated the DPL is considered positive and the patient requires an operation. If blood is not present fluid is run into the abdomen through the catheter and then aspirated and analyzed for the presence of blood [1]. This needle based procedure is charac-

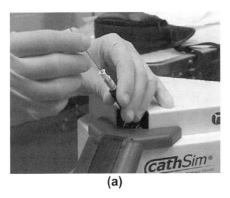
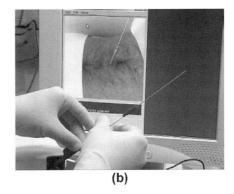

(a)                                                    (b)

**Figure 1.** The SimPL DPL Simulator with the CathSim® haptic needle based platform (a) and the graphical user interface that translates motions on platform to actions on the screen (b).

terized by a well defined "pop" or loss of resistance as the needle passes through both the anterior fascia and the peritoneum.

## 1.2. The SimPL – a DPL Simulator

The *SimPL* is a simulator designed specifically to teach DPL. This simulator couples a CathSim® (Immersion Medical) platform hardware with a graphical and haptic user interface that can be run off a laptop or desktop and is low cost (Figure 1). *SimPL* allows the user to select and perform the proper technique with immediate feedback and terminal reporting. The graphical interface translates performance on the platform with performance on the screen and the haptic interface replicates the sensation of passing the needle through the fascia and the more subtle sensation of passing through the peritoneum [3].

## 2. Methodology

After appropriate institutional review and approval, forty novice (never had seen or performed a DPL) third year medical students were given a thirty item test of their knowledge of DPL prior to any instruction. They were also asked to rate their baseline familiarity, comfort level, and perceived difficulty on a five point Likert scale. The students then received a standardized lecture on the DPL procedure and were randomly divided into two groups of twenty. The first group (pig trained) were trained to perform a DPL on an anesthetized pig with correction and remediation as needed. The second group (*SimPL*) were trained to perform a DPL on the *SimPL* DPL simulator with correction and remediation as needed. Both groups were then tested by performing a DPL on the TraumaMan™ mannequin which is currently used to teach DPL as part of ATLS® . This performance was evaluated by two trauma surgeons who were blinded to the training method. Assessment involved scoring the students on twelve DPL steps and rating the understanding of site selection, indications, complications, technique, and interpretation of results on a five point Likert scale. The students then retook the thirty item test of DPL knowledge as a final test. Differences between groups were assessed using the student t-test with $\alpha$ set at $p<0.05$.

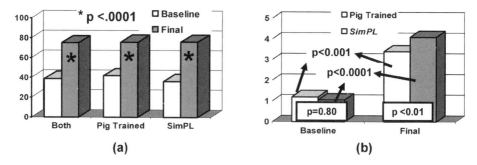

**Figure 2.** The comparison of the baseline and final percentage scores for both groups and each group individually is depicted in (a). The subjects self reported comfort level with DPL (5 = very comfortable, 1 = not very comfortable) is shown in (b).

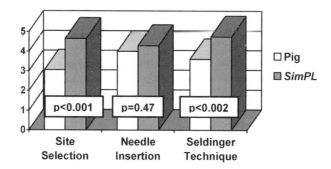

**Figure 3.** Faculty evaluation (5 =excellent, 1 = poor) of the students ability for the skills listed.

## 3. Results

Knowledge level increased significantly ($p < 0.0001$) over base line in both groups (Figure 2a). Students self-reported comfort level with the DPL procedure improved significantly over baseline in both groups ($p < 0.001$) but more so in the *SimPL* group ($p < 0.01$) as shown in Figure 2b. The understanding of the indications, complications, and interpretation of results improved over baseline in both groups with no differences based on training method employed. The students who trained on the *SimPL* had significantly increased performance on site selection ($p < 0.001$) and their ability to perform the Seldinger technique ($p < 0.002$) (Figure 3). The evaluators had an inter-rater reliability of 0.85 and had a greater faith in the ability of the *SimPL* trained students to perform the procedure independently (agree or strongly agree in 90% vs 60%) after this initial training.

## 4. Discussion/Conclusions

The *SimPL* DPL simulator compared favorably with the pig for teaching novices this important procedure. The *SimPL* was superior to the pig in this study for teaching human anatomy/site selection and for teaching the Seldinger technique. The *SimPL* has excellent face, content, and convergent validity. The finding that a simulator is superior to or at least equal to an animal model for teaching an important skill to medical students has profound implications on future training and deserves further study.

## References

[1] Advanced Trauma Life Support for Doctors Student Course Manual, 6th edition. American College of Surgeons. Chicago. IL, pp 165-180, 1997.
[2] Kaufmann C, Zakaluzny S., Liu A. First steps in eliminating the need for animals and cadavers in Advanced Trauma Life Support®. Lecture Notes in Computer Science 1935, Springer. pp. 618-623, 2000.
[3] Liu A, Kaufmann C., Ritchie T. A computer-based simulator for diagnostic peritoneal lavage. Stud. Health Technol. Inform. 2001;81:279-25.

*Medicine Meets Virtual Reality 13*
*James D. Westwood et al. (Eds.)*
*IOS Press, 2005*

# Challenges in Presenting High Dimensional Data to aid in Triage in the DARPA Virtual Soldier Project

A.D. BOYD [a], Z.C. WRIGHT [a], A.S. ADE [a], F. BOOKSTEIN [a], J.C. OGDEN [a],
W. MEIXNER [a], B.D. ATHEY [a] and T. MORRIS [b]

[a] *University of MICHIGAN*
[b] *U.S. Army Medical Research & Material Command,*
*Telemedicine & Advanced Technology Research Center (TATRC)*
*e-mail: adboyd@umich.edu*

**Abstract.** One of the goals of the DARPA Virtual Soldier Project is to aid the field medic in the triage of a casualty. In Phase I, we are currently collecting 12 baseline experimental physiological variables and a cardiac gated Computed Tomography (CT) imagery for use in an prototyping a futuristic electronic medical record, the "Holomer". We are using physiological models and Kalman filtering to aid in diagnosis and predict outcomes in relation to cardiac injury. The physiological modeling introduces another few hundred variables. Reducing the complexity of the above into easy-to-read text to aid in the triage by the field medic is the challenge with multiple display solutions. A description of the possible techniques follows.

## 1. Problem

Most battlefield first responders are not given advanced training for interpretation of physiologic parameters and imagery that could aid in the initial triage and treatment of casualties on the battlefield and far forward areas of care. In the DARPA Virtual Soldier Project (VSP), one of the goals is to prototype new capabilities to aid the battlefield medic in the triage of casualties. Twelve physiological variables, in addition to cardiac gated Computed Tomography (CT), will be used to fit physiological models and applied to Kalman filters to aid in diagnosis and predicting outcome. Detailed physiological modeling adds another few hundred variables to the data stream. In Phase I of the VSP, we are focusing on the consequences of injury on cardiac anatomy and physiology. Reducing the complexity of the models, data, and variables into an easy-to-read graphical user interface is the challenge we face to aid triage by the field medic. Creating a usable and informative interface will minimize health impacts by exploiting preventive measures and controls, by providing forward interim essential diagnosis and treatment of patients prior to strategic evacuation, and provide support to other critical health care support services in theater.

## 2. Methods

Currently field medics are being trained in the art of casualty triage on a conventional battlefield. One of the underlining principals in this training is: "Triage establishes the order of treatment, not whether treatment is given" [1]. There are four priority classifications of treatment: Immediate, Delayed, Minimal, and Expectant. Immediate—casualties demand immediate treatment to save life, such as in the case of airway obstruction. Delayed—casualties have less risk of loss of life or limb: examples are open chest wounds without respiratory distress. Minimal—casualties might be self treated, such as a sprain. The last category, Expectant—casualties is only used if resources are limited. This category of casualty includes those so critically injured that only complicated and prolonged treatment can improve life expectancy. This is meant to give a high level overview of the classifications of triage performed by the field medic; details are beyond the scope of this paper.

The other classification the field medics perform is the Medical Evacuation (MEDEVAC) priority of an individual casualty. The five classifications are Urgent, Urgent-Surgical, Priority, Routine, and Convenience. "Urgent" is a classification for casualties whose status cannot be controlled and have the greatest opportunity for survival. "Urgent-Surgical" are casualties needing far-forward surgical intervention to stabilize the patient. "Priority" casualties are not stable and at risk of trauma-related complications. "Routine" casualties can be controlled without jeopardizing the patient's condition. The "Convenience" classification is for casualties who are evacuated for convenience, not for medical necessity. Further details of the classification of the MEDEVAC priorities of casualties are located in the 91 Whiskey combat medic training manual [1]. Appreciation of the complex decisions made by the field medic will help shape the following discussion of the possible techniques for the presentation of new material. Other variables not mentioned in the above description of field medic triage decision making which need to be taken into account when calculating time to definitive treatment are tactical and environmental situations, such as the number and location of the injured and the evacuation support capabilities available.

Compaq IPAQ handheld computers equipped with the Battlefield Medical Information System Tactical (BMIST) software are currently deployed world-wide in the field by the US Military Medical Corps [2]. These handhelds interface with an electronic dog-tag, or Personal Information Carrier (PIC), also known commercially as the P-TAG. These electronic dog-tags are capable of storing the soldier's entire electronic health record. BMIST is the point-of-care handheld software the field medic uses to record to initiate a field encounter. The data recorded to the PIC is also compatible with the Composite Health Care System II (CHCS II). CHCS II is the medical information system for the military health system. Since this technology is presently deployed with the field medic, we are limited in the presentation of the data listed above to the screen size of the IPAQ. While in the future the deployed handheld systems will have faster CPUs and more memory, portability and limited screen size will continue to be features of the system.

One goal of the VSP is to provide additional decision support information to the field medic to aid the decision making process. Another goal of the project is the creation of a personalized "Holomer structure" a compilation of all imaging and medical data, for each soldier and enable the transmission of this information to the field medic. Although currently all soldiers have a pre-deployment physical exam, additional measurements will need to be collected for the creation of the Holomer. In creating a Holomer, baseline physiological data of each individual will need to be collected. These data are then used to populate the physiological and cardiac models designed by the VSP. Each subject also receives a Computed Tomography (CT) scan. The individual CT scan is processed through an automated segmentation process to define regions of the anatomy. Through the segmentation of the CT scan, personalized parameters of the model can be abstracted [3]. For example, an individual's left ventricular size can be determined through segmentation, and later the individual's left ventricular volume will be integrated into the computer models.

The level of detail and parameters used in the Highly Integrated Physiological (HIP) cardiac models (e.g. elasticity of the ventricle, valve pressure gradients, and baroreceptor firing interval) is beyond the knowledge of clinical care providers [4]. The field medic, while trained in the triage definitions of blood pressure and heart rate, will probably not be familiar with the interplay of pressure gradients across the heart valves used in HIP model calculations. There are over 12 individual measurable parameters that can be fitted to the cardiac physiology models. The measurements the models require can all be obtained non-invasively. While these data may seem large, there are at least 300 outputs from the models, many of which change during a single heart beat cycle.

While the individual HIP models can accumulate experience by model fitting and model design, the VSP has taken an extended statistical approach to obtain population level trends. The method of reducing this high dimensional parameter space uses a Kalman filtering technique running multiple models with varying injury outcomes [5]. The initial number of validation training experiments is too small to be statistical persuasive, and so a Singular Value Decomposition (SVD) of an individual's physiological trends is being employed. A second validation data set will collect sufficient data to validate against a population, and this will provide confidence intervals and time to death estimates. During the whole process we are validating the trends of the expected injuries against test data. From the full data set we will attempt to make a forecast/prognosis of survival, ventricular fibrillation, and level of exsanguination.

In the above description of the VSP, there are several variables that could be of assistance to the field medic. The baseline physiological data of the individual soldier could be helpful for comparison purposes. The current physiological data on the battlefield could be helpful in triage. The HIP models of the individual's physiological state at the time of injury could also be helpful. For example, the outputs of the HIP models could simulate an ICU monitor, or a three dimensional graph of the SVD could be displayed to view the casualties' physiological states.

While all such displays might be relevant, the field medic must be provided with a display that is both useful and usable. The possible designs of these displays can range from simple color coding and a short text display describing the diagnosis and time to death to full functioning graphs and image displays.

Full functioning graphs and image displays of all of the above mentioned variables would provide the field medic with all of the information possible to make an educated decision on the triage and treatment of casualties (see Figure 1 for image of CT on handheld and see Figure 2 for the display of a few relevant variables from the HIP models of an individual). With more advanced training, the field medic might prefer such comprehensive display systems, but these options must always be balanced with the possibilities of information overload, lack of training, or insufficient time to assimilate the information due to battlefield conditions.

The method of displaying only the text of diagnosis, time to death, and confidence interval, relies heavily on the Kalman filter processing. This method would hide most of the models, physiological parameters, and images from the field medic, providing the field medic with just enough information to make informed triage decisions. Predictions become more confident as more data is collected. Alerts will be displayed on the BMIST handheld when a diagnosis reaches a threshold level of confidence (see Figure 3 for display of handheld of statistical results). The benefit of providing diagnosis and time to death allows the field medic to rapidly make critical decisions about a casualty's triage and treatment. However, introducing confidence intervals into a trauma scenario is an entirely new concept. Additional training would be needed to interpret the confidence intervals of the diagnosis, though this training would not be as extensive as that required for more comprehensive data displays.

The third method of displaying the results of the Virtual Soldier Project outputs (e.g. data, models, and predictions) is a simple color spectrum: Green - soldier normal, Yellow - soldier unstable, and Red would mean either severe physiological distress or death (Figure 4). This system has far less detail than the comprehensive system described above, and is similar to the physiological status monitoring research of the military using the classifications of "Alive," "Dead," or "Unknown" [6]. Reducing the data to a single value may reduce the utility of the interface for the complex decision making of a field medic, and may not provide much additional information beyond their current capabilities. For the specific wounds the VSP modeling, such as penetrating wounds to the heart, a field medic will MEDVAC the patient as "Urgent" or "Urgent-Surgical." In the unfortunate condition of "Expectant," the color system would provide limited additional information.

A Plethysmograph measurement of Heart Rate (HR) and Oxygen Saturation (SaO2) could being incorporated into the BMIST system. . From the data being recorded by the Warfighter Physiological Status Monitoring (WPSM) equipment, the additional data presented to the field medic might also include kilo Calorie (kCal) expenditure and respiration rate (RR) measurements (Figure 5). This screen shows how the data could be presented to the field medic (the area of injury is shown by the X on the body.) A pressure tracing of the arterial blood pressure is also shown in the lower left corner. This display is an example of how to integrate multiple data points into simple graphical user interface while providing enough data for the field medic to make an educated decision.

There are many other possible methods of data display, as well as additional combinations of the above descriptions and measurements that could be shown to the medic. Additional input and collaboration from physicians, medics, and interface/usability specialists will be needed to design the ultimate interface. Because of the critical nature of this software, careful analysis of the interface design by employing standard usability techniques such as GOMS (Goals, Operators, Methods, and Selection), cognitive walkthroughs, task analysis, and formal user testing will be necessary. These methods will ensure that the information and interface presented to the field medic is clear and intuitive, especially in the non-ideal and time-sensitive viewing situations that arise on the battlefield.

## 3. Results

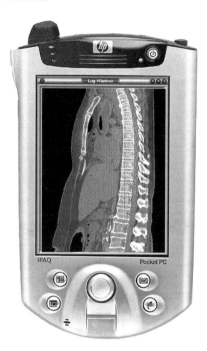

**Figure 1.** Saggital view of Torso CT Scan on hand-held.

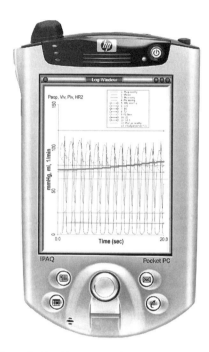

**Figure 2.** Graphing output of the Highly Integrated Physiological (HIP) models on handheld.

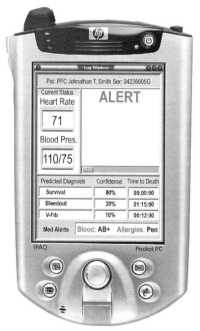

**Figure 3.** Text display of statistical forcast on hand-held.

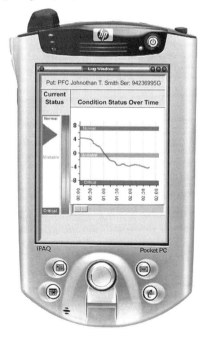

**Figure 4.** Color display of stability of casualty on handheld.

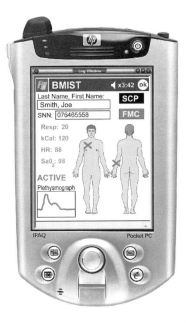

**Figure 5.** Display of the physiology to be collected in the field near term.

## 4. Conclusions/Discussion

The results generated by the DARPA Virtual Soldier Project are a good beginning; however, much of the physiology and statistical information generated to date is too abstract for use by the field medic to triage for treatment or MEDVAC priority. Providing the appropriate information, and an appropriate interface for rapid field use, while allowing the medic to incorporate their own judgment on triage decision-making, is the next step in user interface design. The deployment of this technology will need to be accompanied by additional field medic training. This triage aid system and the additional information provided will need to be integrated into future triage protocols for the field medic's use. A more intuitive method of displaying the uncertainty of each result/prediction is also needed. While most of trauma protocol is binary decision making, allowing one to rapidly run through the triage protocol, the new information generated by the Virtual Soldier Project will need to be integrated in a careful and responsible manner into new protocols. The final system will have to assist the field medic in the critical decisions that will need to be made under difficult battlefield conditions, especially when multiple casualties require prioritization of evacuation. The experimental validation of this modeling and statistical approach will be published elsewhere.

## Acknowledgments

This work was supported by a grant from DARPA, executed by the U.S. Army Medical Research and Materiel Command/TATRC Cooperative Agreement, Contract # W81XWH-04-2-0012.
Special thanks to Marty Cole from the University of Utah for assistance with figure 4.

# References

[1]  Triage Casualties on a Conventional Battlefield 081-833-0080.

[2]  Battlefield Medical Information System – Tactical, www.tatrc.org accessed July 14, 2004.

[3]  Lorensen W, Miller J, Padfield D, Ross J, "Creating Models from Segmented Medical Images" MMVR 2005.

[4]  Neal M, Bassingthwaighte, Usyk T, McCulloch A, Kerckhoffs R, "A Highly Integrated Physiology (HIP) Cardiovascular/Respiratory Model Used to Simulate Cardiac Injury" MMVR 2005.

[5]  Bookstein FL, Cook D, Bassingthwaighte J, "Tracking physiological models by Kalman Filters" MMVR 2005.

[6]  Savell CT, Borsotto M, Reifman J, Hoyt RW, "Life Sign Decision Support Algorithms" MEDINFO 2004, 2004, 1453-1460.

*Medicine Meets Virtual Reality 13*
*James D. Westwood et al. (Eds.)*
*IOS Press, 2005*

# A Web-based Remote Collaborative System for Visualization and Assessment of Semi-Automatic Diagnosis of Liver Cancer from CT Images

Alexandra BRANZAN ALBU, Denis LAURENDEAU,
Marco GURTNER and Cedric MARTEL

*Computer Vision and Systems Laboratory, Laval University, (Qc), G1K 7P4, Canada*
*e-mail: branzan@gel.ulaval.ca*

**Abstract.** We propose a web-based collaborative CAD system allowing for the remote communication and data exchange between radiologists and researchers in computer vision-based software engineering. The proposed web-based interface is implemented in the Java Advanced Imaging Application Programming Interface. The different modules of the interface allow for 3D and 2D data visualization, as well as for the parametric adjustment of 3D reconstruction process. The proposed web-based CAD system was tested in a pilot study involving a limited number of liver cancer cases. The successful system validation in the feasibility stage will lead to an extended clinical study on CT and MR image databases.

## 1. Introduction

Modern virtual environment technologies supporting medical applications are mainly designed for diagnosis, education, training, and rehabilitation purposes. Interactive data visualization techniques are expected to help radiologists and other healthcare professionals in improving the accuracy of image-based diagnosis of various diseases.

The computer-aided diagnosis (CAD) of liver cancer is a powerful alternative to the traditional assessment of this disease. We propose a web-based collaborative CAD system allowing for the remote communication and data exchange between radiologists and researchers in computer vision-based software engineering. Prior to the clinical use of a CAD system for liver cancer, a thorough validation of its reliability is necessary. Therefore, this paper presents a comparison of the semi-automatic segmentation results with the ground-truth manual segmentation performed by an expert radiologist.

The rest of the paper is organized as follows. Section 2 contains a description of our approach. The experimental results are discussed in section 3. Section 4 contains the conclusions as well as a brief discussion about the future work directions.

## 2. Proposed approach

This section begins with a brief technical presentation of the system. Next, the basic principles of the proposed tumour segmentation and 3D reconstruction algorithms are presented. Finally, we describe the validation protocol applied to the CAD interface.

The proposed web-based interface is implemented in the Java Advanced Imaging Application Programming Interface. This environment is compatible with the Internet Imaging Protocol and thus supports client such as laptops to desktops and high-end servers. As shown in Figure 1, the different modules of the interface allow for 3D and 2D data visualization, as well as for the parametric control of the reconstruction process.

The *2D semi-automatic segmentation algorithm* [1] requires the specification of one reference pixel inside the tumour of interest. The lesion is then detected with an algo-

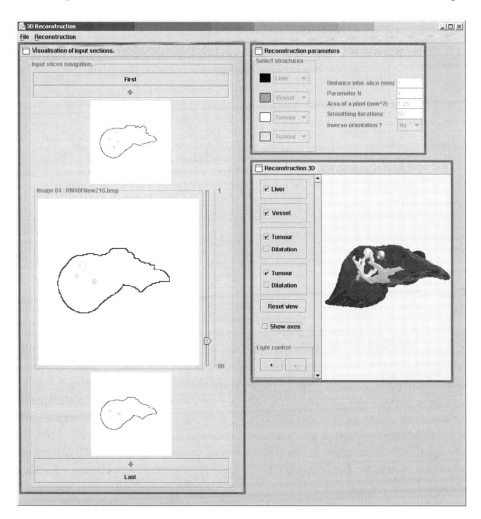

**Figure 1.** The main window of the interface. Left: sub-window for 2D data visualization; Right (upper part): sub-window for the parametric control of the 3D reconstruction; Right (lower part) sub-window for the visualization of the hepatic tumours in their anatomical context.

rithm based on iterative pixel aggregation and local textural information. The limited patient exposure to X-rays results in CT input data with different intra-slice and inter-slice resolutions. Our proposed *3D reconstruction approach* [1] estimates the missing slices using shape-based interpolation and extrapolation. To allow for a context-based visualization, a reconstruction of the liver and the liver vessels from manual segmentations of these structures is also performed, in addition to the tumour reconstruction.

The *proposed validation protocol* uses the 3D reconstructed tumour models from semi-automatic and manual reference segmentations respectively and analyzes the statistical error distribution. The 3D validation technique is implemented in *Polyworks$^{TM}$*, a software dedicated to the inspection of high density point clouds.

## 3. Results

We have tested our method on four CT data sets of liver cancer cases, courtesy of the Radiology Department at the Georgetown University Medical Center (WA, USA). An expert manual segmentation for every dataset was also made available. The anisotropy of the input data (pixel spacing of 0.6 mm along the X and Y direction, and 5 mm along the Z direction) was corrected in the reconstruction process. As shown in Table 1, containing the statistical error distribution for the liver tumour in Figure 2, the validation process was successful. The mean error value for the four analyzed cases was 0.23 mm$^3$.

## 4. Conclusion

The main contribution of our work consists in the design of one of the first CAD systems dedicated to liver cancer and evaluated with a 3D validation protocol. The proposed web-

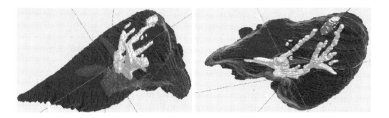

**Figure 2.** Two different views in the visualization of the liver, the tumour, and the major liver vessels.

**Table 1.** Statistical error distribution for the liver tumour in Figure 2.

| Tumour model no. 1 | Semi-automatic segmentation |
|---|---|
| Reference tumour model | Expert manual segmentation |
| Number of points (voxels) | 5135 |
| Mean error (mm$^3$) | 0.1508 |
| StdDev (mm$^3$) | 0.7059 |
| Maximum absolute error (mm$^3$) | 3.3573 |
| Points within +/- (1*StdDev) | 3610 (70.31%) |
| Points within +/-(2*StdDev) | 3795 (93.05%) |

based CAD system was tested in a pilot study involving a limited number of liver cancer cases. The successful system validation in the feasibility stage will lead to an extended clinical study on CT and MR image databases.

The web-based design will allow radiologists to perform the manual segmentation and to compare their diagnosis with the result of the semiautomatic CAD system. Therefore, our system facilitates communication between remote computer vision-based software engineering and medical communities.

The proposed interface allows for visualizing the 3D segmented lesions within the liver and with respect to the major liver vessels. When cryotherapy is a suitable treatment option, the planning of the optimal trajectory of the cryoprobe will consider the 3D liver, tumours, and vessels models provided by the proposed CAD system.

## References

[1]   A. Branzan Albu, D. Laurendeau, C. Moisan and D. Rancourt, "SKALPEL-ICT: Simulation Kernel Applied to the Planning and Evaluation of Image-Guided Cryotherapy", in *Perspective in Image-Guided Surgery*, (T. M. Buzug and T. C. Lueth Eds.), World Scientific, ISBN 981-238-872-9, pp. 295-302.

*Medicine Meets Virtual Reality 13*
*James D. Westwood et al. (Eds.)*
*IOS Press, 2005*

# Heterogeneous Displays for Surgery and Surgical Simulation

Jesus CABAN, BS [a], W. Brent SEALES, PhD [a] and Adrian PARK, MD [b]

[a] *University of Kentucky*
[b] *University of Maryland*

**Abstract.** Instruments and procedures continue to become more complex and challenging, but the display environments to which these technologies are connected have not kept pace. Display real-estate (the size and resolution of the display), the configurability of the display, and the ability for display systems to incorporate, fuse and present diverse informational sources are limiting factors. The capabilities of display technologies are far exceeded by the procedures and instruments that rely on them.

In this paper we show how to break free from display constraints by moving forward with a hybrid, heterogeneous display framework that preserves key characteristics of current systems (low latency, specialized devices). We have engineered a hybrid display and are currently using it to build a surgical simulation and training environment within which we can evaluate both the technology and the performance of subjects using the technology.

## 1. Introduction

Procedures that depend crucially upon instrumentation generating complex visual feedback (e.g., scopes) are now commonplace and have created entirely new areas of research, development, and practice. Traditional endoscopes [1] and more sophisticated stereo endoscopes [3,2] are improving every day to provide the surgeon with high quality imagery. While scopes, lenses, cameras and CCDs are improving, image-guided surgeries are still tightly coupled with single, dedicated display devices that are not integrated with each other. Relevant information such as preoperative medical imaging, CT data, X-rays, patient medical history, and instrument readings can assist during surgery but are largely unavailable because of display constraints.

We believe that multiple, independent, self-contained display devices can be distracting, and place the burden of information integration on the viewer. In response to this problem, we have built a scalable, hybrid display system for surgery and surgical simulation that facilitates device and information integration, providing users with a flexible, unified display space.

## 2. The Hybrid Display

We have constructed a prototype display system that supports a high-resolution, multi-context, hybrid display space to facilitate surgical scenarios. This unified display system

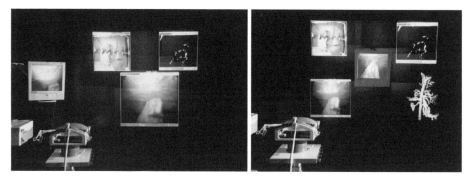

**Figure 1.** (left) A multi-context display system showing scope video, external video and tracking analysis. (right) A hybrid display incorporating an LCD panel.

supports real-time and enhanced video from a variety of sources: scopes, cameras, renderings from 3D datasets, metric assessments, and tracking information. Figure 1 shows a view of this display prototype with multiple contexts available.

The normal 2D video and imagery can be seen in parts of the display, while other areas are enabled for passive, polarized stereo. It is also possible to smoothly incorporate traditional displays devices, such as LCD panels and plasma TVs, creating a hybrid but unified display environment. Figure 1 (right) shows a display system that incorporates an LCD panel connected directly to a scope signal.

Using this environment, we can assemble 3D data, pre-operative CT-scan data, live scope video, procedure slides from a medical image database, metric overlay information, and other important custom data (e.g., stereo reconstruction and identification of anatomy) to create a fused, unified display.

We are experimenting with configurations that provably reduce distractions and streamlines the user's focus of attention under specific constraints in order to better support particular procedures and tasks. Because the display system supports stereo, overlays, scalable resolution, and the potential for side-by-side views to overcome latency issues, we are able to study new configurations that have the potential to improve performance and reduce the onset of fatigue. Additionally, the scalable screen real-estate provides a substrate with which we can integrate features such as remote collaborative consultation and video conferencing on-demand.

## 3. Design

We have created a single and unified display environment by tiling a number of projectors together. Using custom software, this high-resolution display wall is calibrated automatically into a seamless, homogeneous display. At the application level it is viewed as a unified large-scale framebuffer.

The flexible display system uses a scalable number of casually-aligned projectors to create a high-resolution display space (Figure 2a). The areas where the projectors overlap are made to appear seamless through a camera-based warp of geometry and blend of photometrics. After the calibration process, we can display a seamless grid across the complete display (Figure 2b) to show the accuracy of the calibration in terms of

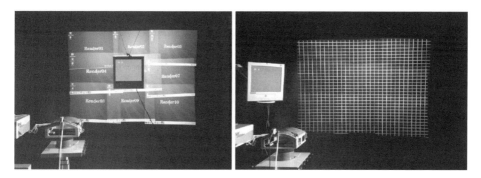

**Figure 2.** (left)A nine-projector display system incorporating a low-latency LCD device (directly connected to a scope) can be calibrated and used as a seamless display device. (right) The grid across the nine-projector display shows calibration results.

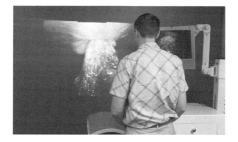

**Figure 3.** A six-projector display used to show scope video.

geometric correction. Also, the display system uses a core low-latency device (commonly an HDTV LCD panel) that is embedded within the projected environment. The LCD device can be programmed to maintain a low-latency core image, while the surrounding pixels are flexibly mapped to any data source, such as video, images from databases, or enhanced views (higher latency) of the core image.

The stereo-enabled portion of the display system is ready to map seamlessly to stereo scopes such as those used by the Da Vinci [2] system and those sold by Vista [3]. Without relying on a specialized headmounted display, the system provides a way to seamlessly integrate the stereo view onto a portion of the screen while all other screen real-estate remains available for other processing. This represents a substantial advantage over other display systems that assume a dedicated posture to support stereo to the exclusion of other important cues.

## 4. Results

Our working prototype consists of any configuration of 9 projectors and a core LCD panel display. Our software system runs on a tightly-coupled computer cluster and drives a rear-projected environment. We use a Stryker laparoscopic training stand in front of the display as a baseline configuration. Cameras, hidden behind the screen, communicate images to the software and automatically configure the display layout. The computer cluster acts as a distributed platform for running simulation code (collision detection, for example) as well as processes that can enhance live video from scopes. The output from multiple scopes can be shown simultaneously without loss of resolution since the 3x3 projected grid has a total resolution of over 9 megapixels.

We believe that the display environment we have demonstrated will provide valuable insight into how best to move beyond the "in-the-box" display systems that have been only incrementally improved over the past 20 years. The display framework removes key constraints on display real-estate (resolution and configuration), embraces the ability to include seamless stereo regions, and still provides the ability to keep information available in a way that is tightly-coupled and potentially less distracting for the surgical team.

## References

[1]  Stryker Corporation. In http://www.stryker.com/.
[2]  SunnyBrook Technologies Inc. In http://www.intuitivesurgical.com.
[3]  Vista medical technologies inc. In http://www.vistamt.com/.

*Medicine Meets Virtual Reality 13*
*James D. Westwood et al. (Eds.)*
*IOS Press, 2005*

# Visualization of Treatment Evolution Using Hardware-Accelerated Morphs

Bruno M. CARVALHO and H. QUYNH DIHN

*Dept. of Computer Science, Stevens Institute of Technology, NJ*
*e-mail: bruno_m_carvalho@yahoo.com; quynh@cs.stevens.edu*

**Abstract.** The observation of the evolution of a course of treatment can provide a powerful tool in understanding its efficacy. To visualize this, we produce animations allowing the visualization, as a function of time, of lesions in an organ. Such animations can be used in teaching or for patient education, influencing a patient's decision of following a course of treatment. The animation produced is a metamorphosis, or morph, describing how a source shape (pre-treatment) gradually deforms into a target shape (post-treatment). We implemented our method using the programming capabilities of current graphics cards (also known as graphics processing units or GPUs), so both visualization of the volumes and morph generation are performed in real-time. We demonstrate our method on data from a patient's liver with lymphoma that was treated with chemotherapy and is currently on remission.

## 1. Introduction

The observation of the evolution of a course of treatment can provide a powerful tool in demonstrating or understanding its efficacy. To perform this, we produce animations allowing the visualization, as a function of time, of lesions in an organ. Such animations can be used in teaching or for patient education, influencing a patient's decision of following a course of treatment.

The animation generated is a metamorphosis, or morph, that describes how a source shape (pre-treatment data set) gradually deforms into a target shape (post-treatment data set). We chose to use implicit morphs, where an implicit function describes the changing geometry and the intermediate shapes are defined by the level sets [5] of the function at different time points. These intermediate shapes are defined by interpolating between signed distance functions (also called distance fields) of the source and target shapes. The magnitudes of these distance fields indicate the distance from the surface of the shape, while the sign indicates where a point is inside (negative) or outside (positive) of the shape.

The fast rate at which the hardware of graphics cards (also known as graphics processing units or GPUs) are evolving, especially the development of their programming capabilities, opened up the possibility of implementing several graphics-related applications using GPUs, thus speeding up their executions. In this paper, we advocate the use of GPU programming to accelerate the visualization and morphing of medical 3D objects, so they can be done interactively in real-time.

## 2. Method

Our method for creating the morph animation is divided in three steps: segmentation of the target organ in the data sets, registration of the data sets, and generation and visualization of the morph.

The method used for segmenting the data sets is the multiseeded fuzzy segmentation of [2], a region growing method, that based on user input, in the form of seed *spels* (short for spatial element), produces a connectedness map that encodes the grade of membership of every spel to the segmented objects. The grade of membership of a spel *c* to an object *m*, a real value between 0 and 1, reflects the confidence that the method's solution has that the spel *c* belongs to the object *m*. This map is then thresholded for the object associated with the target organ/lesions to isolate the objects to be visualized in the morph sequence.

The last two steps of our method are performed using the interface Imorph [3]. In the registration step, the two volumes (pre-treatment and post-treatment) are visualized, so the user can align them and chose correspondence points between them. These correspondence points can then be used to generate a non-linear warping map that is applied to both volumes using dependent textures, in a similar manner as in [8].

The generation of the morph between two shapes *A* and *B* is obtained by cross-dissolving the distance fields (that encode the distance from each point to the surface of the object) of the two shapes, resulting in a linear interpolation between the source and target distance fields [4]:

$$d = (1 - t) \cdot \text{dist}(A) + t \cdot \text{dist}(B),$$

where dist(*A*) is the signed distance field for the shape *A*, dist(*B*) is the signed distance field for the shape *B*, and *d* defines the intermediate shape at time *t*. As *t* is varied, for $0 \leq t \leq 1$, intermediate shapes are extracted where the interpolated distance field *d* evaluates to zero. At the starting time ($t = 0$) the resulting shape is completely defined by the source shape *A*, and at the ending time ($t = 1$) the resulting shape is completely defined by *B*.

To visualize the morph, we modify the volume rendering algorithm of [7] (implemented in [6]) in which the authors use the graphics hardware to perform volume rendering by computing the intersection of planes parallel to the image plane with volumes stored in 3D textures. They then render these textured planes in back-to-front order (from the farthest plane to the closest one). To compute the morph in real-time, we store the distance fields in 3D textures and interpolate between the distance textures of shape A and shape B on every rendering pass using fragment shaders. To extract the volume, we pass only interpolated fragments that are less than or equal to 0 (inside or on the surface).

## 3. Experiment

The experiment shown in Figure 1 depicts the evolution of a liver treatment for a patient that suffers from lymphoma, was treated with chemotherapy, and is currently on remission.

After the data were segmented, the objects of interest in the segmentations (the liver and pre- and post-treatment lesions) were isolated, with the segmentation step taking

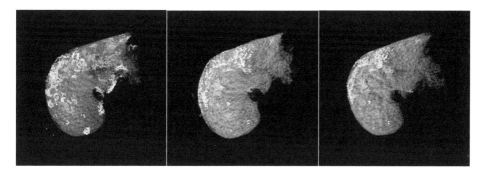

**Figure 1.** Volume rendering of the pre-treatment (left), an intermediate (middle) and the post-teatment (right) stages of a patient's liver affected by lymphoma.

around $60s$ per data set (on a Pentium 4 3GHz). Then, their distance fields were calculated, in a procedure that took around $20s$ for each of the three objects, and stored in three different 3D textures in the memory of an NVidia GeForce FX 5950 graphics card. (It is important to note that the graphics card used in this experiment is an off-the-shelf card that usually is shipped with medium-priced PCs.)

After the segmentation and the initial distance field computation, all other operations are performed in real-time, allowing the user to change the viewpoint during the morph sequence.

## 4. Conclusion

In this paper, we advocate the use of morphs for interactive real-time visualization of the evolution a treatment. This technique allows the user to modify the camera position or the transfer function used to generate the volume rendering and observe in real-time the changes in the morph sequence. The fact that we are using implicit morphing implies that we can model objects whose topology changes over time. Morphing can be a valuable tool that can be used to observe the dynamics of treatments, for example, in tracking the evolution of lesions over time as affected by treatment. Other applications include the interactive visualization of activity in functional imaging and the generation of new data sets from available ones for their use in education [1].

## Acknowledgements

We would like to thank Mitchell Laks for providing the data sets used in this article.

## References

[1] Bergeron, B., L. Sato, and R. Rouse. "Morphing as a Means of Generating Variation in Visual Medical Teaching Files". Comp. in Biol. and Med., 24:11-18, 1994.
[2] Carvalho, B.M., and G.T. Herman. "Multiseeded Segmentation Using Fuzzy Connectedness", IEEE Trans. on Pat. Anal. Mach. Int., 23:460-474, 2001.
[3] Cohen-Or, D., D. Levin, and A. Solomovici. "Three-Dimensional Distance Field Metamorphosis", ACM Trans. on Graph., 17:116-141, 1998.

[4]  Dinh, H.Q., and Carvalho, B.M. "Imorph: An Interactive System for Visualizing and Modeling Implicit Morphs", TR CS-2004-08, Dept. of Computer Science, Stevens Institute of Technology, 2004.

[5]  Payne, B.A., and A.W. Toga, "Distance Field Manipulation of Surface Models", IEEE Comp. Graph. and Appl., 12:65-71, 1992.

[6]  Rezk-Salama, C., Engel, K., and Higuera. F.V. The OpenQVis Project, http://openqvis.sourceforge.net/, accessed in 10/25/2004.

[7]  Westerman, R., and Ertl, T. "Efficiently Using Graphics Hardware in Volume Rendering Applications", Proc. Of SIGGRAPH 98, 169-177, 98.

[8]  Westerman, R., and Rezk-Salama, C. "Real-Time Volume Deformations", Computer Graphics Forum, 20:3, 2001.

*Medicine Meets Virtual Reality 13*
*James D. Westwood et al. (Eds.)*
*IOS Press, 2005*

# Real-time Rendering of Radially Distorted Virtual Scenes for Endoscopic Image Augmentation

M.S. CHEN, R.J. LAPEER and R.S. ROWLAND

*School of Computing Sciences, University of East Anglia, Norwich, UK*
*e-mail: msc@cmp.uea.ac.uk*

**Abstract.** This paper presents a method for rendering radially distorted virtual scenes in real-time using the programmable fragment shader commonly found in many main stream graphics hardware. We show that by using the pixel buffer and the fragment shader, it is possible to augment the endoscopic display with distorted virtual images.

## 1. Introduction

Endoscopes are used to navigate through narrow surgical paths or small openings. Minimal invasive surgical procedures use this technique to provide visual guidance for the surgeon. An endoscope's optics is able to capture a large field of view (FOV) using its small convex lens. However, the lens causes the images to be radially distorted.

Many recent studies have been focusing on methods for accurately calibrating the optics of the endoscope, in order to provide augmented reality based guidance for endoscopic surgery [3,4,6]. For the calibration problem, one can attempt to recover distortion factors up to an infinite number of orders. In practice, camera calibration algorithms such as Tsai's [5] recover the second and fourth orders distortion factors, which are sufficient to accurately model radial distortion of an endoscope.

Graphics rendering API's such as OpenGL, produce images using an ideal perspective projection. Therefore, intrinsic properties such as lens distortion are not directly modeled when using this type of projection. The approach taken by previous research is to correct the distortion in the endoscope images, so that they appear to be captured by an ideal perspective projection. The undistorted endoscope images can then be overlaid by its matching virtual images. We introduce a different method, in which the generated virtual images are distorted in real-time to match the endoscope images. The reason for using this approach is to preserve the distortion in endoscopic images as surgeons are well adapted to the distorted view through years of training and practice. The remaining sections discuss the technique for modeling real-time lens distortion effects.

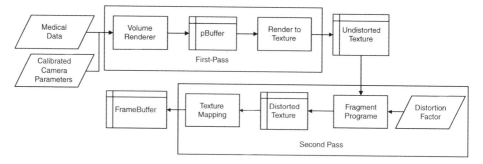

**Figure 1.** A two-pass rendering pipeline for modeling real-time radial distortion.

## 2. Method

### 2.1. Rendering Process Overview

In order to distort the co-ordinate of a pixel, a vector-valued distortion term is computed (Equation 1). The image co-ordinates are then perturbed by this distortion term $\delta\bar{\mathbf{u}}$:

$$\delta\bar{\mathbf{u}} = (\bar{\mathbf{u}}' - \bar{\mathbf{u}}_\mathbf{p})(\kappa_1 r^2 + \kappa_2 r^4) \tag{1}$$

In Equation 1, $\bar{\mathbf{u}}'$ is the undistorted image co-ordinate; $\bar{\mathbf{u}}_\mathbf{p}$ denote the principle point of the optics; $r$ is the distance between a given pixel and the principal point; $\kappa_1$ and $\kappa_2$ are the second and fourth order distortion factors.

Since the distortion only needs to be considered in the image space, it is straightforward to apply the distortion terms for each frame rendered by OpenGL. The complete rendering process consists of two stages as illustrated in Figure 1. The first-pass generates an undistorted scene using the projection matrix from the calibrated camera parameters and stores in a texture unit by using the pixel buffer (*pBuffer*) and the RENDER_TO_TEXTURE extension. In the second-pass the texture containing the undistorted scene is passed to a fragment program that produces a distorted image based on $\kappa_1$, $\kappa_2$ and the principal point $\bar{\mathbf{u}}_\mathbf{p}$.

### 2.2. The Fragment Program

The fragment program written in Cg [1] replaces the standard OpenGL fragment operation. Input to the program is the undistorted texture containing the scene, the centre of distortion $\bar{\mathbf{u}}_\mathbf{p}$, two distortion factors $\kappa_1$, $\kappa_2$ and the texture coordinate $\bar{\mathbf{u}}'$. Since an arbitrary texture size is used, the value of $\bar{\mathbf{u}}'$ and $\bar{\mathbf{u}}_\mathbf{p}$ are expressed in pixel units (i.e. based on the image dimension and its reference frame). It is necessary to normalise the value of $\bar{\mathbf{u}}'$ and $\bar{\mathbf{u}}_\mathbf{p}$, i.e. compute a transformation $\mathbf{M}$ that translates the origin to the centre of the image and scales the pixel coordinates to the range of $[-1, 1]$. Then Equation 1 is applied to calculate the distortion term $\delta\bar{\mathbf{u}}$ for the normalised $\bar{\mathbf{u}}'$. To obtain the distorted image coordinate $\bar{\mathbf{u}}$, we need to de-normalise the result computed from Equation 1 (see Equation 2).

$$\bar{\mathbf{u}} = \mathbf{M}^{-1}(\bar{\mathbf{u}}' + \delta\bar{\mathbf{u}}) \tag{2}$$

The shader then maps the pixel at $\bar{\mathbf{u}}'$ to $\bar{\mathbf{u}}$ in a newly created texture unit that stores the distorted virtual scene.

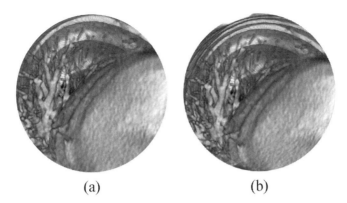

(a)           (b)

**Figure 2.** (a) The undistorted view of the virtual endoscopic lung image; (b) the distorted view of the virtual endoscopic lung image.

## 3. Result and Discussion

The technique mentioned in the previous section is integrated in our volume rendering software ARView [2]. Figure 2(a) and (b) show an undistorted and distorted virtual (CT derived) 'endoscopic' image of a lung. By comparing the two images in Figure 2, we notice that the distorted lung image captures a wider field of view within the same image space.

    The technique presented here takes advantage of the *pBuffer*, which forms the basis of OpenGL's *render to texture* mechanism. If the *pBuffer* is not available, one can still use the standard frame buffer as the rendering target in the first pass. The texture can then be constructed by reading the contents of the frame buffer and uploading it to the texture unit. However, this can significantly degrade the performance because of the expense of using the *glReadPixels* operation for each frame.

## 4. Conclusion

We have presented a method for the real-time rendering of radial distortion effects. This method does not modify any rendering routine currently used for surface and volumetric visualisation. It only diverts the generated image to an intermediate texture, instead of the frame-buffer.

## References

[1] *The Cg Tutorial: The Definitive Guide to Programmable Real-time Graphics.* Addison Wesley, 2003.
[2] R. Lapeer, R. Rowland, and M. S. Chen. PC-based Volume Rendering for Medical Visualisation and Augmented Reality based Surgical Navigation. *IEEE MediViz 2004 Conference Proceeding*, pages 67–72, 2004.
[3] G. Marti, V. Bettschart, J.-S. Billiard, and C. Baur. Hybrid method for both calibration and registration of an endoscope with an active optical tracker. *CARS 2004 Proceedings*, pages 159–164, 2004.
[4] R. Shahidi et al. Implementation, calibration and accuracy testing of an image-enhanced endoscopy system. *IEEE Transactions on Medical Imaging*, 21(12):1524–1535, 2002.
[5] R.Y. Tsai. A versatile camera calibration technique for high-accuracy 3D machine vision metrology using off-the-shelf TV cameras and lenses. *IEEE Journal of Robotics and Automation*, RA-3(4):323–344, 1987.
[6] T. Yamaguchi et al. Camera Model and Calibration Procedure for Oblique-Viewing Endoscope. *LNCS MICCAI 2003 Proceedings*, pages 373–381, 2003.

*Medicine Meets Virtual Reality 13*
*James D. Westwood et al. (Eds.)*
*IOS Press, 2005*

# Tracking the Domain: The Medical Modeling and Simulation Database

C. Donald COMBS, Ph.D. [a] and Kara FRIEND, M.S. [b]

[a] *Founding Co-Director, National Center for Collaboration in Medical Modeling and Simulation Vice President for Planning and Programming Development, Eastern Virginia Medical School*
*e-mail: combscd@evms.edu*
[b] *Research Associate, National Center for Collaboration in Medical Modeling and Simulation Eastern Virginia Medical School*
*e-mail: friendke@evms.edu*

**Abstract.** To foster awareness of the magnitude and breadth of activity and to foster collaboration among the participants, the National Center for Collaboration in Medical Modeling and Simulation (NCCMMS) has created the Medical Modeling and Simulation Database (MMSD). The MMSD consists of two web-based, searchable compilations: one, the Research Database, that contains bibliographic information on published articles and abstracts (where available) and a second, the Companies and Projects Database, that maintains contact information for research centers, development and application programs, journals and conferences. NCCMMS is developing the MMSD to increase awareness of the breadth of the medical modeling domain and to provide a means of fostering collaboration and bringing like-minded organizations and researchers into more frequent contact with each other, thus speeding advancement of medical modeling and simulation.

The terms medical modeling and simulation suggest a myriad of ideas to various people but few people have a definitive idea of what medical modeling and simulation entails. For the purposes of this article medical modeling and simulation is defined as any form of computer or internet-based modeling that is intended to be useful in medical research or training. The field of medical modeling and simulation is rapidly expanding and the data produced by individuals and companies will soon be overwhelming to the casual researcher, and perhaps to those actively working in the field.

Medical modeling and simulation has been the subject of countless studies and articles. These articles, however, are currently spread throughout various sources on the Internet or in print. Similarly, there are hundreds of companies actively researching and creating new modeling and simulation software. Unfortunately, information on these companies is fragmented as well. If researchers could easily contact other researchers working in their field or if scientists knew where to find articles describing the efficacy of specific simulators, new research could be streamlined. To that end, the National Center for Collaboration in Medical Modeling and Simulation (NCCMMS) created the Medical Modeling and Simulation Database (MMSD).

The prototype database was created in ISI ResearchSoft's EndNote (v. 7) [1]. This is a bibliographic database specifically designed for compiling, editing and searching

**Table 1.** The following words were searched in combination with virtual reality, virtual medicine, computers and medicine or computer simulation.

| | | | |
|---|---|---|---|
| Surgery | Computer-aided | Education | Virtual Environments |
| Laparoscopy | Instruction | Remote Medicine | Computer Assisted |
| Endoscopy | Sound | Training Validation | Surgery |
| Telemedicine | Data Display | Telepresence Medicine | Virtual Interface |
| Uteroscopy | Human Factors | Virtual Worlds | Technology |
| Computer Graphics | User Computer | Surgical Simulation | Surgical |
| Medical Applications | Interaction | Haptics | Planning |

**Table 2.** The following search engines were used.

| | |
|---|---|
| Pub Med (NLM) | Dogpile [1] |
| HealthStar (Ovid) | Medline (Ovid) |
| Library of Congress | Various sites will be searched using the search engine associated with the endnote software [4]. |

textual information. It is directly linked to several online libraries, including PubMed and OVID. The program allows the user to search an online database using keywords, dates or author names and download the relevant bibliographic data into the EndNote program. This program then sorts the entries based on the criteria specified by the user. Unfortunately this program was difficult to load on to the Internet. The database was converted to ISI ResearchSoft's Reference Manager (v. 11) as this program has a sub-program that facilitates simple web-publishing [2]. The database is currently located on a dedicated server that has been loaded with the appropriate security measures and is currently available at virtualmedicine.evms.edu.

The initial searches to fill the MMSD were designed to identify as many relevant articles as possible. Available databases were queried through the EndNote or Reference Manager programs and additional searches were performed using several internet search engines. The list of keywords used and websites queried are shown in Tables 1 and 2 respectively. After the search results were loaded into the program the researchers began the arduous task of sorting through the articles to remove any unrelated articles.

When the NCCMMS began this research, several existing catalogs of virtual reality in medicine were discovered. These sites had not been updated since 1999 (at the most recent); however, their data was incorporated into the MMSD for historical purposes. To accommodate various users' interests the database was divided into two parts; the Research Article Database (containing bibliographic data on published articles) and the Companies and Projects Database (containing information on public, private and military research as well as conferences and proceedings).

The Research Article Database contains over 13,000 entries ranging from editorials to reports on scientific experiments. The articles span almost 40 years, although almost 70% of the articles were written from 1995 to the present. The articles are arranged by author, but they can be searched in a variety of ways including journal, year, page number or keyword. Additionally, there are approximately 100 full text articles included in the database. The full text section is available in either Microsoft Word or Adobe Acrobat format. This database can be used for a variety of purposes, including surveying the domain, determining the efficacy of certain simulators, or to determine new developments in one's field of interest.

The Companies and Projects Database contains more than 600 entries detailing information about medical modeling research. This section includes conference informa-

**Table 3.** Virtual Medicine websites.

| |
|---|
| NAS facility at NASA Ames Research Center.<br>http://www.nas.nasa.gov/Groups/VisTech/visWeblets.html#Commercial |
| Waterworth, J. A. (1999). Virtual Reality in Medicine: A Survey of the State of the Art.<br>http://www.informatik.umu.se/~jwworth/medpage.html |
| Emerson, T, Prothero, J, Weghorst, S. (1994). Medicine and Virtual Reality: A Guide to the Literature<br>(MedVR) HITL Technical Report No.B-94-1<br>http://www.hitl.washington.edu/projects/knowledge_base/medvr/medvr.html |

tion as well as links to various research organizations. Some of these organizations are companies specializing in software or virtual reality technology while others are governmentally sponsored medical research. Also included in this section is information on magazines and journals dedicated to virtual reality in medicine. This section is invaluable to those searching for simulators or looking for information about past or planned conferences.

The MMSD will be updated monthly to prevent its obsolescence. The NCCMMS will search the Internet regularly for new publications and new companies. Once the website is fully established there will be links for researchers and developers to contact the site manager to request the inclusion of their article. The MMSD will also accept any information provided by private sector companies, government agencies or research centers. The NCCMMS will maintain the MMSD as an honest broker and will not provide one company more coverage than another except as warranted by the product lines. Not all the products listed on the site have been used or tested; rather, their listing is to provide information to the public for evaluation. The MMSD is designed to help researchers learn what is going on at other research centers and to foster collaboration between centers. This site is designed to be used by researchers, companies and the general public. The default query will search both databases to ensure the best results.

The NCCMMS will continually update the database to guarantee that the most relevant articles are available. Additional abstracts, full text articles or links to existing entries will be added as they become available. The projects section will also be updated on a regular basis including checking the integrity of the links as well as adding information to each company's website. As the database comes online, companies should start volunteering information and writing their own summaries for inclusion. This will not only ensure an accurate appraisal of the company's focus but also help make sure all relevant companies are included in the database.

The NCCMMS hopes that its 14,000 entry database will help to stimulate the field of medical modeling and simulation by allowing better collaboration and communication. While the program is still in its infancy, structural support is already in place to allow the burgeoning field to continue to develop and the MMSD to grow with it. The NCCMMS seeks through this project to ease the growing pains of the medical modeling and simulation field by creating a public forum for discussion and free exchange of ideas. For research centers, the MMSD provides a single location to search through past experiences, and for companies it provides free advertising and a new way to reach thousands of interested clients. The NCCMMS' database is filling the void created by the rapid, fragmented growth of the medical modeling and simulation field by allowing for collaboration and simplifying research.

## Acknowledgement

This study was a collaborative project between the Virginia Modeling, Analysis and Simulation Center (VMASC) at the Eastern Virginia Medical School and Old Dominion University. Funding for this study was provided in part by the Naval Health Research Center through NAVAIR Orlando TSD under contract N61339-03-C-0157, entitled "The National Center for Collaboration in Medical Modeling and Simulation". The ideas and opinions presented in this paper represent the views of the authors and do not necessarily represent the views of the Department of Defense.

## References

[1] For more information about EndNote (v.7), see www.endnote.com.
[2] For more information about Reference Manager (v. 11), see www.refman.com.
[3] Per www.dogpile.com "Dogpile uses innovative metasearch technology to search the Internet's top search engines, including Google, Yahoo, Ask Jeeves, About, Teoma, FindWhat, LookSmart, and many more." Accessed on July 14, 2004.
[4] NCCMMS website, see nccmms.evms.edu. The database is available directly at virtualmedicine.evms.edu.

*Medicine Meets Virtual Reality 13*
*James D. Westwood et al. (Eds.)*
*IOS Press, 2005*

# The ViCCU Project – Achieving Virtual Presence using Ultrabroadband Internet in a Critical Clinical Application – Initial Results

Patrick CREGAN [a], Stuart STAPLETON [a], Laurie WILSON [b], Rong-Yiu QIAO [b], Jane LI [b] and Terry PERCIVAL [b]

[a] *Nepean Hospital, Wentworth Area Health Service, Penrith*
[b] *CSIRO Telecommunications and Industrial Physics, Sydney*

**Abstract.** The ViCCU (Virtual Critical Care Unit) Project sought to address the problems of shortages of Critical Care staff by developing a system that could use the capabilities of Ultrabroadband networks so as to have a Critical Care Specialist virtually present at a distant location. This is not possible in a clinically useful way with current systems. A new system (ViCCU) was developed and deployed. Critically ill or injured patients are now routinely assessed and managed remotely using this system. It has led to a more appropriate level of transfers of patients and the delivery of a quality of clinical service not previously available. This paper describes the history of the project, its novelty, the clinically significant technical aspects of the system and its deployment. The initial results to the end of September 2004 are described

## History

The Metropolitan Hospitals Group of the Greater Metropolitan Services Implementation Group (GMSIG) identified shortages of trained staff particularly in Emergency and Intensive Care as being a major impediment to the provision of care in smaller Sydney suburban hospitals [1]. A similar situation was found in Rural areas by the Rural Group. The CeNTIE (Centre for Networking Technologies in the Information Economy) project coordinated by CSIRO [2], a successful applicant for Federal funding under the BITS (Building on IT Strengths) program had health applications as one of its four principal areas of interest.

The authors conceived a plan (the Virtual Critical Care Unit or ViCCU Project [3]) to address this specialist shortage by leveraging off available specialist expertise in the Principal Referral Hospitals using the capabilities offered by high bandwidth connections being developed as part of the CeNTIE Project. In the Wentworth Area Health Service this need was seen at Blue Mountains District Anzac Memorial Hospital (BMDAMH), which is supported by Nepean Hospital as its Principal Referral Hospital. After Institutional ethics committee approval had been obtained, the project began in early 2002 with the initial development of technical specifications and was first used for patient care on 27 December 2003.

## Novelty

Telemedicine has been in use for many years but has not been used in Critical Care applications beyond talking head videoconferencing consultations and remote monitoring such as VisICU [4]. The ability to provide multiple very high quality television channels by using an ultrabroadband internet connection is what now makes telemedicine possible for critical care use in direct patient care.

## Brief Description of System

A purpose built cart is placed at the foot of the patient's bed in BMDAMH. Using new specifically developed hardware & software five "near broadcast" quality digital television channels derived from cameras on the cart and in the room relay images of the patient, staff and the resuscitation area together with excellent audio, vital signs monitor output, images of patient records, X-rays etc over a 1 Gigabit per second ultrabroadband (second generation internet or I2) Ethernet connection to a specialist in Nepean Hospital who uses the system to directly supervise care of the patient. The Nepean specialist in turn is seen and heard in the BMDAMH using a further channel and displayed on a monitor on the cart so as to be seen by the patient and those around the bed.

## Second Generation / Ultrabroadband Internet

One frame of a high quality television picture is 768 by 1024 pixels in size. For clear, flicker free television it has to be refreshed 25 to 30 times a second. This equates to between 19 and 24 megabits of data per second. If transmitted uncompressed quality is maintained. However, current telemedicine applications use ISDN telephony to transmit data. This means that television images have to be compressed at one end and then decompressed at the other end since ISDN at best only transmits between one and three Mb of data per second and introduces clinically distracting latency. By using ultrabroadband internet based on fibre-optic cable ViCCU is able to transmit 1000 megabits (1 Gigabit) of data per second and hence avoid the problems that compression causes. The fibre-optic cable used is from the NSW State Rail ARGUS network which is the basis of the rail network security system installed for the Olympic Games in 2000 and provides a 1 Gigabit per second Ethernet link.

## Quality of Television

Compression and decompression causes pixilation (where a number of the pixels or tiny coloured dots that make up the image coalesce to make big dots) and blurring / loss of detail (both of which usually occur with movement), and loss of the range of colours necessary to produce skin tones. Additionally, frames can be lost in the process of compression / recompression producing the flickering images frequently seen with conventional ISDN based videoconferencing. Further, the computing time necessary to compress and decompress the image leads to latency or delay in transmission which can be very distracting and compromise the level of communication necessary for safe patient care by

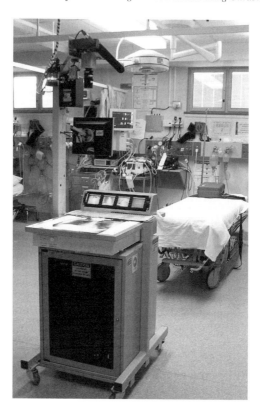

**Figure 1.** The cart.

the team in a resuscitation. By utilizing the bandwidth available over second generation internet connections we are able to avoid compression / recompression and provide "near broadcast" quality television with minimal latency. It is the quality of the television that enables the central clinician to confidently direct patient care at the remote site.

## The Remote end - The Cart

At the heart of the system is a purpose built cart. The actual cart is seen in figure 1.
  It contains:

1. the computers and modems for connection to the fiberoptic network,
2. two of the cameras – Room View and Document
3. connections for the other two cameras – Over patient and Hand held
4. connection for the Vital Signs Monitor
5. inputs for other data sources e.g. ultrasound
6. boom microphone and speakers with sophisticated echo cancellation required due to the harsh audio environment of a resuscitation bay
7. monitor displaying image of the centrally located specialist
8. monitors showing the views being transmitted to the central location
9. display box for X-rays and flat surface for reading the patient's paper based information such as clinical notes.

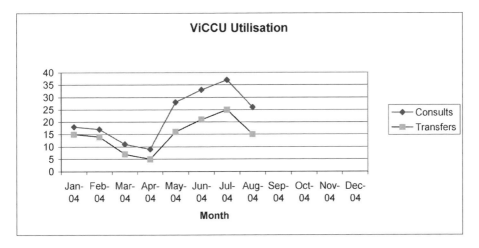

**Figure 2.**

10. a headphone setup to allow private conversation with a member of the remote location team or the patient / relative.

The cart is placed at the foot of the bed in the position usually occupied by the team leader in a resuscitation and is connected to the hospitals internal communications links and thence to the broadband network and the Principal Referral Hospital's work station. The technology was designed to be totally transparent. It is always on and requires only a phone call to ask the Central specialist to go to the work station to activate it.

**Results**

The numbers of patient consultations and transfers are shown in figure 2. There has been a steady increase in the number of activations of the system. Staff has found it easy to use, reliable and it is reassuring for the BMDAMH staff. Unnecessary transfers have been reduced and early, more timely transfers occur for the sickest patients. Further they are better resuscitated for their transfer. The quantification of this is occurring as a case controlled study over the calendar year 2004. An example of this is provided by the case of an 85 year old driver involved in a motor vehicle crash who had a prehospital asystolic cardiac arrest as a result of his injuries. He was resuscitated at BMDAMH by Nepean staff using the ViCCU system and transferred for definitive care. He survived his injuries where the expected mortality in this setting is in excess of 90%.

**Discussion**

The formal evaluation is being concluded over the next six months but the improvement in care is so clear that plans are being developed to extend the system across the whole of the Area Health Service and other Area Health Services, interstate and international interest is such that commercialization is being undertaken at an accelerated rate.

## References

[1]  http://www.health.nsw.gov.au/policy/gap/metro/GMSIGmetro.pdf (last accessed 23 October 2004).
[2]  http://www.centie.org/ (last accessed 23 October 2004).
[3]  http://www3.ict.csiro.au/ict/content/display/0%2C%2Ca16254_b16412_d41654%2C00.html (last accessed 23 October 2004).
[4]  http://www.visicu.com/ (last accessed 23 October 2004).

*Medicine Meets Virtual Reality 13*
*James D. Westwood et al. (Eds.)*
*IOS Press, 2005*

# High Stakes Assessment Using Simulation – An Australian Experience

Patrick CREGAN [a] and Leonie WATTERSON [b]

[a] *Director of Surgery, Wentworth Area Health Service, Sydney, Australia*
[b] *Director, Sydney Medical Simulation Centre, Royal North Shore Hospital, Sydney, Australia*

**Abstract.** The use of simulation for high stakes assessment has been embedded in the New South Wales Medical Practice Act and has been used for high stakes assessment on a number of occasions. Simulation has rarely been used in this manner elsewhere in the world. We outline the use of simulation in particular focussing on its relationship to a performance assessment programme featuring performance focus, peer assessment of standards, an educative, remedial and protective framework, strong legislative support and system awareness.

## Introduction

Medicine truly meets virtual reality when synthetic environments are used or created to meet a specific medical need, for example the education of medical practitioners, the treatment of patients such as treatment of phobias, the use of virtual presence systems to provide high level skills at a distance, or in the assessment of clinical competence and performance which forms the basis of this paper.

## The Problem

Increased accountability is driving a shift in focus away from traditionally self-managed maintenance of standards to favour externally regulated approaches and formal revalidation. The best approach to this is unclear given that no single methodology has high predictive validity for real-world performance. It is generally understood that high stakes assessment should incorporate multiple methodologies; sample from a wide scope of practice; focus on outcomes and use a judicious blend of subjective and objective measures [1]. Several medical licensing bodies have included these principles into their high stakes performance assessment programs and may in due course be expressed in routine revalidation processes [2].

For several reasons however concerns persist that formal performance assessment may be inaccurate or unfair. For example, clinical reviews and ongoing review tools such as CUSUM (Cumulative Sum of Variance) may be used to indicate the presence of a problem or give early warning, but do not necessarily indicate the cause of that problem nor its likely remediation [3]. In retrospect, it is frequently difficult to determine whether

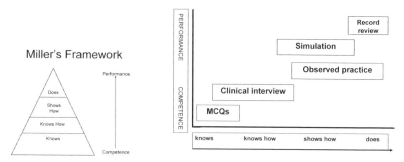

Figure 1.                      Table 1.

an event was due to an accident or failure of competence. This is also a limitation of aggregate measures and outcomes which may fail to adjust for patient characteristics and working context. Direct observation in the field is limited in capturing performance during infrequent events whilst competency assessed under controlled test conditions is limited in assessing higher order functioning such as time-critical decision-making, situation awareness and team behaviours.

This is of particular relevance to the assessment of performance in specialities such as anaesthesia.

## The potential role of simulation

Miller's framework (Figure 1) describes the progression from fundamental knowledge, and applied knowledge to discrete competencies and ultimately to performance which is the successful integration of these [4]. A contemporaneous definition of performance also incorporates "unwatched real world practice" [5]. Table 1 describes the relationship between commonly used assessment methodologies in terms of Millers model and proposes that simulation would have utility in assessing the transition from knows how to shows how [6].

Simulation has the obvious benefits of scheduling rare events, reproducibility and calibration of raters. Thus, it is a medium which can potentially blend the high reliability, content and construct validity achievable under controlled test conditions with the high face validity normally only achieved in field assessment [7]. The validity of simulation assessment has been evaluated and demonstrated in several studies [8–11]. As with more traditional assessment methodologies, performance is not generalisable across different areas of content and accurate assessment is underpinned by sampling a sufficient scope of practice. This requires at least 4 hours of observation and provides one of the strongest arguments that simulation should exist within a broader assessment framework [12,13].

An aspect of simulation-based assessment which has not been sufficiently studied is the role of the debriefing following observed performance. Post scenario debriefing using video replay is a popular educational technique in anaesthesia training and rater assessment of a candidate's capacity to reflect upon his or her performance may serve a number of functions as it affords an opportunity for the rater to explore the candidate's insight, clinical reasoning and mental model of events.

## In defence of simulation

With the exception of one centre in New York, Sydney is the only centre known to the authors which conducts simulation assessments on behalf of a medical licensing board. Without extensive scientific validation concerns will persist about its accuracy and fairness. Despite their excellent safety record, Australian anaesthetists have been responsible for serious and preventable adverse events in a small number of cases and an ethical case for simulation can be argued. It is worth noting that high-stakes assessment is conducted in Australia, Canada, the UK and US irrespective of the fact that no single assessment methodology has yet to be highly validated for this application [14]. It is also evident that in a high proportion of cases practitioners who require assessment are reported to the licensing board by their work colleagues including nurses and surgeons [15]. Assuming robust methods and appropriately selected and trained raters, the simulated environment may in fact offer a more objective and fair approach compared to the judgement of real world colleagues. Lacking content expertise, colleagues may have difficulty distinguishing unusual practice from poor performance or loss of confidence and may suffer from group think.

## N.S.W. Medical Board Performance Assessment Program

New South Wales (NSW) is the largest state in Australia. The Medical Practice Act of 1992 establishes the Medical Board whose functions are defined under section 132. These functions relate to the registration of medical practitioners and in particular to the handling of complaints and notifications concerning professional conduct, impairment and performance. The Board works with the Health Care Complaints Commission, which acts as an investigatory body. There are 25,481 registered medical practitioners in New South Wales and in 2002 – 2003 the Health Care Complaints Commission received 1,129 complaints, of which 126 required significant actions by the Board. These actions may include professional services committee review, a full medical tribunal, counselling, and interviews under a variety of categories. Of note to this paper is that there were 36 practitioners in the performance programme, and 45 of 1,129 complaints referred to competence. Thus only a tiny fraction of all practitioners are in a performance programme, and to date 3 anaesthetists have had simulation used as part of that assessment and remediation programme. Simulation was proposed because, for reasons outlined above, it was deemed that these cases would be otherwise difficult to resolve.

## Simulation Program

The NSW Medical Board refers a sub-group of the anaesthetists enrolled in its Performance Assessment Program to the Sydney Medical Simulation Centre for simulation-based assessment. The assessment is not voluntary. Assessors are protected from legal challenge as part of legislation written into the Medical Practice Act for NSW.

The SMSC program forms one element of a highly integrated, multi-faceted program conducted by the NSW Medical Board. Assessors participate in a number of components to achieve continuity. The simulation program is advised by a group of peers. The program incorporates a variety of assessment exercises including oral viva, standardised patients, review of mock video-based cases and simulations. The candidates undertake a suite of simulated scenarios which are graded from easy to difficult and include routine and crisis events. Each case is presented as a structured interview prior to the scenario being enacted on a high fidelity simulator. A further interview takes place following each scenario.

The raters are trained using previously descried methods for rater training. Rating is achieved with a blend of criteria-based tools and global subjective assessments. Recommended answers are based on published evidence where this exists.

## Case Study

The Report of the New South Wales Medical Board outlines a typical case study:

Dr Y is a 61 year old anaesthctist who was referred to the Board by an Area Health Service on the basis of performance concerns which began with a critical incident, and grew during an extended period of performance management.

As is the program's policy, Dr Y was assessed on site at the public hospital in which she was employed. Given the nature of anaesthetic practice, it was unlikely that the Assessment Team would have the opportunity to observe the practitioner's crisis management skills. However, the onsite assessment provided a valuable opportunity to assess her interaction with patients and other theatre staff. The assessment was supplemented with a full day's assessment at the Sydney Medical Simulation Centre at Royal North Shore Hospital.

In the course of this comprehensive two day assessment, it was apparent that Dr Y's performance was unsatisfactory in her ability to manage complex patients, case planning, particularly the assessment of function and risk in patients with co-existing disease and the management of emergency event situations requiring recognition, decision-making and problem solving.

A Performance Review Panel was convened. Dr Y's performance problems were thought to be so serious that it was necessary to place conditions on her registration, limiting her to working in the position of a supervised trainee.

To her great credit, Dr Y found a position that fulfilled the Board's requirements and undertook 18 months of supervised retraining and study. Her supervisor reported steady improvement in all aspects of her practice, and based on these reports, a reassessment was arranged at the Sydney Medical Simulation Centre.

Dr Y demonstrated a dramatic improvement in her knowledge and confidence. It was determined that her clinical decisions are now correct, but that she needs further practice in time-critical decision making. It is anticipated that she will return to unconditional registration in the near future.

This case illustrates the protective provisions of the Performance Assessment Program. Dr Y's performance problems required strong intervention, but most certainly did not require this to occur in a disciplinary framework. The broad-based assessment that was undertaken allowed the Board to exercise its protective function in a more meaningful way than dealing with the isolated clinical incident would have allowed. Dr Y took responsibility for improving her professional performance and was able to demonstrate her success during her reassessment. (1.)

# Future

Ultimately, simulation may run in the background as measured performance against an ideal standard on a case-by-case basis. Clearly this is going to be easier in anaesthesia than other specialties such as open surgery but still what must be measured is performance, not merely competence. This is best illustrated by an aviation anecdote:

A senior 747 captain had trained regularly in a simulator, and although he knew that a 747 can be flown when the No. 1 hydraulic system has failed, he had rehearsed this many times in a simulator and realised that this was at the edge of his competence. Thus when taking off with a fully laden 747 at 90 knots, just prior to lift-off the No. 1 hydraulic system failed in his aircraft and the pilot took the acknowledged risk of a high speed abort of the take-off rather than take off without the No. 1 hydraulic system and move the edge of his competence. The take off was aborted safely. His performance was therefore exemplary even though his competence in regard to flying without the No. 1 hydraulic system, as assessed in the simulator, was at the limit of his abilities.

The use of virtual reality then in high stakes assessment is established practice now in New South Wales. It is used in the context of a 360 degree assessment of a practitioner's performance and as a potential tool for remediation and training.

# Acknowledgements

Thanks to Drs Michele Joseph and Alison Reid who significantly contributed to the methodology.

# References

[1] Schuwirth LWT, Southgate L, Page GG et al. When enough is enough: a conceptual basis for fair and defensible practice performance assessment. Papers from the 10th Cambridge Conference. Medical Education 2002; 36:925-30.
[2] General Medical Council/ Remedial Doctors http://www.gmc-uk.org/ [Last accessed September 20th 2004].
[3] Bolsin S and Colson M. The use of the Cusum technique in the assessment of trainee competence in new procedures. International Journal for Quality in Health Care 2000; 12(5): 433-38.
[4] Miller GE. The assessment of clinical skills, competence and performance. Acad Med. 1990; 65(9) S63-7.
[5] Rethans JJ, Norcini JJ, Baron-Maldonado M et al. The relationship between competence and performance: implications for assessing practice performance. Papers from the 10th Cambridge Conference. Medical Education 2002; 36:901-9.
[6] Borrowed with permission from Dr Alison Reid, Director, Performance Assessment Program, NSW Medical Board.
[7] Southgate L, Hays RB, Norcine J et al. Setting performance standards for medical practice: a theoretical framework. Medical Education 2001; 35: 474-81.
[8] Weller JM, Robinson P, Larson P, Watterson LM et al. Simulation-based assessment: is it acceptable to anaesthesia trainees?. In press
[9] Gaba DM, Howard SK, Flanagan B. Assessment of clinical performance during simulated crises using both technical and behavioral ratings. Anesthesiology 1998; 89: 8-18.
[10] Forrest FC, Taylor MA, Postlewaite K et al. Use of a high fidelity simulator to deveop testing of the technical performance of novice anaesthetists. BJA 88(3): 338-44.

[11]  J. M. Weller, M. Bloch, S. Young, M. Maze, S. Oyesola, J. Wyner, D. Dob, K. Haire, J. Durbridge, T. Walker, and D. Newble, Evaluation of high fidelity patient simulator in assessment of performance of anaesthetists Br. J. Anaesth. 2003 90: 43-47.

[12]  Newble D, Swanson D. Psychometric characteristics of the objective structured clinical examination. Medical Education 1988; 22: 325-34.

[13]  Van der Veluten C, Swanson D. Assessment of clinical skills with standardized patients: state of the art. Teaching and learning in medicine 1990: 2(2): 58-76.

[14]  Hutchinson L, Aitken P Hayes T. Are medical postgraduate certification processes valid? A systematic review of the published evidence. Medical Education 2992; 36: 73-91.

[15]  http://www.nswmb.org.au/ (Last accessed October 13th 2004).

*Medicine Meets Virtual Reality 13*
*James D. Westwood et al. (Eds.)*
*IOS Press, 2005*

# The Virtual Pediatric Standardized Patient Application: Formative Evaluation Findings

Robin DETERDING [a], Cheri MILLIRON [a] and Robert HUBAL [b]

[a] *Department of Pediatrics*
*University of Colorado Health Sciences Center, Denver, CO*
[b] *Technology Assisted Learning Division*
*RTI International, Research Triangle Park, NC*

**Abstract.** This paper presents formative (i.e., not final project) evaluation data from the use of a responsive virtual human training application by medical students rotating through Pediatrics and by Pediatric medical educators. We are encouraged by the evaluation results and believe the iterative development strategies employed and the subsequent refinements in the scenarios will lead to important instructional and assessment tools for medical educators.

## 1. Problem

Pediatric medical educators face instructional and assessment challenges regarding interaction skills. For instruction, limited faculty observation time of students, variable experiences with pediatric behaviors or problems, and mostly passive curricular material limit students' exposure to and practice with children [1]. The ability to experiment with different interaction strategies with children is restricted to real-world environments that aren't safe places to practice and learn (e.g., mothers don't take kindly to experimenting with different strategies on their ill and irritable children). For assessment, no reliable or valid standardized assessment uses children; as a result, what assessment is conducted is necessarily less authentic than assessment of interactions with adults. Students are frequently required to interact with a "parent" and discuss the child but the child is absent from the assessment. Performance-based pediatric interaction skills cannot be assessed in this manner.

Overall our project aims to study the use of synthetic child characters for training and assessment in pediatric medical education [2]. The goals are to expand cognitive, social, and linguistic models to improve the robustness of student / synthetic child interactions, and address face, content, and construct validity of scenarios.

We describe here work in refining existing scenarios involving a very young girl and her mother and a female adolescent and her father.

## 2. Methods

We iteratively fed results from student and educator surveys and testing into our models. During testing, participants engaged the synthetic characters in dialog in an attempt to check the patient's ears with a virtual otoscope (young girl scenario) or elicit a patient social history (adolescent scenario). Participants' dialog served to improve the depth and breadth of linguistic models. Participants' observed and written reactions served to improve cognitive and social models. A post-usage survey captured participant opinions about validity, performance characteristics, and beliefs on the utility of synthetic character technology for training. We asked:

(i)     Are the scenarios enjoyable?
(ii)    Do the scenarios address important clinical competencies?
(iii)   Do participants view the simulation as a learning tool?
(iv)    Is improved technical fidelity required for authenticity?

### 2.1. Participants

To date we have engaged 52 participants: pediatric experts (n = 14) at the annual Council on Medical School Education in Pediatrics (COMSEP) meeting and novice Colorado medical students (third year medical students before the start of their pediatric clerkship).

### 2.2. Procedures

Pediatric experts and third year medical students, as part of their orientation to the pediatric clerkship, were invited to perform a young child's ear exam and an adolescent social history within synthetic character scenarios. The interactions were recorded for both groups. At the completion of the virtual experience, participants from both sources were given a post-usage survey that asked similar questions but was worded in an appropriate manner to each source. All participants signed consent forms and the University of Colorado IRB approved the study. Quantitative data was analyzed using SPSS (11.0) software and written responses were grouped by themes.

## 3. Results

All of our questions, noted above, were answered affirmatively. Pediatric educators surveyed at COMSEP felt these scenarios address very to extremely important pediatric competencies at which on average only half of their students are competent at graduation. Participating students initially rated response time and overall conversation as only somewhat realistic, and scenarios as only somewhat comparable or adaptable to real world situations; however, subsequent programming refinements improved these ratings. Participants felt that, if limited clinical experiences were available, synthetic characters would be helpful and would allow for more experiential learning. Even at this prototype stage, many students commented that they had already learned valuable lessons from interacting with synthetic characters in these scenarios (e.g., "not to just move to look right away at a child's ear but to try to establish rapport with the child first" or "that a parent needs to be out of the room to get a good social history from an adolescent"). Furthermore, even with sub-optimal fidelity (described next), students and experts enjoyed using the simulations and felt with improved technology they were likely to learn with synthetic characters during their career.

Initially participants clearly felt that the prototype needed improved language and graphic fidelity to enhance authenticity. However, using participant input and performance data with the characters, refinements in the linguistic models have been made and a significant trend toward higher post-usage ratings achieved, especially in the young child ear exam where the language model was more fully defined. Participant input is now better recognized and synthetic character behavior (both children and parents) is improved for both scenarios.

## 4. Conclusion / Discussion

Participants believed even the initial prototype could provide a learning experience and articulated specific concepts learned during their interaction with scenarios. They enjoyed the scenarios and believed these types of applications will be used to enhance their learning in the future. The prototypes were seen as addressing important clinical competencies, skills (i.e., conducting a young child's ear exam and an adolescent social history) that many educators felt were not adequately acquired by medical school graduation. Capturing formative data has been indispensable for enhancing scenarios and creating a refined product, which can now be more rigorously evaluated as an instructional or assessment tool.

Our early evaluation results are encouraging. They suggest that our iterative method of capturing student input and improving linguistic and cognitive models is an appropriate strategy and that virtual pediatric standardized patients may be accepted as an important educational tool with continued technical enhancement. Further development of virtual pediatric standardized patient applications and research in this area is warranted.

## Acknowledgements

Work described in this paper was supported by grant #EIA-0121211 from the National Science Foundation (NSF). Opinions expressed in this paper are those of the authors, and do not necessarily represent the official position of NSF.

## References

[1] Hubal, R.C., Kizakevich, P.N., Guinn, C.I., Merino, K.D., & West, S.L. (2000). The Virtual Standardized Patient: Simulated Patient-Practitioner Dialogue for Patient Inter-view Training. In J.D. Westwood, H.M. Hoffman, G.T. Mogel, R.A. Robb, & D. Stredney (Eds.), Envisioning Healing: Interactive Technology and the Patient-Practitioner Dialogue. IOS Press: Amsterdam.
[2] Hubal, R.C., Deterding, R.R., Frank, G.A., Schwetzke, H.F., & Kizakevich, P.N. (2003). Lessons Learned in Modeling Pediatric Patients. In J.D. Westwood, H.M. Hoffman, G.T. Mogel, R. Phillips, R.A. Robb, & D. Stredney (Eds.) NextMed: Health Horizon. IOS Press: Amsterdam.

*Medicine Meets Virtual Reality 13*
*James D. Westwood et al. (Eds.)*
*IOS Press, 2005*

# The Visible Human and Digital Anatomy Learning Initiative

Parvati DEV [a] and Steven SENGER [b]

[a] *SUMMIT, Stanford University School of Medicine*
[b] *Dept. of Computer Science, University of Wisconsin – La Crosse*

**Abstract.** A collaborative initiative is starting within the Internet2 Health Science community to explore the development of a framework for providing access to digital anatomical teaching resources over Internet2. This is a cross-cutting initiative with broad applicability and will require the involvement of a diverse collection of communities. It will seize an opportunity created by a convergence of needs and technical capabilities to identify the technologies and standards needed to support a sophisticated collection of tools for teaching anatomy.

## 1. Background

The Visible Human and Digital Anatomy areas now have a large number of imaging and learning resources at various stages of development and deployment. At the same time, anatomy teaching faculty at all medicals schools are experiencing cutbacks in teaching hours and staff. This project proposes to develop a broad framework of standards ranging from the storage of media resources through their incorporation into structured lessons. Through the involvement of the diverse group of disciplines represented within the active Internet2 community, the proposed initiative will provide the coordination required to develop the necessary technologies and standards.

### 1.1. Digital Libraries

There are now numerous examples of anatomical data and image sets available around the world. These include the Visible Human Project, the Stanford Visible Female, the Korean and Chinese Humans, the University of Washington Digital Anatomist, the Bassett collection of stereoscopic images, the Carnegie collection of embryo development and teratologic images and new micro-slice images being developed by Stanford. Many of these are not currently organized as libraries, and lack appropriate metadata. This presents an opportunity to involve members of the digital library community in the design of a repository system that can contain the existing anatomical resources and appropriately scale as new resources are developed.

### 1.2. Rich Collaboration

In order to provide a rich learning environment, anatomical resources must be augmented with the ability for students and instructors to collaborate. Two types of collaboration can be envisaged: videoconferencing to link individuals at remote sites, and data sharing within applications in the form of a shared workspace for studying and teaching anatomy. The digital video and shared workspace communities have a significant body of experience in collaborative environments and are natural partners to design enhanced learning environments.

### 1.3. Middleware and Reusable Application Toolkits

Internet2, and related groups, have been active in developing middleware and network performance tools that would supply enabling technology to this initiative. These include Web100 [1], the Shibboleth Project [2], the NMI-Edit components [3] and the Global Network Measurement Infrastructure (E2Epi) project [4]. The technologies will help support the creation of network aware applications that can adapt to prevailing network capabilities between application components.

### 1.4. Enhanced Teaching and Learning

Recent years have seen the creation of numerous systems that use digital anatomical resources to enhance teaching and learning. These include for example the Visible Human Dissector from the University of Colorado [5], labeled segmentations of the Visible Human Female produced by the University of Michigan and the Bassett collection of labeled and annotated stereoscopic images produced by Stanford University. These are in various stages of maturity ranging from demonstration quality to commercial products. The success of these systems demonstrates the existence of an active community interested in using digital resources for anatomical instruction. The applications demonstrate a rich range of possibilities for designing curriculum that utilize these resources in innovative ways. What is lacking is a mechanism in which anatomical resources and applications can be referenced and embedded in structured lessons.

## 2. Proposed Framework

To actually change the practice of instruction in anatomy this project must succeed in seamlessly connecting users to media resources. This project must allow for the creation of structured lessons, that support specific curricular objectives, and that provide users with intuitive access to anatomical data through a range of applications and access methods. We identify four critical layers that require the development of appropriate interface standards (Figure 1).

### 2.1. Anatomical Media Repositories

The media repositories would consist of a federation of servers, distributed across the network, that would store the digital content and also host the appropriate server mechanisms to access the content. Content will span the range from static resources to data dynamically generated through computation and simulation. The repositories would require appropriate metadata information describing the anatomical resources.

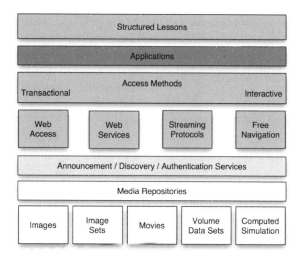

**Figure 1.** Proposed framework for anatomical resources.

## 2.2. Announcement / Discovery / Authentication Services

This layer provides the mechanism for discovering the existence of resources and locating an appropriate repository for a given user. Since "resources" can span a wide range of possibilities there will be a corresponding range of requirements for announcement and discovery. Static resources such as images tend to always be available and can potentially support large numbers of simultaneous users. Other resources, such as collaborative groups of users, may exist for short periods of time. Computationally intense simulations may be able to support only a single user or a small group of simultaneous users.

## 2.3. Applications / Access Methods

Different media types require different access methods. Access methods can be placed on a spectrum depending on the degree of interactivity they provide. At one extreme, access methods such as http are transactional in the sense that a user generates a request, a remote server provides a response and the user spends a period of time working with the response before generating new requests. At the other extreme are highly interactive access methods where a remote server is continually responding to user actions by producing and transporting a stream of data. These two ends of the spectrum are distinguished by the amount of user activity that occurs between requests. The interactive end of the spectrum places significant demands on the intervening network in terms of latency and bandwidth required to produce a good user experience.

## 2.4. Structured Lessons

To support specific curricular objectives it is necessary to combine didactic explanation with a variety of supporting media resources. This combination creates a structured lesson that students can work through as a part of their formal studies. These lessons may take the form of a web page, a dynamically created interactive document, or a real-time, collaborative, videoconference with application sharing, facilitated by an expert anatomist. Individual media resources that require transactional access can be easily included into such lessons. Media resources requiring interactive access, especially where there is an element of navigation or discovery, present a greater challenge to the naïve lesson author, and require additional supporting infrastructure such as a scripting capability within the application.

An interesting alternative exists when the accessing application supports the capture of the stream of data between a group of collaborating peers. In this case, the collaboration data stream can become another kind of media resource. A reference to the captured stream can be included in the lesson. By replaying the captured stream as though it were an active collaborator it is possible to recreate a specific pattern of use in the application.

## 3. Prior Work

Through the NGI and HAVnet projects at SUMMIT [6], Stanford and UW–La Crosse have developed applications that support medical education and require high-performance networks. In the process of developing these applications we have found it necessary to also develop solutions at each level of the proposed framework. Our applications use a range of digital resources including multi-dimensional image sets, volume data sets and computed simulations. The applications focus on highly interactive access methods since these methods place the greatest demands on the network infrastructure.

### 3.1. InformationChannels

To address the need to advertise and discover the availability of various kinds of resources we have created the InformationChannels system. This system allows any component (client, server or peer) of a network-based application to announce its ability to provide or consume a "channel" of information. The system is similar to other announcement/discovery protocols, such as MBONE SDP/SAP [7] and Rendevous [8], in that it uses multicast packets to communicate channel announcements. It differs substantially in that it easily handles a wide range of channel lifetimes. We have found this to be very important for our applications. Some channels, such as specific data resources, are essentially permanently available while others, such as collaboration channels between peers exist for only a brief amount of time. To handle this situation, channel registrations contain an explicit timeout value and we operate a distributed collection of registration servers that listen for channel announcements and maintain the list of currently active channels. Users and application components query these registration servers to discover the available channels of specific types.

We have developed several applications that utilize the InformationChannels system. These include the Remote Stereo Viewer (RSV), Immersive Segmentation (ImmSeg) and the Nomadic Anatomy Viewer (NAV). These applications provide examples of different access methods. Each application uses a client server design. The server announces the availability of the digital resources that it can provide using the InformationChannels system. When a user selects an available resource the appropriate application client is launched. We briefly describe these applications, the digital resources they use and their integration into the InformationChannels system.

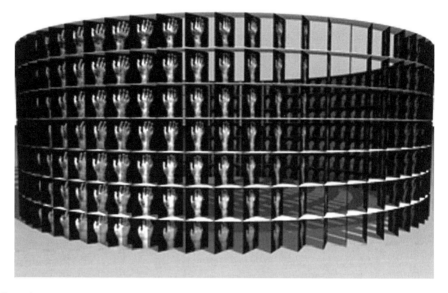

**Figure 2.** Two dimensional image set of a dissected hand organized as a cylinder. The horizontal dimension is rotation about the object. The vertical dimension is level of dissection.

## 3.2. Remote Stereo Viewer

The RSV application provides interactive access using a QTVR style interface to multi-dimensional image sets. Typically an image set is a collection of photographs of some anatomical structure. The collection is organized into a multi-dimensional grid with at least one dimension corresponding to a full rotation of the object and other dimensions corresponding to levels of dissection or some other variation in the image or object (Figure 2). Consecutive images in the rotation dimension are used to produce a stereoscopic view of the object. Typically the image sets are very large and users will only view a small portion of the available images for any particular task. Consequently the application transports images on demand using a UDP layer protocol. The application has the ability to announce and utilize collaboration channels between peers. Collaboration allows one client to control the position in the image set of all other clients in the group. It also has the ability to discover the existence of servers providing annotation labels for the image set. When a label server is available the client presents the user with the option to choose from among the available label sets.

## 3.3. Immersive Segmentation

The ImmSeg application allows the user to visualize and segment volumetric data sets using a stereoscopic immersive interface. It utilizes a remote computational server to render and apply computationally expensive segmentation algorithms to local regions of the data set as steered by the client interface. The server is able to support multiple visualization channels. This allows a small group of users to collaboratively work with the segmentation tools. Figure 3 shows the view of the Visible Male data set provided by two different visualization channels. In addition to the visualization channels the server also announces the ability to utilize a companion client to visualize surface meshes generated

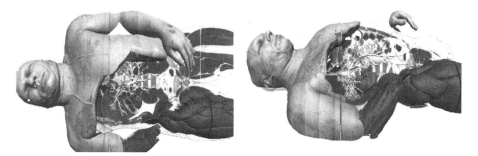

**Figure 3.** Two visualizations from the Immersive Segmentation application. These images are from simultaneously generated streams of the same workspace as the user segments structures of interest.

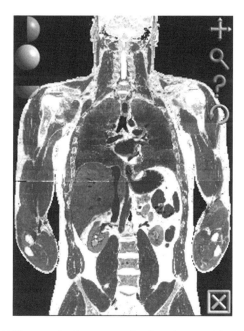

**Figure 4.** NAV screen showing cross section through torso of the Visible Male.

by the user from segmented structures. Also using the InformationChannels systems the client announces its ability to support the use of haptics device to provide input and force feedback from segmented structures.

*3.4. Nomadic Anatomy Viewer*

The NAV application allows the user to view in cross-section volumetric data sets from a handheld computer. The pen-based interface allows the user to translate and rotate the cross-sectional plane within the volume (Figure 4). The application uses the InformationChannels system extensively. The client application can discover of a server offering a structure identification server. This server will provide a structure name corresponding to a given voxel coordinate. Each client can announce the ability to form collaborative partnerships. When connected in a collaborative group one client is able to guide all other clients through the data sets. In addition, there are collaboration recording and playback servers. The recording server watches for the existence of a collaboration channel between peers. When it discovers such a channel it offers to record the data stream being sent over the collaboration channel. These recordings can be replayed at a later time.

## 4. Conclusion

The Digital Anatomy Learning Initiative, within the Internet2 community, seeks to promote the development of standards that will create a uniform framework for providing and using digital anatomical resources over the network. The standards will address issues of distributing repositories of data, announcement and discovery of data resources, a range of access methods and the ability to embed the use of access methods and applications into structured lessons for specific curricular topics. Through the NGI and HAVnet projects, Stanford SUMMIT and UW La Crosse have developed partial solutions at each of these levels.

Internet2, because its membership includes individuals representing diverse disciplines involved in advanced networking projects, is ideally suited to support this effort. We expect the standards to lead to open source implementations of key middleware. We expect both the standards development process and the open source implementation to be overseen by a working group within Internet2.

## Acknowledgements

This work was partially supported by the National Library of Medicine under contracts NO1-LM-3506 and NLM 02-103/VMS.

## References

[1] The Web100 Project, http://www.web100.com.
[2] The Shibboleth Project, http://shibboleth.internet2.edu.
[3] The NMI-EDIT Consortium, http://www.nmi-edit.org.
[4] Internet2 End-to-End Performance Initiative, http://e2epi.internet2.edu.
[5] The Visible Human Dissector, http://www.toltech.net.
[6] SUMMIT HAVnet Project, http://havnet.stanford.edu.
[7] The Internet Engineering Task Force RFC 2974, http://www.ietf.org/rfc/rfc2974.txt.
[8] Zero Configuration Networking, http://www.zeroconf.org.

*Medicine Meets Virtual Reality 13*
*James D. Westwood et al. (Eds.)*
*IOS Press, 2005*

# Laparoscopic Task Recognition Using Hidden Markov Models

Aristotelis DOSIS [a], Fernando BELLO [a], Duncan GILLIES [b], Shabnam UNDRE [a],
Rajesh AGGARWAL [a] and Ara DARZI [a]

[a] *Dept. of Surgical Oncology & Technology, St.Mary's Hospital,*
*Imperial College, London, UK*
[b] *Dept. of Computing, Imperial College, London, UK*

**Abstract.** Surgical skills assessment has been paid increased attention over the last few years. Stochastic models such as Hidden Markov Models have recently been adapted to surgery to discriminate levels of expertise. Based on our previous work combining synchronized video and motion analysis we present preliminary results of a HMM laparoscopic task recognizer which aims to model hand manipulations and to identify and recognize simple surgical tasks.

## 1. Introduction

### 1.1. Preliminary Work

Surgical skills assessment has been paid increased attention over the last few years [1–3]. The reason is that training assessment tools and procedures have traditionally been subjective. Recent literature has commented on the fact that skills evaluation needs to be made more objective [4]. Quantitative systems such as virtual reality and motion analysis have allowed numerical dexterity analysis resulting in more credible feedback and opening a new era for quantitative skills assessment [3,5]. Notwithstanding, they belong to medium level decision-making systems as they lack qualitative analysis and the ability to 'Recognize and Decide'.

We suggest that higher-level-modelling surgical assessment systems should incorporate the 'Recognize and Decide' approach, which is based on stochastic description of the physical environment. The work from Rosen and colleagues can be categorized into this type. They have used Markov and Hidden Markov Models (HMM) to define states according to force/torque data, transitions between states by using video analysis and to show differences between experts and novices [6,7]. Also, recent work from Murphy associated suturing tasks with HMMs using the Da Vinci system [8].

In this paper we study the discrimination performance of a HMM recognizer. The aim was to be able to recognize three laparoscopic tasks, namely: conventional laparoscopic suturing (LS) using the Imperial College Surgical Assessment Device - ICSAD (see [1] for more details on ICSAD), robotic suturing (RS) and robotic rope passing (RRP) using the Da Vinci telemanipulator system.

*1.2. Background Theory*

Hidden Markov Models have been widely used in speech recognition [9]. Briefly, a HMM for discrete symbol observations consists of:

1. $N$ the number of states in the model, where $\{1, 2, \ldots, N\}$,
2. $M$ the number of emissions/signatures $V$ per state. Using speech recognition terminology, $M$ also represents the discrete alphabet, where $V = \{v_1, v_2, \ldots, v_M\}$.
3. The state-transition probability distribution $A = \{a_{ij}\}$ where $a_{ij} = P[q_{t+1} = j \mid q_t = i]$, $1 \leq i, j \leq N$
4. The emission signature probability distribution, $B = \{b_j(k)\}$, where $b_j(k) = P[o_t = v_k \mid q_t = j]$, $1 \leq k \leq M$
5. The initial or prior state distribution $\pi = \{\pi_i\}$, where $\pi_i = P[q_1 = i]$, $1 \leq i \leq N$

The complete notation for HMM is the compact formula $\lambda = (\pi, A, B)$ as described in Rabiner's tutorial [9].

*1.3. Experimental Assumptions*

There were certain assumptions during motion segmentation and modelling. Firstly, we segmented motion data acquired from the right hand which was the dominant hand for all surgeons. Secondly, we assumed that all participants started executing every task from an 'idle' state, that is without executing any movement. Therefore the prior distribution for all states was zero apart from the 'idle' state having 1.

## 2. Methods

*2.1. Experimental Setup*

All laparoscopic and robotic suturing was performed on a suturing bench model by at least 12 surgeons, each one performing several attempts. Surgeons were chosen from all levels of expertise. They were instructed to perform suturing tasks without following any experimental suturing protocol. Thus, a variety of surgical styles has been recorded and used in the HMM training. For the RRP task, surgeons were asked to follow the predefined dotted points on the rope. Data acquisition for the Da Vinci system was setup to be 5Hz using the system's API and 20Hz for ICSAD. It would also be possible to investigate recognition performance between systems with different frequencies.

*2.2. Hand Motion Vocabulary*

The number and type of hand movements in a model is often a matter of judgement and depends on the complexity and precision of the model. Simple hand movements may be represented by their coordinates in 3D space, velocity and angular measurements. It is also important to know which part of the hand/arm is tracked and how many tracking points are available for analysis. All these are essential parameters in order to decide the type of model and to characterize its complexity. An important factor in laparoscopic surgical movements is the effect of endoscopic instruments on hand movements. As the hand manipulates surgical instruments, they become extensions of the arm/hand.

**Table 1.** HMM hand motion alphabet formed by 18 discrete signatures. Each signature is a unique motion feature consisting of XY-plane rotation, elevation and a grip state.

| Rotation | | | Elevation | | | Grip | Signature |
|---|---|---|---|---|---|---|---|
| *(Dextro-)* | *(Levo-)* | *0* | *(+)* | *(−)* | *0* | *Open/Close* | |
|  |  | ☒ |  |  | ☒ | Open | SIG1 |
|  |  | ☒ |  |  | ☒ | Close | SIG2 |
|  |  | ☒ |  | ☒ |  | Open | SIG3 |
|  |  | ☒ |  | ☒ |  | Close | SIG4 |
|  |  | ☒ | ☒ |  |  | Open | SIG5 |
|  |  | ☒ | ☒ |  |  | Close | SIG6 |
| ☒ |  |  |  |  | ☒ | Open | SIG7 |
| ☒ |  |  |  |  | ☒ | Close | SIG8 |
| ☒ |  |  |  | ☒ |  | Open | SIG9 |
| ☒ |  |  |  | ☒ |  | Close | SIG10 |
| ☒ |  |  | ☒ |  |  | Open | SIG11 |
| ☒ |  |  | ☒ |  |  | Close | SIG12 |
|  | ☒ |  |  |  | ☒ | Open | SIG13 |
|  | ☒ |  |  |  | ☒ | Close | SIG14 |
|  | ☒ |  |  | ☒ |  | Open | SIG15 |
|  | ☒ |  |  | ☒ |  | Close | SIG16 |
|  | ☒ |  | ☒ |  |  | Open | SIG17 |
|  | ☒ |  | ☒ |  |  | Close | SIG18 |

In other words, when the arm pulls up, the instrument follows the movement through the endoscopic port.

As in speech recognition, the hand motion vocabulary should consist of primitive movements and be independent of the task performed or any step in the task. For instance, 'dissecting gallbladder' would not be convenient for two reasons. Firstly, it is not a primitive movement and secondly it can only be matched within a laparoscopic cholecystectomy operation. In our experiments we have used the following primitive movements: Dextrorotation, levorotation, positive and negative elevation. If the state of the grip is also encountered, then the hand motion alphabet can be defined as in Table 1.

Dextrorotation and levorotation are calculated on the XY-plane and they have the physical meaning of clockwise and anti-clockwise movements respectively. These are simply identified by calculating the sign of cross-product magnitude between two Cartesian vectors. The elevation principal movement depends on the sign of $dz = z_2 - z_1$ between the consecutive points $P_1$ and $P_2$. When the hand is not moving on the vertical axis, then $dz = 0$. The advantage of these set of signatures is that it can describe primitive movements without any prior Cartesian origin or system recalibration/transformation. Effectively, it has allowed for both ICSAD and robotic data (Da Vinci system) feature extraction without requiring the same Cartesian origin or system.

Taking into account the state of the grip (Open/Close), the hand motion vocabulary is thus represented by a total of $3 \times 3 \times 2 = 18$ feature signatures.

## 2.3. Hidden States

Given the hand motion vocabulary of the previous section, the motion-hidden states of a Markov model were chosen after performing video analysis on the data collected. We

**Table 2.** Hidden Markov Model state description.

| HMM state No | Description |
|:---:|:---|
| 1 | IDLE – No movement with open tip |
| 2 | INSERTING/PUSHING – Positioning away from surgeon with closed tip |
| 3 | PULLING/LIFTING – Positioning closer to surgeon with closed tip |
| 4 | DESCENDING SURVEY- Positioning away from surgeon with open tip |
| 5 | ASCENDING SURVEY – Positioning closer to surgeon with open tip |
| 6 | IDLE HOLDING – No movement or insignificant movement with closed tip |

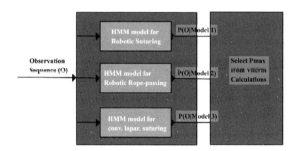

**Figure 1.** HMM task recognition system.

preferred a general description of motion in states in contrast to [8]. This is in order to create task-independent models. Therefore, the states shown in Table 2 can potentially be used in every different task/real operation, including suturing and rope-passing.

The 'IDLE' state exists when there is no movement activity and the tip is opened. We assumed that all tasks started from this state. The second state, 'INSERTING/PUSHING' describes the motion where the tip is closed and the surgeon is either inserting an object e.g. needle or pushing a structure or surveying with closed tip downwards. The third state, 'PULLING/LIFTING' describes the motion where the tip is closed and the surgeon is either lifting an object, pulling a structure or surveying with closed tip upwards. The next state 'DESCENDING SURVEY' describes a descending survey movement with open tip, followed by 'ASCENDING SURVEY' with open tip. Finally, the 'IDLE HOLDING' serves as an idle state with closed tip or as an insignificant movement.

### 2.4. HMM Task Modelling

Motion data were acquired from LS, RRP and RS tasks and initial estimates were calculated for $A$ and $B$ matrices for each one of the three HMM models (LS, RRP, RS). From a total of 57 RRP, 84 RS and 59 LS recorded tasks, 30 RRP, 42 RS, 29 LS were used for training using the Baum-Welch optimization. The remaining data were used for testing and evaluating the recognizer. Figure 1 shows the HMM task recognition system where an 'unknown' observation sequence ($O$) is probabilistically scored by all three HMM task models. The model with the highest likelihood is taken as the most probable source for $O$.

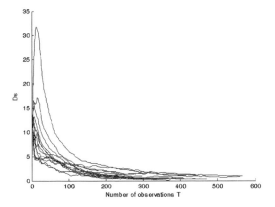

**Figure 2.** Similarity distance measure between RS and RRP signature probability distributions.

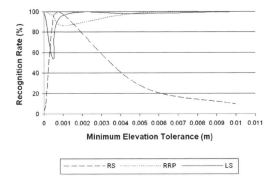

**Figure 3.** Recognition rates for all three models with different minimum elevation tolerance values.

## 3. Results

Initial results showed weak recognition performance between RRP and RS tasks, while the recognizer adequately identified LS. Low performance was caused by the similarity between RRP and RS signature probability distributions as shown in figure 2, where each plot represents a different similarity data set. Let $D(\lambda_1, \lambda_2)$ be a non-symmetric distance measure showing how well a model $\lambda_1$ matches observations $(O)$ with length $T$,

$$D(\lambda_1, \lambda_2) = \frac{1}{T_{O_2}} \Big[ \log P(O_2 \mid \lambda_1) - \log P(O_2 \mid \lambda_2) \Big] \tag{1}$$

and $D(\lambda_2, \lambda_1)$ the reverse non-symmetric formula. According to [9], the symmetric mean

$$D_s(\lambda_1, \lambda_2) = \frac{D(\lambda_1, \lambda_2) + D(\lambda_2, \lambda_1)}{2} \tag{2}$$

The similarity issue was resolved by introducing a minimum tolerance absolute value on both rotation and elevation feature extractions based on the distribution of their values and on the minimum possible distortion. The best recognition performance appeared at a minimum elevation tolerance value of 0.0008m as in Figure 3.

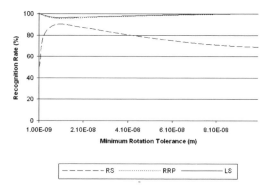

**Figure 4.** Recognition rates against minimum rotation tolerance using an elevation tolerance of 0.0008m.

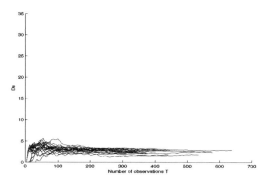

**Figure 5.** Improved similarity distance measure between RS and RRP signature probability distributions.

By fixing the elevation tolerance to 0.0008m we calculated the effect of the minimum rotation tolerance value against the recognition performance of the three tasks (Figure 4).

Recognition rates increased significantly for all tasks. RRP and LS recognition were above 90%, as well as RS having a high peak at $10^{-8}$m. This is explained by the fact that similarity distance measure between RS and RRP has been improved as shown in figure 5.

## 4. Discussion

This paper describes a methodology for developing a HMM task recognizer. Initial results have shown to be promising for simple tasks (RS, RRP and LS) and for different systems. The real value of the recognizer is to identify parts of a procedure such as dissection of cystic duct in laparoscopic cholecystectomy. One of its practical uses includes the detailed activity mapping of an entire operation with its subtasks into a single signal kinematic graph thus providing compact control (instruments and motion activity) for the operation performed.

We have also suggested that principal movements should be as independent as possible. Task-independent models could be used in a variety of procedures providing less effort in HMM configuration and training. In this study, feature parameters such as rotation and elevation were used giving good recognition results. An alternative solution is to redefine the motion alphabet using classic motion terms such as 'yaw', 'pitch' and 'roll'.

Dextrorotation and levorotation were defined in our motion vocabulary to address orientation differences caused by different systems and/or recordings of the same system. For instance, in ICSAD, due to the mobility of the electromagnetic transmitter, 3D Cartesian axes may not have the same origin and alignment in different recordings.

The extraction of hidden states from the current models suggested that further improvement should be carried out on the task models and feature extraction. Validation of the successfully recovered hidden states has been performed via concurrent video and positional analysis. Similarity graphs and recognition rates were not the only validation methods used. In order to insure that our models are closer to the global maximum, a number of HMMs with arbitrary initial parameters were constructed and optimized. Results showed that all models converged to the same point as the original models, indicating that the current HMM parameters maximize the probability for all sequences.

## 5. Conclusions

HMMs have proved to be very powerful in speech recognition and other pattern recognition areas. We believe that they will also play an important role in the area of surgical skills assessment providing stochastic enhancement. We will continue to improve our existing models with the aim of applying the concept to real surgical procedures. Our future work will focus on fine tuning the motion alphabet by finding the most appropriate band-pass filter for the feature extraction part of the recognizer. Another potential area is the change of motion vocabulary to 'yaw', 'pitch', 'roll' and the comparison with the existing vocabulary, performance and hidden states extraction.

## Acknowledgments

BUPA Foundation, UK and Intuitive Surgical, CA, USA.

## References

[1] Datta, V., Gillies, D. F., Mackay, S., and Darzi, A., "Motion Analysis in the Assessment of Surgical Skill," *Computer Methods in Biomechanics and Biomedical engineering*, vol. 4 pp. 515-523, 2004.

[2] Martin, J. A., Regehr, G., Reznick, R., MacRae, H., Murnaghan, J., Hutchison, C., and Brown, M., "Objective structured assessment of technical skill (OSATS) for surgical residents," *Br.J.Surg.*, vol. 84, no. 2, pp. 273-278, Feb.1997.

[3] Sutton, C., McCloy, R., Middlebrook, A., Chater, P., Wilson, M., and Stone, R., "MIST VR. A laparoscopic surgery procedures trainer and evaluator," *Stud.Health Technol.Inform.*, vol. 39 pp. 598-607, 1997.

[4] Darzi, A., Smith, S., and Taffinder, N., "Assessing operative skill. Needs to become more objective," *BMJ*, vol. 318, no. 7188, pp. 887-888, Apr.1999.

[5] Datta, V., Mackay, S., Mandalia, M., and Darzi, A., "The use of electromagnetic motion tracking analysis to objectively measure open surgical skill in the laboratory-based model," *J.Am.Coll.Surg.*, vol. 193, no. 5, pp. 479-485, Nov.2001.

[6]  Rosen, J., MacFarlane, M., Richards, C., Hannaford, B., and Sinanan, M., "Surgeon-tool force/torque signatures evaluation of surgical skills in minimally invasive surgery," *Medicine Meets Virtual Reality - the Convergence of Physical & Informational Technologies: Options for A New Era in Healthcare*, vol. 62 pp. 290-296, 1999.

[7]  Rosen, J., Solazzo, M., Hannaford, B., and Sinanan, M., "Objective laparoscopic skills assessments of surgical residents using Hidden Markov Models based on haptic information and tool/tissue interactions," *Medicine Meets Virtual Reality 2001: Outer Space, Inner Space, Virtual Space*, vol. 81 pp. 417-423, 2001.

[8]  Murphy, T, "Towards objective surgical skill evaluation with Hidden Markov Model-based motion recognition." Master of Science John Hopkins University, 2004.

[9]  Rabiner, L. R., "A Tutorial on Hidden Markov-Models and Selected Applications in Speech Recognition," *Proceedings of the Ieee*, vol. 77, no. 2, pp. 257-286, Feb.1989.

*Medicine Meets Virtual Reality 13*
*James D. Westwood et al. (Eds.)*
*IOS Press, 2005*

# Intraoperative Augmented Reality: The Surgeons View

Georg EGGERS [a], Tobias SALB [b], Harald HOPPE [c,d], Lüder KAHRS [c],
Sassan GHANAI [a], Gunther SUDRA [b], Jörg RACZKOWSKY [c],
Rüdiger DILLMANN [b], Heinz WÖRN [c], Stefan HASSFELD [a]
and Rüdiger MARMULLA [a]

[a] *Department of Cranio-Maxillofacial Surgery, University of Heidelberg, Germany*
*e-mail: georg.eggers@med.uni-heidelberg.de*
[b] *Department for Computer Science – IRF, Universität Karlsruhe (TH), Germany*
[c] *Institute for Process control and Robotics, Universität Karlsruhe (TH), Germany*
[d] *Stryker Leibinger GmbH & Co KG, Freiburg, Germany*

**Abstract.** Augmented Reality (AR) is a promising tool for intraoperative visualization. Two different AR systems, one projector based, one based on see-through glasses were used on patients. The task was the transfer of preoperative planning into the intraoperative reality, or the visualization of space occupying lesions, respectively. The intraoperative application of both systems is discussed from the surgeons point of view.

## 1. Introduction

In the collaborative research centre "Information Technology in Medicine - Computer- and Sensor-Aided Surgery", one main topic is the transfer of preoperative planning into the intraoperative situation. Besides robotic surgery [1], two alternative systems for augmented reality, one projector based, one based on see-through glasses, have been developed. In extensive preclinical testing either system has proven its functionality and tests with volunteers had been performed successfully, based on MRI imaging [2,3]. The first clinical experience with both systems based on patient cases are reported.

## 2. Materials and Methods

The AR-system "Projector Based Augmented Reality in Surgery" uses a video projector and video cameras for surface registration, tracking of the patient and for the projection of augmented reality information onto the patients surface. [4,5] The INPRES system uses tracked head-mounted see-through glasses for the display of augmented reality in the surgeons field of view. Tracking of patient and surgeon is performed using an infrared tracking system [6–11].

Preoperative planning for both systems was performed based on CT image data. For the projector based system, the surfaces, which would later be used for registration and for projection, were segmented, as well as the information to be projected. For the see-through system, the information to be projected was segmented, and the fiducial markers were preregistered in image data [2,13,14].

For clinical evaluation, the systems are used to assist surgical treatment of patients. The systems were used to transfer osteotomy planning onto the skull (Projector Based Augmented Reality in Surgery) or to visualize cysts in the mandible for guided osteotomy (INPRES). Intraoperatively, the use of the systems was always assessed by two surgeons.

## 3. Results

Both systems proved their functionality under OR conditions in patient care: Augmented reality information could be visualized with both systems. The accuracy was sufficient for the surgical task. None of the systems inhibited the surgical workspace. However, a few limitations occurred:

In preclinical trials, wearing the glasses during all the time of an operation had been proven to be too cumbersome. Hence, the surgeon would put on and calibrate the glasses at the time when they are needed intraoperatively [15]. In mandible cyst surgery the glasses were used after conventional surgical exposure of the bone. The glasses were put on the surgeons head by an assistant and the calibration was performed by the surgeon within minutes. Now the osteotomy for the exposure of the cyst was performed AR-guided using conventional instruments.

The projector based system was used for tracking of the patient and providing AR-information. The skin surface was used without problems for the registration of the patient to the image data. Then, after conventional surgical exposure, the planned osteotomies were projected onto the bone surface to guide the osteotomy using conventional instruments. However, the system could only be used as long as a preoperatively defined surface - be it bone or skin - remained intact and clean for registration and projection respectively.

## 4. Discussion

The two presented systems complement one another in clinical use. The advantage of the projector based system is, that there is no need for the surgeon to calibrate or wear any equipment. Furthermore, the system would register and track the patient automatically. Every member of the surgical team can see the projected information. The absence of additional hardware near the surgeon is important for acceptance.

The advantage of the see-through glasses is the higher flexibility. Information can be visualized without the need for a surface, that maintained its preoperative shape. A virtual stereoscopic image can be set up wherever and whenever intended.

## 5. Conclusion

The projector based system is more comfortable and integrates better into the surgical workflow. However, surface-related restrictions limit the scope of interventions that can be supported by this system. In such cases, or when stereoscopic augmented reality is desired, the see-through glasses are the AR-system of choice.

# References

[1] Engel D, Raczkowsky J, Wörn H: A safe robot system for craniofacial surgery. In International Conference On Robotics And Automation (ICRA), 2020-2024, Seoul, Korea, June 2001.

[2] Hoppe H, Eggers G, Heurich T, Raczkowsky R, Marmulla R, Wörn H, Hassfeld S, Moctezuma JL: Projector Based Visualization for Intraoperative Navigation: First Clinical Results. Proceedings of the 17th International Congress and Exhibition on Computer Assisted Radiology and Surgery (CARS) 2003.

[3] Salb, T, Brief, J, Welzel, T, Giesler, B, Hassfeld, S, Muehling, J and Dillmann, R: The INPRES System – Augmented Reality for Craniofacial Surgery Proceedings of Conference: SPIE Electronic Imaging – Stereoscopic Displays and Applications XIV, Santa Clara, CA, January 2003.

[4] Hoppe H, Däuber S, Raczkowsky J, Wörn H, Moctezuma JL: Intraoperative Visualization of Surgical Planning Data using Video Projectors. Proceedings of Conference: Proceedings of Conference: Medicine Meets Virtual Reality (MMVR), Newport Beach, CA, 2001.

[5] Hoppe H, Kübler C, Raczkowsky J, Wörn H, Hassfeld S: A Clinical Prototype System for Projector-Based Augmented Reality: Calibration and Projection Methods. Proceedings of the 16th International Congress and Exhibition on Computer Assisted Radiology and Surgery (CARS) 2002.

[6] Salb, T., Brief, J., Burgert, O, Hassfeld S, Mühling J, Dillmann R: An Augmented Reality System for Intraoperative Presentation of Planning and Simulation Results. Proceedings of 2nd Workshop: European Advanced Robotic Systems Development - Medical Robotics, Pisa, Italy, September 1999.

[7] Salb T, Brief J, Burgert O Hassfeld S, Dillmann R: Intraoperative Presentation of Surgical Planning and Simulation Results using a Stereoscopic See-Through Head-Mounted Display. Proceedings of Conference: Stereoscopic Displays and Applications, Part of Electronic Imaging / Photonics West (SPIE), San Jose, CA, January 2000.

[8] Brief J, Hassfeld S, Salb T, Burgert O, Muenchenberg J, Pernozzoli A, Grabowski H, Redlich T, Raczkowsky J, Krempien R, Kotrikova B, Wörn H, Dillmann R, Mühling J, Ziegler C: Clinical Evaluation of a See-Through Display for Intraoperative Presentation of Planning Data. Proceedings of : Israeli Symposium on Computer-Integrated Surgery, Medical Robotics and Medical Imaging (ISRACAS), Haifa, May 2000.

[9] Salb T, Burgert O, Gockel T, Giesler B, Dilmann R: Comparison of Tracking Techniques for Intraoperative Presentation of Medical Data using a See-Through Head-Mounted Display. Proceedings of Conference: Medicine Meets Virtual Reality (MMVR), Newport Beach, CA, January 2001.

[10] Salb T, Brief J, Burgert O, Gockel T, Hassfeld S, Mühling J, Dillmann R: INPRES: INtraoperative PRESentation of Surgical Planning and Simulation Results. Proceedings of the 16th International Congress and Exhibiton on Computer Assisted Radiology and Surgery (CARS) 2001.

[11] Salb T, Brief J, Burgert O, Gockel T, Hasssfeld S, Mühling J, Dillmann R: Evaluation of INPRES – Intraoperative Presentation of Surgical Planning and Simulation Results Proceedings of Conference: Medicine Meets Virtual Reality (MMVR), Newport Beach, CA, January 2003.

[12] J. Brief, S. Hassfeld, C. Haag, J. Münchenberg, O. Schorr, S. Daueber, D. Engel, R. Krempien, M. Treiber, H. Wörn and J. Mühling Clinical evaluation of an operation planning system in the field of cranio–maxillo-facial surgery. In: H.U. Lemke, M.W. Vannier, K. Inamura, A.G. Farman, K. Doi (eds.): Computer Assisted Radiology and Surgery. Proceedings of the 15th International Symposium and Exhibition on Computer Assisted Radiology and Surgery. CARS 2001 Berlin, June 27th – 30th 2001, pp. 1230-1231.

[13] Lorensen WE, Cline HE: Marching cubes: A high resolution 3D surface construction algorithm. International Conference on Computer Graphics and Interactive Techniques: Proceedings of the 14th annual conference on Computer graphics and interactive techniques 163 - 169, 1987 ISSN:0097-8930.

[14] Schorr O, Brief J, Haag C, Raczkowsky J, Hassfeld S, Muhling J, Wörn H. Operationsplanung in der Kopfchirurgie. Biomed Tech (Berl). 2002;47 Suppl 1 Pt 2:939-41.

[15] Ghanai S, Salb T, Eggers G, Dillmann R, Mühling J, Marmulla R, Hassfeld S: Calibration of a stereo see-through head-mounted display, Workshop Medical Robotics, Navigation and Visualization, Remagen, 2004.

*Medicine Meets Virtual Reality 13*
*James D. Westwood et al. (Eds.)*
*IOS Press, 2005*

# A Vision-Based Surgical Tool Tracking Approach for Untethered Surgery Simulation and Training

James ENGLISH, Chu-Yin CHANG, Neil TARDELLA and Jianjuen HU
*Energid Technologies Corporation*
*124 Mount Auburn Street, Suite 200 North, Cambridge, MA 02138, USA*
*Tel: 888 5474100, e-mail: {jde,cyc,nmt,jjh}@energid.com*

**Abstract.** This paper presents progress in the development of an untethered surgery simulation and training system. A surgical trainee interacts with the simulation in the most natural way possible—using standard, untethered surgical tools and hands. This natural interface requires innovations in tracking, haptic feedback, and visualization. This article describes the approach used for tool tracking with color cameras. A novel tracking algorithm is used to identify the type of tool, its position, and its orientation. Integration of the vision system with the tissue deformation and visualization modules is also discussed.

## 1. Introduction

Laparoscopic procedures are tethered and have been successfully simulated using tethered robotic systems and haptic devices [1–3], where the positions of surgical tools are tracked by motion encoders, optical sensors (such as Optotrak) or magnetic sensors (such as Polhemus). Open surgeries, in contrast, are typically untethered, complicating simulation. A key component to untethered surgery simulation is determining the type, position, and orientation of the tool being used by the trainee in an unobtrusive way. The significance of our research lies in having established a method for doing this using just color cameras.

With our approach, tool tracking is performed through spatial processing that analyzes each video frame in isolation [4] and temporal processing that combines spatial output over time. Novel components include a harmonic approach to template matching and real-time model matching using PC graphics cards. The result is a system that allows trainees to interface to a simulation in the most natural and cognitively correct manner—through free-moving, untethered surgical tools. In this article, we introduce our visual tracking approach and describe its integration into an untethered surgery simulator.

This paper presents the development of an untethered surgery simulation and training system, a cooperative effort for the Army by personnel from Energid Technologies, Massachusetts General Hospital, and the MIT Touch Lab. It introduces the framework of the simulation system, the visual tracking method, and results of the visual tool tracking. A proof-of-concept example is provided to demonstrate the approach's feasibility.

## 2. Framework of Surgery Simulation System

### 2.1. System Top Level Framework

Figure 1 shows the top-level framework for the surgical trainer. We capture information on tools using the tracker and use that information for visualization and performance assessment. There are six principal modules in the system: visual tool tracking (spatial processor & object tracker), tissue deformation, visualization, haptics, metrics (used for real-time quality assessment through a database of "expert" values), and a database of surgery procedures.

### 2.2. Key Components

By designing the interface generically through an Extensible Markup Language (XML) based language, it is straightforward to swap out hardware and software components as newer technologies become available. We are exploring hardware alternatives for the optical sensors, visualization devices, and the haptic feedback system. The exchangeable system components are listed below and illustrated in Figure 2.

- *Tissue Deformation Models.* We are developing simplified tissue deformation models and a meshless computationally efficient algorithm using a technique called MFS (method of finite spheres) [5].

Visual Motion Capture

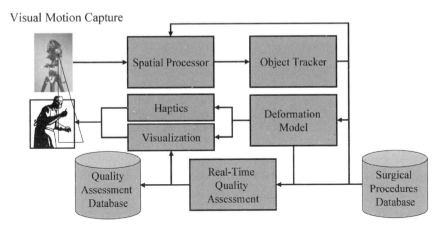

**Figure 1.** Top Level Framework for the Surgical Trainer.

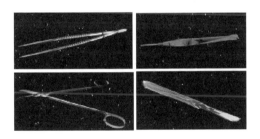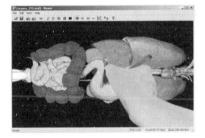

**Figure 2.** Sample CAD models for surgical simulation (left), and hand/tool/tissue rendering (right).

- *Visual Tool Tracking.* We have developed a model based visual tool tracking algorithm for surgery simulation. This will be discussed in detail in section 3. *This article addresses primarily this component.*
- *Visualization.* We have developed a fast OpenGL based rendering engine that handles stereo image generation, and supports several standard CAD formats. We plan on supporting the NIH Digital Human models in the upcoming year.
- *Haptic Feedback.* We are in the process of developing an untethered Maglev-based haptic system for open surgery simulation.
- *Surgery Procedure.* Energid is developing scenario based surgery simulation procedures through collaboration with surgeons.
- *Metrics.* A collection of metrics are being developed. Metrics are needed for assessing training procedures and validating the system capability and simulation quality.

## 3. Visual Tracking

For untethered simulation, tools must be tracked without a physical connection. Visual identification and tracking, though simple and intuitive for a human brain, is challenging for a computer implementation. In fact, only recently has it been possible with low-cost computer hardware. Energid Technologies is applying object-tracking techniques it has developed for the Air Force, NASA, and the Missile Defense Agency to identify and track surgical tools.

### 3.1. Tracking Software Organization

The organization of the tool-tracking software is shown in Figure 3. Video from a color camera is preprocessed to remove sensor anomalies (such as nonfunctioning pixels), then analyzed sequentially by any number of tracker-identifiers. Each tracker-identifier can suppress the tracker-identifiers below it and provide the track information to the

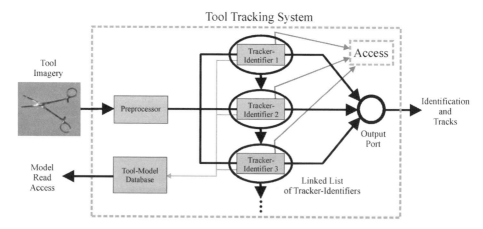

**Figure 3.** The tool-tracking system is composed of a preprocessor, a tool-model database, and a list of prioritized trackers. All components are configured using XML.

simulation. This approach allows different algorithms to be used in different surgical scenarios—one implementation might be better for tools, while another is better for hands.

Each tracker-identifier shown in Figure 3 is organized into spatial and temporal processing. The spatial processor analyzes a single image and forms hypotheses of what tools are present, and the temporal processor combines these results over time.

## 3.2. Spatial Processing

Spatial processing uses three stages: 1) segmentation, 2) Initial Type, Pose, and Geometry (ITPG) estimation, and 3) Refined Type, Pose, and Geometry (RTPG) calculation, as shown in Figure 4. *Geometry* refers to shape change, as when forceps are opened and closed.

### 3.2.1. Image Segmentation

The image segmentation module (Stage I in Figure 4) isolates the tools from the background. It uses edge detection and thresholding to first find the pixels that may be part of a tool. These pixels are grouped into blobs, with the larger blobs representing potential surgical tools. Each blob is bound by a rectangular box for output, as illustrated in Figure 5 below.

### 3.2.2. ITPG

The second module in Figure 4 creates an initial estimate of the tool type and configuration using matched filtering (or template matching). This visual-identification approach has been successfully applied to quickly detect objects [6]; identify the pose of objects

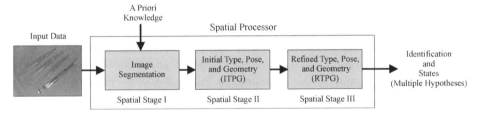

**Figure 4.** The spatial processor uses three stages. First, tools are segmented from the background. Then the type, pose, and geometry of all tools in the image are estimated in the ITPG module. Finally, refined type, pose, and geometry are calculated in the RTPG module.

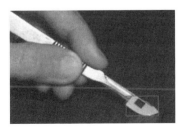

**Figure 5.** Image segmentation creates a bounding rectangle around the portion of the tool being tracked.

[7]; and discriminate between them [8], including those in confusing environments [9, 10]. Energid Technologies has a novel way to create template images, and applying this algorithm to tool tracking is a unique part of our approach.

We condense synthetic images using an image subspace that captures key information. Three degrees of freedom each in orientation and position, and any number of degrees of freedom in geometry can be included through the template-matching framework shown in Figure 6. This framework uses an offline system to calculate template images, measurement images, and the measurements of the template images. These results are used online as the simulation executes to match segmented tools against the templates.

### 3.2.3. RTPG

The third module in Figure 4 is the RTPG processor, which finds precise states of tools given initial conditions from the ITPG module. It uses a local search with 3D model matching. Synthetic images of the tool are created and compared to the sensed data in real time.

To run in real time, the RTPG module exploits low-cost PC graphics cards. PC graphics cards give high-performance processing, driven largely by the video game industry. A function of orientation, distance, and articulation is defined as a metric on the difference between the captured image and a synthetic image. The synthetic image is created using a model that is looked up in the tool-model database shown in 3. This metric is minimized using Nelder and Mead's algorithm [11], with the orientation, distance, and articulation giving the minimum metric value chosen as the best estimate of truth.

### 3.3. Temporal Processing

For temporal processing, we use a variant of the Multiple Hypothesis Tracking (MHT) algorithm. There are two broad classes of MHT: hypothesis centric and track centric. The original MHT algorithm proposed by Reid [12] uses a hypothesis-centric approach, where hypotheses are scored and these scores are propagated. Track scores are calculated from existing hypotheses. Track-centric algorithms score tracks and calculate hy-

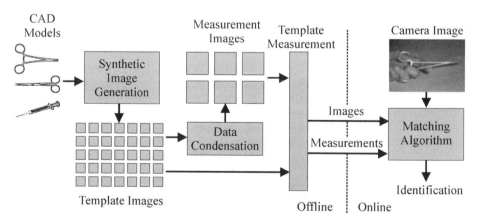

**Figure 6.** Initial type, pose, and geometry recognition has an offline and an online process. The offline process (left of the dashed line) creates measurement images using CAD models of the tools. It is run once during algorithm generation. The online process uses the templates to implement the ITPG module shown in Figure 4.

pothesis scores from the track scores. Our variation on MHT we call measurement centric. Because we have detailed spatial information on the type, position, and orientation of the tool, we are able to eliminate undesirable tracks quickly and improve tracking performance.

## 3.4. Visual Tracking Examples

In the example shown on the left of Figure 8, the marked blade of the scalpel shown in Figure 5 is tracked. For tracking this part, first a CAD model of the marked blade was used to calculate 40 32×32 measurement images constructed with six-degree increments. This was used with a 40-step Nelder-Mead optimization process to refine each match.

The right side of Figure 8 illustrates the recreation of a virtual scene. The image was created by tracking an electrocautery pen with a webcam and replaying the motion in a virtual environment. The location of the tool was automatically tracked and placed in the scene.

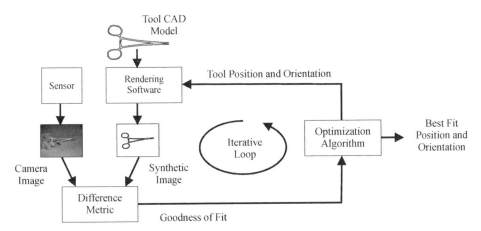

**Figure 7.** RTPG calculation uses three-dimensional object matching. A measure of the difference between the captured image and a graphics-hardware-generated synthetic image is optimized over type, orientation, distance, and articulation. The initial conditions for the numerical optimization come from the ITPG module.

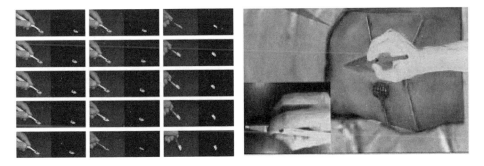

**Figure 8.** On the left are results from tracking the scalpel shown in Figure 5 through a video sequence (top to bottom ordering). The right image shows one frame of vision-based tool tracking.

## Acknowledgements

The authors gratefully acknowledge collaboration with Dr. Janey Pratt, a surgeon at Massachusetts General Hospital for her contribution to the project planning and main idea of the open surgery simulation design. We also would like to thank Dr. James Biggs at MIT Touch Lab for his contribution to tissue modeling and James Bacon at Energid for software design. This work was done under contract the U.S. Army's Telemedicine and Advanced Technology Research Center, through the direction of Mr. Harvey Magee.

## References

[1]  A. Liu, F. Tendick, K. Cleary, and C. Kaufmann, "A Survey of Surgical Simulation: Applications, Technology, and Education," *Presence,* vol. 12, issue 6, Dec. 2003.

[2]  S. Dawson, M. Ottensmeyer, "The VIRGIL Trauma Training System", *TATRC's 4th Annual Advanced Medical Technology Review*, Newport Beach, CA, Wednesday, January 14, 2004.

[3]  J, Kim, S. De, M. A. Srinivasan, "Computationally Efficient Techniques for Real Time Surgical Simulations with Force Feedback," *IEEE Proceedings for 10th Symp. On Haptic Interfaces For Virtual Environments & Teleoperator Systs.* 2002.

[4]  C.-Y. Chang, *Fast Eigenspace Decomposition of Correlated Images,* Ph.D. Dissertation, Purdue University, 2000.

[5]  C. Basdogan, S. De, J. Kim, M. Muniyandi, H. Kim and M.A. Srinivasan, "Haptics in Minimally Invasive Surgical Simulation and Training", *IEEE Computer Graphics and Applications*, March 2004.

[6]  I. Reed, R. Gagliardi, and L. Stotts, "Optical Moving Target Detection with 3-D Matched Filtering," *IEEE Transactions on Aerospace and Electronic Systems*, vol. 24, no. 4, July 1988.

[7]  H. Murase and S.K. Nayar, "Parametric Eigenspace Representation for Visual Learning and Recognition," *Geometric Methods in Computer Vision II*, SPIE, vol. 2031, 1993, pp. 378–391.

[8]  S.K. Nayar, S.A. Nene, and H. Murase, "Real-Time 100 Object Recognition System," *Proceedings of the 1996 IEEE International Conference on Robotics and Automation,* April 1996.

[9]  W.A.C. Schmidt, "Modified Matched Filter for Cloud Clutter Suppression," *IEEE Transactions on Pattern Analysis and Machine Intelligence*, vol. 12, no. 6, June 1990.

[10] M. Hiroshi and S.K. Nayar, "Detection of 3D Objects in Cluttered Scenes Using Hierarchical Eigenspace," *Pattern Recognition Letters,* vol. 18, 1997, pp. 375–384.

[11] J. Nelder and R. Mead, "A Simplex Method for Function Minimization," *Comp. J.*, v. 7, 308-313, 1965.

[12] D.B. Reid, "An Algorithm for Tracking Multiple Targets," *IEEE Transactions on Automatic Control*, AC-24(6), pp 843-854, December 1979.

*Medicine Meets Virtual Reality 13*
*James D. Westwood et al. (Eds.)*
*IOS Press, 2005*

# Haptic Simulation of the Milling Process in Temporal Bone Operations

Magnus ERIKSSON, Henrik FLEMMER and Jan WIKANDER

*Mechatronics Lab, Department of Machine Design,*
*The Royal Institute of Technology, Stockholm, Sweden*
*e-mail: magnuse@md.kth.se*

**Abstract.** A VR-simulation system for educating surgeons of the temporal bone milling processes is presented in this paper. E.g. the milling process that occurs during the removal of certain cancer tumors in the brain. The research project is recently started up and this paper is an introduction to the bone milling simulation topic. We present how the graphical rendering of the temporal bone is done. Acquired data are managed using the Marching cubes algorithm to perform a visual representation. A re-production of iso-surfaces will represent the material removal occurred during the milling process. Force models are discussed and will be implemented in the H3D API, which is used to control the virtual simulation and collision detection. Equipment, implementation and future work are also presented in the paper.

## 1. Introduction

For removal of cancer tumors in certain locations of a human head, the surgeon has not only to open up a hole in the temporal bone, a path along the inside of the temporal bone must also be made. Today, the surgeon mills this path very carefully with a small hand held mill such that the tumor can be reached without affecting the brain more than necessary and not to damage other vital parts of the head located close to the tumor. Typically, this path is located in a region where the temporal bone is geometrically complicated and is surrounding neurons, brain tissue and critical parts of the nervous system. Hence, the milling phase of an operation of this type is difficult, safety critical and very time consuming. Reduction of operation time by only a few percent would in the long run save society large expenses.

In order to reduce operation time and to provide surgeons with an invaluable practicing environment, this paper discusses the introduction of a simulator system to be used in both surgeon curriculum and in close connection to the actual operations.

In earlier research [1], a prototype master slave system for introduction of telerobotic surgery in the described task was developed. The work presented in this paper describes an extension to that system in terms of development of a simulator system based on a virtual reality representation of the human skull from which both haptic and visual feedback to the surgeon is generated. The visual and haptic implementations are two major steps to reach the over all goal with this research project, to get an appropriate haptic and virtual reality system to train and educate surgeons practicing bone milling.

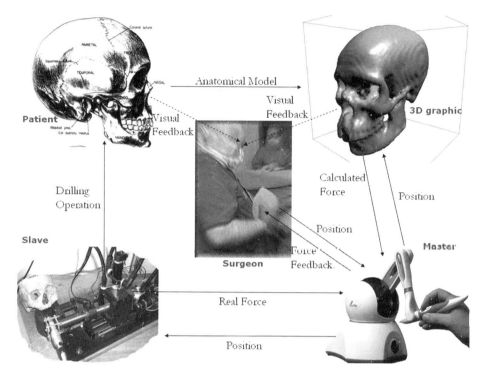

**Figure 1.** The complete telerobotic and VR-system.

Another future goal is to connect the VR system with the already developed telerobotic surgery system to control a real operation situation with the help of using VR interaction. The complete system is presented in figure 1.

The overall research focus is here put on modeling the haptic forces due to the milling process and implements them into the system. This is a challenging problem caused by stability problems occurring when two stiff objects collide and the force model to describe a milling process is more complex than other common force models used for haptic simulations. This paper focuses on the graphical implementation of the human skull and also to describe the components and equipment used in the VR-system for simulation of the bone milling process.

## 2. Visual representation of temporal bone

For the temporal bone representation we use data acquired from CT-scan, which is the most qualitative way to perform highly detailed images of bone structures for surgeons. The image representation consists of a dataset of the spatially varying x-ray attenuation values. To cut away material from the temporal bone object in real-time simulation is a challenging problem. To represent the volume as a surface-based empty shell is not sufficient for this purpose. Instead the idea of using the attenuation values from the CT-scan as a description of the internal structure of the volume is applied. The data set from the CT is implemented in a matrix and then the Marching cubes algorithm [2] is used to manage this data and perform a 3D model of the skull bone based on a predefined

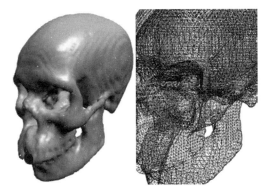

**Figure 2.** 3D model of a skull bone using the Marching cubes algorithm (filled and wire).

iso-value. For the time being, the Marching cubes algorithm is tested and implemented in the SenseGraphics H3D API for visual representation. Figure 2 shows a 3D model of a skull bone using the Marching cubes algorithm and an attenuation value-based method to calculate the normals of the surface.

After collision is detected, the material removal during the milling process will be illustrated via that the voxels density-values will be regenerated at the local volume where the interaction between the burr and the skull bone takes place and a new surface will be rerendered at this level. The visual rendering handles an updating rate of 30 Hz and a latency of less than 300 ms to give a realistic visual impression.

## 3. Force modeling and equipment

The haptic loop, updated at 1000 Hz, consists of two different parts. First, collision detection between the drill and skull bone surface and then generation of force feedback to the haptic device. The H3D API handles the collision detection and controls which forces to send to the haptic device. Different contact models will be developed and implemented in the API. The basic spring-damper contact model is today implemented in the API, this method is suitable to give a good feeling of contact with a stiff surface, but the model is insufficient to describe the milling process. To do a mathematical description of the burr-bone interaction is complicated because it involves changing of an inhomogeneous surface when the rotating burr is cutting material away. It also deals with the impact of two stiff materials colliding, which often leads to instability of the dynamical system.

An energy-based approach will be used to determine how much material that is removed from the skull bone during the milling process.

The SenseGraphics H3D API is used for graphical representation of the scene and control of the haptic rendering. The API is a dual licensed product, both available for open source users and commercial applications. The H3D API scene graph is connected to Sensables OpenHaptics for dynamical control of the PHANToM Omni haptic device. In the API, the graphics and the haptic information are modeled in the same scene graph and visual and force modeling will be implemented in the same software environment and sharing the same data.

## 4. Conclusion and future work

In this paper a complete VR-training system for temporal bone surgery has been introduced. The focus is put on graphical representation of the skull bone and modeling of contact forces occurring during the milling process. For the time being, the graphics are implemented and future work will focus on modeling contact forces.

## References

[1]  Flemmer, H, "Control Design and Performance Analysis of Force Reflective Teleoperators – A Passivity Based Approach", Doctoral Thesis 2004, KTH Stockholm Sweden, June 2004.
[2]  Lorensen, W.E. et al. "Marching Cubes: A High Resolution 3D Surface Construction Algorithm", Computer Graphics, 21(4), July 1987, pp. 163-169.

Medicine Meets Virtual Reality 13
James D. Westwood et al. (Eds.)
IOS Press, 2005

# Soft Tissue Deformation using a Nonlinear Hierarchical Finite Element Model with Real-Time Online Refinement

Alessandro FARACI, Fernando BELLO and Ara DARZI

*Department of Surgical Oncology and Technology, St. Mary's Hospital,
Faculty of Medicine, Imperial College London*

**Abstract.** Simulating soft tissue deformation in real-time is a requirement for realistically rendering the VR interaction between human organs and surgical tools. Finite Element Model (FEM) describes complex mechanical and physiological behaviour but it is computationally too demanding especially when a nonlinear model is to be implemented. For this reason, we introduce a multiresolution approach to FEM that only employs the region of the object under deformation to find the solution of the differential equations of motion. In order to increase the quality of the deformation, refinement of the original mesh is performed with the insertion of new surface nodes in real-time in the region of interaction. To guarantee the stability of the nonlinear model, the presence of flat tetrahedra (slivers) has to be avoided; therefore a sliver elimination technique has been implemented resulting in a more stable simulation.

## 1. Introduction

Several surgical simulators are currently available for training and rehearsing surgical skills. Although they have reached a considerable level of realism, great improvement will come from a highly precise simulation of soft tissue deformation and from the integration of force feedback or haptics. In order to achieve a satisfactory immersion in the virtual environment, the simulation requires at least 30 frames per second for graphics. For haptics 1-KHz is a common rate, although there are no firm rules. This rate is an acceptable compromise allowing presentation of complex objects with reasonable stiffness. Higher frequencies can provide crisper contact and texture sensations, but at the expense of reduced scene complexity [1].

Various methods have been proposed for real-time simulation of soft tissue deformation, such as Mass Spring Models (MSM) [2,3] and the Finite Element Method (FEM) [4–6]. MSM achieve real-time but lack in accuracy when precise modelling of physiological behaviour is needed. FEM is more accurate for rendering the mechanical characteristics of human organs but it is more computationally expensive. Multiresolution techniques have been proposed as a way of solving the problems that these two methods carry with them. Multiresolution approaches apply different levels of detail to the mesh that approximates the object: a higher resolution in the region where the deformation takes place; a lower resolution far from the region of contact. Increasing the number of points in the contact region improves the simulation of the biomechanical behaviour. Less nodes where no deformation occurs concentrates the computational workload where is needed. In order to take advantage of this approach for real-time simulation the same mesh at two different levels of detail can be pre-computed as proposed in [7] for an application of implicit FEM. Unfortunately, pre-computation does not allow implementing cutting or any other interaction which implies modifying the topology of the mesh. One solution can be the online refinement of the original mesh as proposed in [8] for a volumetric MSM or as described in [9] for explicit FEM.

This paper presents a multiresolution approach to the simulation of soft tissue deformation combining FEM accuracy in rendering mechanical and physiological properties with the concentration of the computational workload in the region of contact. We call this approach *Hierarchical Finite Element Model* (HFEM). This method does not take into account tetrahedra that do not deform or deform marginally, allowing for the incorporation of a nonlinear elastic model with greater complexity and easier integration of force feedback. A nonlinear FEM that allows for large deformations with second Piola-Kirchhoff stress and Green-Lagrange strain according to Hook's law has been chosen.

Since the stability of a nonlinear FEM is affected at each time step by the quality of the deformed mesh [10], ensuring a mesh of good quality at each time step is vital. For this reason, the advantages of online Delaunay-refinement of the mesh have been studied and a procedure to eliminate flat tetrahedra during simulation that incorporates a Delaunay test for quality is presented.

The VR environment has been recreated using a desktop VR Reachin System [11], which incorporates stereo vision with haptics co-location via a Phantom force feedback device [12]. The user is immersed in the virtual environment and interacts with it sitting in front of a computer and looking down at a mirror where the graphical rendering is projected. To perceive the virtual object through the sense of touch, the haptic device is used to interact in real-time, providing the inputs to calculate the deformation of the volume (the amount of force, direction and point of application) and communicating in output the response of the virtual object in the form of force feedback.

## 2. Volumetric Nonlinear HFEM

As shown in [14] an elastic material description for large deformation analysis is obtained by generalizing the Hookean linear elastic relations to the total Lagrangian formulation:

$$S_{ij} = C_{ijrs}\varepsilon_{rs}$$

where $S_{ij}$ and $\varepsilon_{rs}$ are the components of the second Piola-Kirchhoff stress and Green-Lagrange strain tensors and the $C_{ijrs}$ are the components of the constant elasticity tensor. Considering three-dimensional stress conditions, we have:

$$C_{ijrs} = \lambda\delta_{ij}\delta_{rs} + \mu(\delta_{ir}\delta_{js} + \delta_{is}\delta_{jr})$$

where $\lambda$ and $\mu$ are the Lamé constants and $\delta_{ij}$ is the Kronecker delta. We implemented the central difference scheme [13], a time-explicit integration method whose main shortcoming lies in the severe time step restriction for stability which requires the time step

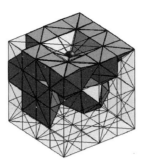

**Figure 1.** Active tetrahedra during deformation of a cube.

$\Delta t$ to be smaller than a critical time step $\Delta t_{crit}$ [14]. Whereas in a linear analysis the stiffness properties remain constant, in a nonlinear analysis these properties change during the response calculations. Therefore, $\Delta t$ needs to be decreased if the system stiffens so that $\Delta t_{crit}$ is valid at all times. An adaptive time step dependent also on the geometry of the object has to be calculated: a different $\Delta t$ smaller than $\Delta t_{crit}$ is selected when the portion of the object under deformation changes. Each time a tetrahedron is added or deleted from the subset of deforming tetrahedra the time step is updated, ensuring a more homogenous behaviour of the deformation along the entire mesh.

A hierarchical mesh of an object is defined as its tetrahedral mesh subdivided into regions of interaction. A region of interaction is a portion of the mesh that is deforming under the contact of a surgical tool and may be refined by adding new internal and/or external nodes. Only the tetrahedra in a region of interaction are considered for the integration of the equations of motion. This is illustrated in Fig. 1 where a cube is deforming under a force load applied at the top. At any given time step, only a subset of tetrahedra is deforming.

A geometrical explicit FEM has been implemented to solve the equations of motion. Instead of building the system matrices (stiffness, damping and mass matrices) and integrating for the whole object in one step, in geometrical explicit FEM the equations of motion are solved at the element level for each tetrahedron independently and the nodal displacements are calculated by summing the displacement contribution of each tetrahedral element [15]. This is possible by considering the damping matrix and the mass matrix as diagonal so that the mass and the damping effects can be concentrated on the vertices of the mesh. This simplification increases the speed of the simulation as the solution does not involve the triangular factorization of a matrix. Geometrical explicit FEM allows for taking into account only the tetrahedra affected by the propagation of internal forces and for dynamic tetrahedra selection and deselection. An active node has been defined as a point of the mesh whose internal force vector's norm has a magnitude large enough to change the configuration of neighbouring tetrahedra, i.e., if it is higher of a certain threshold value. Active nodes are also the ones having an external force applied to them. Thus, a tetrahedron is called active if at least one of its four nodes is active. When the nodes of an active tetrahedron present very small displacements, velocities and accelerations, the tetrahedron becomes inactive and its nodal displacements, velocities and accelerations are set to zero.

## 3.  Remeshing and Refinement

Refinement of a mesh consists in adding new nodes. Whenever a mesh is refined, a remeshing technique is needed to create new tetrahedra after the insertion of a new node. Remeshing can also be applied when the configuration of the mesh has to be changed (e.g. cutting). We have implemented a remeshing technique for recovering a mesh of good quality and a surface refinement procedure. As seen in [16], employing a Delaunay mesh improves the stability of the simulation because of the presence of good quality tetrahedra. Computing a new stiffness matrix at each time step from a changed tetrahedral mesh carries numerical problems. If the quality of the mesh has degraded as a result of the deformation, the stiffness matrix creates errors that make the simulation unstable. In order to maintain the quality of the mesh in a nonlinear model, a Delaunay-*remeshing* procedure has to be performed at each time step. If the quality of the deformation has to be increased, new nodes are inserted in the region of contact of the original mesh modifying the existing Delaunay structure that can be recovered by a local Delaunay-remeshing.

To increase the resolution of the simulation a new surface node is added. The longest edge **L** connected to the closest external node to the point of contact is split by adding a new node at its midpoint. The two external faces that share **L** are divided as the underlying tetrahedra, generating at least two new tetrahedra per refinement step. Not all edges are eligible for splitting as some of them can become too short decreasing the quality of the mesh and generating numerical errors in the integration algorithm. Therefore, the length of the edges is checked and if the split edges are shorter than a threshold value the node is rejected for insertion.

Adding surface nodes improves the external mesh resolution at the cost of a less homogeneous density of points, therefore it would be desirable to also add internal nodes. Surface refinement is easily implemented online without decreasing the frequency of the simulation. In the future we will extend our work to the online insertion of internal nodes while ensuring real-time simulation.

## 4.  Sliver Elimination Process (SEP)

In a nonlinear model the deformed mesh affects the numerical integration and large forces can generate slivers (flat tetrahedra) leading to numerical errors and instability. To address this problem we have implemented a Sliver Elimination Process (SEP) which consists of a Delaunay remeshing procedure that deletes slivers and locally recovers a mesh of good quality to ensure stability to the nonlinear model under the interaction of high forces. A local Delaunay-refinement technique allows for maintaining the initial number of nodes as numerous slivers can form during deformation and their elimination would decrease the quality of the simulation. Our SEP consists of three basic steps:

1. *Elimination of the sliver*: one of the internal points of the sliver is replaced by the closest point among the remaining vertices forcing the sliver to 'collapse' to a face. Other tetrahedra will be reduced to a face as well and these degenerated tetrahedra (and the sliver) are removed (Fig. 2(a)).
2. *Insertion of a new node*: a node is inserted in the centroid of the largest tetrahedron amongst the tetrahedra sharing at least one vertex with the "collapsed"

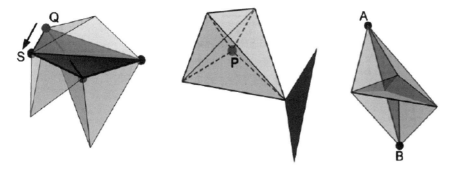

**Figure 2.** SEP Illustration: Sliver collapsing to a face (a); Node insertion (b); Face flipping (c).

sliver. This node is then joined to the other vertices splitting into 4 the tetrahedron (Fig. 2(b)).

3. *Flipping of faces*: if a face of the split tetrahedron is not locally Delaunay and if the two tetrahedra that share this face form a convex hexahedron, the face is flipped and three new tetrahedra are formed replacing the two pre-existing ones as shown in [8] (Fig. 2(c)).

## 5. Experiments

We carried out a series of experiments to demonstrate the relevance of SEP. While they were performed offline and without haptics, the results obtained showed that SEP is applicable online and with force feedback. A 5*cm*-edge-cube with 139 nodes and 473 tetrahedra, Elastic Modulus = 4*KPa*, Poisson's ratio = 0.475, damping = 200, density = 1050Kg/m$^3$ was considered and $\Delta t = 0.0005sec$. A perpendicular force was applied on top of the cube (Fig. 1) for 75 time steps and the simulation continued until the cube returned to the rest configuration at time step 110. Under a force of 2*N*, as a sliver formed, the simulation became unstable and SEP was applied. SEP was studied considering the application of: *a)* step 1; *b)* step 1 and 2; *c)* full SEP. The results obtained were as follows:

*a)* The sliver becomes a face deleting 1 node and 7 tetrahedra. The mesh is locally coarser.

*b)* The number of nodes reverts as at the beginning and 4 new tetrahedra are formed.

*c)* The number of tetrahedra increases after flipping the faces of the split tetrahedron.

Let $minV$ = (*smallest volume in the mesh*), $Q$ = (*circumradius-to-shortest edge ratio*) defining the quality of the mesh [16] and $seim$ = (*shortest edge in the mesh*). We considered $minV$, $Q$ and $seim$ over time to evaluate the SEP implementation.

Having defined the Energy Norm as $EN = \frac{\|\mathbf{u}-\mathbf{u}'\|}{\|\mathbf{u}'\|}$, where $\mathbf{u}$ and $\mathbf{u}'$ are the displacement vectors of the simulation without and with approximation, Fig. 3(a) illustrates $EN$ for the three cases under consideration. A full SEP affects the quality of the deformation the most, decreasing the energy of the system and increasing the oscillations of the deforming object. Cases *a)* and *b)* do not differ considerably. For all three cases, differences are more noticeable during equilibrium under the force load and decrease after releasing the force.

The changing in $minV$ is shown in Fig 3(b). SEP was applied at time step 17 with an immediate increase in the volume for cases *a)* and *b)* and a time step later for case *c)*.

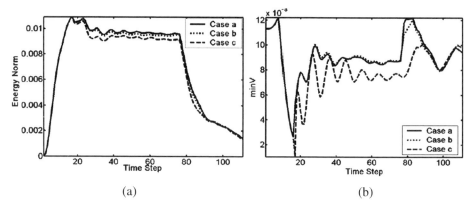

(a)                                                    (b)

**Figure 3.** EN for each of the cases studied (a). Minimal volume in the tetrahedral mesh (b).

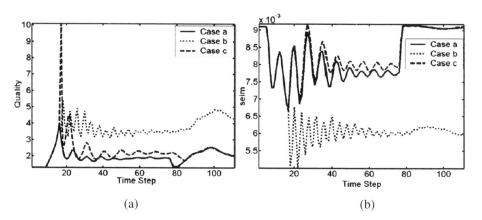

(a)                                                    (b)

**Figure 4.** Quality of the mesh during deformation (a). Lower values indicate better quality. Shortest edge in mesh (b). Higher values are preferred.

$minV$ does not decrease in the following time steps, suggesting that slivers do not form anymore. SEP succeeds in all three cases, but in particular for cases $a)$ and $b)$. Case $a)$ is not acceptable since we are trying to maintain the same number of nodes throughout the entire simulation. Therefore, case $b)$ is the more effective in eliminating the sliver.

Fig. 4(a) shows $Q$ when applying SEP. Although $minV$ from the previous figure suggests that case $b)$ is preferable to case $c)$, this figure highlights the importance of the flipping step. The quality of the mesh for case $c)$ is far better than case $b)$: we therefore consider more valuable case $c)$ as what we are concern with is primarily the quality of the mesh. Fig. 4(b) confirms the importance of flipping since it increases considerably $seim$, which is linked to the $\Delta t$ needed for the numerical method to converge. If $seim$ decreases too much, $\Delta t$ has to be decreased to ensure stability. These experiments demonstrate SEP useful for stability and that is an effective method for local remeshing, improving the quality of the mesh and increasing its shortest edge.

## 6. Conclusions and Future Work

We have presented a nonlinear FEM running in real time with a high number of nodes allowing surface refinement that improves the simulation of soft tissue deformation. A sliver elimination technique has been shown to increase its stability.

The advantages of the proposed method are: nonlinear model running in real time; application of the numerical solution only to the deforming tetrahedra and refinement by insertion of a high number of points in the region of contact without affecting performance or stability. This has shown to be suitable for implementation in real time with integration of force feedback: the time spent for internal refinement of the mesh has been recorded offline using MATLAB and had demonstrated to maintain a satisfactory high frequency in the simulation.

We are currently working on the implementation of tool-tissue interactions in real time feeding back the real force produced by the model when the tool touches or pushes on the soft tissue or when it pulls it in one point after grasping. We are also studying problems occurring in the real interaction with a haptic device, especially the presence of unwanted oscillations arising from the haptic interface.

Our further work will include a quality controlled refinement that will allow for improved stability and online insertion of a larger number of nodes enabling topology modifying interactions such as cutting.

## References

[1]   Salisbury, K.; Conti, F., & Barbagli, F. (2004). Haptic rendering introductory concepts. Computer Graphics and Applications, IEEE, 24(2), 24-32.
[2]   Xavier Provot. Deformation Constraints in a Mass-Spring Model to Describe Rigid Cloth Behavior. Wayne A.Davis and Przemyslaw Prusinkiewicz. In Proceedings of Graphics Interface '95, pages 147-154. 1995. Canadian Human-Computer Communications Society.
[3]   U.Kühnapfel, H.K.Çakmak, and H.Maaß. 3D Modeling for Endoscopic Surgery. Oct. 1999.
[4]   S.Roth, M.Gross, S.Turello, and F.Carls. A bernstein-bézier based approach to soft tissue simulation. Proceedings of the Eurographics '98 (Lisbon, Portugal, September 2-4, 1998), COMPUTER GRAPHICS Forum, Vol. 17, No. 3, C285-C294. 1998.
[5]   M.Bro-Nielsen and S.Cotin. Real-time volumetric deformable models for surgery simulation using finite elements and condensation. Computer Graphics Forum, 15(3):C57–C66, C461. Sept. 1996.
[6]   D.Bielser and M.Gross. Open surgery simulation. In Proc. of Medicine Meets Virtual Reality. 2002.
[7]   Xunlei Wu, Micheal S.Downes, Tolga Goktekin, Frank Tendick. Adaptive Nonlinear Finite Elements for Deformable Body Simulation Using Dynamic Progressive Meshes. Computer Graphics Forum 20, 3, pages 349-358. 2001.
[8]   Celine Paloc, Fernando Bello, Richard I.Kitney, and Ara Darzi. Online Multiresolution Volumetric Mass Spring Model for Real Time Soft Tissue Deformation. Proc. of MICCAI, pages 219-226. Oct. 2002.
[9]   Gilles Debunne, Mathieu Desbrun, Marie-Paule Cani, and Alan H.Barr. Dynamic Real-Time Deformations using Space and Time Adaptive Sampling. Computer Graphics Proceedings. Aug. 2001. ACM Press / ACM SIGGRAPH. Annual Conference Series.
[10]  Shewchuk, J. (1997). Delaunay Refinement Mesh Generation. PhD thesis, School of Computer Science, Carnegie Mellon University, Pittsburgh, Pennsylvania.
[11]  http://www.reachin.se.
[12]  http://www.sensable.com.
[13]  Young W.Kwon and Hyochoong Bang. The finite element method using MATLAB, Boca Raton, FL; London : CRC Press, 2nd ed. 2000.
[14]  Klaus-Jurgen Bathe. Finite Element Procedures. Prentice-Hall, Inc., London, 1996.

[15] César Mendoza (2003). Soft Tissue Interactive Simulations for Medical Applications including 3D Cutting and Force Feedback. PhD thesis, Institute National Polytechnique de Grenoble, France.

[16] Celine Paloc (2003). Adaptive Deformable Model (allowing Topological Modifications) for Surgical Simulation. PhD thesis, Bioengineering Department, Imperial College London, UK.

*Medicine Meets Virtual Reality 13*
*James D. Westwood et al. (Eds.)*
*IOS Press, 2005*

# Modeling Biologic Soft Tissues for Haptic Feedback with an Hybrid Multiresolution Method

Antonio FRISOLI, Luigi BORELLI and Massimo BERGAMASCO

*PERCRO Scuola Superiore Sant'Anna Pisa*

**Abstract.** The simulation of realistic surgical procedures requires specialized optimized algorithms for the models of organs and tissues, which should comply both with accuracy of results and run-time computation. This paper provides a numerical method for implementing deformation of soft tissues for haptic feedback that makes use of a hybrid pre-computation scheme.

## Introduction

Multiresolution FEM methods [1] are promising methods in terms of speed and accuracy for the simulation of soft tissues. These methods solve a FEM model by splitting its solution into two problems, one based on a coarse mesh representing the global deformation of the whole model, and another one computing more accurately the deformation only in the contact area through a finer mesh. However the update of the local model can still be computationally expensive, especially when complex non-linear model are adopted to simulate a realistic response of the material, e.g. Mooney-Rivlin or other rheologic models. To overcome these limitations, in this paper we propose a new hybrid method, that combines a pre-computation scheme with a multi-resolution technique.

## 1. Methods

A discretized mesh is generated from the model of the body and constraints and loads are applied to its nodes. We assumed that the shape of the local deformation is not much influenced by the topological characteristics of the model, but only by the mechanical properties of material and by the size of the surgical tool; under this assumption, in the contact area, the finer FEM local model has been replaced by a pre-computed solution obtained from an accurate FEM model. The global coarser model used as first-attempt is a quasistatic model mass-model with the general non-linear law supporting large deformations and implementing the algorithm presented in [2]:

$$F_i = \sum_{j \in \sigma i} K_{ij} \left( \|x_i x_j\| - l_{ij}^0 \right) \frac{x_i x_j}{\|x_i x_j\|} = \sum_{j \in \sigma(i)} K_{ij} \left( 1 - \frac{l_{ij}^0}{\|x_i x_j\|} \right) \widehat{x_i x_j}$$

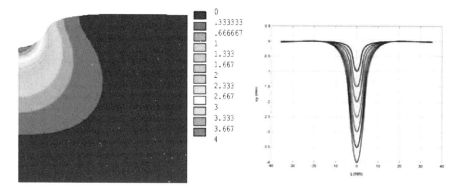

**Figure 1.** Results from the indentation analysis simulated by a FEM method.

The displacements of each node $x$ under a given load are computed as the superimposition of both local and global effects $u(x) = u_L(x) + u_G(x)$ where $u$ is the total displacement and $u_L$ and $u_G$ are respectively the local and global displacement for each node.

When a displacement $u_P$ is applied to a given node $P$, it is split into a local and global component according to two weights $\alpha_L$, $\alpha_G$ associated to it, such that $u_L = \alpha_L(x_P)u_P$, $u_G = \alpha_G(x_P)u_P$ and $\alpha_L + \alpha_G = 1$. A set of weights $\alpha_L$, $\alpha_G$ is associated to each node of the body and has been pre-computed through a FEM analysis, conducted by imposing explorative unitary loads on each node and evaluating the mutual coefficients of influence for nodal displacements. The more a node is close to a constraint, the more its local coefficient $\alpha_L$ will tend to 1; the more a node is placed on a compliant area of the body, the more $\alpha_L$ will tend to 0.

Afterwards the displacement $u_L(x_P)$ is input into a pre-computation model that generates the displacements for all the nodes in the neighborhood of the contact area. The displacement $u_G(x_P)$ is instead provided as input to the coarse mass-spring model to generate the displacements for all the nodes in the model. Then the total displacements are computed for each node $x$ as $u(x) = u_L(x) + u_G(x)$.

## 1.1. Derivation of a pre-computation function

A correct measure of the deformation and of the state of strain of the material is not always achievable from in-vivo experiments on biological tissues. In order to derive a pre-computation function for the displacements, we implemented an accurate FEM model of the contact between the tool and the organ. The model was made of a hyperelastic Neo-Hookean material with $W = (\mu/2)(I_1 - 3) + (\kappa/2)(J - 1)^2$ and data corresponding to SilGel612 that are consistent with properties of biologic tissues ($\mu = 1600 \ N/m^2$, $\kappa = 10^7 \ N/m^2$ ) [3].

## 2. Results

From the analysis of the FEM simulation, it resulted that the local deformation is weakly influenced by the local geometry of the body, in the case of bulky bodies.

**Table 1.** Dimensionless coefficients $\xi_{ai} = a_i/R_e$ as a function of $\xi_d$ for SilGel612.

| $\xi_d$ | $\xi_{a1}$ | $\xi_{a2}$ | $\xi_{a3}$ | $\xi_{a4}$ |
|---|---|---|---|---|
| 0 | 0 | 0 | 0 | 0 |
| 1 | 0,0431 | 0,0197 | 0,4959 | 0,3621 |
| 2 | 0,0639 | 0,0645 | 2,6750 | 2,4079 |
| 2,5 | 0,0481 | 0,1076 | 4.30110 | 3,9574 |
| 3 | 0,0130 | 0,1562 | 6,2433 | 5,8175 |
| 3,5 | 0,0100 | 0,1927 | 8,4936 | 7,9874 |
| 4 | 0,01326 | 0,224 | 10,7440 | 10,1570 |

**Table 2.** Dimensionless coefficients $\xi_{ci} = c_i/R_e$ as a function of $\xi_d$ for SilGel612.

| $\xi_d$ | $\xi_{c1}$ | $\xi_{c2}$ | $\xi_{c3}$ | $\xi_{c4}$ |
|---|---|---|---|---|
| 0 | 0 | 0 | 0 | 0 |
| 1 | 0,8588 | 1,7120 | 0,3241 | 0,2843 |
| 2 | 0,9830 | 1,6234 | 0,4291 | 0,4108 |
| 2,5 | 0,9913 | 1,5627 | 0,4732 | 0,45748 |
| 3 | 1,0617 | 1,5245 | 0,5115 | 0,4976 |
| 3,5 | 2,1157 | 1,6378 | 0,5422 | 0,5569 |
| 4,3 | 1,697 | 1,6645 | 0,5728 | 0,5613 |

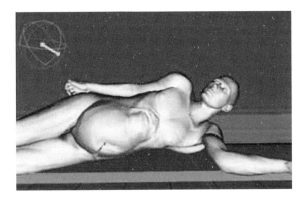

**Figure 2.** Application of the presented algorithm in a paracentesis simulator.

The deformation of the local area can be predicted through the superimposition of Gaussian distributions with shape given by $u_y = \sum_{i=1}^{n} a_i\, e^{-(s/c_i)^2}$.

The results have been set into a dimensionless format, by introducing the variables $\xi_d = d/R_e$ and $\xi_F = F/\mu a^2$ with the equivalent curvature radius $R_e$ defined as by the contact theory (it depends of principal curvatures of both the tool and the body), where $a$ is the width of the contact area, and $d$ is the indentation tool displacement. The obtained values for the coefficients of the Gaussian interpolating functions have been expressed in dimensionless format for generality and are reported in table 1 and 2.

## 3. Conclusions

The simulation of a paracentesis training session with a force feedback device confirmed the validity of the presented algorithm for modeling the behavior of biologic tissues. The FEM analysis showed that convex bulky bodies of soft material with curvature varying up to 10 times do not present noticeable differences in their deformation, that so can be considered as a local phenomenon, with extinction radius independent on the indentation of the tool. Global deformation effects should be taken into account in slim bodies or parts that exhibit flexional behavior. The presented algorithm allows to cope with bodies subjected to stress that exhibit both local and global deformation patterns.

## References

[1]  O. R. Astley and V. Hayward. Real-time finite-elements simulation of general visco-elastic materials for haptic presentation. In Workshop on Dynamics Simulation: Methods and Applications, IROS'97, pages 1–6, 1997.

[2]  L.F. Borelli A. Frisoli and al. Simulation of real-time deformable soft tissues for computer assisted surgery. The International Journal of Medical Robotics and Computer Assisted Surgery, 1(1):107–113, 2004.

[3]  M. Kauer (2001). Inverse Finite Element Characterization of Soft Tissues with Aspiration Experiments. Ph.D. thesis, Swiss Federal Institute of Technology.

*Medicine Meets Virtual Reality 13*
*James D. Westwood et al. (Eds.)*
*IOS Press, 2005*

# Control of Laparoscopic Instrument Motion in an Inanimate Bench Model: Implications for the Training and Evaluation of Technical Skills

David GONZALEZ, MSc [a], Heather CARNAHAN, PhD [a],
Monate PRAAMSMA, MSc [a], Helen MACRAE, MD [b]
and Adam DUBROWSKI, PhD [b]

[a] *Department of Kinesiology, University of Waterloo, Waterloo, Ontario, Canada*
[b] *Surgical Skills Centre, Department of Surgery, University of Toronto, Toronto,
Ontario, Canada*
*e-mail: adam.dubrowski@utoronto.ca*

**Abstract.** Laparoscopic surgery requires new methods of technical competency evaluation, as well as training. The first purpose was to assess the differences in motion characteristics between the tip of the instrument and the wrist. The second purpose was to determine whether similar control strategies are used to move instruments in virtual reality and bench model environments.

Surgically naive participants were required to tap a laparoscopic instrument between two targets that differed in size and separation distance.

Large amplitude movements were controlled with the movements of the wrist and small amplitude with the wrist and the fingers (p<.001). Participants utilized the flexibility of the skin of the laparoscopic trainer to facilitate their movements.

These results suggest that monitoring the motions of the instrument tip is a more precise indication of its motions than are motions of the wrist when movements of small amplitudes are produced. Moreover, in order to increase fidelity, VR trainers should simulate the flexibility of the real structures around the insertion of the instrument.

## 1. Introduction

Technical surgical skills can be assessed by subjective qualification by an expert surgeon [1], and by objective quantification of a surgeon's wrists movements [2–4]. In this study, we address the suitability of this second method in the evaluation of performance of a precision task using laparoscopic instruments. The first purpose of this study was to investigate whether direct tracking of the tip of a laparoscopic grasper, rather than tracking of the motion of the wrist, reflected more accurately the task demands.

Virtual reality (VR) trainers became a logical training tool for laparoscopy. They use a joystick-like design to simulate laparoscopic instruments that enable limited degrees of freedom (the number of planes or dimensions in which the movement can be controlled). Non-VR training scenarios may provide additional degrees of freedom because the skin around the trocar, where the instrument enters the body, is elastic and allows some flexibility and stretching. The second purpose was to investigate whether simulated skin elasticity is utilized during novice laparoscopic performance on a simulated, real-life inanimate bench model.

## 2. Materials and Methods

### 2.1. Apparatus

An Optotrak (Northern Digital, Canada) system tracked small (2 mm) markers (200 Hz, 15 Hz dual Butterworth filter), along forward-backward, side-to-side, and up-and-down axes. A laparoscopic needle driver was inserted into a trainer (Auto Suture ENDO DIS-SECT) with a clear cover. Instrument positioning resulted in a $50^O$ angle between the grasper and the floor (25 cm height) of the trainer along the forward-backward axis, and $80^O$ along the side-to-side axis. Markers were placed on the tip and heel of the laparoscopic grasper, and on the wrist.

Undergraduate students (N=11, naïve to the task [5]) performed 10 taps alternately touching two targets on a paper. Each set comprised three different Indexes of Difficulty (IDs). ID was described by: $ID = Log^2 (2A/W)$: A=movement amplitude in cm, W=target width also in cm (**C1**: A=1, W=.05, ID = 2, **C2**: A=2, W=1, ID=2, **C3**: A=2, W=.5, ID=3, **C4**: A=4, W=1, ID=3, **C5**: A=2, W=.25, ID=4, **C6**: A=4, W=.5, ID=4).

### 2.2. Dependent Measures and Analyses

Movement time, tapping accuracy, and peak velocity were calculated for all three markers based on the displacement and velocity profile of each tap. Accuracy was expressed as the percentage of taps landing within the targets. Spatial displacements in the forward-backward, side-to-side, and up-down axes were correlated for the tip to heel and tip to wrist.

The data were analyzed in 3 ID (2,3,4) × 3 marker (tip, heel, wrist), as well as 6 condition × 3 marker (tip, heel, wrist) analyses of variance (ANOVAs). The tip to heel and tip to wrist correlations were subjected to separate 6 condition × 3 direction (X, Y, Z) ANOVAs. Effects significant at p < .05 were further analyzed using the Tukey HSD method.

## 3. Results and Discussion

Fitts' Law was replicated in a remote laparoscopic environment. Movement time increased as a function of ID (Figure 1a). Furthermore, accuracy data showed that the movements made to the more difficult targets were less accurate than those made to the easier targets (ID 2 = 95% +/− 2.2; ID 3 = 94% +/− 4.0; ID 4 = 85% +/− 8.1). Therefore as the task difficulty increased by tapping to small targets that were separated by large distances, not only did the movement times increase but also the accuracy decreased, suggesting that laparoscopic performance constitutes a highly complex motor challenge.

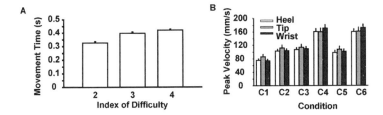

**Figure 1.** The relationship between Movement Time and Index of Difficulty (ID) collapsed across wrist, heel, and tip (A). The effects of condition (Table 1) on the peak velocity of the wrist, heel of the instrument, and tip of the instrument (B).

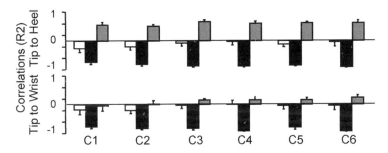

**Figure 2.** Tip to heel and tip to wrist correlations for all three movement components across the six conditions (White bars: forward-backward, black: side-side, grey: up-down).

Figure 1b shows that the wrist moved at the highest velocity in comparison to the tip and heel for conditions 4 and 6 (p<.001) when movement amplitudes were large. In all other conditions, requiring smaller movement, the tip of the grasper moved more quickly. Thus, for making large movements, the wrist or arm is largely involved; however, for making smaller movements, the wrist or arm moves less, and movements of the fingers are responsible for generating movements of the instrument tip. This indicates that monitoring motions of the tip of the grasper rather than the wrist motion involved in moving the instrument presents a more precise representation of the actual performance, specifically for small amplitude movements.

The correlational analysis of both the tip to the heel and the tip to the wrist revealed statistically significant interactions of condition-by-direction (p<.001). Figure 2 shows that the tip to heel correlations were relatively large and positive in the up-down direction, and large and negative in the side-to-side direction; and finally, smaller negative correlations were seen in the forward-backward direction. By contrast, the correlations of tip to wrist in the up-down directions were negligible for conditions 1 and 2, and positive but small for conditions 3 to 6; however, the correlations in the side-to-side direction were large and negative, similar to the tip to heel analysis; and, finally, correlations in the forward-backward direction were negative and smaller than the correlations on the side-to-side direction. This suggests that reciprocal tapping movements performed with a laparoscopic instrument inside an inanimate model utilize surrounding tissue flexibility. In order to increase the realism of the design, the instrument-trainer interface should simulate the flexibility of the simulated skin surrounding the virtual trocar, thus increasing the potential for learning the technical aspects of laparoscopic procedures.

# References

[1] Martin JA, Regehr G, Reznick RK, MacRae H, Murnaghan J, Hutchison C, Brown M (1997) Objective structured assessment of technical skills (OSATS) for surgical residents. Br J Surg 84: 273-278.
[2] Datta V, Mandalia M, Mackay S, Chang A, Cheshire N, Darzi A (2002) Relationship between skill and outcome in the laboratory based model. Surgery; 131(3): 318-323.
[3] Taffinder N, Sutton C, Fishwick RJ, McManus IC, Darzi A (1998) Validation of virtual reality to teach and assess psychomotor skills in laparoscopic surgery: results from randomized controlled studies using the MIST VR laparoscopic simulator. Stud Health Technol Inform; 50: 124-3.
[4] Torkington J, Smith SG, Rees BI, Darzi A (2001) Skill transfer from virtual reality to a real laparoscopic task. Surg Endosc; 10: 1076-9.
[5] Munz Y, Moorthy K, Bann S, Shah J, Ivanova S, Darzi SA. (2004) Ceiling effect in technical skills of surgical residents. Am J Surg. 188(3): 294-300.

*Medicine Meets Virtual Reality 13*
*James D. Westwood et al. (Eds.)*
*IOS Press, 2005*

# Tearing of Membranes for Interactive Real-Time Surgical Training

Johannes GRIMM

*Institute for Computational Medicine, University of Mannheim*

**Abstract.** Tearing for interactive real-time surgical training is a problem rarely discussed in scientific publications. In this paper, an approach is presented to model the tearing of membranes. Based on a mesh of mass nodes connected by springs and triangles tears propagate along the springs of the mesh. Springs and triangles at the crack are divided up between both sides, keeping the number of triangles constant. Node stress indicates when and where the membrane tears. Tear threshold of a node depends on the node's location in the mesh. Edge nodes tear more easily than internal nodes. Nodes at the end of a crack have the lowest threshold to favor the propagation of already created cracks. Compared to a straightforward solution of the problem, the deletion of overstretched springs, the approach has some advantages. The presented algorithm shows a more plausible result for small resolutions that are used by the real-time simulation of stiff materials. On high-resolution meshes, there is only little difference between both approaches. Two training modules for the ophthalmosurgical simulator EYESI use the presented tearing method to model realistic membrane tearing.

## Introduction

Virtual Reality simulators for surgical training need realistic tissue models to create plausible scenarios. A lot of research is done to simulate the deformations of organs in order to provide a realistic interaction between surgeon and tissue. In some cases, surgeons must learn to control the tear propagation of tissue. Therefore, a realistic tearing model is needed. The paper describes and discusses an algorithm developed to model the tearing of two membranes located inside the human eye.

## Previous Work

Models for tearing of tissue must solve two problems. First a suitable indicator must be found do decide where and when a crack begins and in what direction it propagates. Second, topological changes must be modeled and considered by the simulation under the real-time constraint. Modeling the tearing of tissue is a subject often neglected. However, there are two well-discussed problems arguing with these questions. The problem of cutting during surgical simulation also requires the modeling of topological changes under the real-time constraint. The animation of fracturing deals with the problem of indication start and propagation of cracks.

*Cutting of tissue*

Cotin et. al. [1] developed the tensor-mass model to allow topological changes in volumetric bodies in real-time. Cutting is modeled by removing tetrahedron elements from the mesh. This leads to unrealistic holes in the simulated body. Therefore, local mesh refinements of cutting area are introduced [2,3]. However, refinement leads to increased calculation times and may cause numerical instabilities. Nienhuys et. al. [4] adapts the mesh to the cut without changing the resolution.

*The animation of fracturing*

Neff et. al. [5] use a descriptive model to animate fracturing. In their approach, they distinguish between the creation and propagation of a crack. Crack propagation is considered much more likely. O'Brien et. al. [6] animate the fracture of brittle material. Their model is based on continuums mechanic. They use a Finite Element Discretization and analyze the stress tensor of each element to determine where, when and in what direction the body tears. Müller et. al. [7] use a hybrid approach to achieve real-time performance in their fracture and deformation model. They use rigid body simulation to calculate the movement of the objects. At collision events, a quasi-static FEM approach provides deformations and indicates the fracture.

## Methods

The presented approach is based on a mesh of mass nodes connected by triangles and springs. The springs are located at edges of the triangles and used for biomechanical simulation. In order to allow topological changes in real-time a mass-spring simulation with explicit integration methods calculates the deformations of the tissue. The triangles are needed for visualization.

*Topological changes*

Tear propagation is considered to take place along the springs of the mesh to keep the number of triangles constant. Tearing is modeled by duplicating the node and the spring that tear. Springs and triangles connected to the torn node must be divvied up between original and doubled node depending on what side of the crack they are located. Figure 1 illustrates modeling of tear propagation. Two additional cases need a special treatment. When a crack reaches an edge node, the mesh parts must be separated (see figure 2). The creation of a new crack needs the doubling of two springs in order to create a hole (see figure 3).

*Tear Criteria*

The presented approach uses tear criteria based following observations:

- Tearing is caused by elongation of tissue. Compression of a membrane does not lead to tearing.
- Tear propagation is much more probable than creation of a new crack.

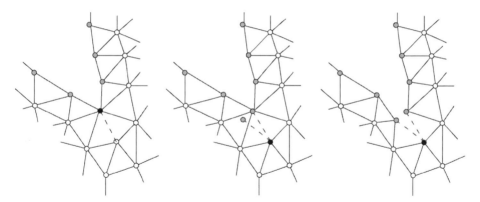

**Figure 1.** Tear propagation is modelled in two steps illustrated from left to right. From the left to the middle figure, the black coloured node and the dashed spring are doubled. From the middle to the right figure, the existing springs and triangles are divvied up between old and new node.

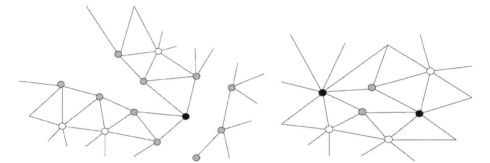

**Figure 2.** When the crack reaches an edge node (black), the two parts of the mesh must be separated.

**Figure 3.** The creation of a new crack required the doubling of one node and two springs.

- It is likely that a new crack starts at an edge of the membrane.
- The membrane is inhomogeneous: Weak areas exist that tear more probably than others do.

The model distinguishes three kinds of nodes: edge nodes, interior nodes, and sprouts. Sprouts are edge nodes located at the end of a crack. In the figures 1 to 3 sprout nodes are colored black, edge nodes are colored grey and the interior nodes are colored white. The mesh structure is analyzed to determine the node type. Edge nodes are nodes connected to an edge spring. Edge springs are springs bordering only one triangle. If a node is not connected to an edge spring, it is an internal node. Edge nodes must be further analyzed. An edge node is a sprout if one of its two neighboring edge nodes was created through doubling of the other neighboring edge node during a tear step before. This is indicated through identical initial positions of the nodes. Algorithm 1 shows how the node type is determined from the structure of the mesh, with $S(n_i)$ and $T(n_i)$ are the sets of springs respectively triangles connected with node $n_i$. $N(t_i)$ is the set of nodes connected with triangle $t_i$ and $N(s_i)_j$ is the j-th node of spring $s_i$. The actual implementation uses an edge flag for the nodes to speed up the algorithm.

```
Algorithm 1 type DetermineNodeType(nᵢ)
 1: edgeNeighbor1 = 0
 2: edgeNeighbor2 = 0
 3: for all sᵢ ∈ S(nᵢ) do
 4:    if IsEdgeSpring(sᵢ) then
 5:       for all nⱼ ∈ N(sᵢ) do
 6:          if not nⱼ = nᵢ then
 7:             if edgeNeighbor1 = 0 then
 8:                edgeNeighbor1 = nⱼ
 9:          else
10:                edgeNeighbor2 = nⱼ
11:             break
12: if edgeNeighbor1 == 0 then
13:    return IS_INTERIOR_NODE
14: else if edgeNeighbor1.initialPosition == edgeNeighbor2.initialPosition then
15:    return IS_SPROUT_NODE
16. else
17:    return IST_EDGE_NODE
```

```
Algorithm 2 bool IsEdgeSpring(sᵢ)
 1: n₁ = N(sᵢ)₁
 2: n₂ = N(sᵢ)₂
 3: counter = 0
 4: for all tᵢ ∈ T(n₁) do
 5:    for all nᵢ ∈ N(tᵢ) do
 6:       if nᵢ = n₂ then
 7:             ++counter;
 8: if counter == 1 then
 9:    return true
10: else
11:    return false
```

Stress in every node is analyzed to determine when and where tearing takes place. Node stress is defined proportional to the sum of the stresses of the elongated springs connected with the node. Stress of compressed springs is not considered, as compression does not lead to tearing. Every node has a tear factor weighting the node stress to map inhomogeneous structures to the membrane model. The three classes of nodes have different stress thresholds increasing from the sprouts to the edge nodes and to the interior nodes. Therefore, less local stress is necessary for tear propagation than for creation of a new crack that starts at an edge of the mesh. The creating of a new hole like in figure 3 needs the most node stress. In all three cases, the direction in which the mesh tears is determined by the spring with minimum relative length.

*Remarks*

Since a crack can only propagate along a spring direction, the mesh structure must reflect the tearing that may occur. A hexagonal mesh structure is better suited to model isotropic tearing than a square structure as the tear may propagate along six directions instead of four. For simulation involving radial and tangential tearing, a radial mesh like the ones in figure 4 and 5 are a good choice.

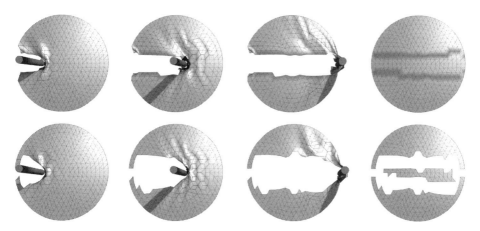

**Figure 4.** A mesh with 272 nodes, 758 springs, and 486 triangles tears when a cylinder is moved through it. Screenshots from the presented approach are displayed in the first row. The results of the straightforward method can be seen in the second row. The first three columns show the simulation after different time-steps. One can see that the results of the presented approach are close to the results with the high-resolution mesh displayed in figure 5. The last column shows the meshes after the tearing with all nodes reset to their initial position. The straightforward approach leads to considerable reduction of triangles.

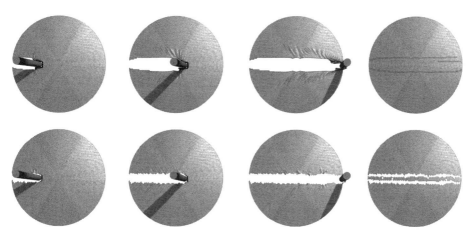

**Figure 5.** The figure shows the same simulation as figure 4 but with a mesh of 8587 nodes, 25440 springs, and 16854 triangles. The results of the two approaches are similar if the mesh has a high resolution.

Giving the springs an initial tension enables the modeling of brittle material. The spring elongation leads to initial stress in the nodes. If the stress is higher than the threshold for the sprout nodes but to low to tear an internal node the material is stable until a first tear is created for some reason. Then the tear propagates quickly through the whole mesh.

## Results

To rate the presented tearing method it is compared to a straightforward approach: The deletion of the springs that exceed a maximum length. Triangles connecting both nodes of the spring must also be removed to keep the consistency of the mesh.

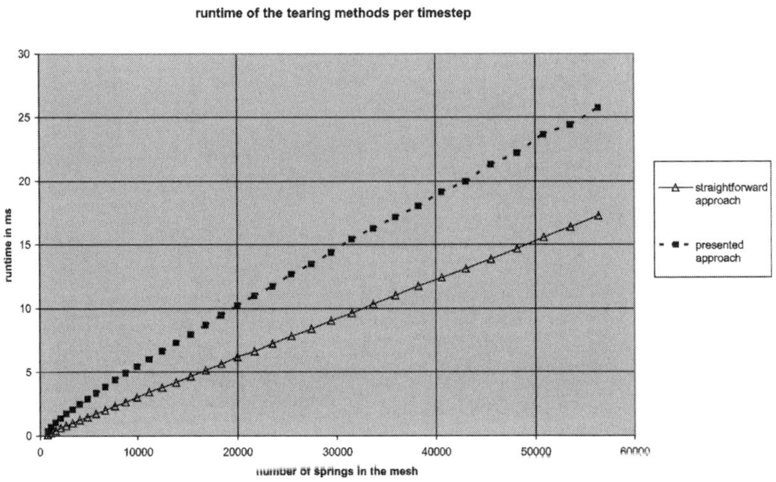

**runtime of the tearing methods per timestep**

**Figure 6.** Approximately, the runtime of both approaches is increased linear with the number of springs in the mesh. The presented method is slower than straightforward tearing.

A circular mesh with different resolutions is used to compare the approaches. A cylindrical object is causing the tearing by moved through the mesh. Movement of the object was recorded prior to the simulation to provide equal conditions. The time for the tissue calculation is measured and screenshots are captured during simulation. All measurements were made on a Pentium 4 system with 2.8 GHz under WindowsXP.

Figure 4 and 5 shows the tearing of the two approaches with different mesh resolutions. The two models show different behavior with a low-resolution mesh. Straightforward tearing leads to a reduction of triangles and frayed edges with low-resolution meshes. On high-resolution meshes, the differences are not so apparently. The presented approach behaves similar with both resolutions.

The diagram in figure 6 compares the runtimes of both approaches. They increase approximately linear with the number of springs in the mesh increasing. The straightforward approach is faster than the presented approach.

Based on the tearing approach described above and the simulation algorithm discussed in [8] two training modules were developed for the ophthalmosurgical simulator EYESI [9]: the peeling of the Internal Limiting Membrane and the Capsulorhexis procedure. Surgeons validating the training modules describe the tearing of the virtual membranes as realistic.

## Discussion

The presented tearing approach is suited and used for modeling membranes during interactive real-time surgical training. With low-resolution meshes, the tearing is more plausible compared with the straightforward approach. When the resolution of the mesh is increasing, both approaches show more and more similar behavior. The new algorithm is slower than the straightforward tearing. However, it is well suited to modeling stiff membranes. Stiff tissue require a lot of calculation time for the simulation to achieve numerical stability. The cost for the tearing can than be neglected.

# References

[1]  Cotin, Stephane; Delingette, Herve; Ayache, Nicholas: A Hybrid Elastic Model allowing Real-Time Cutting Deformations and Force-Feedback for Surgery Training and Simulation. 16 No 8 (2000), S. 437–452.

[2]  Bielser, Daniel; Maiwald, Volker A.; Gross, Markus H.: Interactive Cuts through 3-Dimensional Soft Tissue. In: Brunet, P. (Hrsg.); Scopigno, R. (Hrsg.): Computer Graphics Forum (Eurographics '99) Bd. 18(3), The Eurographics Association and Blackwell Publishers, 1999, S. 31–38.

[3]  Mor und Kanade 2000 Mor, Andrew B.; Kanade, Takeo: Modifying Soft Tissue Models: Progressive Cutting with Minimal New Element Creation. In: MICCAI, 2000, S. 598–607.

[4]  Nienhuys, Han-Wen; Stappen, A. F. d. A Delaunay approach to interactive cutting in Triangulated Surfaces. 2002.

[5]  Neff, Michael; Fiume, Eugene: A Visual Model For Blast Waves and Fracture. In: Graphics Interface, 1999, S. 193–202.

[6]  O'Brien, James F.; Hodgins, Jessica K.: Graphical modelling and animation of brittle fracture. In: Proceedings of ACM SIGGRAPH 1999, ACM Press/Addison-Wesley Publishing Co., August 1999. – ISBN 0–201–48560–5, S. 137–146.

[7]  Müller, Matthias; McMillan, Leonard; Dorsey, Julie; Jagnow, Robert: Real-time simulation of deformation and fracture of stiff materials. In: Proceedings of the Eurographic workshop on Computer animation and simulation, Springer-Verlag New York, Inc., 2001. – ISBN 3–211–83711–6, S. 113–124.

[8]  Grimm et al. 2004 Grimm, J.; Wagner, C.; Männer, R.: Interactive Real-time Simulation of the Internal Limiting Membrane. In: International Symposium on Medical Simulation. Cambridge, MA, June 2004, S. 153–16.

[9]  Wagner et al. 2002 Wagner, Clemens; Schill, Markus A.; Männer, Reinhard: Intraocular Surgery on a Virtual Eye. In: Communications of the ACM 45 (2002), July, Nr. 7, S. 45–49.

Medicine Meets Virtual Reality 13
James D. Westwood et al. (Eds.)
IOS Press, 2005

160

# Interactive Real-Time Simulation of an Endoscopic Polyp Removal

Johannes GRIMM

*Institute for Computational Medicine, University of Mannheim*

**Abstract.** The paper describes methods used for an interactive real-time training simulation of an endoscopic procedure: the removal of a colon polyp. Biomechanical simulation of the polyp is provided by a Finite Element approach. A combination of animation and simulation models the flexing, retraction and deployment of the used instrument, a wire sling. The presented method enables a training simulation of the surgery, based on the endoscopic simulator EndoSim.

## Introduction

Interactive real-time modeling of non-rigid bodies is a challenging field in the development of Virtual Reality simulators for medical surgery training. The simulated tissue must respond to the user's actions in a plausible way. The real-time constraint demands fast algorithms. Frame rates above 25 Hz leave 40 ms computation time per time-step for collision detection, simulation, and visualization. Since the human sense of touch can perceive frequencies up to about 1 kHz, the available computation time per time-step for force feedback systems is even more limited. To enable cutting and tearing of the simulated body, topological changes must also be applicable to the model within a single time-step.

   Due to the unfamiliar view and the difficult control of the instruments, endoscopic procedures need a lot of experience and permanent practice. Virtual Endoscopy may replace diagnostic endoscopies in many cases. However, when endoscopic invasions become necessary for therapeutic reasons, the physician lacks the practice of the diagnostic invasions. The endoscopic simulator EndoSim [1] enables the surgeon to train endoscopic invasions virtually. A training simulation developed for EndoSim is the removal of a colon polyp. The surgery is performed in the following steps:

1. The surgeon moves the tip of the endoscope through the colon to the location of the polyp.
2. A wire sling is wrapped around the polyp.
3. An electric current through the wire sling cuts off the polyp from the colon wall and seals the veins to prevent bleeding.
4. The polyp is grasped with forceps, torn apart and pulled out of the colon.

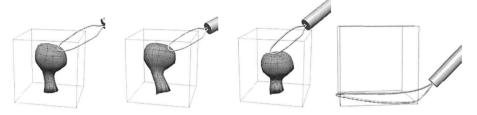

**Figure 1.** The deformations of the polyp and the wire sling are modeled with a Finite Element approach using linear elasticity and an implicit Houbolt integration.

## Previous Work

Many approaches exist to model soft tissue. The most common are Mass-Spring models and the Finite Element Method (FEM). FEM is an accurate method based on continuums mechanics. Combined with an implicit integration scheme it is unconditional stable. On the other hand it needs a lot of calculation time especially when the mesh's topology is changed to model cutting or tearing. Many approaches exist to speed up FEM like Condensation [2] or hybrid approaches that combine a local FEM with a pre-calculated model [3] or a rigid body simulation [4]. To handle topological changes in real-time the Tensor-Mass [3] model uses mass-lumping and an explicit integration scheme, which lacks the unconditional stability of an implicit approach. When simulated objects encounter large rotations, simplification of a linear elasticity approximation becomes noticeable. The volume of the simulated body is increasing which is an unrealistic behavior. Nonlinear approaches [5,6] solve the problem but increase the calculation time necessary to calculate the forces.

## Methods

A Finite Element approach and a Catmull-Rom spline animation technique calculate deformations of polyp and the wire sling.

### Deformation and tearing of the polyp

The simulation approach is based on the theory of linear elasticity. A mesh consisting of 4-node tetrahedron Finite Elements models the simulated body. Linear elasticity and the used Finite Elements are for example described in [3]. The implicit Houbolt approach [7] is used as integration scheme because of its stability. Figure 1 shows examples of the deformed polyp.

During the intervention, the only topological change is the tearing of the polyp. Although the polyp is torn apart by pulling with the forceps, the location of the crack is determined before, when the current is send through the wire sling. This enables us to generate separate meshes for the two parts of the torn polyp and to do the necessary pre-processing before the tearing starts. Calculations are processed in a background thread to ensure a continuous simulation. When the tearing starts, the simulation of the whole polyp is stopped and the actual positions, velocities, and accelerations of the nodes are copied to the meshes of the polyp parts. Then the simulations of the two parts start. To

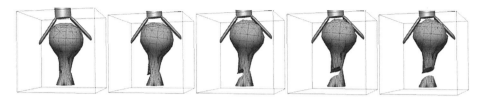

**Figure 2.** The two parts of the polyp are simulated separately.

animate the tearing process the two parts are "glued" together by setting the positions of two corresponding nodes of the two parts to a common value. This is done every time-step until a certain distance is reached. Figure 2 shows the tearing of the polyp.

*Flexing, retraction and deployment of the wire sling*

During surgery, the wire sling is first deployed then wrapped around the polyp and re-tracted again to better enclose the polyp. Physicians sometimes flex the wire sling by pressing the loose end of the sling at the colon wall to wrap the sling around the polyp. A Catmull-Rom [8,9] spline animates the retraction and deployment of the wire sling. Unlike a Bezier spline, the Catmull-Rom curve passes through all control points, which makes it easy to control the curve. A set of control points describe the curve of the wire sling. A Catmull-Rom spline is used to construct the sling out of the control points. Re-traction and deployment of the sling is modeled by moving the control points. Therefore, an additional Catmull-Rom spline is defined for every control point describing the tra-jectory of the point during deployment. The Finite Element approach described above is used to simulate the flexing of the sling (see figure 1).

**Results and Discussion**

A simulation was developed to train the endoscopic removal of a colon polyp. Since the Finite Element approach is based on an implicit integration algorithm, it is numerically stable. A Catmull-Rom spline animation enables modeling of retraction and deployment of a wire sling in real-time. On the test system (Pentium4 HT 2.8 GHz), simulation and animation together need about 11 ms calculation time per time-step to model polyp (1500 tetrahedrons, 396 nodes) and wire sling (600 tetrahedrons, 404 nodes). That is fast enough for smooth visualization. For force feedback, the algorithm would require further improvements. Currently, EndoSim does not support force-feedback for the instrument channel. Tearing of the polyp is modeled in background. Generation and preparation of the simulation meshes for the two polyp parts need about 437 ms computation time on the test system. This is sufficient since the user must change the instruments before the tearing starts. Switching the simulation from the whole polyp to the polyp parts needs less than one ms. Accuracy of the simulation is limited by the assumption of linear elas-ticity. This is a problem when deformable objects encounter large rotations. However, the accuracy of the model is sufficient to enable training simulations under the limited conditions of an endoscopic surgery.

# References

[1]  Körner, O., Männer, R.: Implementation of a Haptic Interface for a Virtual Reality Simulator for Flexible Endoscopy. In Hannaford, B., Tan, H., eds.: 11th Symposium on Haptic Interfaces for Virtual Environment and Teleoperator Systems, IEEEVR2003, Los Angeles, USA (2003) 278–284.

[2]  Bro-Nielsen, Morten; Cotin, Stephane: Real-time Volumetric Deformable Models for Surgery Simulation using Finite Elements and Condensation. In: Computer Graphics Forum 15 (1996), Nr. 3, S. 57–66.

[3]  Cotin, Stephane; Delingette, Hervé; Ayache, Nicholas: A Hybrid Elastic Model allowing Real-Time Cutting Deformations and Force-Feedback for Surgery Training and Simulation. 16 No 8 (2000), S. 437–452.

[4]  Müller, Matthias; McMillan, Leonard; Dorsey, Julie; Jagnow, Robert: Real-time simulation of deformation and fracture of stiff materials. In: Proceedings of the Eurographic workshop on Computer animation and simulation, Springer-Verlag New York, Inc., 2001. – ISBN 3–211–83711–6, S. 113–124.

[5]  Picinbono, G.; Delingette, Herve; Ayache, Nicholas: Real-Time Large Displacement Elasticity for Surgery Simulation: Non-linear Tensor-Mass Model. In: MICCAI, 2000, S. 643–652.

[6]  Wu et al. 2001 Wu, X.; Downes, M.s.; Gotektekin, F: Adaptive nonlinear finite elements for deformable body simulation using dynamic progressive meshes. In: Eurographics Volume 20 Bd. 20, 2001, S. 349–358.

[7]  Bathe, K.J.: Finite-Elemente-Method. Springer (1990).

[8]  Catmull, E., Rom, R.: A class of local interpolationg splines. Barnhill R.E. and R.F. Riesen ed (eds.), Computer Aided Geometric Design (1974).

[9]  Faux, I., M.J., P.: Computational geometry for design and manufacture. Barnhill R.E. and R.F. Riesen ed (eds.), Computer Aided Geometric Design (1979).

164

*Medicine Meets Virtual Reality 13*
*James D. Westwood et al. (Eds.)*
*IOS Press, 2005*

# Surgical Robot Setup Simulation with Consistent Kinematics and Haptics for Abdominal Surgery

Mitsuhiro HAYASHIBE [a], Naoki SUZUKI [a], Asaki HATTORI [a], Shigeyuki SUZUKI [a], Kozo KONISHI [b], Yoshihiro KAKEJI [b] and Makoto HASHIZUME [b]

[a] *Institute for High Dimensional Medical Imaging, Jikei Univ. School of Medicine, 4-11-1, Izumihoncho, Komae-shi, Tokyo 201 8601 Japan*
[b] *Center for Integration of Advanced Med. and Innovative Technology, Kyushu University Hospital, 3-1-1, Maidashi, Higashi-ku, Fukuoka 812-8582 Japan*

**Abstract.** Preoperative simulation and planning of surgical robot setups should accompany advanced robotic surgery if their advantages are to be further pursued. Feedback from the planning system will plays an essential role in computer-aided robotic surgery in addition to preoperative detailed geometric information from patient CT/MRI images. Surgical robot setup simulation systems for appropriate trocar site placement have been developed especially for abdominal surgery. The motion of the surgical robot can be simulated and rehearsed with kinematic constraints at the trocar site, and the inverse-kinematics of the robot. Results from simulation using clinical patient data verify the effectiveness of the proposed system.

## 1. Preface

Useful robotic operation systems such as the da Vinci$^{TM}$ surgical system of Intuitive Surgical Inc. [1] and ZEUS$^{TM}$ of Computer Motion Inc., which realize minimally invasive surgery with increased dexterity, are presently available. In the operating room, surgeons have to prepare and set up an environment where the robot is able to have adequate degrees of freedom for motion so the function of the robot can be fully performed for each clinical case. An optimal set up will vary with the type of interventions and the equipment used in the operation. An adequate placement of the trocar ports maximizes the movability of a robot, and significantly influences the success of an operation. Moreover, the region in which the robot can reach and be maneuvered is restrained by the fixed point at the trocar sites; therefore, in each case these sites have to be carefully chosen for the particular patient.

## 2. Preoperative setup simulation for robotic surgery

Some research groups have developed a setup simulation system and an image guided navigation system for robotic surgery [2,3]. Optimized port-placement planning for cardiac surgery was addressed in [2] where a mathematical algorithm was implemented.

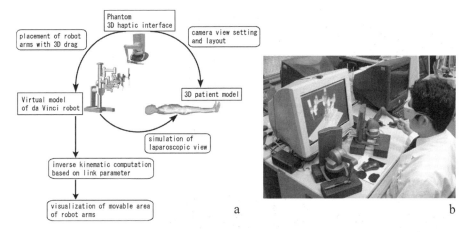

**Figure 1.** (a) System Configuration. (b) This system provides stereoscopic vision of virtual laparoscopic image using liquid crystal shutter glasses and quad buffering. Surgeons can push and drag the arms of the virtual surgical robot which has same kinematics as the real one.

A Data-Fusion system in which an inner structure virtual model is superimposed onto the live laparoscopic image according to the direction of scope was developed in [3]. In this paper, we have developed a robot setup simulation system with kinematic and haptic function for appropriate trocar site placement for abdominal surgery. The motion of the surgical robot can be simulated and rehearsed in advance with the computation of collisions between the robot arms, the constraints at the trocar site, and the inverse-kinematics of the robot. Being integrated with a haptic interface, surgeons can push and drag the arms of the virtual surgical robot which has same kinematics as the real one. Each link shape and distances between links of the da Vinci surgical system were measured in detail, and the geometric model was then created and reconstructed in a 3D CAD software. Each link is described with the information including the child-parent relationship based on Denavit-Hartenberg notation. This system mainly consists of this da Vinci geometric model, typical 3D patient model and haptic device as shown in Fig.1 (a). The typical patient model of a whole body structure was reconstructed from MRI images scanned at 4mm intervals. For gastroenterological surgery, there are patient models of stomach, liver, intestines, and kidney along with texture information. This typical model can be used for general planning and in educational trials. Indeed, for clinical use and fine planning, the preoperative CT/MRI image data of each patient should be segmented.

Once the trocar site has been determined, the manipulator makes a pivoting motion around the incision point. The arm's movable range, which depends on the fixed point, is shown in the planning window. Setup planning can be conducted as the way in which an endoscope is first inserted and then forceps are guided with reference to the virtual stereo laparoscopic images. This system provides stereoscopic vision using liquid crystal shutter glasses and quad buffering like in Fig.1 (b) to help spatial perception.

## 3. Planning for laparoscopic cholecystectomy using clinical data

The initial pose of the surgical robot and the incision site of the robot arm in laparoscopic cholecystectomy have been be discussed and planned in this developed system. Fig.2 (a)

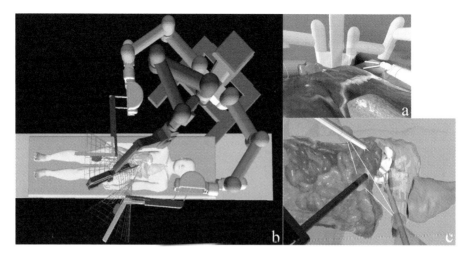

**Figure 2.** (a) Laparoscopic camera view is depicted in subwindow. (b) Surgical robot setup simulation for cholecystectomy. (c) Port placement was examined for patient model of cholecyst and hepatic duct.

shows the appearance of a da Vinci setup simulation. For clinical planning, the preoperative CT/MRI image data of each patient should be segmented. Suitable acquisitions have to therefore be performed on each patient. The MRCP images of the patient, who was actually operated on with a da Vinci system, were used and processed for clinical evaluation. ICP registration was conducted to replace the liver model of a typical whole body model with the particular patient liver model. Fig.2 (b) depicts the results of the setup simulation. The triangle shows the positional relationship of the two forceps ports and the camera port. We could confirm the feasibility of the surgical robot setup simulation which reflects each patient's structure information by using preoperatively scanned images.

## 4. Conclusion

A surgical robot setup simulation system for abdominal surgery has been developed with kinematic and haptic function. The motion of the surgical robot could be simulated and rehearsed preoperatively with the constraints at the trocar site, and the inverse- kinematics computation of the surgical robot providing a haptic sensation.

## References

[1]  G. S. Guthart and J. K. Salisbury, "The Intuitive Telesurgery System," Proceedings of the IEEE International Conference on Robotics and Automation, pp.618-621, 2000.
[2]  L. Adhami and E. Coste-Maniere, "A versatile system for computer integrated mini-invasive robotic surgery," Lecture Notes in Computer Science 2488: MICCAI2002, pp 272-281, 2002.
[3]  A. Hattori, N. Suzuki, M. Hashizume, T. Akahoshi, K. Konishi, S. Yamaguchi, M. Shimada, M. Hayashibe, "A robotic surgery system (da Vinci) with image guided function System architecture and cholecystectomy application," Medicine Meets Virtual Reality 11, IOS Press, pp.110-116, 2003.

Medicine Meets Virtual Reality 13
James D. Westwood et al. (Eds.)
IOS Press, 2005

# Development of a Navigation Function for an Endosocopic Robot Surgery System

Asaki HATTORI [a], Naoki SUZUKI [a], Mitsuhiro HAYASHIBE [a], Shigeyuki SUZUKI [a], Yoshito OTAKE [a], Hisao TAJIRI [b] and Susumu KOBAYASHI [c]

[a] Institute for High Dimensional Medical Imaging, The Jikei Univ.
School of Med., 4-11-1 Izumihoncho, Komae-shi 201-8601, Tokyo, Japan
[b] Dept. of Endoscopy, The Jikei Univ. School of Med., 3-25-8
Nishishinbashi, Minato-ku 105-8461, Tokyo, Japan
[c] Dept. of Surg., The Jikei Univ. School of Med., 3-25-8
Nishishinbashi, Minato-ku 105-8461, Tokyo, Japan

**Abstract.** An endoscopic robot system that we reported at MMVR11 is able to perform various surgical procedures in the stomach by using two manipulators. However, it is difficult for surgeons to recognize the 3D location and the direction of the endoscope's tip in the abdominal region during robotic surgery. In this research, we have developed a navigation function that enables image-guided surgery by superimposing the patient's abdominal organ structure onto the endoscopic image. In this paper, we describe the overview of the navigation for the robot system and the result of an animal experiment done while applying the system.

## 1. Purpose

We have been developing an endoscopic robot system for abdominal surgery. The robot system has two forceps type manipulators located beside the tip of the endoscope. The robot is inserted through the mouth and enables the surgeon to perform various surgical procedures in the abdominal region without making any incisions on the body surface. Because of the flexibility and the narrow field of view of the endoscope, it is difficult for the surgeon to understand the 3D location and the direction of the robot during the surgery. Therefore, we have developed a navigation function for the robot system. The function superimposes the patient's 3D organ models onto the endoscope's image according to the endoscope's movement in real-time. We will describe the system's overview and the result of an animal experiment that we performed using this system.

## 2. Methods

This system consists of an endoscopic robot system and a data fusion system. Figure 1 shows the system's outline. The left part shows the endoscopic robot system, and the right part shows the data fusion system. The endoscopic robot system is a master-slave device and two forceps type manipulators are attached to the endoscope (Figure 2). The

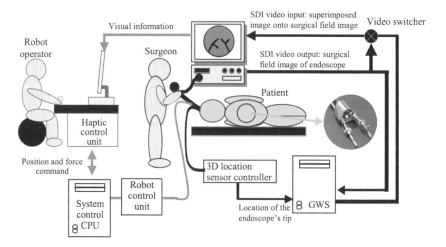

**Figure 1.** Outline of the system. Left side is a component of the endoscopic robot system. Right side shows a setup of the navigation function.

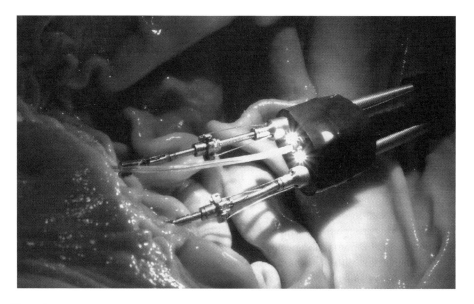

**Figure 2.** An appearance of the endoscopic robot. Two forceps type manipulators are attached to a tip of the endoscope. These manipulators enable to perform various surgical procedures in a stomach.

detail of the robot system was reported at MMVR11. The data fusion system consists of two devices. One is a graphic workstation (GWS: OCTANE MXE, Silicon Graphics Inc.) that captures the endoscopic image, superimposes a 3D organ model onto the image and outputs to the monitor of the endoscope. The other device is the magnetic location sensor (miniBird, Ascension Technology Co.) that is attached to the endoscope's tip (Figure 3) and tracks the location and the direction of the endoscope. We use titanium to a component that fixes the manipulators to the endoscope, because a metal object that has a large volume affects the magnetic sensor's accuracy.

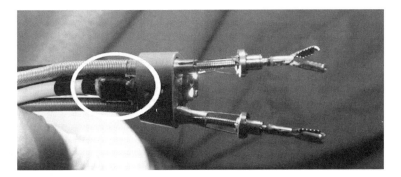

**Figure 3.** The magnetic location sensor that is attached to the bottom of the endoscopic robot.

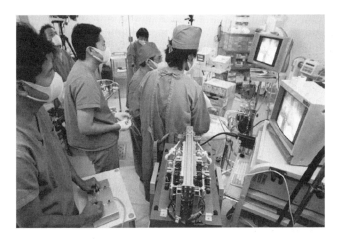

**Figure 4.** A scene of the animal experiment. The surgeon (center) and the robot operator (left) performed EMR procedures by their cooperative work.

Before we apply the data fusion system to the endoscopic robot system, two measurements are required. First, the endoscope's optical parameters have to be determined to project the 3D organ model on a computer display. We measured the parameters by capturing an endoscopic image of a reference board that previously measured squares are printed. The second procedure is a registration to transform the organ model coordinate system into a surgical field coordinate system. We determined these coordinate systems by measuring some locations on the actual body surface and pointing the same locations on the organ model from the GWS display.

After these measurements, GWS transforms the coordinate system of the 3D organ model to the surgical field coordinate system and renders the 3D organ model image by using the positional data of the location sensor.

## 3. Results

We applied this system to an endoscopic mucosal resection (EMR) of a pig. Before the experiment, we measured the inner structures of the pig by X-ray CT. The body surface, spine, ribs, liver and liver artery models were reconstructed from the dataset. Figure 4

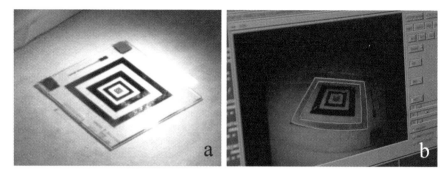

**Figure 5.** A scene of the measurement for the endoscope's optical parameter. The endoscope's image of the reference board (a) was captured and processed on the GWS (b).

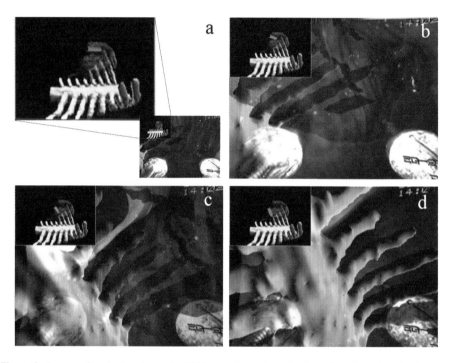

**Figure 6.** A scene of navigation during the EMR procedure. Figure 6a shows the sub window that indicates the current location of the endoscope's tip in the coordinate system of the organ models. The organ models are superimposed onto the endoscope's image. According to the endoscope movement (in this figures b-d, the endoscope moves from right to left while looking down to the spine), the superimposed organ models follow the movement.

shows a scene of the animal experiment. We measured the endoscope's optical parameter (Figure 5) and registered the coordinate system by pointing to the same position of the actual body surface and the organ model. After the measurement, the endoscopic robot was inserted into the stomach and the organ models were superimposed onto the endoscopic image. The results of the navigation are illustrated at figure 6. The top left sub window indicates the current location of the endoscope's tip in the coordinate system of the organ models (Figure 6a). The surgeon was able to change the viewpoint of this window interactively and identify the location of the endoscope. The spine, ribs and hepatic artery models were superimposed onto the endoscopic image. The images b-d show the results when the endoscope moved from right to left. As the endoscope moved, the organ models were transformed to a proper location of the endoscopic image in real-time. According to the situation of the surgical field, the surgeon can switch the normal endoscopic video image to the navigation video image using a video switcher.

## 4. Conclusion

The surgeon was able to perform EMR procedures applying the navigation function to the endoscopic robot surgery system with that followed the endoscope movement. The navigation function enabled the surgeon to understand the 3D orientation of the endoscope in the abdomen during the surgery.

We are trying a new surgical method that performs surgical procedures to other abdominal organs by the robot system that penetrates a stomach wall and approaches the abdominal cavity. At the trial, we found the navigation function was necessary to approach the targeted organs safety and quickly. In the current system, it is difficult for the surgeon to know the distance between the endoscope's tip and organ model. Therefore, we are going to develop a more suitable display method for the endoscopic robot system.

## References

[1] Suzuki N, Sumiyama K, Hattori A, Ikeda K, Murakami EAY, Suzuki S, Hayashibe M, Otake Y, Tajiri H. Development of an endoscopic robotic system with two hands for various gastric tube surgeries. Medicine Meets Virtual Reality 11 2003: 349-53.
[2] Hattori A, Suzuki N, Hashizume M, Akahoshi T, Konishi K, Yamaguchi S, Shimada M, Hayashibe M. A robotic surgery system (da Vinci) with image guided function. Medicine Meets Virtual Reality 11 2003: 110-6.

*Medicine Meets Virtual Reality 13*
*James D. Westwood et al. (Eds.)*
*IOS Press, 2005*

# Development of a 3D Visualization System for Surgical Field Deformation with Geometric Pattern Projection

Mitsuhiro HAYASHIBE [a], Naoki SUZUKI [a], Susumu KOBAYASHI [b],
Norio NAKATA [a], Asaki HATTORI [a] and Yoshihiko NAKAMURA [c]

[a] *Institute for High Dimensional Medical Imaging, The Jikei Univ. School of Medicine*
*4-11-1, Izumihoncho, Komae shi, Tokyo 201-8601 Japan*
[b] *Department of Surgery, The Jikei Univ. School of Medicine*
*3-25-8, Nishishinbashi, Minato-ku, Tokyo 105-8461 Japan*
[c] *Department of Mechano-Informatics, University of Tokyo*
*7-3-1, Hongo, Bunkyo-ku, Tokyo 113-8656 Japan*

**Abstract.** Intra-operative navigation in which the target position is provided to assist an intuitive understanding of the surgical field has been studied and applied in many clinical areas. Position measurement of a surgical field is usually performed with a magnetic sensor, a marker type optical position sensor. For navigation of hard tissue, the measurement of several markers dispersedly located on the surface is enough to detect the position of an object that can be assumed as a rigid body. However, for the navigation of soft tissue such as skin and liver, a sensor that can measure the deformation of the object surface time-sequentially would be essential. We have developed a 3D visualization system for surgical field deformation with geometric pattern projection. In an animal experiment, the registration of preoperative 3D organ model could be done with the time-sequentially updated surface deformation data. In the video image of surgical field, the inner structure model of organ could be superimposed successfully.

## 1. Introduction

In recent years, intra-operative navigation in which the target position is provided to assist an intuitive understanding of the surgical field has been studied and recently applied in many clinical areas. This image-guided surgery is mainly introduced for orthopedics and neuro surgery. Position measurement of a surgical field is usually performed with instruments such as a magnetic sensor [1,2] and a marker type optical position sensor [3,4]. For navigation of hard tissue such as bone, the measurement of several markers dispersedly located on the surface is sufficient to detect the position of an object that can be assumed as a rigid body. However, for the navigation of soft tissue such as skin and liver, a sensor that can detect the deformation of the object surface time-sequentially is required. In this study, a PC generated geometrical pattern projected on the object surface is captured by digital video (DV) cameras from multiple angles. This system is easily set up in an operation room and can visualize the 3D deformation and texture of the living body.

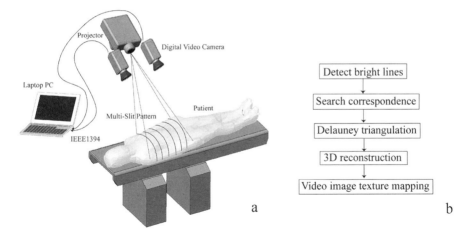

**Figure 1.** (a) System configuration. (b) Computation routine.

## 2. Method

In this system, a multi-slit pattern generated by a PC is projected on the body of the target, and synchronous photography is carried out by two sets of commercially available DV cameras. The system configuration is illustrated in Fig. 1 (a). The real-time image capture is carried out via an IEEE1394 interface of a laptop computer using DirectX, and areas with high luminosity are segmented by image processing. Next, corresponding points on the two images are searched using epipolar geometry. Then, Delaunay triangulation is carried out on the left 2D image coordinate system of a point set that has a corresponding point on the right image; finally, 3D coordinates are calculated using the solved camera parameter. Further, texture coordinates are also computed from the relationship of the correspondence with an original color image, and texture mapping is performed from the video image of the surgical field. The procedure for this system is summarized in Fig. 1 (b). Acquisition and visualization of a 3D surface form and its texture on an area of interest need to be achievable by equipment such as this that can be set up easily in an operating room; not just in a huge and expensive facility designed for the purpose.

For camera calibration, a checkered board is used and is simultaneously captured with two cameras while the posture of the board is changed for a period of time just before measurements are made. This instantly solves the internal parameter of each of the two cameras and the position relation between the two external camera parameters. This is a very useful way to calibrate parameters and can be executed quickly and easily during an operation. For details of the calculations and algorithms, other literature [5,6] should be referred to. Fig. 2 is the graph of the differential error between the detected corners of the checker board on the real picture and the re-projected corners in the computed projection matrix on the image plane. The calibration was performed at about 700-800mm distance, being the distance of an object placed in an actual clinical situation. (a) is the result when the resolution is 360×240 and (b) when it is 720×480. The RMS error for the resolution of 360×240 was 0.1157 pixel and for 720×480 was 0.107 pixel. 35 points of the grid per one frame were used for this calibration, and 16 frames were captured in this case. It is considered that both results show sufficient accuracy to undertake 3D reconstruction. Although the accuracy of the reconstruction in the case of 720×480 is

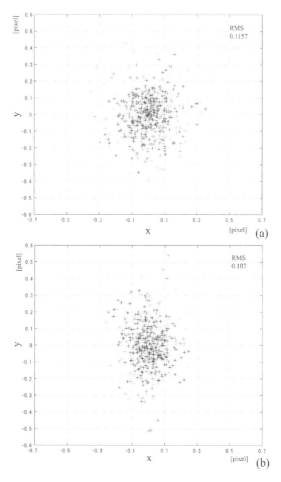

**Figure 2.** Reprojection error in camera calibration (a) For a resolution of 360×240 (b) For a resolution of 720×480.

good, judgment should be made considering the balance of accuracy with reconstruction processing speed.

## 3. Visualization of a deforming hand

Fig. 3 shows the result of measuring the change of the form of a hand. The 3D surface form and the texture of the hand at the time of moving from a to d was able to be visualized in 9 fps for the 360×240 image resolution and at 2 fps for the 720×480 image resolution. PC specification is listed as follows: (CPU: Dual Xeon Processor 2.8GHz, Memory: 2GB RAM, Video Card: $nVidia^{TM}$ Quadro FX1000).

Here, the wire frame of the generated polygon is also depicted to show the sampled resolution. To make a concavo-convex situation understandable, a reconstructed 3D form is rotated and displayed from a slanting direction.

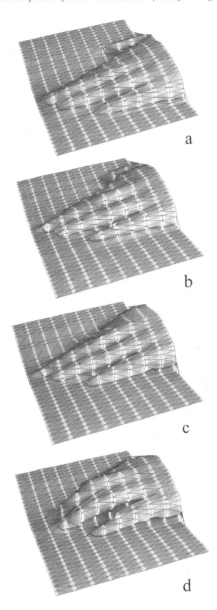

**Figure 3.** Result of the visualization of a deforming hand. The 3D surface form and the texture of the hand at the time of moving from a to d could be visualized at 9 fps.

## 4. In-vivo experiment and volumetric Data-Fusion

The system was verified for the body surface and liver of an anesthetized pig. The experiment in-vivo set up is shown in Fig. 4 (a). Fig. 4 (b) shows the visualized 3D surface map of the abdominal surface. To demonstrate that it can measure a surface with some unevenness, a hand in a surgical glove was placed on the body surface. With this system, since the 3D surface data of an object can be obtained almost instantly, it becomes possible to perform registrations reflecting the latest deformation of a body surface or

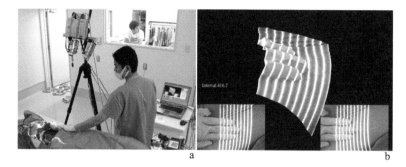

**Figure 4.** (a) A picture of the in-vivo experiment with an anesthetized pig. (b) The visualized 3D surface map of the abdominal surface. A hand in a surgical glove is placed on the body surface.

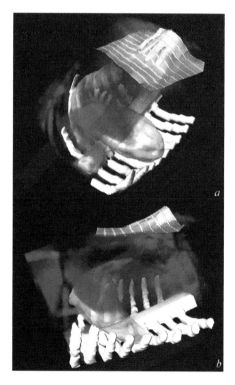

**Figure 5.** (a) Full view of the volumetric navigation of the inner structure based on the scanned skin surface. Volume data of abdomen was rendered as blue MIP image along with segmented surface data of pig's liver, hepatic vein and ribs. (b) Side view of this scene. Green line shows the angiographic catheter used for contrast enhancement.

elastic organs. Here, a point-based method [7,8] previously applied in other research for navigation in brain and orthopedic surgery was used and confirmed the registration of preoperative CT images. The preoperative model was segmented and created for the body surface, bones, and the liver and its blood vessels based on CT scans with contrast enhancement. Data-Fusion navigation was performed by registration of the preoperative model to intra-operatively scanned data, and visualizing the volume data of the original CT images by fusion as shown in Fig. 5.

## 5. Conclusion and Discussion

A system for 3D visualization of a surgical field deformation that can easily be set up in an operating room was developed. This system enables simultaneous measurement and visualization of a 3D form and its texture at 9 fps using the real-time capture of a geometrical pattern projected from a PC projector. The in-vivo experiment was conducted and the feasibility of this system to a living body was confirmed. This information can be applied and utilized for surgical navigation that can respond to soft tissue deformation. The navigation of present position to the volume data of trunk was able to be performed. Evaluation and verification of this system is going to be performed applying for clinical cases.

## References

[1] POLHEMUS Inc. FASTRAK. http://www.polhemus.com/, 2004.
[2] Ascension Technology Corporation. miniBIRD. http://www.ascension-tech.com/, 2004.
[3] Northern Digital Technology Inc. Polaris. http://www.ndigital.com/polaris.html, 2004.
[4] Northern Digital Technology Inc. Optotrak. http://www.ndigital.com/optotrak.html, 2004.
[5] Z. Zhang, "A flexible new technique for camera calibration," IEEE Transactions on Pattern Analysis and Machine Intelligence, Vol.22, No.11, pp.1330-1334, 2000.
[6] R. Y. Tsai, "A versatile camera calibration technique for high accuracy 3D machine vision metrology using off-the-shelf TV cameras and lenses," IEEE J. Robotics Automat., Vol.RA-3, No.4, pp.323-344, 1987.
[7] KS Arun, TS Huang, and SD Blostein, "Least-squares fitting of two 3-d point sets," IEEE Trans Pattern Anal Mach Intell, Vol.9, pp.698-700, 1987.
[8] BKP Horn, "Closed-form solution of absolute orientation using unit quaternions," J Opt Soc Am A, Vol.4, No.4, pp.629-642, 1987.
[9] M Hayashibe, N Suzuki, A Hattori, Y Nakamura, "Intraoperative Fast 3D Shape Recovery of Abdominal Organs in Laparoscopy" Proceedings MICCAI. Volume 2489 of LNCS, Springer, pp.356-363, 2002.

*Medicine Meets Virtual Reality 13*
*James D. Westwood et al. (Eds.)*
*IOS Press, 2005*

# In Vivo Force During Arterial Interventional Radiology Needle Puncture Procedures

Andrew E. HEALEY [a,e], Jonathan C. EVANS [a], Micheal G. MURPHY [a],
Steven POWELL [a], Thien V. HOW [c], David GROVES [b], Fraser HATFIELD [b],
Bernard M. DIAZ [d] and Derek A. GOULD [b]

[a] *Dept of Radiology, Royal Liverpool University Hospital, Prescot St,
Liverpool L7 8XP, UK*
[b] *Dept of Medical Imaging, University of Liverpool, Brownlow Hill,
Liverpool, L69 3GB, UK*
[c] *Dept of Clinical Engineering, University of Liverpool, Prescot St,
Liverpool L7 8XP, UK*
[d] *Dept of Computer Science, University of Liverpool, Peach St,
Liverpool L69 7ZF, UK*
[e] *Cook/Medtronic Fellow*

**Abstract.** To adequately simulate the forces generated during interventional radiological (IR) procedures, non intrusive in-vivo methods must be used. Using finger
tip mounted, non intrusive capacitance force sensor pads (PPS, Los Angeles, California) we have been able to measure the forces involved in interventional radiology without a change in procedure technique. Data acquired during the process
of calibration of the capacitance pads in conjunction with extensive in-vitro needle
puncture force measurement using a commercially available tensile tester (Nene
Industries, UK) are presented here.

## 1. Introduction

Interventional Radiology is minimal access surgery using manipulation of needles, wires
and catheters. IR procedures generally commence with placement of a needle and demand for these procedures is increasing, yet there is a shortage of radiologists both in
the UK and worldwide. Apprenticeship training relies on straightforward, invasive diagnostic studies in patients under supervision, but such cases are being replaced by non
invasive imaging methods (CT and MR) and alternative training paradigms are required.
Models for needle puncture training lack robustness and are destroyed by repeated punctures. Animal models have anatomical differences [1], a lack of pathology and, in the UK,
of political acceptability. Virtual reality (VR) simulator models using real CT and MR
data have the potential to simulate many procedures, though there is a lack of VR models
of arterial needle puncture for interventional radiological procedures. Some models of
venepuncture (eg: using the Immersion, Cathsim device [2]) exist, as do lumbar puncture

and liver biopsy simulations [3–5] but force feedback in existing virtual reality simulators is typically based on mathematical models and the subjective assessment of experts. Incorporation of empirical data measured during procedures on patients should improve the feel of a simulated procedure and enhance the authenticity of the simulator [6]. Tissue deformation, and cutting and friction forces, during *in vitro* prostate needle placement have been investigated [7] as well as needle forces in cadaveric dog prostate [8] and a soft tissue phantom [9]. In developing realistic simulation of IR needle puncture procedures in virtual environments, it is important to have accurate models of instrument-tissue interaction [10,11], though the complexity of these forces requires direct measurement of tissues *in vitro* and, owing to differences of tissue physical properties in life, *in vivo* [12]. Our literature searches have, however, revealed no references to *in vivo*, human vascular needle force measurement and indeed there has been a dearth of unobtrusive devices, which might be used to measure instrument forces in the sterile, *in vivo* environment. Measurement systems for *in vitro* studies [7–9] have allowed a high degree of accuracy but were generally cumbersome and not easily applicable to the *in vivo* scenario. The development of flexible capacitance pads presents a novel opportunity to collect these data *in vivo* [12].

## 2. Materials and Method

### 2.1. Calibration

Static testing was initially completed using a laboratory test rig. Fixed masses were used to establish a maximal range of sensor output voltage over the estimated range of in-vivo forces to be measured. Voltages were measured using a digital voltmeter. Masses were applied to the sensors over a range of surface areas to establish that true force, and not pressure, was being measured. The sensors were then subjected to masses increasing by 50g amounts to a maximum of 1050g, the mass was then reduced serially to zero. This process was repeated to establish linear behaviour with increasing force upon the sensor.

Dynamic testing using a test rig consisting of a manufactured finger jig, on which a capacitance sensor could be mounted, was performed using a tensile tester (Nene Industries, UK). A spring was compressed to different forces driven by the tensile tester and held at that force to allow capacitance sensor output to be measured. Output from the capacitance pads was measured using a laptop PC (Dell Computers, USA) via a USB analogue-to-digital converter (Measurement Computing, PMD-1208LS, USA). This testing demonstrated excellent reproducibility in force measurement, the voltage output of the capacitance pads was found not to be linear with respect to applied force but could be modelled accurately using a third order polynomial equation [13].

Further dynamic testing was carried out using tissue substitutes (plasticine, polystyrene, Playdough, cardboard, silastic rubber). Correlation between input force, as measured and applied by the tensile tester, and output voltage from the capacitance sensor pads following translation using the polynomial calibration equation were evaluated and found to be satisfactory.

Dynamic frequency response testing was completed using a high frequency low amplitude bench oscillator with square wave input. This showed responsiveness far in excess of that required to measure physiological systems.

## 2.2. In-Vitro

### 2.2.1. Liver

Ox liver with time minimised from slaughter to laboratory use was used for in-vitro estimation of liver needle puncture force. Liver was chosen as the initial test substrate because it has a homogenous tissue structure lacking macroscopic anatomical variation in its peripheral parenchyma. Ox liver was chosen as the specific test medium to provide sufficient depth of tissue in the organs homogeneous periphery during needle puncture. A range of needles were mounted on the tensile tester finger jig and were driven into the tissue at a fixed rate, 500mm per minute, an approximation of the speed of needle insertion during interventional radiological procedures. Needle orientation was normal to the liver surface being punctured, depth of puncture was 6cm. Output force data from the tensile tester and the capacitance pad output voltage were continuously measured. Punctures were repeated to obtain an average and a range of forces involved. Output from the capacitance pads was measured using a laptop PC via a USB analogue-to-digital converter.

Needles used for puncture included Chiba needle (Cook, Europe), co-axial biopsy trocar needle (Temno, Allegiance Heathcare Corp, USA), uni-axial biopsy needle (Temno, Allegiance Heathcare Corp, USA), Kellett needle (Rocket Medical, UK), Kimal needle (Kimal, UK), Rita radiofrequency ablation needle (Rita, UK), Radionics radiofrequency needle (Radionics, UK), spinal needle (Steriseal, UK), vascular access one part needle (Cook Europe, Denmark) and vascular access two part needle (Cook Europe, Denmark).

### 2.2.2. Kidney

Pig kidneys with time minimised from slaughter to laboratory use, were used for in-vitro estimation of kidney needle puncture force. Kidneys do have macroscopic variation in their structure but this variation has conformity across the specimen where the needle puncture path is normal to the capsule of the organ. Pig kidney was chosen as the specific test medium because of the similarity between porcine and human anatomy. A range of needles (see above in the liver in-vitro methodology) were mounted on the tensile tester finger jig and were driven into the tissue at a fixed rate, 500mm per minute, an approximation of the speed of needle insertion during interventional radiological procedures. Needle orientation was normal to the surface of the kidney being punctured; a depth of puncture of 6cm was used. Output force data from the tensile tester and the capacitance pad output voltage were continuously measured. Punctures were repeated to obtain an average and a range of forces involved.

### 2.3. In-Vivo arterial needle puncture

Following Local Research Ethics Committee approval, measurement was made of forces generated during arterial needle puncture during vascular interventions in ten adult patients (8 male, 2 female, mean age 69 yrs, range 42 to 83 yrs). Following a surgical hand scrub a single sensor pad was mounted on the operator's right thumb, the sensor pad was lightly taped to the operator's thumb, beneath a sterile surgical glove. During the needle puncture procedure, the operator's thumb was positioned such that the sensor pad was centred over the needle hub, allowing normal forces to be measured. Static and dynamic forces were then measured throughout the arterial needle puncture procedures. Patients undergoing evaluation were routine listed patients undergoing standard investigation for peripheral vascular disease. Vascular access was obtained by puncture of the common femoral artery. Ultrasound guidance was used to determine the anatomical location of the needle tip while a sensor generated force profile was obtained. The needle advancement was effected under ultrasound guidance with the needle hub normal to and centred on the force pad, allowing forces to be measured throughout arterial needle puncture. Data were sampled at a rate of 100Hz and saved to a PC. The whole procedure was video taped to establish a time line to correlate force fluctuations to physical manoeuvres.

## 3. Results

### 3.1. Calibration

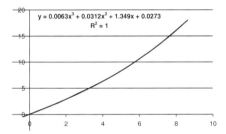

**Figure 1.** Calibration curve with the calibration equation to convert from capacitance pad voltage output to force in Newtons. X axis is Volts and Y axis is force (Newtons).

### 3.2. In-Vitro

Our data demonstrates the influence on force of needle gauge, needle design and the tissue being punctured.

### 3.2.1. Liver

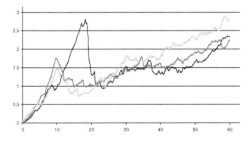

**Figure 2.** Comparison of force required for in-vitro liver puncture all needles are 18 gauge, light grey trace biopsy needle, dark grey trace, spinal needle, black trace, Kimal needle. X axis is displacement (mm) and Y Axis is force (Newtons).

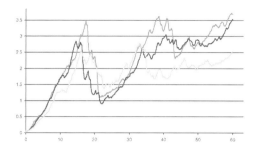

**Figure 3.** Comparison of force required for in-vitro liver puncture. All needles are coaxial biopsy trocar needles, the light grey trace is a 19 gauge needle (thinnest calibre), the dark grey a 15 gauge needle (thickest calibre) and the black a 17 gauge needle (mid calibre). The X axis is displacement (mm) the Y axis is force (Newtons).

### 3.2.2. Kidney

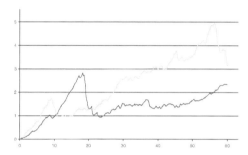

**Figure 4.** Comparison of force required for in-vitro puncture of liver, black trace and kidney, grey trace using a Kimal needle. X axis is displacement (mm) and Y axis is force (Newtons).

### 3.3. In-Vivo arterial needle puncture

The capacitance sensors were found to be unobtrusive during *in vivo* studies with no adverse clinical events recorded. Voltage output range 0.066 to 2.706 Volts, was equivalent to 0.13 to 8.89 Newtons (mean 3.76, SD: 3.32) required to puncture the arterial wall. Fig. 5 shows sensor output over a 55 second period during ultrasound guided needle puncture. The elevated baseline is due to the compressive force of the surgical gloves. There is a low amplitude periodic waveform recorded during needle / vessel wall contact (commencing at black arrow in fig. 1) with periodicity correlating to the patient's pulse rate (72 beats / min). Just prior to vessel lumen entry there are two peaks of sensor output, the second being the maximum at 3.9 V which is equivalent to 5.1 Newtons. The final reduction in sensor output corresponds to the observation of vessel wall penetration by ultrasound imaging with an arterial blood jet from the needle (white arrow in fig. 5).

Fig. 6 shows a 24 second period of sensor output during arterial puncture in this case. This again shows a periodic waveform during needle / vessel wall contact, followed by progressive increase in sensor output, up to 2.9 V (equivalent to 3.8 Newtons) immediately preceding entry into the vessel lumen. The final reduction in sensor output corresponds to the observation of vessel wall penetration during ultrasound imaging, with a simultaneous arterial blood jet from the needle.

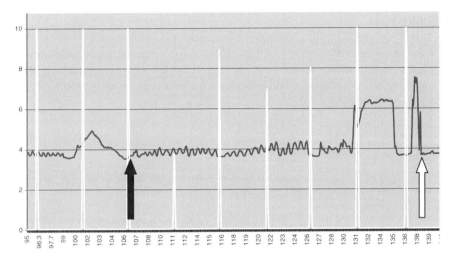

**Figure 5.** Sensor output shown in Volts (black trace). Baseline as time (seconds) with 5 second time points (white trace). Wall contact at black arrow. White arrow indicates vessel entry.

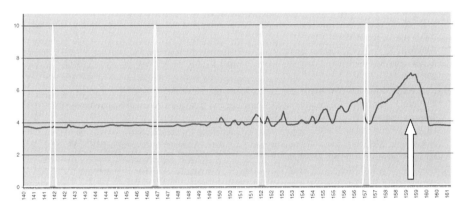

**Figure 6.** Sensor output shown in Volts (black trace). Baseline as time (seconds) with 5 second time points (white trace). White arrow indicates vessel entry.

## 4. Conclusions

Using the capacitance force sensor pads single degree of freedom force measurement can be performed in-vivo in the sterile clinical environment and without significant interference with the operator's 'feel' encountered during the procedure. These preliminary data show feasibility of using these unobtrusive sensors during any IR invasive procedure in order to model instrument-tissue forces intra-operatively. The sensor responses are reproducible, with the output being related to force rather than pressure. During arterial puncture, a periodic waveform during needle–wall contact was equivalent in rate to the observed pulse, and is likely to represent force transmitted by the needle due to arterial pulsation. This method does not distinguish cutting from friction / clamping effects [9], and cannot capture rotational and lateral forces. Nonetheless such techniques should provide a suitable method of authenticating haptic output forces in simulator models.

## 5. Future Work

We are continuing to acquire data on the needle force involved during IR procedures. In-vitro and *in vivo* puncture force data is being incorporated into new simulations and we are exploring and developing novel techniques for measurement of the forces involved in IR [13].

## References

[1]  Dondelinger RF, Ghysels MP, Brisbois D, *et al.* Relevant radiological anatomy of the pig as a training model in interventional radiology. European Radiology. 8(7):1254-3,1998.

[2]  http://www.immersion.com.

[3]  Dodd A, Riding M and John NW. Building Realistic Virtual Environments using Java and VRML Third Irish Workshop on Computer Graphics, 2002, Dublin, Ireland, pp.53-61.

[4]  John NW, Riding M, Phillips NI, *et al.* Medicine. Web-based Surgical Educational Tools, Meets Virtual Reality 2001, Studies in Health Technology and Informatics, IOS Press, 2001, ISSN: 0926-9630, ISBN 1-58603-143-0, pp.212-217.

[5]  Moorthy K, Jiwanji M, Shah J *et al.* Validation of a web based training tool for lumbar puncture. Medicine Meets Vitual Reality 11, J.D.Westwood et al (Eds). IOS press, 2003, 219-225.

[6]  Gerovichev O, Panadda M and Okamura A. The effect of visual and haptic feedback on manual and teleoperated needle insertion, Medical Image Computing and Computer Assisted Intervention MICCAI 2002, Tokyo, Japan, pp.147-154.

[7]  Alterovitz R, Pouliot J, Taschereau R, *et al.* Simulating needle insertion and radioactive seed implantation for prostate brachytherapy. Medicine Meets Virtual Reality 11. J.D.Westwood et al (Eds). IOS press, 2003. 19-25.

[8]  Kataoka H, Toshikatsu W, Kiyoyuki C *et al.* Measurement of the tip and friction force acting on a needle during penetration, Medical Image Computing and Computer Assisted Intervention MICCAI 2002, Tokyo, Japan, September 2002. pp. 216-223.

[9]  DiMaio SP and Salcudean SE. Needle insertion modelling for the interactive simulation of percutaneous procedures, Medical Image Computing and Computer-Assisted Intervention MICCAI 2002, Tokyo, Japan, September 2002 pp. 253-260.

[10] Brouwer I, Ustin J, Bentley L, *et al.* Measuring *In Vivo* Animal Soft Tissue Properties for Haptic Modelling in Surgical Simulation. Medicine Meets Virtual Reality 2001. J.D.Westwood et al. (eds) IOS Press. 69-74.

[11] O'leary MD, Simone C, Washio T, *et al.* Robotic Needle Insertion: Effects of Friction and Needle Geometry. Proceedings of the 2003 IEEE Iinternational Conference on Robotica and Automation, Taipei, Taiwan, pp. 1774-1780.

[12] Healey AE, Evans J., Murphy M. *et al.* Challenges realising effective radiological interventional virtual environments: The *CRaIVE* approach. In Medicine Meets Virtual Reality 12 Jan. 2004, IOS Press, pp.127-129.

[13] www.craive.org.uk

*Medicine Meets Virtual Reality 13*
*James D. Westwood et al. (Eds.)*
*IOS Press, 2005*

# The Virtual Terrorism Response Academy: Training for High-Risk, Low-Frequency Threats

Joseph V. HENDERSON, MD

*Institute for Security Technology Studies, Dartmouth College, Interactive Media*
*Laboratory, Dartmouth Medical School, Hanover, New Hampshire, USA, 03755*

**Abstract.** The Virtual Terrorism Response Academy is a reusable virtual learning environment to prepare emergency responders to deal with high-risk, low-frequency events in general, terrorist attacks in particular. The principal learning strategy is a traditional one: apprenticeship. Trainees enter the Academy and travel through its halls, selecting different learning experiences under the guidance of instructors who are simultaneously master practitioners and master trainers. The mentors are real individuals who have been videotaped according to courseware designs; they are subsequently available at any time or location via broadband Internet or CD-ROM.

The Academy features a Simulation Area where trainees are briefed on a given scenario, select appropriate resources (e.g., protective equipment and hazmat instruments), then enter a 3-dimensional space where they must deal with various situations. Simulations are done under the guidance of a master trainer who functions as a coach, asking questions, pointing out things, explaining his reasoning at various points in the simulation. This is followed by a debriefing and discussion of lessons that could be learned from the simulation and the trainee's decisions.

## 1. Introduction

### 1.1. The Problem of High-Risk and Low-Frequency

California Highway Patrol Captain Gordon Graham speaks nationally about risk management in the public safety professions. To a wide range of audiences—including police and fire chiefs, first responders, and FBI Academy students—he stresses the importance of preparing for high-risk, low-frequency events. He elaborates on the classic risk-frequency analysis shown in Figure 1. "Everything we do can be put into one of the four boxes." [1]

> "I have no worries when you get involved in high frequency—HF—events, as RPDM kicks in. Recognition-Primed Decision Making[1] is your friend and will be of great assistance to you."

---

[1]Referring to the RPD model developed by Gary Klein [2] (see next section). The model is widely accepted among military and emergency response decision theorists. It is a basis for incident command training at the National Fire Academy and the Emergency Management Institute.

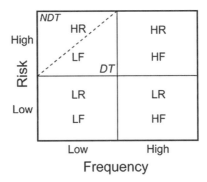

**Figure 1.** Classic risk/frequency analysis.

"The principles of RPDM are as follows. Consider your mind as a 'hard drive. . .' Your daily experiences help you load this drive. . . Everything you do and experience is loaded into your hard drive. When you get involved in any task or incident, your magnificent brain quickly scans your hard drive and looks for a close match. . .

"RPDM allows people with experience to do things right. However, if you have not experienced the task you have now encountered, or do not experience it on a regular basis, then your brain cannot quickly locate a match. Without a match you are en route to problems. It is the low frequency events that cause us grief.

"I get very worried when you get involved in incidents that fall in the top left box. This is where problems occur. Note that this box has been split into two triangles, the DT and NDT tasks. DT is discretionary time; it means you have time to think things through. NDT is non-discretionary time; you have to do the task now."

Graham is talking about risk management in general, but his reasoning is very applicable to terrorism preparedness. Terrorist events, especially those involving weapons of mass destruction (WMD), will clearly fall into the LF/HR quadrant. When they happen, some tasks will fall into the NDT triangle and require quick action. Some tasks need to be thought through before acting: there is discretionary time, but not a lot of it. *Before* they happen, it's *all* discretionary time. Plans and procedures can be thought through and put in place. And we can *train* our public safety personnel.

### 1.2. Training for High-Risk, Low Frequency Threats

Applying RPDM depends on having our mental "hard drives" loaded with appropriate experiences. We need to provide training that approximates the situations and circumstances that can accompany a WMD attack. It helps to know pertinent facts and rules, and to be familiar with applicable plans and procedures. But doing the right thing in a timely manner requires more. And, as Gary Klein, developer of the Recognition-Primed Decision model, notes, it requires training that is more than technical in nature, regardless of how systematically it's presented.

"This [technical training] strategy makes sense for simple, procedural tasks. Especially in high-turnover jobs, with minimally educated workers, the strategy allows for efficient instructional programs. Systems approaches to training were an improvement over anarchy. Nonetheless, they were not designed to teach people to gain higher levels of expertise or to make better judgments and decisions. . .

"Presenting the procedures to trainees gives them a false sense of progress. This confidence dissipates when novices realize that applying the procedures depends on *context* and that no one can *tell* them what context is. Judgment and decision tasks in natural settings are rarely straightforward..." [3]

"If you want people to size up situations quickly and accurately, you need to expand their experience base." [4] [Emphases added.]

Klein advocates use of simulations and story telling as ways of expanding that experience base. He also speaks of "annotated examples" in which a teacher presents "a core set of examples to serve as analogues," experiences that can be applied to a broad range of situations:

"For each example, the teacher could describe the choice points in the solution where someone might have taken the wrong path... The teacher could explain the cues the expert used in avoiding these traps. In that way, learners get the advantage of the examples along with guidance on the principles the have to learn to safely apply the examples." [5]

At Dartmouth Medical School's Interactive Media Laboratory, we are developing a virtual learning environment, the Virtual Terrorism Response Academy, that combines these concepts. It provides technical training in support of facts, plans, and procedures (e.g., those connected with WMD-hazmat response). It also provides guided simulations that can "load the mental hard drives" of local emergency responders with experiences that can serve as analogues for a range of situations associated with terrorist events. A mentor provides cues, explains reasoning, points out traps, and explains principles immediately before, during, and immediately after each simulation. Story telling is an intrinsic element of the simulations and of interviews with emergency responders who have experienced terrorist attacks. The Academy is described in the next section.

## 2. The Virtual Terrorism Response Academy

### 2.1. General Description

The Virtual Terrorism Response Academy (VTRA) is a reusable virtual learning environment to prepare emergency responders to deal with high-risk, low-frequency events in general, terrorist attacks in particular. The principal learning strategy is a traditional one: apprenticeship. The Academy applies Dartmouth's Virtual Practicum model, which has been described previously.[2] [6]

VTRA presents information in a modular form, using a variety of media including motion video, sound, still and animated graphics, and text. It employs multiple instructional modes, including complex simulations (with immersive, 3-D interfaces based on the Quake 2 engine) accompanied by after-action reviews; conventional talks; interactive talks; computer-based activities; and interviews with experienced practitioners who relate "war stories" and lessons learned.

Trainees enter the Academy and travel through its halls, selecting different learning experiences under the guidance of instructors who are simultaneously master practition-

---

[2]http://iml.dartmouth.edu/education/pubs/vpract-intro.html/

ers and master trainers.[3] Note that nearly all elements in the Academy are virtual. The mentors are real individuals who have been videotaped according to courseware designs; they are subsequently available for training at any time or location.

The architecture also provides for access to synchronous and asynchronous web-based resources that are provided by others. The Web Room presents a portal to online resources, including course schedules, relevant documents, and the Web sites of organizations (e.g., members of the Domestic Preparedness Consortium) that provide hands-on training. The Academy's Conference Room offers access to real-time training via web-conferencing.

The Virtual Terrorism Response Academy is constructed to run on older computers (Pentium II, 600 MHz), with a low-bandwidth Internet connection or no connection. It can be used without CD-ROM if a broadband Internet connection is available. Thus, most jurisdictions already have the technological infrastructure to use courseware built using the VTRA infrastructure.

It should be noted that, though the program is designed to be used via broadband Internet without CD-ROM, the program is not Web- or HTML-based. It requires installation of an application file and other program resources on the local machine, as is the case for many of today's computer games. The VTRA installer can be accessed via a Web-site.[4] Video and audio can then be streamed from a central server on demand with very low latencies and good quality. Performance is equivalent to having the media on a CD-ROM in the trainee's computer.

The VTRA infrastructure supports reconfiguration and reuse to address the training needs of different audiences on any number of topics. We are constructing an integrated development environment (IDE) that draws on and extends existing open source tools and engines including wxWidgets and the Quake 2 game engine. This IDE, which we call "Tamale," will be made available to other developers who may wish to create courseware using the VTRA designs and infrastructure. Tamale will be released as an open source initiative under general public license from Dartmouth College.

## 2.2. First Application of the Academy

We are also developing the first "course" to run in the Academy: *Ops-Plus for WMD-Hazmat*. Principal audiences are first responders in law enforcement, fire service, and emergency medical services who are already trained in general hazmat response at the Operations Level (NFPA 472 and OSHA 1910.120). *Ops-Plus* extends this training to address the hazmat aspects of attacks by terrorists using chemical, biological, radiological, nuclear, and explosive weapons. That is, the program stresses the application of existing hazardous materials policies, procedures, and competencies to terrorist incidents, and extends the capabilities of Ops-level responders to respond to WMD threats. The program also serves as an instantiation of the Academy, providing a model for other developers that they can adopt, adapt, and extend.

We are developing *Ops-Plus* with assistance from the Center for Domestic Preparedness, the New Mexico Institute of Mining and Technology, the Nevada Test Site; the

---

[3]Mentors for the *Ops-Plus* course are well known among emergency responders: for fire fighters, Chief Alan Brunacini; for law enforcement, Captain Gordon Graham; and for EMS, Chief James O. Page. For hazmat-specific content, all trainees work under the mentorship of Chief John Eversole and Greg Noll.

[4]Several of IML's completed programs can be accessed and run this way. Visit http://iml.dartmouth.edu.

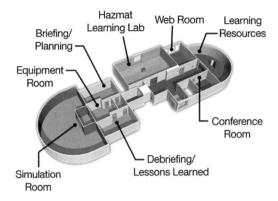

**Figure 2.** Virtual Terrorism Response Academy configured for its first course, *Ops-Plus for WMD-Hazmat.*

National Fire Academy, the FBI Hazardous Materials Response Unit, and the FBI Hazardous Devices School. There is also an advisory board consisting of representatives from the target professions; this is in addition to the experts appearing in the program itself. Development of the VTRA infrastructure, development tools, and the *Ops-Plus* courseware is funded by the Office for Domestic Preparedness, Department of Homeland Security, via a grant to Dartmouth's Institute for Security Technology Studies.

Fig. 2 provides an overview of the general VTRA configuration, set up to support the *Ops-Plus* course. There are two "wings." The right wing has four rooms. The largest is the Hazmat Learning Lab. It provides reviews of a variety of hazmat principles, via a combination of computer-based activities and presentations. Topics include the use of instruments and protective equipment, triage and casualty care, crime scene management, etc. It also contains a final exercise that the trainee must pass (demonstrating an adequate grasp of fundamentals) to get a key to the Simulation Area of the Academy.

The Web and Conference Rooms were described previously. The Learning Resources Room contains interactive talks on topics not covered in the Hazmat Learning Lab, such as the nature of the terrorist threat, communicating with the media and the public, and post-traumatic stress. This is also where we find previously-mentioned interviews with individuals who have direct experience with terrorism and/or WMD.

The left wing of the Academy is the Simulation Area, which consists of a suite of rooms. Trainees travel through the area getting briefings, selecting protective equipment and instruments, then entering a 3-D space where they must deal with various situations related to WMD Hazmat. Simulations are done under the guidance of Greg Noll, a master hazmat trainer, who functions a as , asking questions, pointing out things, explaining his reasoning at various points in the simulation. This is followed by a debriefing and discussion of lessons that could be learned from the simulation and the trainee's decisions.

## 3. Conclusion

A key advantage if the Virtual Terrorism Response Academy is that it can deliver training at any time or location to public safety professionals, helping them learn to deal with low-frequency, high-risk threats, including terrorist attacks. This training can be used to prepare individuals for "hands-on" training at special facilities or mobile training units brought to regional centers. This could shorten training cycles and the time trainees must spend away from their communities, preserving emergency response manpower and reducing training costs. It can also be used for sustainment training to maintain knowledge and skills once the trainee has returned to his or her community.


Supported under Award No. 2000-DT-CX-K001 from the Office for Domestic Preparedness, U.S. Department of Homeland Security.

Points of view in this document are those of the author and do not necessarily represent the official position of the U.S. Department of Homeland Security.

## References

[1]  Graham, G. Risk Management Workshop for the Vermont Career Fire Chiefs Association, May 20-21, 2004, Fairlee, VT.
[2]  Klein, G. *Sources of Power: How People Make Decisions.* Cambridge: MIT Press, 1998.
[3]  *Ibid.* pp. 168-169.
[4]  *Ibid.* p. 42.
[5]  *Ibid.* p. 209-210.
[6]  Henderson, J. Comprehensive, Technology-based Clinical Education: the "Virtual Practicum." Int'l J. Psychiatry in Medicine, 28(1): 41-79, 1998.

Medicine Meets Virtual Reality 13
James D. Westwood et al. (Eds.)
IOS Press, 2005

# Real-Time Ultrasonography Simulator Based on 3D CT-Scan Images

Alexandre HOSTETTLER, Clément FOREST, Antonello FORGIONE,
Luc SOLER and Jacques MARESCAUX

*Ircad/EITS, Stasbourg, France*

**Abstract.** A new method for real-time simulation of ultrasonography is presented. This method uses directly 3D enhanced helical CT-scan images. The originality of this method is that it can be run directly on real patient data with no need of any pretreatment.

## 1. Introduction

Ultrasonography is a non invasive technique that is widely used in a large range of applications, such as tumor detection or intra operative guiding. However, this technology is challenging to master for young residents, due to the difficulty of interpretation of resulting images. The aim of this research is to provide a little expensive ultrasonography simulator based on real patient CT-scan. Using real patient data instead of a doll or a set of pre-generated 3D models is interesting because it increases the amount of available exercises, especially since it is possible to use the patient's CT scans directly without any pretreatment. The drawback of our method is that the use of CT-scans makes it improper for prenatal ultrasonography. For this reason, we focus our application on digestive diagnosis and intra-operative ultrasonography.

## 2. Previous work

Real time simulation of ultrasonography remained for a long time a difficult challenge, essentially due to computer limitations. Indeed, strict computation of ultrasonic waves remains a complicated topic and is still far from allowing interactivity. The most common way to simplify the real time requirement is to use a reconstructed 3D ultrasound volume [1–4]. Once the volume has been pre-processed to suppress position-dependent artifacts such as shadows, gain or focus artifacts, it is possible to generate the simulated image by slicing the 3D volume according to probe position and orientation. Finally, this slice is modified in order to recreate those position-dependant artifacts. It is even possible to take deformations generated by the probe pressure [5] into account. Another known method is to use a reconstructed geometry of the body and to simulate the ultrasound propagation within this model [6], allowing to simulate artifacts such as multi echos. Both methods give good results but require strong prerequisites which are the acquisition of the 3D ultrasonic image or the organ segmentation and mesh generation.

## 3. Description of the method

The originality of this work is to use directly 3D enhanced helical CT-scan images with no need of any pretreatment. To optimize the computation of the image, ultrasound propagation is modelled as a one-dimensional problem. Therefore, the first step of our method consists in a volumetric ray-tracing directly inside the 3D scan to retrieve all voxels that are within the plane of the probe. Each possible direction of the ultrasound wave corresponds to a line of the resulting 2D image. This image is then analyzed in order to get two different informations. On the one hand, the acoustic behaviour of each pixel is estimated, and on the other hand the intersected interfaces are detected and labeled (soft tissues, bones, gas, ...). Note that these studies can be done off-line directly in the 3D CT-scan.

Using these data, three images are created. The first one is the *multiple echo image*, which is created using the knowledge of the nature and position of the interfaces between organs. With this image, multiple echos are detected and represented. The second image is the *absorbtion image*, which represents the accumulation of absorbtion caracteristics of materials along the ultrasonic wave. The third image is the *texture image*, which is generated combining the value read from the CT-scan and the information related to the nature of the corresponding tissues and its accoustic behaviour. The texture image is also blurred using a generated noise. Finally, those three images are merged in order to obtain the simulated image, which is mapped in a texture and displayed on the screen.

The choice of all inner constants has been validated by ultrasonography specialists. We are currently able to represent different organs satisfactorily such as the portal vein, bowels, bones and kidneys. We have also modelled several ultrasound artifacts: reverberation, shadowing and enhancement. The whole method has been patented.

## 4. The radiofrequency simulator

The simulator is planed to be integrated into a larger tool whose goal is to plan and to train radiofrequency manipulations [7]. The idea is to provide students with two force feedback devices: one for the needle and one for the ultrasonograph. It would then be possible to simulate the operation on real patient data. Currently, only the ultrasound part of the simulator is part of our simulator prototype, integration of the needle penetration is planed for early 2005.

The simulator includes a force feedback device in order to ease the probe location according to the virtual patient position. The skin geometry is automatically detected from the 3D CT-scan with a simple level set method and a mesh is generated which is used to compute the force feedback interactions. The whole simulation process is computationally cheap as it works well on a simple laptop.

## 5. Conclusion

We proposed a new method for real-time simulation of ultrasound. The realism of our simulator is sufficient to identify different structures: organs, bones, tumors, and even needles in the case of an ultrasound-guided radiofrequency tumor ablation.

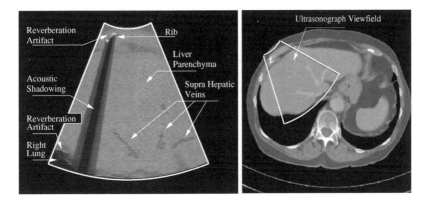

**Figure 1.** A simulated ultrasonography of the liver and the corresponding 3D scan cut.

Next steps of the development will consist in the validation of our method first by comparing real and simulated images from a same patient and secondly by evaluating its contribution to the average learning curve of trainees. These studies will be done in early 2005 in the IRCAD institute. Other studies are currently beeing carried in order to take the effects of respiration and cardiac movements and blood propagation into account.

## References

[1] P. Baier, A. Scharf, and C. Sohn. New ultrasound simulation system: a method for training and improved quality management in ultrasound examination. *Z Geburtshilfe Neonatol.*, 205(6):213– 217, Nov-Dec 2001. in German.

[2] C. Terkamp, G. Kirchner, J. Wedemeyer, A. Dettmer, J. Kielstein, H. Reindell, J. Bleck, M. Manns, and M. Gebel. Simulation of abdomen sonography. evaluation of a new ultrasond simulator. *Ul- traschall in Med*, 24:239–244, July 2003.

[3] D Henry, J. Troccaz, and J-L Bosson. Virtual echography: simulation of ultrasonographic exami- nations. In *Proceedings of MMVR'4*, pages 176–183, Jan 1996.

[4] Dror Aiger and Daniel Coher-Or. Real-time ultrasound imaging simulation. *Real-Time Imaging*, 4(4):263– 274, 1998.

[5] D. Henry, J. Troccaz, J.L. Bosson, and O. Pichot. Ultrasound imaging simulation: Application to the di- agnosis of deep venous thromboses of lower limbs. In *Proc. Intl. Conf. Medical Image Computing and Computer-Assisted Intervention (MICCAI)*, volume 1496 of *LNCS*, pages 1032–1040, 1998.

[6] Wibaux L. and Chaillou C. Construction d'images échographiques pour des simulateurs médicaux. In *5èmes journées AFIG*, Décembre 1997.

[7] C. Villard, L. Soler, A. Gangi, Mutter D., and Marescaux J. Toward realistic radiofrequency ablation of hepatic tumors 3d simulation and planning. In *Proceeding of SPIE*, volume 5367 of *Medical Imaging*, pages 586–595, 2004.

*Medicine Meets Virtual Reality 13*
*James D. Westwood et al. (Eds.)*
*IOS Press, 2005*

# Fuzzy Classification: Towards Evaluating Performance on a Surgical Simulator

Jeff HUANG, Shahram PAYANDEH, PhD,
Peter DORIS, MD and Ima HAJSHIRMOHAMMADI, BSc
*Simon Fraser University and Surrey Memorial Hospital, Vancouver, Canada*

**Abstract.** Computer-based surgical simulators such as the MIST-VR (www.mentice.com) are able to provide scoring metrics such as time taken to complete a task, number of errors made, and economy of movement. Using MIST-VR's basic metrics, we explored the possibility of classifying skill levels using fuzzy logic. Our objective was to create a fuzzy classifier capable of classifying the performance of a subject training on a surgical simulator into 1 of 3 categories: Novice, Intermediate, and Expert. To accomplish this, we needed to establish a baseline skill level for each category. We had four laparoscopic surgeons, four surgical assistants/residents and four non-surgical staff/students with no laparoscopic experience perform two basic tasks on the simulator involving the placement of a ball into a box. We have found, through this preliminary study, that the results were inconclusive. We suspected a number of issues such as the size of our sample space used to train our classifier, and the difficulty of the chosen tasks adversely affected our results.

## 1. Introduction

Laparoscopy, despite being beneficial to the patient when done properly, is more difficult than open surgery. The surgeon is working in a relatively confined space and has only a two-dimensional view of the patient's anatomy through a video screen, rather than a direct three-dimensional view. This increases the chance of complications. The introduction of laparoscopic cholecystectomy (LC) was associated with an increased number of complications; more precisely, there were three times as many complications than in traditional cholecystectomy [8]. More alarming is that the number of injuries does not seem to be decreasing with time [8]. Olsen has found that these injuries are still being reported 6 years after the introduction of LC [5]. He found that the majority of injuries were the result of misidentification of anatomy, which is preventable. The need to reduce the number of injuries related to laparoscopic procedures has lead to a review of how surgeons are trained.

All surgeons are taught laparoscopic techniques through the use of tools such as mechanical box trainers, inanimate models, animals, and surgical simulators. In residency programs, trainees are evaluated using In Training Evaluation Reports (ITERs) over a number of years. ITERs are completed at periodic intervals during training. These reports consist of oral and written examination, and comments from the overseeing surgeon; however, they do not include an objective assessment of technical skill, preventing a standard from being established [1]. Without a standard, newly certified surgeons may emerge without the necessary level of surgical proficiency.

One part to a complete solution would be enhancing the VR simulators to evaluate the trainee. The evaluation would be objective in nature, as the metrics are based on actual performance and not perception. Current simulators can only provide a few basic metrics such as time taken to complete a procedure, the number of errors made, and the efficiency of movements. We want to extend these metrics to the point where we can determine where the subject's skills lie in comparison to those in the general laparoscopic surgical community. These simulators would allow more practice time for surgeons, and advise them of their current skill level.

Fuzzy logic can be applied to achieve our goals. Operative procedures can be divided into a number of tasks, and each task can be evaluated according to criteria set out by an expert surgeon. Ota outlines how the task of dissecting a blood vessel can be evaluated by fuzzy logic [4].

Hence, this paper explores the possibility of extending the performance evaluations offered by a surgical simulator with the ability to compare the trainee's performance with general levels of skill. We propose the use of a fuzzy-based if-then rule system known as a fuzzy inference system (FIS) [3], or more specifically a fuzzy classifier, to promote objective assessment. A FIS is a system that maps an input to an output using fuzzy logic. Neural networks can be used to train and generate rules from the input data. These rules are the foundation of the fuzzy classifier.

Fuzzy classification has many applications and has been used in various automated medical diagnostic areas including breast cancer tumour diagnosis and prognosis by Hoffman [1]. Hoffman constructed a classifier using a breast cancer data set containing features such as the texture, smoothness and radius of cell nuclei from a breast lump. Each instance in the data was classified as malignant or benign, according to actual, known diagnosis of the patient. Using 15 if-then rules, a 95% correct classification resulted for the testing data set.

For our surgical simulator application, a fuzzy classifier can be constructed to evaluate a trainee's skill level based on their performance on surgical tasks in a VR trainer. This particular classifier evaluates the trainee in tasks mainly involved with the dominant hand.

## 2. Method

The general approach is to conduct a user study to get performance metrics from people of different skill levels. The data from the study will then be used to build our classifier.

### 2.1. Experimental Setup

In order to create a fuzzy classifier, we conducted a user study at Surrey Memorial Hospital in B.C., Canada. Our setup (see Figure 1) consisted of an isolated room with a 19" eye-level LCD monitor, a two-handed laparoscopic device with needle-driver handles (Virtual Laparoscopic Interface, by Immersion Inc.), and a dual Intel Xeon 2.8Ghz computer.

The simulator used for our study was the Minimally Invasive Surgical Trainer – Virtual Reality (MIST-VR) by Mentice AB. This simulator has been shown to transfer skills

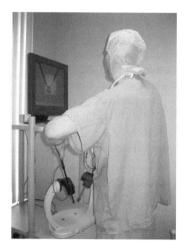

**Figure 1.** The Experimental Setup.

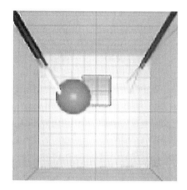

**Figure 2.** An image of AcquirePlace & TransferPlace.

from virtual reality into the operating room [7]. MIST-VR offers a number of tasks, combined within two modules: Coreskills and Suturing. The Coreskills module focuses on familiarizing the trainee with basic laparoscopic skills. It includes tasks focusing on target manipulation and placement, transferring objects between instruments, and diathermy. The Suturing module trains the surgeon to manipulate a needle and perform suturing. MIST-VR keeps track of the user's performance through a number of metrics. These metrics will be explained in the next paragraph.

The tasks used in our study were AcquirePlace and TransferPlace. Both tasks involved the manipulation of a ball with grippers. AcquirePlace consist of grasping the ball with a gripper, manipulating the ball into a 3-dimensional cube, and releasing it within the cube. TransferPlace is similar to AcquirePlace and consists of grasping the ball with one gripper, transferring the ball to the other gripper, manipulating the ball into a 3-dimensional cube, and releasing it within the cube. Both of these use the following metrics: the time taken to complete a task, the number of errors made, the economy of the user's movements, and the user's overall score. Some possible errors are touching tools together, dropping the ball, and removing the ball from the cube without releasing it. The economy of movement is the ratio of actual tool movements during the task to the optimal calculated movement of the tools necessary to complete the task. These ratios are set by Mentice, and are unknown to us. The best results are the ones that approach the value of 1. The overall score is the sum of all the other metrics multiplied by their respective weights, which are set by the administrator of the simulator. For this study, all weights were set to 1. Hence, the overall score was simply the sum of all other metrics for the task. A sample of the scoring for a trial from the task AcquirePlace is shown in Table 1.

## 2.2. Experimental Design

Three groups of people were selected based on the following definitions: novices (little or no laparoscopic experience), intermediate (1-2 yrs of laparoscopic experience) and experts (people with 2+ years of laparoscopic experience). Our novices consisted of 1 SFU

**Table 1.** This is an example of the AcquirePlace metrics. It shows the performance for each hand for one trial.

|  | Scores | |
| --- | --- | --- |
|  | **Left Hand** | **Right Hand** |
| **Time** | 33.2 | 22.0 |
| **Errors** | 29.0 | 27.0 |
| **Economy of Movement** | 2.2 | 2.6 |
| **Total Score** | 117.8 | |

**Table 2.** This is a detailed breakdown of the test groups.

|  | Group A | Group B |
| --- | --- | --- |
| **First Task** | AcquirePlace | TransferPlace |
| **Second Task** | TransferPlace | AcquirePlace |
| **# of Experts** | 2 | 2 |
| **# of Intermediates** | 2 | 2 |
| **# of Novices** | 2 | 2 |

student and 3 operating room nurses; our intermediate group consisted of 4 surgical residents/assistants; and our experts consisted of 4 laparoscopic surgeons. We split our subjects into two groups in order to vary the task order. Group A did AcquirePlace first, then TransferPlace while group B did TransferPlace first, and then AcquirePlace. Two subjects from each classification were placed in each group. The group compositions are outlined in Table 2.

For each task, the presenter introduced the subject to the task, played a video of an error-free trial of the task, and explained what constituted as errors. The subject was then given two practice trials before performing 4 trials which were counted in the results. Each trial consisted of starting the task with the left hand, and then the right hand. At the end of the task, they were allowed to view their performance data.

## 2.3. Fuzzy Classifier Design

The purpose of the user study was to gather data necessary to create the classifiers for each task. We needed data from subjects that fit our three categories of skill. This data would be split in equal halves in order to form two representative data sets. One would be used for training, and the other would be used for testing the classifier. We created our classifier using Matlab's Fuzzy Toolbox's Adaptive Neuro-Fuzzy Inference System (ANFIS), which uses neural networks in order to train the classifier. ANFIS applies the learning abilities of neural networks [2] to detect trends in the training data. From these trends, ANFIS can generate the fuzzy if-then rules of the classifier. The benefit of using ANFIS is that if we do not have a conceptual view of what our system, membership functions and rules should be, ANFIS can create this for us automatically. The resulting system will be adapted to the data, and accommodate any variations [3].

ANFIS is limited to using Sugeno systems. In order to generate our classifier, we loaded our training data set and used subtractive clustering with the following parameters: *Range of Influence = 1; Squash Factor = 1.25; Accept Ratio = 0.5; and Reject Ratio = 0.15*. The benefit of using subtractive clustering is that it keeps the number of rules relatively low, requiring less computation. We then trained the FIS using the hy-

**Table 3.** Breakdown of our training and testing data sets.

| Training Data Set | Testing Data Set |
|---|---|
| 1 Group A Expert | 1 Group A Expert |
| 1 Group B Expert | 1 Group B Expert |
| 1 Group A Intermediate | 1 Group A Intermediate |
| 1 Group B Intermediate | 1 Group B Intermediate |
| 1 Group A Novice | 1 Group A Novice |
| 1 Group B Novice | 1 Group B Novice |

**Table 4.** Samples of vectors in a data set. A class of '1' represents an expert, '2' represents an intermediate, and '3' represents a novice.

| Economy of Movement | Time | # of Errors | Score | Class |
|---|---|---|---|---|
| 4 | 9.4 | 2 | 15.4 | 1 |
| 2.4 | 9.5 | 0 | 11.9 | 2 |
| 5.2 | 19.7 | 3 | 27.9 | 3 |

brid learning rule [2] for 200 epochs. A testing set is used to evaluate the validity of the trained classifier.

## 3. Results

### 3.1. Organizing the Resulting Data

In total, we had 12 participants who came in on a drop-in basis. This yielded 12 full sets of data. We first separated the data from AcquirePlace and TransferPlace. The data for each task was organized into 48 vectors in total (12 subjects who did 4 trials each). Each vector contained the performance metrics for the trial.

Then, the data had to be reorganized to exclude non-dominant hand scores. This involved removing extra data (all the data related to the non-dominant hand in each trial) and recalculating the score for just the dominant hand. Note that MIST calculates the scores using metrics for *both hands*. Since we were only interested in the dominant hand, we recalculated the scores using the metrics for only the dominant hand.

Next, we formed our training and testing data sets. Each data set contained 2 subjects per skill level category. For each of the two subjects, one was taken from group A and the other from group B. This is clarified in Table 3. Each subject did 4 trials, so s/he has 4 vectors associated with him/her; hence, each data set had 24 vectors: 8 experts, 8 intermediates, and 8 novices. For each vector, we added an extra tag called Class to indicate the correct classification. A class of '1' represents an Expert, a '2' represents an Intermediate, and a '3' represents a Novice. This is shown in Table 4.

### 3.2. The Resulting Classifiers

The plots in Figure 3 and Figure 4 show the plots for the classifiers. The •'s in the plots represent our desired output, which is the Class of each vector. The actual output of our classifier is represented by the *'s. Optimal results would be indicated by minimal separation between desired output points and their corresponding actual output points.

## 4. Discussion

By inspection of the classifier plots in Figure 3 and Figure 4, it is evident that our classifier does not offer the optimal results. In AcquirePlace, only 1 vector (#12) was

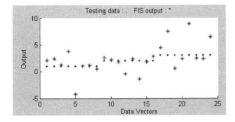 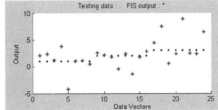

**Figure 3.** The AcquirePlace fuzzy classifier plot. The output (y-axis) represents the classification of the vector (x-axis).

**Figure 4.** The TransferPlace fuzzy classifier plot. The output (y-axis) represents the classification of the vector (x-axis).

correctly classified. The remainders were haphazardly classified into categories not defined.

However, TransferPlace offers some positive hopes. At least eight vectors are close enough to be considered classified correctly. Also, most vectors were within the defined classes 1, 2, or 3. This suggests that the classifier is having trouble distinguishing between our categories of skill level. Using more training data may correct this problem.

The underlying hypothesis for this study was that a fuzzy classifier could be used to properly distinguish various users and their levels of expertise. A number of factors influenced the conclusions in this paper: sample size and grouping methods; organization of the training and testing data sets; task selection; task difficulty; and formulation of the fuzzy classifier. Varying these factors in further studies may serve to provide more positive results.

## 5. Conclusion and Future work

Although the classifiers for the tasks AcquirePlace and TransferPlace were not accurate, there is still more variations and improvements to be made to produce a successful classifier. In our case, we believe a major factor affecting our result is that our sample did not represent the performance variation of our three categories of people. A larger sample size will be necessary for further studies. Using more difficult tasks may also improve chances of a working classifier by providing a larger skill gap between the classifications.

We are conducting further studies to collect data to be used for an improved classifier, focusing on suturing and knotting tasks, which is a difficult skill for laparoscopic practitioners. Tasks such as *StitchStart* and ContinuousSuture have metrics such as the distance between the actual needle hit point and the hidden target point, and a stitch deformation metric will present a larger gap between the categories of skill levels, and present the opportunity to create a working classifier.

Traversing beyond MIST-VR, there are other surgical simulators in progress. SFU is developing the Laparoscopic Training Environment (LTE) [6], in which other metrics can be built into tasks such as suturing. In this case, we could integrate the fuzzy inference system into the software. Also, the LTE supports a haptic-feedback laparoscopic device, which would give the subject a more realistic training experience.

## References

[1] Hoffmann F. Boosting a genetic fuzzy classifier, IFSA/NAFIPS 2001, Vancouver, Canada.

[2] Jang JSR, Sun CT. Neuro-fuzzy modeling and control. *The Proceedings of the IEEE*. March 1995; 83; 378-406.

[3] The MathWorks. (2002). *Fuzzy Logic Toolbox User Guide*. The MathWorks, Inc.

[4] Ota D *et al*. Virtual reality in surgical education. Computers in Biology and Medicine. 1995; 25; 2; 127-137.

[5] Olsen D. Bile duct injuries during laparoscopic cholecystectomy. Surgical Endoscopy. 1997; 11; 133-138.

[6] Payandeh S *et al*. LTE: A multi-modal training environment for surgeons, In *Proc. of ACM Fifth International Conference on Multi-Modal Interface*.
2003; 301-302.

[7] Seymour NE *et al*. Virtual reality training improves operating room performance. Annals of Surgery. 2002; 236(4); 458-464.

[8] Walsh RM *et al*. Trends in bile duct injuries from laparoscopic cholecystectomy. 1997 Americas Hepato-Pancreato-Biliary Congress, Miami, Fla.

[9] Wanzel KR, Ward M, Reznick RK. Teaching the surgical craft: from selection to certification. Curr Prob Surg 2002; 39; 573-660.

*Medicine Meets Virtual Reality 13*
*James D. Westwood et al. (Eds.)*
*IOS Press, 2005*

# Structural Flexibility of Laparoscopic Instruments: Implication for the Design of Virtual Reality Simulators

Scott HUGHES, James LARMER, Jason PARK, Helen MACRAE
and Adam DUBROWSKI

*Surgical Skills Centre at Mt. Sinai Hospital, Department of Surgery,*
*University of Toronto, Toronto, Ontario, Canada*
*e-mail: adam.dubrowski@utoronto.ca*

**Abstract.** In accordance with the Practice Specificity Theory, training on models that closely resemble real life scenarios is most beneficial to learning. Research in the virtual reality (VR) simulation, as a potential teaching and evaluation tool, concentrated on the design of trainers to resemble operating room (OR) conditions. The purpose of the present investigation was to determine the structural flexibility of laparoscopic instruments of different materials and diameters under a wide range of stresses. Incorporating the mechanical properties of these instruments into the algorithms can prove to further increase the fidelity of VR simulators. The amount of deviation from pre-stress position in the instruments' shaft was measured with infrared markers and used as the index of structural flexibility. All instruments deviated considerably with the largest deviations observed for the small disposable, and lowest for the large reusable instruments. There was a linear relation between the stress and deviation for all instruments, which varied as a function of diameter. Similar instrument deviations were observed during cholecystectomy performed on porcine liver. Our findings show that laparoscopic instruments are not rigid bodies and are prone to significant deviations during standard laparoscopic procedures. This suggests that the structural flexibility of laparoscopic instruments should be modeled in the design of VR simulators.

## 1. Introduction

The VR simulators allows surgeons to hone their skills in an environment much more forgiving to mistakes than clinical settings. The Practice Specificity Theory states that training on models that closely resemble real life scenarios is most beneficial to learning [1]. Many efforts have been made to increase the fidelity of virtual reality models. Figure 1 depicts factors that can be manipulated to increase the fidelity of these simulators.

With advances in computer graphics technology, the simulators are constantly improving in the degree of presentation of virtual tissues. In addition, to convey realistic touch, models have been developed to mimic the non-linear mechanical properties of biological tissues [2–5]. However, replicating the mechanical properties of laparoscopic instruments remains problematic. At present the instruments behave as rigid bodies but a better understanding of how applied forces effect the integrity of laparoscopic tools

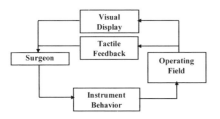

**Figure 1.** Factors affecting the fidelity of VR simulators. First is the quality of visual and haptic feedback information about the operating filed (e.g., visual displays and haptic representations of the textures), and second is the behavior of the instruments used (e.g., their structural flexibility).

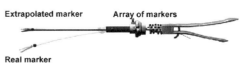

**Figure 2.** Stress was applied to the tip of the instrument in a perpendicular direction in 0.1N increments (Max 10N). The distance between the application of force and where the instrument exited the trocar was 170 mm and 190 mm for the 5mm and 10mm instruments respectively. Markers were placed at the tip of the instrument and the handle of the instrument and their deviations were tracked using OPTOTRAK system (v. 3020; Northern Digital Inc., Waterloo, ON, CA). (RMS accurate to 0.1 mm, resolution to 0.01 mm, sampling frequency 200 Hz).

would further strengthen the fidelity of laparoscopic simulators. Therefore, the purpose of the present investigation was to determine the structural flexibility of various laparoscopic instruments, and to determine the amount of bend during a cholecystectomy performed on porcine liver.

## 2. Methods

### 2.1. Experimental Materials

The flexibility of four laparoscopic instruments: 2 reusable (metal) with 5 mm (Stryker), and 10 mm diameters (Ethicon Inc.), and two disposable (plastic) with 5 mm (Tyco – AutoSuture endograsp), and 10 mm diameters (AutoSuture endobabcock) was examined in this study.

### 2.2. Experimental Design

The variables included instrument bend at 10N, and the relationship between stress and bend as described by the line of best fit. For each instrument an equation was derived that best described this line ($Y = AX + B$, where Y was the bend, A = slope, X = stress, and B = intercept). $R^2$ were also analyzed.

NDI 6D Architect (Northern Digital Inc., Waterloo, ON, CA) was used to create rigid body files for two instruments (5mm reusable, and 5mm disposable). The coordinates of the tip of these instruments were extrapolated (Figure 2), and a real marker was placed at the same coordinates to allow tracking the bend during 30 attempts of cholecystectomy on a porcine liver.

### 2.3. Statistics

All measures were analyzed in a separate two-factor mixed analysis of variance (ANOVA) with 2 materials (metal, plastic), and 2 diameters (5, 10 mm) as factors. Effects at $p < 0.05$ were analyzed using the Tukey HSD post hoc method for comparison of means.

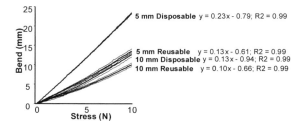 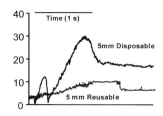

**Figure 3.** Left panel: Bend to stress functions and SD for each of the four types of instruments. Right panel: Bend as a function of time during a porcine cholecystectomy.

## 3. Results

As seen in Figure 3 the 5mm disposable instrument bend more than the other three instrument types (p = .002). The same trend was seen when the slopes were analyzed (p = .002). The correlation coefficient for the 10mm instruments was less that of the 5mm instruments (p = .002). Based on the analysis of the intercepts of the lines bend was the same for all instruments at no stress.

Figure 3 also represent bend as a function of time of a 5mm disposable and 5mm reusable instrument during a porcine cholecystectomy. The 5mm disposable instrument bent significantly more during the procedure than did the 5mm reusable instrument (Maximum bend averaged over 30 trials: Disposable mean = 24.3mm; Reusable mean = 9.3mm).

## 4. Discussion

Contrary to traditional view, laparoscopic instruments are not rigid bodies and are susceptible to bends during surgical procedures. We observed significant bend in all types of laparoscopic instruments during static loading. The amount of bend was a function of the instrument material and diameter. The relationship between bend and stress was nearly linear, subsequently facilitating the derivation of an algorithm that would simulate instrument flexibility in a virtual simulator. We further validated or data by demonstrating bends in two laparoscopic instruments during separate cholecystectomies on a porcine liver model. VR simulators have yet to take into account the bend of laparoscopic instruments when striving to create the highest fidelity model for laparoscopic practice.

## References

[1] Schmidt RA, Lee TD. *Motor control and learning: A behavioral emphasis.* Champaign, IL: Human Kinetics. 1999.
[2] Basdogan C., Ho C., Srinivasan M., Small S., Dawson S. Force interactions in laparoscopic simulations: haptic rendering of soft tissues. *Stud Health Technol Inform* 50: 385-391, 1998.
[3] Bholat O., Haluck R., Kutz R., Gorman P., Krummel T. Defining the role of haptic feedback in minimally invasive surgery. *Stud Health Technol Inform* 62: 62-66, 1999.
[4] Ottensmeyer M., Ben-Ur E., Salisbury J. Input and output for surgical simulation: devices to measure tissue properties in vivo and a haptic interface for laparoscopy simulators. *Stud Health Technol Inform* 70: 236-242, 2000.
[5] Radeztky A., Nurnberger A., Pretschner D. Elastodynamic shape modeler: a tool for defining the deformation behaviour of virtual tissues. *Radiographics* 20(3): 865-881, 2000.

Medicine Meets Virtual Reality 13
James D. Westwood et al. (Eds.)
IOS Press, 2005

# A Networked Haptic Virtual Environment for Teaching Temporal Bone Surgery

Matthew HUTCHINS [a], Stephen O'LEARY [b], Duncan STEVENSON [a],
Chris GUNN [a] and Alexander KRUMPHOLZ [a]

[a] CSIRO ICT Centre, Australia
[b] University of Melbourne Department of Otolaryngology, Australia
e-mail: Matthew.Hutchins@csiro.au

**Abstract.** This paper describes a computer system for teaching temporal bone surgery using networked haptic workbenches. The system enables an instructor and student to collaboratively explore and drill a volumetric bone model including significant anatomical features. Subjective evaluations by otologists have been favourable, and experimental trials are planned.

## 1. Introduction

This paper describes a computer system for teaching temporal bone surgery using virtual reality technology. The temporal bone, located in the base of the skull, houses the delicate organs of the middle and inner ear that contribute to hearing and balance. Safe surgical drilling in the region requires excellent knowledge of the complex 3D anatomy, confidence in the correct technique and approach to the procedure, and physical dexterity and tool handling skills. Training in temporal bone drilling is challenging; in particular, it is becoming more difficult to obtain access to the large number of human bone samples required to achieve competence.

From a technologist's point of view, there is a satisfying match between the requirements of temporal bone surgery training and the capabilities of certain types of virtual reality environments. For instance: stereo microscopy that is similar to current methods of presentation of interactive 3D graphics; tool use that is a good match in workspace and force to currently available haptic devices; the use of rigid bony models that are easier to segment from CT and simulate dynamically than many soft tissues.

Several groups have reported on previous and ongoing development of temporal bone trainers [1–6]. Our system adds to the growing body of research in this area, while at the same time taking a different approach on some of the key problems. Technically, we have chosen a hybrid volume/surface approach to graphical and haptic rendering of an erodable bone model. In terms of training, we have chosen to implement a networked system that allows a mentor to interactively observe and guide a trainee through the steps of a procedure. Our system is superficially similar to that recently reported by Morris et. al. [6], but is unrelated, and differs in the implementation details. Our aim is to demonstrate the effectiveness of this sort of training through experimental trials.

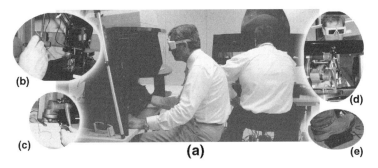

**Figure 1.** The Haptic Workbench configured for temporal bone surgery training. (a) Instructor and student seated at networked haptic workbenches. (b) One hand uses a haptic device for drilling. (c) The other hand uses a haptic device for suction, or 6DOF input device to orient the bone. (d) Active stereo shutter glasses generate 3D views. (e) A foot pedal controls the drill speed.

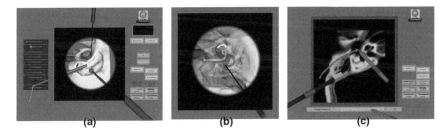

**Figure 2.** Screen captures of the system in operation. (a) A student drills the bone in the simulated microscope view, with guidance from the instructor. (b) The bone is made transparent to show the anatomical landmarks beneath. (c) The instructor annotates a slice from the CT scan of the bone.

## 2. System Overview

Our system uses the haptic workbench environment [7], with two Phantom haptic devices from SensAble Technologies [8], and a foot pedal to control drill speed, as shown in Figure 1. The software was developed using the Reachin API [9], and makes use of our previously reported software tools and approach to developing collaborative haptic surgical training systems [10–12]. Although the system can be used by a trainee alone, one of our main aims is to explore how networked virtual reality systems can be used for surgical mentoring, both within the same room, and tele-collaboratively over long distances. Thus, the system allows two users at separate haptic workbenches, typically an instructor and student, to share a common view of the procedure, and interact equally. Depending on the hardware configuration, there may be as many as four tools active in the scene simultaneously (two hands for each user). As an example of use, the instructor might demonstrate the drilling, then reset the model and observe the student perform the same task.

The primary view provided by the system is of a simulated stereo microscope, with a temporal bone model placed centrally (Figure 2). Several tools are available for selection in either hand, including a drill handle, sucker, facial nerve stimulating probe, marker, eraser, and networked haptic guiding hand. The drill handle can be loaded with cutting or polishing burrs in a range of sizes. The bone models for the system are volumetric, derived from CT scans. We also model, as polygonal surfaces, some of the major anatomical landmarks in the bone, including the dura, the sigmoid sinus, the carotid artery, the facial nerve, the labyrinth, the eardrum and lining of the external ear canal, and the ossicles.

## 3. Preliminary Evaluation

Our first significant experimental trials, designed to measure training transfer, will be conducted in November 2004. In March 2004 the system was demonstrated at the annual scientific conference of the surgical specialty in Australia, and at an associated hospital-based temporal bone drilling course, in order to gather qualitative feedback about the acceptability of the system to educators and trainees, and to record suggestions for future improvements. We asked attendees to experience the demonstration and fill out a short questionnaire, ranking the acceptability of various aspects of the system on a five point scale and providing written comments on other areas.

Feedback from the questionnaire was strongly in favour of the concept we presented, and also helped us to identify key ways we can improve the system for future trials. For example, 54 out of 55 respondents ranked the concept as "acceptable" (3) or better for teaching surgical anatomy, and 51 respondents ranked the concept as "acceptable" or better for teaching surgical planning and approach. 16 out of 16 respondents who experienced remote mentoring across a network ranked the mentoring concept as 4 or 5 out of 5.

## 4. Future Work and Conclusion

Our system has been designed with a strong emphasis on the requirements of teaching safe temporal bone surgery, with less weight given to physical simulation realism. Thus, the initial use will be in teaching surgical anatomy and surgical planning and approach. We hope to soon be able to demonstrate a measurable improvement in surgical technique, at least in the bone drilling lab, after students use our system. This will add value to the existing training, and may enable a reduction in the number of human bone samples that are required to achieve safe competence.

## Acknowledgement

This work was funded under the CeNTIE project. The CeNTIE project is supported by the Australian Government through the Advanced Networks Program of the Department of Communications, Information Technology and the Arts.

## References

[1] Mary Rasmussen, Theodore P. Mason, Alan Millman, Ray Evenhouse and Daniel Sandin. "The virtual temporal bone, a tele-immersive educational environment." *Future Generation Computer Systems*, volume 14, pages 125 – 130, 1998.
[2] Gregory J. Wiet, J. Bryan, E. Dodson, D. Sessanna, D. Stredney, P. Schmalbrock and B. Welling. "Virtual temporal bone dissection simulation." In proceedings of *Medicine Meets Virtual Reality*, 2000, IOS Press.

[3]   Nigel W. John, Neil Thacker, Maja Pokric, Alan Jackson, Gianluigi Zanetti, Enrico Gobbetti, Andrea Giachetti, Robert J. Stone, Joao Campos, Ad Emmen, Armin Schwerdtner, Emanuele Neri, Stefano Sellari Franceschini, and Frederic Rubio. "An integrated simulator for surgery of the petrous bone." In proceedings of *Medicine Meets Virtual Reality*, 2001, IOS Press.

[4]   Marco Agus, Andrea Giachetti, Enrico Gobbetti, Gianluigi Zanetti, Antonio Zorcolo, Nigel W. John, and Robert J. Stone. "Mastoidectomy simulation with combined visual and haptic feedback." In proceedings of *Medicine Meets Virtual Reality*, 2002, IOS Press.

[5]   Bernhard Pflesser, Andreas Petersik, Ulf Tiede, Karl Heinz Höhne and Rudolf Leuwer. "Volume cutting for virtual petrous bone surgery." Computer Aided Surgery, volume 7, number 2, pages 74 – 83, 2002.

[6]   Dan Morris, Christopher Sewell, Nikolas Blevins, Federico Barbagli, and Kenneth Salisbury. "A collaborative virtual environment for the simulation of temporal bone surgery." In proceedings of *Medical Image Computing and Computer-Assisted Intervention – MICCAI 2004*, Lecture Notes in Computer Science, volume 3217, pages 319 – 327, 2004, Springer-Verlag.

[7]   Duncan R. Stevenson, Kevin A. Smith, John P. McLaughlin, Chris J. Gunn, J. Paul Veldkamp, and Mark J. Dixon. "Haptic Workbench: A multisensory virtual environment." In proceedings of *SPIE – The International Society for Optical Engineering*, volume 3639, pages 356 – 366, 1999.

[8]   SensAble Technologies. Web site: http://www.sensable.com (visited October 2004).

[9]   Reachin Technologies AB. Web site: http://www.reachin.se (visited October 2004).

[10]  Chris Gunn, Matthew Hutchins, Matt Adcock and Rhys Hawkins. "Trans-world haptic collaboration". In proceedings of *SIGGRAPH (Sketches and Applications)*, 2003.

[11]  Chris Gunn, Matthew Hutchins, Matt Adcock and Rhys Hawkins. "Surgical training using haptics over long distances." In proceedings of *Medicine Meets Virtual Reality*, 2004, IOS Press.

[12]  C. Gunn, D. Stevenson, A. Krumm-Heller, S. Srivastava, P. Youngblood, L. Heinrichs, and P. Dev. "An interactive master class in remote surgery." In proceedings of *OZCHI*, 2004 (to appear).

Medicine Meets Virtual Reality 13
James D. Westwood et al. (Eds.)
IOS Press, 2005

208

# Real-Time Haptic Interface for VR Colonoscopy Simulation

Dejan ILIC [a], Thomas MOIX [a], Nial MC CULLOUGH [a], Lindo DURATTI [a],
Ivan VECERINA [b] and Hannes BLEULER [a]

[a] *Laboratoire de Systèmes Robotiques (LSRO), EPFL,
Chemin des Machines, ME.B3, 1015 Lausanne, Switzerland*
[b] *Xitact S.A., Rue de Lausanne 45, 1110 Morges, Switzerland*

**Abstract.** Colonoscopy is an endoscopic medical procedure where the colon of the patient is examined. This minimally invasive technique is performed with a colonoscope, a long tube with an integrated imaging device at its tip. The doctors performing these procedures require high skills in multiple domains such as hand-eye coordination, visualization, safety and ease at guiding flexible endoscopes. The importance of training colonoscopy procedures rises with the growth of variety of colon diseases.

In order to safely train surgeons to these procedures, a computer-assisted haptic simulator is proposed. This paper describes both the haptic hardware interface and virtual reality software that compose the training system. A high friction belt is used to render the required forces and to insure the absence of slippage. A differential drive actuated with two DC motors enables to set the system into translation and rotation. A virtual reality environment has been developed to provide real-time visualisation and force feedback.

## 1. Introduction

### 1.1. Colonoscopy

Colonoscopy is an endoscopic procedure performed to inspect the inner lining of the rectum and entire colon (large intestine). It is carried out with a colonoscope, which is a long flexible tube that carries a miniaturized wide-angle camera installed at its tip. A colonoscopy is generally recommended to patients who complain of rectal bleeding, a change in bowel habits, or other unexplained abdominal symptoms, but also as a regular check-up for patients at risk for colon cancer. It allows diagnosing, assessing and sometimes treating intestinal inflammation, ulcerations, bleeding, colitis, colon polyps or cancers.

During the procedure, a well-lubricated flexible colonoscope is inserted and guided through the colon. To clear the intestine doctors may pump in some air. If there is blood or excessive secretions that obstruct the field of view, they can be suctioned out. The entire length of the colon can be examined in similar manner. If suspicious growths are observed, the doctor can perform a biopsy. In such case, a polyp sample is taken and sent to the laboratory for analysis. Small polyps can also be directly removed through the colonoscope. At the end of the examination, the colonoscope is slowly withdrawn. The complete procedure lasts from 30 minutes to 2 hours depending on how easy it is to navigate the colonoscope [1].

## 1.2. Colonoscopy Challenges

A physician performing a colonoscopy procedure faces several difficulties: the moving viewpoint makes hand-eye coordination challenging; the vision field is very limited, tactile sensations are weakened due to the length of the instruments and the encountered friction forces. Another major difficulty is to prevent and reduce the looping of the tip of the colonoscope. The endoscopist must be taught the principles of loop formation and the techniques to safely reduce the loops while performing a procedure. All trainees should also understand the need for frequent withdrawal of the colonoscope by applying clockwise torque [2].

## 1.3. Colonoscopy Training

Extensive training is required before a physician can safely perform complicated colonoscopy procedures on real patients. Practicing on cadavers or animals is of limited effectiveness, since tissue properties and the anatomy are different and some pathologies are difficult to find.

A computer-assisted training system provides a cost-efficient and more ethical alternative. Such systems consist of a virtual reality (VR) environment simulating an anatomy and the interaction of the surgical instruments. However, existing systems [3,4] fail to accurately reproduce the force and torque dynamic experienced during a real procedure. Some studies show that the maximal force obtained in colonoscopy is up to 44N in translation and 1Nm in rotation [5]. Other groups [6,7], reported haptic interfaces for colonoscopy with maximal translational force of 8N.

## 2. A Haptic Interface for Colonoscopy Simulation

## 2.1. Requirements

During a typical procedure the colonoscope is inserted along and rotated around an axis entering the colon. The tip of the colonoscope can be angled, according to two perpendicular planes, to select the correct orientation inside the colon. An accurate simulation requires the control of four degrees of freedom:

- Translation and rotation of the colonoscope
- X-Y planar bending of the tip.

Estimated forces and torques for a procedure performed with a regular size colonoscope are respectively in range of about ±44N and ±1Nm with resolutions of 0.45N and 0.09Nm [8].

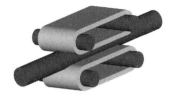

**Figure 1.** The Friction Belt Drive.

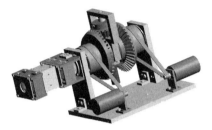

**Figure 2.** The Differential Gear Arrangement with Actuators.

## 2.2. The Proposed Interface

This paper focuses on the development of the unit that handles a colonoscope. The instrument is held between two rubber coated belts mounted on four cylinders as illustrated in Figure 1. The belts and cylinders are notched to permit an accurate control of the advance of the flexible tube. The tube can be set in translation with the rotation of the cylinders that are mounted into the structure of the device. The rotation is obtained through the rotation of the structure into which the cylinders are mounted.

The contact forces between the apparatus and the colonoscope need to be particularly high in order to reach the required maximum of 44N. A high friction belt spreads the area on which the force is applied over a greater surface. Therefore, the system can achieve the required forces without destroying the colonoscope. In the case of a colonoscope coated with polytetrafluoroethylene (PTFE) a dynamic friction coefficient of 0.3 with the rubber can be observed. This will require a contact force of 146N in order to insure absence of slippage, even in case of high insertion forces. The system adapts to diameters varying from 9 mm to 25 mm. A spring mechanism preloads the surface of the belt insuring a sufficient contact force between the belt and the colonoscope, independently of its diameter.

In order to actuate the translational movement of the interface, a motor can be mounted directly onto the belt system. In that case the added weight and the inertia would hinder the dynamical behaviour of the system. Thus, a conical gear system is proposed to set the system into rotation and translation in an indirect and external way. This arrangement enables the control of both the rotation and translation of the colonoscope with a differential drive presented in Figure 2. The inner wheel of the gear rotates around its own axis advancing the belt and thus setting the colonoscope into the translation. When the two outer wheels are rotating at identical speeds, the gear will rotate around the axis of the entire system enabling the control of the rotation of the colonoscope. Both the rotation and translation are controlled by two DC motors. The forces that must be exerted upon the system have been determined and the motors chosen to satisfy the force requirements as closely as possible.

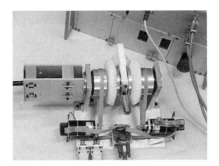

**Figure 3.** The Haptic Interface for Colonoscopy Simulation.

## 2.3. VR Simulation Environment

The virtual reality model that has been developed provides real-time visualization and force feedback of the colon and the colonoscope. The model of the colon was extracted from the database of the *Visible Human Project* by the *Computer Vision Laboratory (BIWI)*, ETHZ (Zurich, Switzerland). The colon is modelled by a two-dimensional mesh and a skeleton composed of spheres and links. The mesh nodes are connected to the closest skeleton element. Each skeleton element has a bounding box and is surrounded by the mesh. Bounding boxes limit the area where a collision of the colon with the colonoscope can occur (9). Hence, the speed of the overall collision detection algorithm is greatly improved. Collisions with the mesh are computed only for particles of the colonoscope that are outside of any bounding box. The deformations of the colon are computed in two steps. Local small deformations are handled by the mesh. The mesh is modified according to the applied pressure. Global deformation is computed with the skeleton elements. The links of the skeleton are given stiffness. A new sphere is added to the skeleton when a particle of the colonoscope is still outside of any bounding box but a collision with the mesh occurs. The mesh nodes where the collision occurs transmit forces to their links on the skeleton. A spring mass-model is used to compute the new dynamic position of the spheres [10].

The colonoscope is modelled as a chain of segments linked by joints whose positions are computed using the inverse kinematics [11]. The motion of the colonoscope measured by the hardware is reflected in the simulation and its trajectory is computed based on the collisions with the colon and the internal constraint limitations of the instrument. Contact forces are summed up to compute the haptic force feedback. The rotation of the camera attached to the colonoscope is simulated by rotating the camera view.

## 2.4. The Realized Prototype

The realized prototype of the haptic hardware interface for colonoscopy is presented in Figure 3. Forces and torques that are rendered reach respectively 44N and 2.2Nm with resolutions of 21.5mN and 0.5mNm. Optical encoders provide tracking with a resolution of $\pm 0.03°$ in rotation and $\pm 13 \mu m$ in translation.

The system has been integrated with the existing control and measurement electronics that had been developed in our institution for previous haptic interfaces.

The proposed VR environment runs on a standard PC (PIII, 866 MHz, 256 MB RAM) equipped with a 3D graphic card (NVidia GeForce3). A frame rate of around

25 Hz is reached with a scene composed of a colon anatomy (16000 triangles) and a colonoscope of 200 particles.

## 3. Conclusion

A computer-assisted training system for colonoscopy has been developed to improve the current state of the art by delivering realistic sensations. The simulation framework includes a VR environment, a 3D anatomy, a rendering and physics engine adapted to the procedure.

Further work focuses on improving the device that is handling the tip of the colonoscope. Force sensors are being integrated in to the current prototype to further enhance the accuracy of the haptic sensations. On the software side, rendering is being improved and enhancements to the interaction models will raise the overall performance of the complete system.

## Acknowledgement

This research is supported by the Swiss National Science Foundation within the framework NCCR CO-ME (COmputer aided and image guided MEdical interventions).

## References

[1] E. Huang and J. Marks. "The diagnostic and therapeutic roles of colonoscopy", Surgical Endoscopy, vol.15, no. 12, pp. 1373-1380, Dec. 2001.

[2] C. Viala, M. Zimmerman, D. Cullen and N. Hoffman, "Complication rates of colonoscopy in an Australian teaching hospital environment", Internal medicine journal, vol. 33, no. 8, Aug. 2003.

[3] R. E. Sedlack and J. C. Kolars, "Colonoscopy curriculum development and performance-based assessment criteria on a computer-based endoscopy simulator", In progress reports, www.simbionix.com.

[4] T. Grantcharov, A. Eversbuch, P. Funch-Jensen, "Teaching and testing surgical skills on a VR endoscopy simulator-learning curves and impact of psychomotor training on performance in simulated colonoscopy", GI Mentor validation studies, SAGES, 2004, Denver, Colorado.

[5] M. Appleyard, C. Mosse, T. Mills, G. Bells, F. Castillo, and C. Swain, "The measurment of forces during colonoscopy," Gastrointestinal Endoscopy, vol. 52, no. 2, Aug. 2000.

[6] O. Körner and R. Männer, "Implementation of a haptic interface for a virtual reality simulator for flexible endoscopy," in 11th Symposium on Haptic Interfaces for Virtual Environment and Teleoperator Systems (IEEE-VR2003), Los Angeles, CA, 2003, pp. 278–284.

[7] K. Ikuta, M. Takeichi, and T. Namiki, "Virtual endoscope system with force sensation," in Lecture Notes in Computer Science, MICCAI'98, vol. 1496, 1998, pp. 293–304.

[8] H. Tan, B. Eberman, M. Srinivasan, and B. Cheng, "Human factors for he design of force-reflecting haptic interfaces," Dyn. Sys. Cont., vol. 55, no. 1, 1994.

[9] M. Vollenweider "High quality virtual systems with haptic feedback", Ph. D. dissertation, EPFL, Lausanne, Switzerland, 2000.

[10] U. Spaelter, L. Duratti, D. Ilic, T. Moix, and H. Bleuler, "The Virtual Patient: Surgery Simulation and Virtual Reality Modelling", in 21$^{th}$ CADFEM User's Meeting, Berlin, Germany, November 2003.

[11] P. Baerlocher, R. Boulic, "Combining Multiple Tasks with Different Priorities for Human Posture Control", to appear in The Visual Computer 20, summer 2004.

*Medicine Meets Virtual Reality 13*
*James D. Westwood et al. (Eds.)*
*IOS Press, 2005*

# Computational Simulation of Penetrating Trauma in Biological Soft Tissues using the Material Point Method

Irina IONESCU [a,b], James GUILKEY [a,c], Martin BERZINS [a,d],
Robert M. KIRBY [a,d] and Jeffrey WEISS [a,b]

[a] *Scientific Computing and Imaging Institute*
[b] *Department of Bioengineering*
[c] *Department of Mechanical Engineering*
[d] *School of Computing, University of Utah*

**Abstract.** The objective of this research was to develop realistic computational models for soft tissues subjected to finite deformation and failure, and to test these models in the context of numerical simulations of penetrating trauma injuries. A transversely isotropic hyperelastic model with strain-based failure criteria was used to represent the behavior of anisotropic soft tissue. The constitutive model was implemented into an existing numerical code based on the Material Point Method (MPM). The penetration of a low-speed bullet through a myocardium material slab was simulated and several wounding scenarios were analyzed and compared. The material symmetry, the type of contact modeled between the bullet and the soft tissue and the bullet speed were shown to have a significant influence on the wound profile.

## 1. Introduction

Injuries due to penetrating trauma from bullet or knife wounds represent a significant healthcare problem [1]. An improved understanding of the factors that control the extent of tissue damage from these wounds can provide the means to improve diagnosis and treatment. Soft tissue failure (skeletal and cardiac muscle, ligament and tendon, nerve) typically represents a large part of the damage resulting from penetrating trauma [2]. However, the detailed three dimensional prediction of soft tissue failure is complicated by the highly anisotropic nature of the materials as well as the lack of appropriate failure models.

The objective of this research was to develop realistic computational models for soft tissues subjected to finite deformation and failure and to implement and test these models in the context of numerical simulations of penetrating trauma injuries.

## 2. Methods

The current research focused on modeling penetrating injuries to an analog of the myocardium. A "two-surface" strain-based failure criterion was incorporated into a hyperelastic constitutive model of the myocardium. The myocardium was represented as a composite of matrix and collagen fibers, each failing by different strain-driven failure mechanisms. Bullet penetration simulations of myocardial material slabs were performed using the Material Point Method (MPM) with explicit time integration [3].

## 2.1. Constitutive model and Failure Criteria

A strain-based failure model was developed for transversely isotropic hyperelastic soft tissues. The myocardium was modeled as a transversely isotropic hyperelastic material, comprised of an isotropic Mooney-Rivlin matrix reinforced by a single fiber family [4]. The local fiber direction was described by a unit vector $\mathbf{a^0}$ that changes direction and length as the material deforms, so that:

$$F \cdot a^0 = \lambda a, \tag{1}$$

where $\lambda$ denotes the local fiber stretch and $\mathbf{F}$ is the deformation gradient tensor. The strain energy function $W$ was written in terms of the matrix and fiber response, respectively:

$$W = F_1(I_1, I_2) + F_2(\lambda), \tag{2}$$

where $I_1$ and $I_2$ are the first and second invariants of the right Cauchy-Green deformation tensor. The matrix was modeled using a Mooney-Rivlin model, while the elastic response of collagen fibers was considered exponential in the toe region and linear subsequently [5]:

$$F_1(I_1, I_2) = c_1(I_1 - 3) + c_2(I_2 - 3)$$

$$\lambda \frac{\partial F_2}{\partial \lambda} = \begin{cases} 0, & \lambda < 1 \\ c_3 e^{c_4(\lambda-1)-1}, & \lambda \le \lambda^* \\ c_5 \lambda + c_6, & \lambda > \lambda^* \end{cases} \tag{3}$$

The five material coefficients to define the transverse isotropy of the above described material have been chosen as follows. The Mooney-Rivlin constants for the matrix were taken as $c_1 = 2.1$. KPa, $c_2 = 0$. The elastic fibers were characterized by a constant to scale the exponential stresses in the toe region $c_3 = 0.14$ KPa, the rate of fiber uncrimping $c_3 = 22$, and the modulus of the straightened collagen $c_5 = 100$ Kpa [4]. The stretch at which the collagen fibers straighten was assigned a value of $\lambda^* = 1.4$ [4]. The constant $c_6$ was determined from the condition that the collagen stress is continuous at $\lambda^*$. The material was considered as nearly incompressible, with a bulk:shear modulus ratio of 47.62. To represent the type of material symmetry exhibited by the myocardium, the fiber direction $a^0$ was varied through the thickness of the slab so that fibers rotated clockwise 180° from epicardial to endocardial surface (Fig. 1a).

A strain-based failure criterion was developed to quantify failure resulting from the wounding. The myocardium can be seen as a composite material whose phases, matrix and fibers, have different ultimate strains, the collagen fibers withstanding a higher tensile strain than the matrix. Two modes of failure were represented: matrix failure under shear (Fig. 1b) and fiber failure under tension (Fig. 1c); hence the failure criterion was defined in terms of two failure surfaces. With these assumptions, the Cauchy stress was decomposed as:

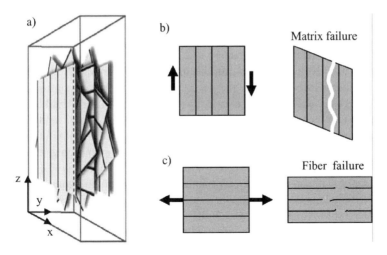

**Figure 1.** a) Material symmetry of the myocardial slab. The local fiber direction rotated 180 degrees through thickness of the slab. Failure modes: b) matrix failure via shear strain and c) fiber failure via elongation along the fiber direction.

$$\sigma = \sigma_{\text{volumetric}} + \sigma_{\text{matrix}} + \sigma_{\text{fibers}} \tag{4}$$

The matrix material was considered to fail locally if the maximum shear strain at a point exceeded 50% strain [6] and the matrix contribution to the stress was annulled:

$$\gamma_{\text{matrix}} > 50\% \;\Rightarrow\; \sigma_{\text{matrix}} = 0, \; \sigma_{\text{volumetric}} = 0 \tag{5}$$

If the fiber stretch $\lambda$ exceeded 40% [5] strain at a point, the fiber was considered failed and its contribution to the total state of stress was annulled:

$$\varepsilon_{\text{fibers}} > 40\% \;\Rightarrow\; \sigma_{\text{fibers}} = 0 \tag{6}$$

If both of the above conditions were fulfilled locally, the material point exhibited total failure.

At each material point, the strains in the matrix and fibers were compared with the assigned failure values. A failure flag was defined at each of the particles in the model, to record if and what particular type of material failure may occur. The type of failure and the distribution of failed particles helped to interpret the wound profile.

## 2.2. Numerical Discretization with Material Point Method

The equations of motion were discretized in space using the Material Point Method (MPM) [3]. Explicit time integration was used. MPM is a particle method for simulations in computational mechanics that is implemented within the Uintah computational framework, a software infrastructure for large-scale numerical simulations [7]. Like other quasi-meshless methods, MPM offers an attractive alternative to traditional finite element (FE) methods [8] because it simplifies the modeling of complex geometries, large deformations and fragmentations that are typical of penetrating trauma to the torso or its components.

## 2.3. Test problems

To test the failure model, the penetration of a bullet through a slab of myocardium was simulated. A $50 \times 10 \times 50$ mm myocardial slab was considered (Fig. 1a). The $x-y$ and $y-z$ side boundaries were fixed, while the $x-z$ faces were free of constraints. A 9 mm diameter bullet was modeled as an elastic-plastic material with neo-Hookean elastic material properties (properties used: bulk modulus $K = 117$ GPa, shear modulus $\mu = 53.8$ GPa, yield stress 422.6 MPa, hardening modulus 53.8 MPa). The simulations consisted of $1.6 \cdot 10^6$ material points, distributed in a $4 \times 4 \times 4$ spacing in each grid cell.

Simulations of a bullet wound to a myocardial tissue sample were performed using several material symmetry models and wounding scenarios. Simulations were performed for bullet velocities in the 'low-speed' range, i.e. less than 1000 ft/s. Low speed projectiles have been shown to produce most of their damage by crushing the tissue, and almost no damage due to cavitation. Two initial bullet velocities were considered: 150 m/s and 50 m/s. To study the effects of anisotropy on wound profile, an isotropic material slab was also considered and results were compared to that obtained for the anisotropic case. Frictional contact with a coefficient of friction of 0.08 was considered between the bullet and the soft tissue. The matrix, fiber, or total tissue failure were recorded for the each of the simulations.

## 3. Results

The wound profile in each of the cases showed the damage from the bullet as it passed through the myocardial sample. The wound profile for the case of a bullet with an initial speed of 150 m/s and an anisotropic slab is presented in Fig. 2.

In all cases the entrance wound had a clean appearance and an approximate circular shape. Total tissue failure was observed in the immediate vicinity of the bullet tract, zones of matrix and fiber failure surrounding the inner total tissue failure zone (Fig. 2). The wound tract diameter increased uniformly from entrance to exit. The exit wound appeared to be elliptic, the fiber alignment in the slab outer layer perhaps influencing its regular shape. The phenomenon of cavitation of the bullet was not observed, due primarily to the small thickness of the slab.

The wound profiles and shape of the exits wounds were different between the anisotropic and isotropic cases (Fig. 3). The shape of the exit wound was elliptic for the case of anisotropic material symmetry (Fig. 3a) and circular for the case of isotropic material symmetry (Fig. 3b).

## 4. Discussion

The results of the test problems are encouraging and can be interpreted in terms of the physics of the bullet penetration.

The wound profile (Fig. 2) showed an approximate circular central area of complete tissue disruption in the bullet path presenting a diameter increase from entrance to exit, as bullets were reported to produce [1]. The adjoining area of 'injured' soft tissue, presented a layered failed particle distribution. As the bullet penetrated the slab, it transferred its

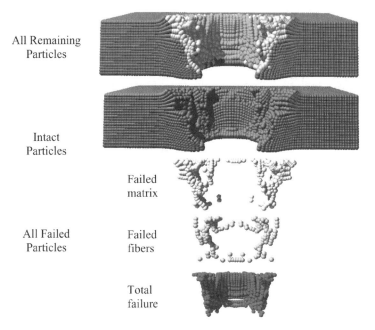

All Remaining
Particles

Intact
Particles

Failed
matrix

All Failed
Particles

Failed
fibers

Total
failure

**Figure 2.** Wound profile and failed particles for a myocardium slab in which material fibers rotate 180°
through thickness. The failed particles are separated by the type of failure undergone: matrix, fiber or total
tissue failure.

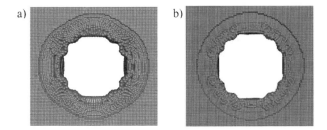

a)    b)

**Figure 3.** Effects of anisotropy on the wound profile (exit wound view): a) anisotropic slab; b) isotropic slab
(initial bullet speed 50 m/s).

energy to the surrounding tissue producing damage. Closest to the wound tract, a layer
of particles recording total tissue failure was observed, surrounded by a layer of particles
with fiber failure and matrix failure. The damage dissipated with the distance from the
bullet tract, as physically expected [1].

Fiber reinforcement was shown to make a difference even for very slow speeds (50
m/s) to the wound appearance (Fig. 3). The isotropic case presented a totally symmetric wound pattern, whereas in the anisotropic case the collagen fibers contribute to the
asymmetry of the wound profile.

The jaggedness of the exit wound (Fig. 3) is most likely a result of projecting a circular object (the bullet) to a cartesian mesh. This artifact becomes less prominent with
increasing grid resolution. Future work will investigate the use of higher order interpolation, which is also likely to improve the results.

It is understood that the predictions of failure from these simulations will clearly depend on the assumptions associated with the failure model. Future research will consider alternative myocardial material models [9] and failure properties. Beyond this, the approach of using MPM with constitutive models that explicitly represent failure in composites may be useful for large-scale simulations of injuries to the torso that affect multiple organs. Preliminary large-scale simulations of the entire torso, including bones and soft tissue organs, have yielded encouraging results. Others have reported on the use of MPM for modeling material failure and accommodating structural failure under impact [10]; this research demonstrates the feasibility of using MPM for computational modeling of soft tissue failure associated with penetrating wounds.

## Acknowledgement

This work was supported by a grant from the DARPA, executed by the U.S. Army Medical Research and Materiel Command/TATRC Cooperative Agreement, Contract # W81XWH-04-2-0012.

## References

[1] Bartlett CS, *'Clinical Update: Gunshot Wound Ballistics'*: Clin Orth and Rel Research, 2003; 408:28-57.
[2] Eisler RD, Chatterjee AK, Burghart GH, *'Simulation and modeling of penetrating wounds from small arms'*: Stud Health Technol Inform, 1996; 29:511-22.
[3] Sulsky D, Chen Z, Schreyer HL, *'A particle method for history dependent materials'*: Comp Meth Appl Mech Eng, 1994, 118:179-196.
[4] Humphrey JD, Strumpf RK, Yin FC, *'Determination of a constitutive relation for passive myocardium: II. Parameter estimation'*, J Biomech Eng., 1990; 112(3):340-346.
[5] Weiss JA, Maker BN, Govindjee S., *'Finite element implementation of incompressible, transversely isotropic hyperelasticity'*: Comp Meth Appl Mech Eng, 1996; 135:107-128.
[6] Hunter PJ, McCulloch AD, ter Keurs HE, *'Modelling the mechanical properties of cardiac muscle'*: Prog Biophys Mol Biol, 1998; 69:289-331.
[7] Parker S, *'A Component-based Architecture for Parallel Multi-Physics PDE Simulation'*: Intl Conf on Comp Science (ICCS2002) Workshop on PDE Software, 2002, April 21-24.
[8] Chen Z, Brannon R, *'An Evaluation of the Material Point Method'*: Sand Report, SAND2002-0482.
[9] Guccione JM, McCulloch AD, Waldman LK, *'Passive material properties of intact ventricular myocardium determined from a cylindrical model'*: J Biomech Engng, 1991; 113:42-55.
[10] Chen Z, Hu W, *'Recent Advances in First-Principle Simulation of the Transition from Continuous to Discontinuous Failure under Impact'*, 16th Eng Mech Conf of the ASCE, Seattle, Washington, 2003, July 16-18.

*Medicine Meets Virtual Reality 13*
*James D. Westwood et al. (Eds.)*
*IOS Press, 2005*

# Adaptive Soft Tissue Deformation for a Virtual Reality Surgical Trainer

Lenka JERABKOVA [a], Timm P. WOLTER [c], Norbert PALLUA [c]
and Torsten KUHLEN [a]

[a] *Center for Computing and Communication, RWTH Aachen University*
*e-mail: jerabkova@rz.rwth-aachen.de*
[c] *Department of Plastic and Reconstructive Surgery, Hand Surgery – Burn Center,*
*University Hospital Aachen*

**Abstract.** Real time tissue deformation is an important aspect of interactive virtual reality (VR) environments such as medical trainers. Most approaches in deformable modelling use a fixed space discretization. A surgical trainer requires high plausibility of the deformations especially in the area close to the instrument. As the area of intervention is not known a priori, adaptive techniques have to be applied.

We present an approach for real time deformation of soft tissue based on a regular FEM mesh of cube elements as opposed to a mesh of tetrahedral elements used by the majority of soft tissue simulators. A regular mesh structure simplifies the local refinement operation as the elements topology and stiffness are known implicitly. We propose an octree-based adaptive multiresolution extension of our basic approach.

The volumetric representation of the deformed object is created automatically from medical images or by voxelization of a surface model. The resolution of the volumetric representation is independent of the surface geometry resolution. The surface is deformed according to the simulation performed on the underlying volumetric mesh.

## 1. Introduction

Real time tissue deformation is an important aspect of interactive virtual reality (VR) environments such as medical trainers. Most approaches in deformable modelling use a fixed space discretization. A surgical trainer requires high plausibility of the deformations especially in the area close to the instrument. As the area of intervention is not known a priori, adaptive techniques have to be applied. Although our main focus lies on virtual surgery, the approach we present can be used for arbitrary 3D objects.

## 2. Related Work

[1] discuss a level of detail (LOD) technique, which uses independently defined meshes representing the simulated object at different resolutions. The deformable body can be simulated by combining fine LOD at the area of interest with coarser LODs. [2] propose a dynamic extension of the progressive mesh (PM) concept. The dynamic progressive meshes (DPM) allow selective online refinement at the area of interest. Geometric and

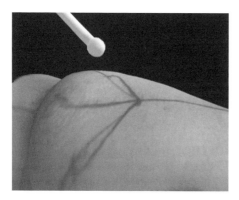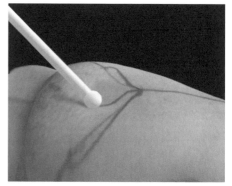

**Figure 1.** An interactive deformation of a female breast.

finite element parameters are precalculated offline for each level of the hierarchy. [3], [4] and [5] describe hybrid techniques that use different computational models for the area of interest and for the remaining parts. [6] use a hierarchical particle representation. An octree structure is used to store the uniform space samples at each level. The proposed method offers an automatic adaptive resolution.

## 3. Method

We present an approach for real time deformation of soft tissue based on a regular finite elements method (FEM) mesh of cube elements as opposed to a mesh of tetrahedral elements used by the majority of soft tissue simulators. The volumetric representation of an object is created automatically from segmented medical images or by voxelization of a given surface model. The original mesh is deformed according to the simulation performed on the underlying volumetric mesh.

Most FEM approaches in medical simulation use the decimated surface to generate tetrahedral representation of the volume closed by the surface. A tetrahedra mesh generally approximates a volume better than a cubic mesh with elements of similar size. The boundary faces of the FE model are identical to the triangles of the geometry surface, which makes the update of the geometry surface simple. However, to achieve a good visual quality a high resolution surface is required, whereas a plausible deformation can be achieved with coarser elements. Furthermore, as the tetrahedra geometries are different, the local subdivision of the finite elements requires computing and saving of all element stiffness matrices separately.

A regular mesh structure simplifies the local refinement operation as the elements topology is known implicitly. The size of the finite elements is independent of the resolution of the deformed surface. Since all elements have the same geometry, their stiffness matrices only depend on material properties. Thus, only one stiffness matrix per material as opposed to one per finite element has to be generated.

The deformed surface intersects the finite elements, but the surface faces and vertices do not exactly match with the finite elements or nodes. Each FEM element stores a list of intersecting faces that have to be updated when the element is deformed. The deformation is computed for the FEM mesh. The vertex displacements are then computed using trilinear interpolation of the displacements of the surrounding FEM nodes (Figure 1).

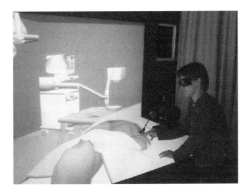

**Figure 2.** A VR Surgical Trainer Application on a Holobench.

A realistic tissue deformation at the area of intervention is of high importance for a surgery training system. At the same time, a real time response to user actions in an interactive virtual environment is crucial. Organizing the cube elements in an octree structure enables an adaptive refinement of the mesh at the area of interest. The simulation starts at a default resolution level. Once the user interacts with the object, the mesh is gradually refined using a fine resolution at the area of interaction and coarse resolutions at distant areas.

## 4. Results

The approach described in this paper is integrated in a virtual reality environment for the training of plastic surgeons. The VR surgery trainer offers a new instrument for shortening the learning curve of medical students. The first operation we simulate is breast reduction as it is one of the most common interventions of medium complexity in plastic surgery. Basic manipulations are performed with force feedback using the PHANToM haptic device. The visual display is accomplished on a two sided Holobench (Figure 2).

## 5. Discussion

We present an adaptive method for real time soft tissue deformation. Our approach is based on a hierarchical structure of cubic FEM elements. We use the described technique in a VR environment for training of plastic surgeons, which requires topological changes (cutting) of the manipulated geometry. Tissue cutting has an immediate impact on the structure of the FE mesh and has to be integrated in our concept.

## References

[1]  Debunne, G., Desbrun, M., Cani, M. P., Barr, A. H., Adaptive simulation of soft bodies in real-time. *Proceedings of Computer Animation*, 2000.
[2]  Wu, X., Downes, M. S., Goktekin, T., Tendick, F., Adaptive nonlinear finite elements for deformable body simulation using dynamic progressive meshes. *Proceedings of Eurographics, vol. 20/3*, 2001.

[3] Wu, W., Sun, J., Heng, P. A., A hybrid condensed finite element model for interactive 3D soft tissue cutting. *Proceedings of Medicine Meets Virtual Reality*, 2003.

[4] Kim, J., De, S., Srinivasan, M. A., Physically based hybrid approach in real time surgical simulation with force feedback. *Proceedings of Medicine Meets Virtual Reality*, 2003.

[5] Faraci, A., Bello, F., Darzi, A., Soft tissue deformation using a hierarchical finite element model. *Proceedings of Medicine Meets Virtual Reality*, 2004.

[6] Debunne, G., Desbrun, M., Barr, A. H., Cani, M. P., Interactive multiresolution animation of deformable models. *Proceedings of Eurographics Workshop on Computer Animation and Simulation*, 1999.

Medicine Meets Virtual Reality 13
James D. Westwood et al. (Eds.)
IOS Press, 2005

# Simulation of Color Deficiency in Virtual Reality

Bei JIN, Zhuming AI and Mary RASMUSSEN

*Virtual Reality in Medicine Lab, College of Applied Health Sciences,*
*University of Illinois at Chicago*
*e-mail: {bjin1,zai,mary}@uic.edu*

**Abstract.** Color deficiency protanopia is simulated in a virtual home environment. A color database is created to set the corresponding relation between each color for normal vision and for protanopia. Based on this database, a second texture system is set up for the home model. The proper texture system is used according to the user's choice on the interactive menu.

## 1. Introduction

Color deficiency is a common eye disease caused by absorption spectra shift of different cones (anomalous trichromacy), or the total lack of one or more kinds of cones (dichromacy). The theory of transformation function between normal vision and dichromacy is often applied to 2-dimensional print and Web content, both to educate the public and make design legible for color deficient users. We have expanded this work to simulate color deficiency protanopia in 3 dimensions, giving doctors, patient family members, and general public with normal vision a unique opportunity to "experience" color blindness in an immersive and familiar setting.

## 2. Method

A fundamental color space based on the spectral sensitivity function in the human visual system has been found, and a transformation function was set up between the color percept of normal vision and color deficiency [1]. On a uniform chromaticity diagram, there is a single confusion point for each type of color deficiency. Colors that are confused lie on straight lines radiating from this point. For protanpia, the point is at u=0.61, v=0.51, very close to the far red corner. There is an axis for each type of dichromacy, and all confused colors will collapse onto this axis. For protanopes, the ends of the axis are 473nm and 574nm (Fig 1).

Based on this special relationship, each color in a computer RGB color system (the area inside the triangular) is converted into CIE u', v' chromaticity coordinates. In this space, the intersection point of the major axis (dashed line in Fig 1) for each type of dichromacy and the confusion line (radiate line in Fig 1) that connects the original color and the confusion point for the same dichromacy is found. This intersection is the color

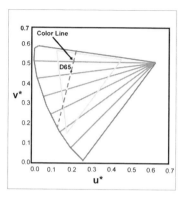

**Figure 1.** The CIE Yu¹v¹ color space, with confusion lines for prtanopes.

that a colorblind person will actually see. We then convert the resulting color back to RGB coordinates. In this way, a database can be calculated for the corresponding color pair.

We have built a 3-dimensional polygonal model of a typical Chicago house and furnishings, and added navigational functions to allow users to "walk" through the virtual home. When the house model is rendered, the colorblind database is also loaded. The whole virtual reality scene is a huge tree structure in Performer (a virtual reality development tool from SGI); each branch of it is searched from top to bottom level by level until reaching the ultimate leaf pfGeoSet (pfScene → pfChannel → pfGroup→ pfNode → pfGeode → pfGeoSet). pfGeoSet has texture information with it. Read the image from the original texture; look into the database and find the proper transformation color to establish a new texture for the colorblind condition. In this way, establish a texture list for each kind of texture found in the whole model, set the original texture as the default choice in the list, while list the new texture as the choice for color-blindness. According to the menu choice, navigate the tree branch again to set the proper texture active in the list.

In this house model, each polygon has texture applied, and the texture has priority to display over the material color. So the color in the model is purely from the texture, but not from a mixture of the texture and the material, or from the material alone. So in this color deficiency simulation, the change is applied only to the texture. If both texture and material are considered here, the different mix computation method between them will complicate this problem, so this transformation is simplified in the texture level alone. This limitation will be an area for future improvement.

Using these techniques, a picture of the world as seen by color deficient observers can be synthesized (Fig 2 and Fig 3).

## 3. Result

Since protanopia is a kind of 'red-green defect', colors with the same ratio of red and green components will look alike. Different pseudo-isochromatic plates are used in clinical settings to test for certain kinds of color deficiencies. Patterns on the plates are vis-

---

[1]Full color images can also be found at www.ahs.uic.edu/ahs/php/section.php?id=301.

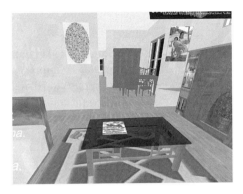

**Figure 2.** Normal Color Vision.

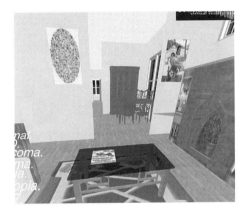

**Figure 3.** Color Vision For Protanopia.

ible to color normals, but invisible to dichromats. In the house model, such a pseudo-isochromatic plate is hung on the wall as a painting to show the result of a color deficiency simulation. After the menu choice, the number 5 on the plate is mixed with the background, and can't be discerned, and the tone of the whole house becomes more pale yellow (Fig 3). The transformations for other kinds of dichromacy have been also tried directly on other 2-dimensional pseudo-isochromatic plates and color spectra images, causing the similar chromatic aberrations and pattern confusion.

## 4. Conclusion

This color transformation theory has mainly been used in improving 2-dimensional computer graphic display and website design. This simulation in a virtual reality environment is a new attempt, and has wider application. Since many eye diseases have chromatic vision aberrations, this application lays the groundwork to simulate these diseases, and can help to improve medical education and interior design for patient safety.

## 5. Discussion

The large color database requires considerable time to load into memory. For this reason, only protanopia is realized in this application. Future improvements in data structure should make the memory usage more efficient. In this model, only the texture color can be changed, and the factors of material color and light color are not considered here, and are left for future development.

## References

[1]  Gary Meyer and Donald Greenberg: Color-Defective Vision and Computer Graphics Displays. IEEE Computer Graphics & Applications, September 1988.

*Medicine Meets Virtual Reality 13*
*James D. Westwood et al. (Eds.)*
*IOS Press, 2005*

# Improving the Visual Realism
# of Virtual Surgery

Wei JIN [a], Yi-Je LIM [a], Xie George XU [a], Tejinder P. SINGH [b] and Suvranu DE [a]

[a] *Department of Mechanical, Aerospace, and Nuclear Engineering,*
*Rensselaer Polytechnic Institute, Troy, NY 12180*
[b] *Department of Surgery, Albany Medical College, Albany, NY 12208*

**Abstract.** In this work we focus our attention on improving the visual realism of virtual surgery. A synthetic solution by innovative use of various image-based rendering methods is presented for realistic rendering of virtual surgery scenes. We have, for the first time, developed a methodology for generating virtual surgery scenes with realistic glistening effects by a combination of various image-based rendering techniques, including image mosaicing and view-dependent texture mapping. Realistic examples are presented to showcase the results.

## 1. Introduction

Thanks to the chip-at-the-tip technology, today's endoscopes offer unprecedented optical resolution [1]. For instance, the rigid EL2-R410 and flexible EL2-TF410 from Fujinon have a 410 Megapixel resolution [1]. Not only are the images of high resolution, the display quality is also superb. While only 350 lines of horizontal resolution are used in consumer grade video monitors, the ones for laparoscopic surgery have about 700 lines [2]! It is therefore essential that current surgical simulators deliver the best possible visual realism for effective training.

Photorealistic rendering of virtual surgery scenarios is complicated by the irregularity of visceral organ geometry, the presence of a pervasive mucous membrane, the frequent deformation of the anatomical objects and the rich texture of the reticulated peritoneum [3]. Classical texture mapping, the method of choice for most realistic simulators developed to date, suffers from some major drawbacks which delimit its use in a fully realistic simulation. The results of texture maps obtained by cropping images of surgical procedures are usually visually unappealing as they fail to capture the global illumination properties of the scene: radiosity, shadows and varying amounts of illumination from one part of the scene to the other. Even if the results are convincing from one viewpoint, the scene does not look realistic as one navigates around it since the same pixel values are mapped onto the scene regardless of the view. This lack of realism is commonly referred to as the "painted shoebox effect" [3]. In this paper we investigate and provide promising solutions for this very important problem.

## 2. Methods and tools

Image-based rendering (IBR) [4] is a promising set of techniques that tackles the problem of realistic rendering by innovative draping of actual images on the scene. While some IBR techniques are useful in the presence of a background model, others are not. The observation that the surgical tools interact with polygon-based models of the organs (the foreground) while the background is more or less invariant, allows us to develop a novel methodology based on a combination of conventional texture mapping, image mosaicing [5], view dependent texture mapping (VDTM) [6], and light source shading techniques as a synthetic solution to create realistic surgery scenes with excellent glistening effects.

### 2.1. Creating realistic background with glistening effects

The background of a laparoscopic scene is usually complex due to

1) the presence of various types of organs and soft tissues, veins and the peritoneum,
2) a variety of colors and textures, and
3) dynamic glistening of the mucous membrane under the illumination of the head light attached to the laparoscopic camera.

At the same time, the background is more or less invariant compared to the foreground (except when the laparoscope is panned). It is, therefore, computationally effective not to generate separate 3D geometric models for the objects in the background. While static texture mapping is ineffective as we have pointed out, a collection of images, obtained from videos of actual laparoscopic surgeries, with very few geometry primitives may be used to render novel views using the principles of IBR.

### 2.1.1. Generation of Background-specific Texture using Image Mosaicing

Digitized video recorded with the laparoscopic camera is a rich source of information about surgical scenarios, which can be used in IBR. Each second of video usually contains 15-30 frames, which is a large amount of information (The "average" video bit rate is around 4 Mbps) [7], and how to utilize this information in IBR is an issue. The viewport of the laparoscopic camera is very narrow and each frame of the video captures only a small part of the surgical scene. Image mosaicing [5], an IBR technique, is well adapted to create the background texture from the segmented video frames. The main steps of image mosaicing include

1) Correcting geometric deformations using image data.
2) Image registration using image data.
3) Eliminating seams from image mosaics.

Commercial mosaicing software such as ER Mapper® [8] and Geomatica Ortho-Engine® Productivity Tools [9] can be used to perform image mosaicing. Custom-written programs, using standard image editors are preferable to attain greater control and more precise application-specific results. An example of how the background may be created using image mosaicing is presented in Figure 1.

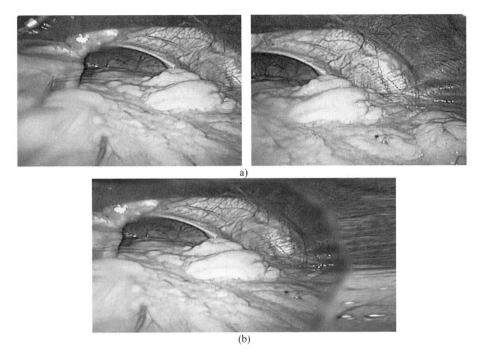

**Figure 1.** Generating background-specific texture using image mosaicing. (a) Two images extracted from laparoscopic surgical video and (b) the composite background image.

### 2.1.2. Generation of glistening effects of the background using VDTM

It is difficult to capture visual effects such as highlights, reflections, and transparency using a single texture-mapped model. Light source shading is a good method to create these effects, but in OpenGL model, various light source effects depend on a number of geometric surfaces that absorb and reflect light and each surface is assumed to be composed of a material with various properties. A material might scatter some incoming light in all directions, and it might reflect some portion of incoming light in a preferential direction (such as a shiny surface) [10]. However, as we have stated above, it is not computationally worthwhile to create various geometric models of the background and assign them different material properties; hence the use of light source shading is not advisable. Instead we propose to use view dependent texture mapping (VDTM) [6], another IBR method, to generate the glistening background seen in surgical videos.

### 2.1.3. Generation of glistening effects of the background using VDTM

It is difficult to capture visual effects such as highlights, reflections, and transparency using a single texture-mapped model. Light source shading is a good method to create these effects, but in OpenGL model, various light source effects depend on a number of geometric surfaces that absorb and reflect light and each surface is assumed to be composed of a material with various properties. A material might scatter some incoming light in all directions, and it might reflect some portion of incoming light in a preferential direction (such as a shiny surface) [10]. However, as we have stated above, it is not computationally worthwhile to create various geometric models of the back-

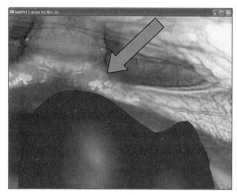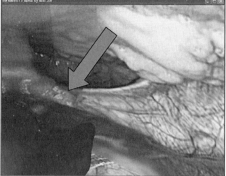

**Figure 2.** Using VDTM to create glistening effect of a realistic virtual surgery scene as the camera moves.

ground and assign them different material properties; hence the use of light source shading is not advisable. Instead we propose to use view dependent texture mapping (VDTM) [6], another IBR method, to generate the glistening background seen in surgical videos.

Developed for rendering architectural models [6], in the VDTM method, actual video images can be draped on an underlying geometry. In principle this technique is quite close to the texture mapping idea. However, rather than using one single texture map per polygon several view-dependent images, originally captured from different angles, are smoothly warped and blended (using weights) to provide a new view.

The motivation of using VDTM for the glistening effect of the background is from the observation of the surgery scene. Tissues appear to glisten when the relative position of the laparoscopic camera changes. Since the real light source is attached to the end of the camera, the displacement of the light source is identical to the change in viewpoint. Thus we sample a few images with different glistening effects from video sequences of actual surgical procedures, and selectively blend between the original images. As a result, the view-dependent texture mapping approach allows the renderings to be considerably more realistic than static texture-mapping. The rendering of the background in Fig. 2 was created in real time using this technique.

## 2.2. Creating realistic foreground with glistening effects

For the foreground, which undergoes frequent changes in topology (due to the interaction with surgical tool), conventional texture mapping is used to couple with light source shading [10] to generate glistening.

When building the lighting model in OpenGL, we create the light source as a spotlight, attach it to the viewpoint position, and enable it in the local viewer mode. We also need to properly set the ambient, diffuse, specular properties as well as the spotlight exponent and attenuation parameters of the light source.

In OpenGL lighting model, each surface that reflects light is assumed to be composed of a material with various properties. Therefore, after applying the light source, we have to define the material properties such as diffuse, ambient and specular reflection correctly.

Putting it all together, the following represents the entire lighting calculation of n-multiple light sources in RGBA mode in OpenGL:

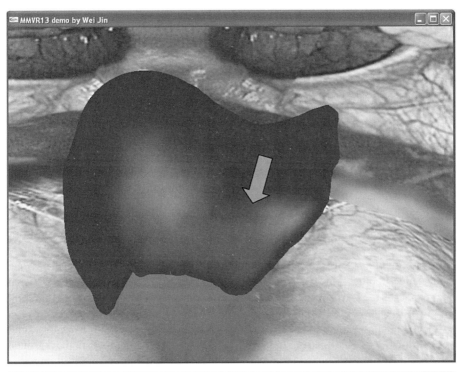

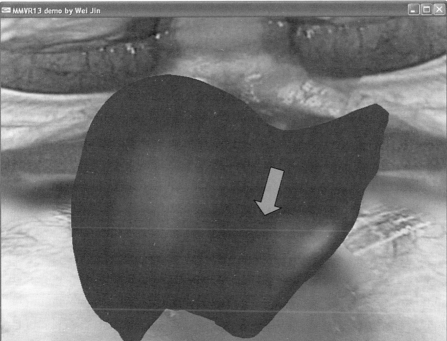

**Figure 3.** Snapshots of the foreground with light source shading.

$$vertexColor = emission_{\text{material}} + ambient_{\text{light}} \times ambient_{\text{material}} +$$

$$\sum_{i=0}^{n-1} \left( \frac{1}{k_c + k_l d + k_q d^2} \right)_i \times (spotlightEffect)i \times [ambient_{\text{light}} \times ambient_{\text{material}} +$$

$$\left( \max\{\mathbf{L} \cdot \mathbf{n}, 0\} \right) \times diffuse_{\text{light}} \times diffuse_{\text{material}} +$$

$$\left( \max\{\mathbf{s} \cdot \mathbf{n}, 0\} \right)^{\text{shininess}} \times specular_{\text{light}} \times specular_{\text{material}}]i$$

where $d$ is the distance between the light's position to the vertex, $k_c$, $k_l$, $k_q$ are attenuation coefficients, $\mathbf{L}$ is the unit vector that points from the vertex to the light position, $\mathbf{n}$ is the unit normal vector at the vertex, $\mathbf{s}$ is a normalized vector sum for the specular term.

## 3. Results

In our preliminary results shown in Figures 2 and 3, we use a human liver model, obtained from Visible Photographic Man, or VIP-Man [11] using the segmented Visible Human data set [12] as the foreground. By using the different approaches for the background and foreground, we have developed a realistic virtual surgery scene.

The simulator was implemented in C++ using OpenGL on a 3.00Ghz Pentium® 4 PC with 2.00GB RAM. Using only 38 triangles we created the realistic background. The liver model consists of 8654 triangles, which is considered sufficient for illumination and haptic simulation. The model is fully interactive through a haptic interface device (Phantom).

## 4. Discussion

In this work we have, for the first time, developed a methodology for generating realistic virtual surgery scenes with glistening effect using a combination of various image-based rendering methods, including image mosaicing and VDTM. The visually realistic models are coupled to a physically-based computational scheme. This computational scheme has been presented in [13]. Realistic examples are presented to showcase the results.

## Acknowledgements

This work was supported by grant R21 EB003547-01 from NIH/NIBIB.

## References

[1]  B. Meltzer, "The Laparoscopic revolution", Outpatient Surgery, February, 2003.
[2]  D. Denziel, "The SAGES Manual: Fundamentals of Laparoscopy and GI endoscopy", Chapter 9, Carol E. H. Scott-Conner Ed., http://www.sages.org/.
[3]  C. E. Prakash, J. Kim, M. Manivannan, M. A. Srinivasan, "A new approach for the synthesis of glistening effect in deformable anatomical objects displayed with haptic feedback", Proceeding of MMVR Conference, pp.369-375, 2002.

[4]   H.-Y. Shum, S. B. Kang, "A review of image-based rendering techniques", IEEE/SPIE Visual Commu-
      nications and Image Processing, pp.2-13, 2000.
[5]   R. Szeliski, "Image mosaicing for tele-reality applications", Proceeding of IEEE Workshop on Applica-
      tions of Computer Vision, pp.44-53, 1994.
[6]   P. E. Debevec, Y. Yu, G. D. Borshukov, "Efficient view-dependent image-based rendering with projective
      texture-mapping", Eurographics Rendering Workshop, pp.105-116, 1998.
[7]   J. Taylor, "DVD Demystified, 2nd edition", McGraw-Hill Professional, 2000.
[8]   ER Mapper® official site, http://www.ermapper.com/.
[9]   Geomatica OrthoEngine® official site, http://www.pcigeomatics.com/.
[10]  OpenGL Architechture Review Board, D. Shreiner, J. Neider, M. Woo, T. Davis, "OpenGL programming
      guide: the official guide to learning OpenGL, Version 1.4", Addison-Wesley, 2003.
[11]  X. G. Xu, T. C. Chao, A. Bozkurt, "VIP-Man: An image-based whole-body adult male model constructed
      from color photographs of the visible human project for multi-particle Monte Carlo calculations", Health
      Physics, 78(5), pp.476-486, 2000.
[12]  M. J. Ackerman, "The Visible Human project", Proceeding of MMVR Conference, pp.5-7, 1994.
[13]  S. De, J. Kim, and M. A. Srinivasan, "A meshless numerical technique for physically based real time
      medical simulations", Proceeding of MMVR Conference, pp.113-118, 2001.

*Medicine Meets Virtual Reality 13*
*James D. Westwood et al. (Eds.)*
*IOS Press, 2005*

# ChiroSensor – An Array of Non-Invasive sEMG Electrodes

E.A. JONCKHEERE [a], P. LOHSOONTHORN [a] and V. MAHAJAN [b]

[a] *Dept. of Electrical Engineering–Systems, University of Southern California,*
*Los Angeles, CA 90089-2563*
*e-mail: jonckhee@usc.edu; lohsoont@hotmail.com*
[b] *Department of Biomedical Engineering, University of Southern California,*
*Los Angeles, CA 90089-2563*
*e-mail: vikram.mahajan@usc.edu*

**Abstract.** It is shown that the statistical analysis of the sEMG signals recorded by the ChiroSensors along the paraspinal muscles during Network Spinal Analysis (NSA) provides objective confirmation of the physiological reality as perceived by the practitioner as it relates to levels of care and spinal injury recovery.

## 1. Problem

The *problem* is to develop objective confirmation, via statistical analysis of the sEMG signals recorded along the paraspinal muscles, of the existence of the so-called Network Spinal Analysis (NSA) wave, and, probably most importantly, the amount of recovery of a spinal injury patient receiving NSA care. So far, this has been left to the subjective judgment of the practitioner, who was relying for the most part on visualization of the rocking motion of the spine.

## 2. Background

The spinal cord is pivotal in the movement of the human body, and as such it needs to be kept in proper alignment. Chiropractors have developed solutions for people suffering from back pain and injuries, among other disorders. Network Spinal Analysis (NSA) is one such technique [5–7], which has been demonstrated to relieve physiological stress by generating a somatosensory wave along the spine. This wave originates in the cervical and sacral areas, where the dural-vertebral attachments [2] at C2-C4 and the attachment of the filum terminale to the coccyx create sensory-motor loops, which by digital contact elicit oscillations, first localized in the neck and sacral areas, and then propagating along the whole spine in a rocking, involuntarily-controlled movement, accompanied by the respiratory wave. This evolution is concomitant with increased burstyness of the sEMG signals [4,7]. The NSA wave, while primarily located in the spinal region, bears some commonality with the cycling style repetitive motion that produced some Central Nervous System (CNS) regeneration in the well-publicized case of Christopher Reeve [9]. In fact, as a recent study has shown, a patient who had sustained an injury similar to that of Reeve did recover some sensory and motor function after NSA care [6]. Both cases are *activity based* recovery programs with the difference that in the Reeve case the activity is generated by the Functional Electric Stimulation (FES) bicycle, whereas with NSA the body is entrained to reactivate a Central Pattern Generator (CPG).

## 3. Methods

The *method* consists in acquiring sEMG signals from an array of non-invasive electrodes at the C, T, L, and S levels during NSA entrainment. The raw signal is recorded by an Insight Millenium machine, sampled at a rate of 4000 sec$^{-1}$ by a DAS16/16 board and stored on a PC compatible computer. Then various analyses are performed: (ia) The spatio-temporal analysis [6], which correlates the signals at various points along the spine in order to positively establish a traveling wave settling in a stationary wave, as already called up by the practitioner; (ib) For a spinal injury patient [6], the correlation is measured on sEMG signals across the injury area; (ii) Dynamical modeling of the neck signals revealing structural changes [7], called up by the practitioner as changes in the level of care, that is, number of rhythmically entrained spinal oscillators (sacral, cervical, and thoracic-sternal).

## 4. Results

The *results* are (ib) 99% confidence level correlation between signals across injury area for a quadriplegic patient who has been under NSA care, and observation of an extra phase shift in the correlation involving signals across injury area [6]; it is however unclear what kind of regeneration this points to. (ii) Objective confirmation of practitioner's visual evaluation of NSA wave by dynamical modeling of sEMG signals as examplified

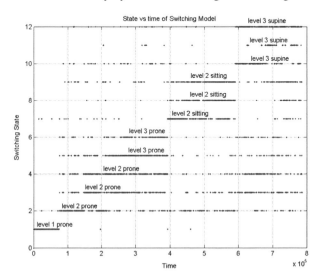

**Figure 1.** Best fit mathematical model of cervical sEMG signal versus progression towards entrainment. The abscissa is the entrainment time and the ordinate is the ARIMA model chosen among 12 of them.

by the staircase diagram of best fitting ARIMA model of cervical sEMG signal versus progression through NSA entrainment [5].

## 5. Discussion

Since the NSA wave has been objectively confirmed by mathematical analysis, it appears the time has come to correlate the visual observation with the motor pathways involved.

The cutaneous cervical receptors receive sensory input from the skin and reach the cervical plexus at level C2-C3. The cervical plexus at level C2 sends motor outputs to the accessory nerve and the sternomastoid muscle of the neck and at level C3-C4-C5 sends motor output to the phrenic nerve, which innervates the diaphragm (which is one of the major muscles of inspiration). The accessory nerve in turn innervates the sternomastoid muscles of the neck and the trapezius muscle of the shoulders. These sensory-motor pathways explain the NSA wave to the extent of involvement of the neck and shoulder muscles which may give rise to the somatosensory wave in the spinal cord and the diaphragm muscles which may give rise to the respiratory wave. It is conjectured that the sensory-motor loop closes via the dural mechanoreceptors [1,3,8].

From another point of view, the electrophysiological bursts at the neuronal level [4] appear to synchronize to produce the bursts at the sEMG level [7]. It is also observed that the accrued burstyness under neurotransmitters at the neuronal level appears similar to the one at the sEMG level at higher levels of care.

## 6. Conclusions

The spinal wave pattern that can be observed during NSA has been confirmed by statistical analysis of the signals and a tentative explanation of the wave as a sensory-motor loop oscillation has been proposed.

## References

[1] Bove GM and Moskowitz MA. Primary afferent neurons innervating guinea pig dura. *J Neurophysiol* 77: 299-308, 1997.
[2] Breig A. Adverse Mechanical Tension in the Central Nervous System. JohnWiley and Sons, New York, 1987.
[3] Burstein R, Yamamura H, Malick A, and Strassman AM. Chemical stimulation of the intracranial dura induces enhanced responses to facial stimulation in brainstem trigeminal neurons. *J Neurophysiol* 79: 964-982, 1998.
[4] Grattarola M, Chiappalone, M, Davide, F, Martinoia, S, Tedesco, MB, Rosso, N, and Vato, A. Burst analysis of chemically stimulated spinal cord neuronal networks cultured on microelectrode arrays, Neural and Bioelectronic Technoloy Group, University of Genoa, Italy, 2004.
[5] Jonckheere EA, Lohsoonthorn P, and Boone R, Dynamic modeling of sEMG activity during various spinal conditions, *ACC'2003*, Denver, CO, June 4-6, 2003, WA-13-3, pp. 465-470.
[6] Jonckheere EA and Lohsoonthorn P. Spatio-temporal analysis of an electrophysiological wave phenomenon, *MTNS'2004*, Leuven, Belgium, July 5-9, 2004.
[7] Lohsoonthorn P and Jonckheere EA, Nonlinear switching dynamics in sEMG of the spine, *Physics and Control*, St. Petersbourg, Russia, August 21-23, 2003, pp. 277-282.
[8] Levy D and Strassman AM. Mechanical response properties of A and C primary afferent neurons innervating rat intracranial dura. *J Neurophysiol* 88: 3021-3031, 2002.
[9] McDonald JW, Becker D, Sadowsky C, Jane J A, Conturo TE, and Schultz L. Late recovery following spinal cord injury. *J. Neurosurgery (Spine 2)* 97:252–265, 2002.

*Medicine Meets Virtual Reality 13*
*James D. Westwood et al. (Eds.)*
*IOS Press, 2005*

# Multiple Contact Approach to Collision Modelling in Surgical Simulation

Bhautik JOSHI, Bryan LEE, Dan C. POPESCU and Sébastien OURSELIN
*CSIRO ICT Centre, BioMedIA Lab*
*Cnr Vimiera & Pembroke Rds, Marsfield NSW 2122, Australia*

**Abstract.** In this paper we present a technique for the modelling of realistic collisions between arbitrary rigid surgical tools and deformable geometry that is independent of the resolution of colliding objects. We use a spatial hash table to provide an efficient narrow-phase collision detection and modelling backend. This is combined with previous work on collision modelling in our surgical simulation environment to model realistic collisions and collision response at haptic rates.

## 1. Introduction

Collision modelling has received much attention recently, notably for its use in surgical simulation for collision between rigid surgical tools and soft deformable organs. However, the computational restrictions that are introduced by performing this modelling at haptic rates has only allowed for the modelling of relatively simple surgical tools [2,4].

In our surgical simulator, we represent surgical tools as a rigid collection of points which penetrate deformable objects on collision. To model collision, these individual penetrations are redistributed to nodes on the deformable object, and an appropriate collision response (force feedback and geometry deformation) is modelled.

To enable the collision modelling to operate at haptic rates, it is necessary that the underlying point penetration calculations run at the same rate. Penetration calculation can be made more efficient by pre-computation; however, this is not always practical with deformable objects. Teschner *et. al* [9] have proposed an optimised spatial hashing technique which can be used for both collision detection and to efficiently store deformable objects and perform penetration depth calculations efficiently.

In this paper we present a new technique for modelling realistic collisions between arbitrary rigid and deformable objects, where the geometric resolution of colliding objects can differ. We make use of a dynamic spatial hash table to provide an efficient collision detection and penetration calculation backend; this extends our previous work on contact modelling with haptic feedback, by integrating a discrete rigid tool of arbitrary shape.

We demonstrate our technique with several tetrahedralizations of geometric primitives, and examine the performance of the algorithm within the context of our surgical simulation environment at the BioMedIA Lab. We have been able to run the complete collision modelling loop at haptic rates and validate our collision modelling technique in the context of a finite element surgical model [8].

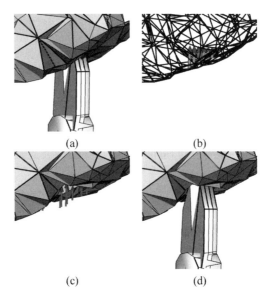

(a)                          (b)

(c)                          (d)

**Figure 1.** Point penetration depth calculation of a tool into a virtual organ. A virtual tool collides with and penetrates a virtual organ (a). The set of point penetrations from the tool are determined (b) and redistributed to the nodes on the surface of the organ (c), and an appropriate collision response is modelled (d).

## 2. Background

A common problem in collision detection is the computation time needed to calculate the penetration depth of a point. Pre-processing algorithms such as BSP-trees or oct-trees can help reduce the computational load; however, they are not very tolerant to deformation of the geometry being queried.

Collision detection can be made easier by breaking down the mesh into simpler spatial components. Tetrahedral meshes automatically meet such criteria, but the number of tetrahedra can be quite large. It is therefore necessary to reduce the number of elements that are compared against to achieve real-time rates, by surrounding smaller elements with shapes that can be queried quickly for intersection.

One such technique that can be used is Oriented Bounding Boxes (OBB's). It uses a series of rectangular prisms which are translated, rotated and scaled to tightly fit the object until it is completely covered [5]. A less precise, but much less computationally demanding process is to use Axis-Aligned Bounding Boxes (AABB's) to cover the object. Hierarchical AABB's have been proven to be effective for handling collision detection in deformable meshes [3].

A newer approach uses graphics hardware to accelerate collision detection [1,7]. The viewing frustum of an OpenGL camera can be transformed to match an OBB; if there is any geometry present when the scene in the camera has rendered, a collision is detected.

Teschner *et al.* have proposed a technique which places volume elements which may span many AABB's into an optimised spatial hash table [9]. They have demonstrated that the resulting data structure can be updated easily when geometry changes. It is ideally suited to storing tetrahedral meshes which may deform, and serves as the core to our proposed point penetration depth algorithm for collision modelling.

Collision modelling is a key aspect in a surgical simulator; see Basdogan *et al.* [2] for a recent review on the major issues of this complex topic, including interaction with soft tissue. In general, this interaction can be described by the three major components of collision detection, collision modelling and collision response.

## 3. Method

For our collision modelling to operate at haptic rates, it is sufficient to treat rigid surgical tools as a rigid group of points. This can easily be achieved by using the points on the surface mesh of the tool. When the tool collides with a deformable organ, the points penetrate the object along the axis defined by the movement of the tool. The first stage of the algorithm makes use of a spatial hash table to store information about the deformable organ. This data can be queried to return the point penetrations caused by the surgical tool.

Deformable organs are represented as discrete meshes, and the accuracy of the modelling is dependent on the resolution of the discrete representation. However, modelling penetrations that involve the surface of the organ but do not make contact with the mesh nodes requires a contact modelling algorithm.

In the case of deformable objects, contact modelling uses detection of information from the point penetrations to determine the shape of the area of contact. We have previously proposed a general algorithm of contact modelling for deformable objects, which redistributes an arbitrary field of displacements, located anywhere on the surface of a deformable object, into an equivalent field of displacements located at the discrete nodes of the deformable mesh [6]. This allows us to generate an appropriate collision response, namely haptic feedback and deformation of the organ.

### 3.1. Point Penetration Depth Calculation

To enable the collision modelling to operate at haptic rates, an efficient collision detection and point penetration depth algorithm was required. We chose a spatial hash table because it both effectively stores our deformable tetrahedral meshes and can be extended to perform the needed mesh query algorithms.

Spatial hashing reduces the search space for queries on a surface or volume mesh by subdividing space into equal sized addressable cells where elements of the mesh are placed. A hash function based on the cell address maps cells covering all of space to a finite number of cells. We propose extensions to Teschner's optimised spatial hashing technique by introducing early rejection tests to minimise redundant queries and allow for fast point penetration depth calculation.

Spatial hashing rasterises an object with respect to the volume grid it generates, as shown in Fig. 2. If the element is poorly aligned with the grid or has a low dimension (such as a line or a triangle) the element will occupy many wasted cells. This potentially increases query time. Combined with early rejection tests, tightly rasterising elements and minimising wasted cells can help improve hash query time.

Point depths are determined by intersecting lines through the tool points situated inside the mesh with the surface of the mesh. The direction of the line is set to the query direction. The hash cells that lie along the line starting at the query points are queued

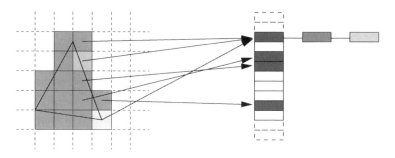

**Figure 2.** Adding an element to the spatial hash. When an element, such as a triangle, is added to the spatial hash, it is rasterised with respect to the spatial grid (left). The ID of the triangle is added to the hash bucket corresponding with each spatial cell to which it belongs (right).

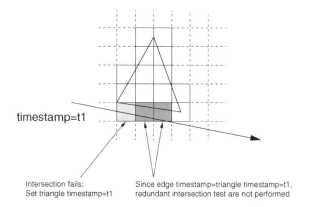

timestamp=t1

Intersection fails;          Since edge timestamp=triangle timestamp=t1,
Set triangle timestamp=t1    redundant intersection test are not performed

**Figure 3.** Timestamping to reduce computation. Each query has a unique timestamp, and when an element is queried, it acquires this timestamp. If it re-acquires the same timestamp, the query has already occurred and it returns automatically with no action.

and the elements in each cell are tested successively for intersection with the line. When an intersection occurs, the distance between the intersection and corresponding point on the tool gives the point penetration depth.

Each depth query test has a unique sequence number, or timestamp. When a line segment is tested against an element in the spatial hash, the element acquires that timestamp. If the depth query comes across an element with the same timestamp as itself, the element has already been tested is not tested again. Fig. 3 shows one such query, which reduces redundant queries when an element spans multiple hash cells.

## 3.2. Collision Modelling

Our method for determining multiple point penetrations integrates naturally with the multiple point contact modelling method we have presented in [6]. The contact modelling technique solves the problem of interaction between objects of different resolutions by redistributing a field of point penetrations, located anywhere on the surface of a deformable organ, into an equivalent field of displacements located strictly at the nodes of the discrete representation of the mesh. It avoids situations where a small-sized or thin

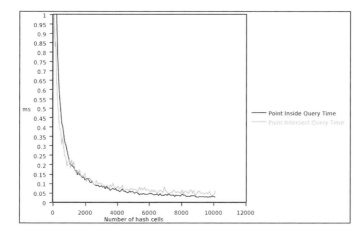

**Figure 4.** Hash Timings vs. Hash Table Size. The number of hash cells is proportional to the hash query time, and hash query times can be pushed well below 0.1ms per point by choosing a sufficiently high number of cells. This is demonstrated in the graph above with a tetrahedral mesh consisting of 40,000 tetrahedra.

rigid surgical tool could "pass through" a virtual organ, without making contact, because of the relatively large size of the triangles on the surface.

This equivalent field of displacements can then be used to accurately drive the collision response – deformation plus haptic feedback – for example, in conjunction with a finite element method. Our technique is accurate but also efficient: by using a divide and conquer strategy, the computational complexity depends on the size of the touched area, but not on the overall size of the mesh representing the organ.

## 4. Results

Our experiments show that complex mesh queries such as penetration depth calculation for arbitrarily shaped objects can be carried out at haptic (1kHz) rates. We have this method integrated into the BioMedIA Lab surgical simulator. Using a wide variety of test meshes, we demonstrate that on a 2.8 GHz desktop PC, point depth queries can be carried out at 10-20kHz for meshes consisting of 40,000 tetrahedra.

Our experiments also confirm Teschner's result that the hash table is optimised when the hash cell size is close that of the mesh edge length. Fig 4 demonstrates that by choosing a suitable value for the number of hash cells (in practice, about 0.25 times the number of tetrahedra) the time for an individual query can be kept well below 0.1ms, allowing for query rates of above 10kHz.

We chose a deformable organ model of a tumour consisting of 1200 tetrahedra and performed our complete collision loop on it with various tool interactions. The average time for each loop and its components (depth determination and collision modelling) are shown in table 1.

## 5. Discussion and Further work

We have developed our technique for use in a haptic surgical simulation. The haptic device we are using is a 3-DOF device, and, as such, 6-DOF haptic effects such as torque

**Table 1.** Timings for various tool penetrations into a deformable organ model consisting of 1200 tetrahedra on a 3GHz Intel PC running linux. Overall time was kept at or below the required haptic cutoff of 1kHz.

| # points | Depth Determination (ms) | Contact Modelling (ms) | Total Time (ms) |
|---|---|---|---|
| 16 | 0.7 | 0.3 | 1.0 |
| 12 | 0.55 | 0.27 | 0.82 |
| 10 | 0.51 | 0.27 | 0.78 |
| 8 | 0.42 | 0.24 | 0.66 |

on the tool are not modelled. However, it could easily be implemented by summing the cross-product of the forces at points on the surface of the tool to the vector from the point of action of the tool to the points of contact.

In our future work we plan to investigate collision modelling with several deformable objects. Also, whilst point depth determination is valuable, potential exists to extend the point depth algorithm to determine the minimum separation distance (polyhedral penetration depth) between two overlapping arbitrary meshes.

## References

[1] S. Aharon and C. Lenglet. *Collision Detection Algorithm for Deformable Objects Using OpenGL*, MIC-CAI(2), pages 211–218, 2002.
[2] C. Basdogan, S. De, J. Kim, M. Muniyandi, H. Kim, and M. Srinivasan. *Haptics in Minimally Invasive Surgical Simulation and Training*, IEEE Comp. Graphics and Applications, 24(2):56–64, 2004.
[3] G. van den Bergen. *Efficient Collision Detection of Complex Deformable Models using AABB Trees*, Journal of Graphics Tools, 2(4):1–14, 1998.
[4] C. Forest, H. Delingette, and N. Ayache. *Surface Contact and Reaction Force Models for Laparoscopic Simulation*, In International Symposium on Medical Simulation 2004, pages 168–176, June 2004.
[5] S. Gottschalk, M.C. Lin, and D. Manocha. *OBBtree: A Hierachical Structure for Rapid Interference Detection*, In Proceedings of ACM SIGGRAPH '96, pages 171–180, 1996.
[6] B. Lee, D.C. Popescu, and S. Ourselin. *Contact Modelling Based on Displacement Field Redistribution for Surgical Simulation*, In The Second International Workshop on Medical Imaging and Augmented Reality, volume 3150 of LNCS, pages 337–345, Beijing, China, August 2004. Springer Verlag.
[7] J.C. Lombardo, M.P. Cani, and F. Neyret. *Real-time Collision Detection for Virtual Surgery*, In Computer Animation, pages 33–39, Geneva, Switzerland, May 1999.
[8] D.C. Popescu and M. Compton. *A Method for Efficient and Accurate Interaction with Elastic Objects in a Haptic Virtual Environment*, In Proceedings of Graphite 2003, pages 245–250, Melbourne, Australia, 2003. ACM Press.
[9] M. Teschner, B. Heidelberger, M. Mueller, D. Pomeranets, and M. Gross. *Optimized Spatial Hashing for Collision Detection of Deformable Objects*, In Proceedings of Vision Modeling and Visualization 2003, pages 47–54, Munich, Germany, November 2003.

Medicine Meets Virtual Reality 13
James D. Westwood et al. (Eds.)
IOS Press, 2005

# Visualization of Surgical 3D Information with Projector-based Augmented Reality

Lüder Alexander KAHRS [a], Harald HOPPE [b], Georg EGGERS [c],
Jörg RACZKOWSKY [a], Rüdiger MARMULLA [c] and Heinz WÖRN [a]

[a] *Institute of Process Control and Robotics, Universität Karlsruhe (TH), Germany*
*e-mail: kahrs@ira.uka.de*
[b] *Stryker Leibinger GmbH & Co KG, Freiburg, Germany*
[c] *Department of Cranio-Maxillofacial Surgery, University of Heidelberg, Germany*

**Abstract.** For visualizing surgical information (operation plans) directly onto the
patient a projector-based augmented reality system is used for cranio-maxillofacial
surgery. A prototype is introduced which has been evaluated in the first clinical
cases. In a new setup with a second video projector it is now possible to give additionally 3D information for localization and orientation (6DoF). With this method
the repositioning of a bone segment is intuitive and exact applicable.

## 1. Introduction

### 1.1. Clinical Prototype of a Projector-based Augmented Reality System

In the collaborative research centre "Information Technology in Medicine - Computer-
and Sensor-Aided Surgery" of the German Research Foundation a projector-based augmented reality system is developed and has been tested in some first clinical experiments.
The system consists of a video projector, an airproof enclosure for the projector, air supply and exhaust tubes, two cameras, four lamps (cp. fig. 1a), a mounting and a notebook
[1,2]. Predefined operation plans [3] are projected onto the patient with high accuracy.
Tracking and registration are realized with this system too.

### 1.2. Projection of 3D Information

One of the main problems in projector-based augmented reality is the reduction of the
dimensionality from 3D to 2D during the projection onto an object. Points, which are not
placed on the illuminated surface, can not be augmented. This becomes important when
e.g. a bone segment should be repositioned (fig. 1b/c). With one projector and without
wearing i.e. red-green glasses it is not possible to define the position and orientation.
A method for the solution of this problem will be specified in the following.

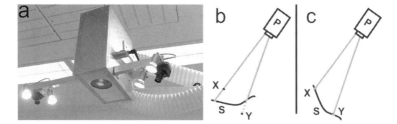

**Figure 1.** a) The clinical prototype of the projector for augmented reality in surgery. In figure b) and c) the same points onto the surface (or bone segment) S are illuminated by the projector P. The position and orientation of S is not defined.

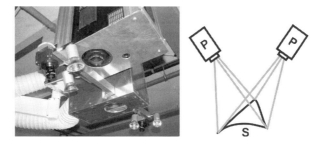

**Figure 2.** Two projectors illuminate the scene. The left picture shows the laboratory setup. In the background the prototype of the projector-based augmented reality and in the front the additional video projector are located. In the right pictures the projection-based localisation concept for a bone segment is shown.

## 2. Method

In a new initial setup with the clinically used prototype and another video projector (see figure 2) this experiment for visualization of 3D information is done. The algorithms of the projector-based augmented reality system is extended for the usability with more than one projector. The projectors were calibrated in the same coordinate system looking on the same calibration object. Hence, the possibility exists to project redundantly as well as to locate an object with its orientation in 3D. In fact, with the double projection of at least three points the determination of six degrees of freedom (6DoF) for an object is fixed. These are the same requirements on the output side (LCD/DLP) like on the input side (CCD/CMOS). This analogon at the I/O concept appears during the calibration too [4].

## 3. Results

After the calibration of both projectors they are able to augment the scene redundantly. In figure 3 an augmented operation plan on a phantom head is displayed with two projectors. The lines over the forehead and the nose are only projected to give the surgeon trust into the system. In the left picture the lines on the cheek visualize the segment in the correct location. In the right picture the lines are not overlapping in the correct way. The paper sheet symbolizes the position of a potential implant or a bone segment. In the image

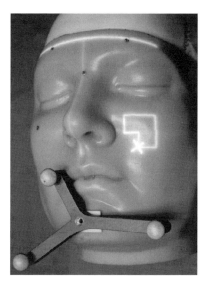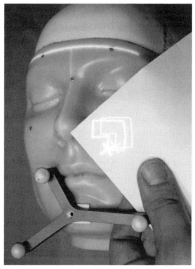

**Figure 3.** Visualization of an operation plan with two projectors. The left picture shows the redundant projection. The right picture shows the projected deviation of a segment (simulated with the sheet), which is not at the right position.

the planed insertion is below the correct position and the system shows intuitively the direction of movement towards the true location. Occlusions aroused by the surgeon can be avoided with projectors illuminating the scene from different directions. The number of used projectors is only limited by the possible number of different VGA/DVI ports.

## 4. Discussion and Conclusion

With the described novel approach it is possible to give the surgeon 3D information nearly like with glasses-based augmented reality. The localization of a bone segment with the determination of 6DoF is possible. Other projector-based augmented reality systems [5,6] are able to easily inherit this functionality. The next steps will be to minimize the projection technology and test the double projection in the operating room.

## References

[1] Hoppe H, Däuber S, Raczkowsky J, Wörn H, Moctezuma JL: Intraoperative visualization of surgical planning data using video projectors. Stud Health Technol Inform 2001;81:206-8 (ISSN: 0926-9630).
[2] Salb T, Hoppe H, Eggers G, Marmulla R, Raczkowsky J, Hassfeld S, Wörn H, Dillmann R: Augmented Reality in Surgery: Clinical Studies, CURAC, Nuernberg, Germany, 2003 (http://curac.org/curac03/download/abstracts/sfb-9.pdf).
[3] Schorr O, Eggers G, Haag C, Hassfeld S, Wörn H: Operation Planning and its Automation in Cranio Maxillofacial Surgery, CURAC, Nuernberg, Germany, 2003 (http://curac.org/curac03/download/ abstracts/sfb-7.pdf).
[4] Hoppe H, Däuber S, Kübler C, Raczkowsky J, Wörn H: A New, Accurate and Easy To Implement Camera and Video Projector Model. Studies in Health Technology and Informatics, Medicine Meets Virtual Reality (MMVR) 2002, IOS Press, pp. 204-206.

[5] Bantiche O, Coste-Manière E, Devernay F, Viéville T: A video-projector-mono-camera stereoscope for surgical planning transfer. In Surgetica CAS, pp 158-163, Grenoble, France, 2002.

[6] Glossop N D, Wang Z: Laser Projection Augmented Reality System for Computer-Assisted Surgery. H U Lemke et al. (Editoren), Proceedings of the 17th International Congress and Exhibition Computer Assisted Radiology and Surgery (CARS) 2003, pp. 65-71, Elsevier, 2003.

*Medicine Meets Virtual Reality 13*
*James D. Westwood et al. (Eds.)*
*IOS Press, 2005*

# Facial Plastic Surgery Planning Using a 3D Surface Deformation Tool

Zacharoula KAVAGIOU [a], Fernando BELLO [a], Greg SCOTT [a],
Juian HAMANN [a] and David ROBERTS [b]

[a] *Department of Surgical Oncology and Technology, Imperial College London*
*e-mail: f.bello@imperial.ac.uk*
[b] *ENT Department, Guy's Hospital, London*

**Abstract.** The range of facial malformations that plastic surgeons are asked to alter is wide. Even a subtle deformity may strongly affect both the way a person perceives herself as well as her quality of life. Moreover, the changes achieved during craniofacial surgery often result in dramatic differences on the face of the patient. Consequently, both surgeons and patients would benefit from the visual approximation of the outcome of the operation provided by adequate three dimensional planning tools. In this paper we propose a three-dimensional texture-mapped surface deformation tool as part of a planning system for rhinoplasty.

## 1. Introduction

When planning craniofacial surgical procedures a surgeon might be in need of multiple and complex data gathered from different sources, such as clinical examination, radiological and intra-operative data. This heterogeneity makes the therapeutic decision difficult and the development of several types of three-dimensional surgical analysis, simulation and planning software important.

Computer aided surgical planning has been investigated by many researchers over the past decade [1–9]. Their purpose is to offer better surgical results with fewer procedures, especially the ones that are successive and aim to refine the initial result. The time in the operating room decreases, as does the risk patients face due to infections or lack of precision of a technique.

Surgical planning systems typically consist of the following steps: *data acquisition* from the patient is performed first. If different modalities are used, *registration* is employed to combine information. The data is *segmented* into different types of tissue or bone and image processing techniques help to remove artefacts. Meshes of the different tissues are then produced and decimation algorithms are used to reduce the computational load of the *deformation model*. These meshes are used for visualization and interaction in the process of surgical simulations. The cycle of surgical planning closes with the *validation* of errors when the post-operative result is compared to the pre-operative simulations [6,9].

While significant advances have been made in computer aided surgical planning systems, their intrinsic complexity renders them unsuitable for routine use in the clinic.

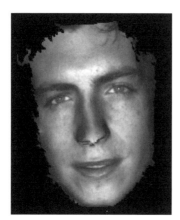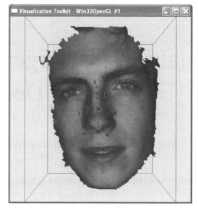

**Figure 1.** The 3D surface deformation tool: (a) Sample image data. (b) Control points.

Instead, two-dimensional warping tools such as WinMorph have recently been used to perform rhinoplasty planning [3]. Such 2D planning aids are less than ideal as both the surgeon and patient would prefer a full three-dimensional system that allows for more control of the deformation as well as different views. We have developed a 3D deformation tool that allows the surgeon to interact with a 3D texture-mapped surface model of the face by specifying a series of control points on and along the nose anatomy. These control points can then be used to perform a controlled deformation of the nose and its surrounding tissue. The system is intuitive and straightforward to use giving the surgeon the opportunity to discuss the procedure with the patient and to compare the pre- and expected post-operative views and precisely plan the procedure.

## 2. Methods

### 2.1. Data Acquisition

The data acquisition was done with the aid of a video-based surface reconstruction system provided by *VisionRT Ltd.* [11]. The patient is positioned at a certain distance in front of a multiple-camera assembly. A structured light pattern is aimed at the patient. The cameras are calibrated and this calibration affects the coordinates of the surface model that is later produced. Typical values of acquisition parameters are 25fps and up to 60 captures for each model. The reconstruction of the surface model is based on the video images from the cameras. The output of the system includes a polygonal surface mesh that represents the geometry of the face of the patient, texture coordinates, and a grey-scale bitmap file; the texture image. Fig. 1(a) shows a typical facial surface acquired by the system.

### 2.2. Deformation Tool

We chose a Free-Form Deformation (FFD) technique for our tool due to its versatility and ability to make the deformation more intuitive and interactive by dissociating the underlying geometric model from the interaction surface. A recent approach proposed by

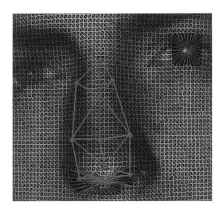 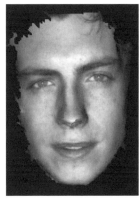

**Figure 2.** (a) Underlying Control Mesh *B*. (b) Locally deformed face.

Kobayashi and Ootsubo known as *t-FFD* [10] was implemented. This method allows the Free-form Deformation of a large-scale polygonal mesh or point-cloud with the aid of a control mesh. Let *M* be the original shape/object and *M'* the deformed shape. Control mesh *B* is constituted of a set of triangles of arbitrary topology and geometry, including cases when these triangles are disconnected or intersected with each other. These triangles are selected by the user or can be automatically generated by the system that is used for the implementation. If the control mesh *B* covers and affects the whole extent of *M*, then the deformation performed is global. Otherwise, a local deformation is achieved. For our purposes, *B* is automatically generated from a list of 10 control points specified by the user at the start of the planning session (Fig. 1(b) ). These points correspond to positions that are critical when it comes to deforming the nose both virtually as well as during a rhinoplasty.

## 3. Results

We have developed a 3D deformation tool that allows the surgeon to interact with the 3D texture-mapped surface model of the face by specifying a series of control points on and along the nose anatomy (Fig. 2(a)). These control points can then be used to perform a controlled deformation of the nose and its surrounding tissue (Fig. 2(b)). The system is intuitive and straightforward to use giving the surgeon the opportunity to discuss the procedure with the patient, to compare the pre- and expected post-operative views and precisely plan the procedure. At present the system is undergoing further testing and refinement prior to its use in the ENT clinic.

## 4. Conclusions and Future Work

When planning surgical resection and/or reconstruction of lesions or deformities of the face, anxiety prior to the procedure is common. This is to a large extent due to apprehension regarding the postoperative outcome. The lack of adequate surgical planning technology makes it difficult for the patient to communicate to the surgeon the desired outcome following surgery. The surgeon is consequently unable to precisely plan the procedure to meet the patient's requirements. The 3D deformation tool presented here is intended to facilitate the surgeon-patient discussions that take place prior to an operation. Together with 3D scanning at follow-up consultations, it could also allow the changes following surgery to be monitored. This would generate valuable information that could be used in the future to further modify surgery as necessary.

## References

[1]  Zachow, S., T. Hierl, and B. Erdmann, *On the predictability of tissue changes for osteotomy planning in maxillofacial surgery: a comparison with postoperative results.* International Congress Series - Elsevier, 2004. **1268**: p. 648-653.

[2]  Schmidt, J.G., et al., *A Finite Element based Tool Chain for the Planning and Simulation of Maxillo-Facial Surgery.* European Congress on Computational Methods in Applied Sciences and Engineering (ECCOMAS 2004), 2004.

[3]  Özkul, T. and M.H. Özkul, *Computer simulation tool for rhinoplasty planning.* Computers in Biology and Medicine, 2004.

[4]  Koch, R.M., et al., *Simulating Facial Surgery Using Finite Element Models.* Proceedings of SIGGRAPH 96, 1996: p. 421-428.

[5]  Teschner, M., S. Girod, and B. Girod, *Direct Computation of Nonlinear Soft-Tissue Deformation.* Vision, Modeling, and Visualization (VMV'00), 2000.

[6]  Bettega, G., et al., *A Simulator for Maxillofacial Surgery integrating 3D Cephalometry and Orthodontia.* Computer Aided Surgery, 2000. **5**: p. 156-165.

[7]  Bockholt, U., et al., *Rhinosurgical Therapy Planning via Endonasal Airflow Simulation.* Computer Aided Surgery, 2000. **5**: p. 175-179.

[8]  Honrado, C.P. and W.F.J. Larrabee, *Update in Three-Dimensional Imaging in Facial Plastic Surgery.* Current Opinion in Otolaryngology & Head & Neck Surgery, 2004. **12**(4): p. 327-331.

[9]  Montgomery, K., M. Stephanides, and S. Schendel, *Development of a Virtual Environment for Reconstructive Surgery.* Computer Aided Surgery, 2000. **5**: p. 90-97.

[10]  Kobayashi, K.G. and K. Ootsubo, *t-FFD: Free-Form Deformation by using Triangular Mesh.* Proceedings of the 8th ACM Symposium on Solid Modeling & Applications, 2003: p. 226-234.

[11]  www.visionrt.com.

Medicine Meets Virtual Reality 13
James D. Westwood et al. (Eds.)
IOS Press, 2005

# The Haptic Kymograph: A Diagnostic Tele-Haptic Device for Sensation of Vital Signs

Youngseok KIM and T. KESAVADAS

*Virtual Reality Laboratory,*
*809 Furnas Hall, Department of Mechanical and Aerospace Engineering,*
*The State University of New York at Buffalo, Buffalo, NY 14260*
*e-mail: {ykim5,kesh}@eng.buffalo.edu*
*url: http://www.vrlab.buffalo.edu*

**Abstract.** The kymograph is device for measuring and presenting pressure-based signals, such as human heart beat and artery volume pressure. The Haptic Kymograph is a haptically-enhanced tele-medicine system which is used to acquire human vital signs and then to transform these signs into sensible, scalable and ubiquitous media so that a user can easily comprehend subtle and ambiguous signals in a remote place. In an experiment setup a patient's artery pressure pulse was captured at 200 Hz of sampling rate, transmitted via TCP/IP network, and replicated in a remote place using a PHANToM haptic device coupled with a real-time visual interface. In this paper we report our recent progresses in developing a low-cost input system, network interfaces and haptic replication of the human artery volume pulse signal.

**Keywords.** VR, telehaptics, kymograph, diagnostics, vital signs, telemedicine, artery volume pressure pulse.

## 1. Introduction

The complexity of human body and multivariate situations of medical diagnostics usually make symptoms very hard to recognize. This is especially true in physical examination of vital signs, such as touching and feeling pulsation of artery volume pressure. Because patients often have weak pulses in their body, the ambiguity and subtlety somtime gives doctors problems during capturing and evaluating conditions of a patient.

The Haptic Kymograph is a novel telehaptics and telemedicine application. It captures and transforms human vital signs into sensible, scalable and ubiquitous media so that doctors can easily comprehend subtle and ambiguous signals from human body (Figure 1). We developed the fundamental framework of the Haptic Kymograph in an earlier work [1], and this paper reports recent progresses focused on its usability, such as low-cost piezoelectric pulse sensor and performance test using common Internet connection.

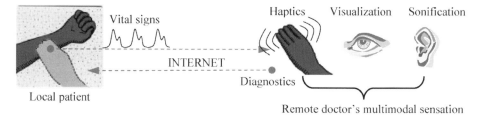

**Figure 1.** Multimodal diagnostics by the Haptic Kymograph.

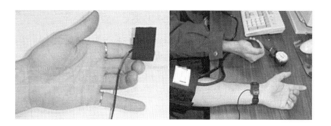

**Figure 2.** Low-cost piezoelectric sensor.

## 2. The Haptic Kymograph System

The system of the Haptic Kymograph acquires and transforms abstract data (pulses, for example) into various human sensations in a real-time remote environment. The separation of haptic and graphical rendering loops makes the real-time interface possible (1kHz for haptic, 30fps for visualization). For the readiness in data acquisition, distribution and replication, the system adopts relatively inexpensive sensor and hardware, and common platform-independent software: A piezoelectric sensor for pulse sensing (Figure 2), a NI-DAQ 1200 PCMCIA card of National Instrument, LabVIEW 7.0 as a data acquisition and processing [2,3]. For the remote site, we used PHANToM Desktop for haptic interface, GHOST SDK for haptic device control, TCP/IP network interfaces, Open Inventor for real-time graphics [4], MS Visual C++ 6.0 for integrative software development in two Pentium III 1.0 GHz PCs in Microsoft Windows 2000 operating system.

## 3. Implementation and Results

### 3.1. Haptic Replication using PHANToM

The Haptic Kymograph simulation was implemented in a network environment (Figure 3). A set of sphygmomanometer and stethoscope were also used for simulating the use of human auditory channel. This served as a supplementary cue and will be replaced by sound recreation device in the future. To achieve smooth feeling along with digitized step pulses [5], digitized data was processed at 200 Hz, and transmitted via Internet, and replicated in the remote site within our research institution. By placing the virtual hand on the leaping disk with PHANToM stylus, the remote user could feel the patient's pulse.

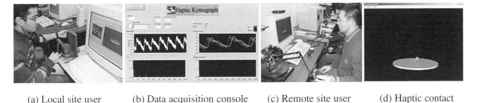

(a) Local site user     (b) Data acquisition console     (c) Remote site user     (d) Haptic contact

**Figure 3.** The simulation of the Haptic Kymograph.

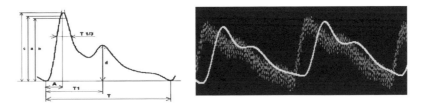

**Figure 4.** Comparison of the pulse shapes: using sophisticated equipment (left) and a low-cost piezoelectric sensor.

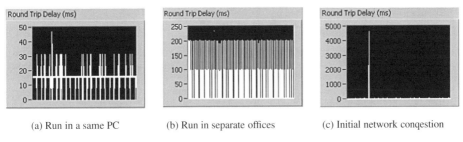

(a) Run in a same PC     (b) Run in separate offices     (c) Initial network congestion

**Figure 5.** The round trip delay for the two network sites of the Haptic Kymograph.

## 3.2. Validity of Low-cost Piezoelectric Sensor

The low-cost piezoelectric sensor captured reasonably good data about human arterial pulse when compared with more sophisticated and expensive equipment [6] (Figure 4). This pulse was successfully processed, transferred, and replicated at the remote site haptic device.

## 3.3. Network Performance

The Haptic Kymograph uses TCP/IP [7] for better quality of service (QoS) [8,9]. We measured the network performance in two cases: running on a single PC and in two separate PC at two different locations. Round trip delay showed the average of 16 msec in the case of running on a single PC (less than 30 msec with a hop at 47 msec). The test in two separate offices showed initial inherent TCP/IP network congestion for 4.8 seconds [10]. After this period, round trip delay was measured at the average of 100 msec (less than 200 msec). A network buffer was devised for data qualification and device safety of the PHANToM. For 200 Hz of data sampling rate and haptic replication, minimum 5 seconds of initial delay was recommended for the remote site. With adaptive network traffic control, the initial network delay was reduced to 900 msec at 60 Hz of data transmission rate.

## 4. Conclusion and Future Work

Cost-effective and reliable telehaptics technologies of the Haptic Kymograph can lead remote diagnostics thus taking the benefits of telemedicine to people irrespective of their location. Furthermore, the ability to manifest subtlety and ambiguity can also provide training to a novice or present new insights into the mysteries of the oriental medicine.

High-end networking technologies, such as multi-threaded adaptive network traffic control and predictive algorithms are being developed to makeup for loss of data in the network. We are adding multimodal cues such as signal sonification, and also developing low-cost, compact vibrotactile stimulator which will contribute to portability of the proposed telemedicine system.

## References

[1]  Kim, Y. and Kesavadas, T., Haptic Kymograph: Towards transmission of diagnostic vital signs. in *Proceedings of the Eurohaptics 2004*, (Munich, 2004).
[2]  Olansen, J.B. and Rosow, E. *Virtual Bio-Instrumentation*. Prentice Hall, Upper Saddle River, NJ, 2002.
[3]  Chugani, M.L., Samant, A.R. and Cerna, M. *LabVIEW Signal Processing*. Prentice Hall, Upper Saddle River, NJ, 1998.
[4]  Wernecke, J. *The Open Inventor Mentor*. Addison Wesley, Reading, MA, 1994.
[5]  Burdea, G.C. Haptic sensing and control. *Force and Touch Feedback for Virtual Reality. Chapter 2*. John Wiley & Sons, New York, NY, 1996.
[6]  Korpas, D., Halek, J. and L., C. Surface artery volume pulse wave measurement - Verification of a new method. *Biomed Papers*, 147(2). 181-184.
[7]  Tanenbaum, A.S. The Internet Transport Protocols, Performance Issues: TCP, *Computer Networks*. Prentice Hall, Upper Saddle River, NJ, 2003. 532-572.
[8]  Fukuda, I., Matsumoto, S., Iijima, M., Hikichi, K., Morino, H., Sezaki, K. and Yasuda, Y. A robust system for haptic collaboration over the network. in McLaughlin, M.L., Hespanha, J.P. and Sukhatme, G.S. eds. *Touch in Virtual Environments, IMSC*, Prentice Hall, Upper Saddle River, NJ, 2002, 137-157.
[9]  Singhal, S. and Zyda, M. *Networked Virtual Environments; Design and Implementation*. Addison & Wesley, New York, NY, 1999.
[10] Niemeyer, G. and Slotine, J. Toward Bilateral Internet Teleoperation. in Goldberg, K. and Siegwart, R. eds. *Beyond Webcams: An Introduction to Online Robots*, MIT Press, Cambridge, MA, 2001, 293-213.

*Medicine Meets Virtual Reality 13*
*James D. Westwood et al. (Eds.)*
*IOS Press, 2005*

# A Study of the Method of the Video Image Presentation for the Manipulation of Forceps

Soichi KONO [a], Toshiharu SEKIOKA [b], Katsuya MATSUNAGA [a],
Kazunori SHIDOJI [a] and Yuji MATSUKI [a]

[a] *Dept. of Intelligent Systems, ISEE, Kyushu University, 6-10-1 Hakozaki,
Higashi-ku Fukuoka 812-8581, Japan*
*e-mail: {konos,matsnaga,shidoji,matsuki}@brain.is.kyushu-u.ac.jp*
[b] *Panasonic ITS, 2-5-15 Shin-yokohama, Minatohigashi-ku Yokohama 222-0033, Japan*
*e-mail: sekiot@brain.is.kyushu-u.ac.jp*

**Abstract.** Recently, surgical operations have sometimes been tried under laparo-scopic video images using teleoperation robots or forceps manipulators. Therefore, in this paper, forceps manipulation efficiencies were evaluated when images for manipulation had some transmission delay (Experiment 1), and when the convergence point of the stereoscopic video cameras was either fixed and variable (Experiment 2). The operators' tasks in these experiments were sewing tasks which simulated telesurgery under 3-dimensional scenography. As a result of experiment 1, the operation at a $200 \pm 100$ ms delay was kept at almost the same accuracy as that without delay. As a result of experiment 2, work accuracy was improved by using the zooming lens function; however the working time became longer. These results seemed to show the relation of a trade-off between working time and working accuracy.

## 1. Introduction

Recently, surgical operation has sometimes been tried under laparoscopic video images using teleoperation robots or forceps manipulators. It is also expected that teleoperation could be done via networks. When the information is transmitted via networks, there could be a transmission delay which might cause a lowering of work efficiency [1]. In surgical operations, wide lens images would be necessary to get the surrounding information. On the other hand, when fine operation was required, high resolution images would be necessary [2]. Therefore, in this paper, forceps manipulation efficiency was evaluated when images for manipulation had some transmission delay (Experiment 1), and when images were taken through narrow and wide lenses (Experiment 2).

## 2. Experiment 1 : The evaluation of the effects of the transmission delay

### 2.1. Method

An experimental system was set up with two video cameras (Sony: DFW-VL500 with zoom lens) and two forceps manipulators (Johnson and Johnson: 5DSG). Stereoscopic

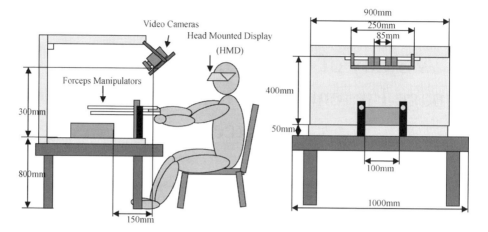

**Figure 1.** Experimental environment.

images were displayed using the head mounted display (Olympus: Mediamask MW601). Video images were displayed as stereoscopic. The elevation angle of the cameras was −47 degrees and the viewing angle of lenses was 17degrees.

The task was to sew a piece of the cloth using two forceps manipulators under the stereoscopic video images. The subjects were required to insert a needle in to the cloth on which five marks were painted. The respective delay times of the transmission of the video signal were 200ms ± 100ms, 300ms ± 100ms, and none. The subjects were six people who have normal stereoscopic vision.

## 2.2. Experimental Procedure

The subjects were required to insert a needle in to the cloth on which five marks were painted. This task was done with the procedure of 1 to 4 of the following.

1) A subject held a needle with the forceps manipulator in his right hand.
2) He held a cloth with the forceps manipulator in his left hand.
3) He penetrated the point with the needle.
4) He held the needle top with the forceps manipulator in his left hand.

The subjects were required to sew all five marks during this procedure five times and under three different kinds of condition. We measured the completion time, the numbers of corrections of insertions, and differences between the distance of insertion points from marked points. The complete time was from the time when the subject first held a needle to the time when he has sewn all five points.

## 2.3. Results and Discussion

The mean completion times of the five needle insertions were 309.5s (SD = 125.9s) under the non delay conditions, 565.2s (SD = 361.2s) under delay conditions of 200ms± 100ms, and 712.3s (SD = 399.7s) under delay conditions of 300ms ± 100ms. Analysis of variance and multiple comparisons showed that the mean completion time under non delay conditions was significantly shorter than the others ($F(2, 10) = 12.4$, $p<0.05$).

The mean number of corrections to insertions was 0.27 times under non delay conditions, 0.39 under $200\pm100$ms, and 0.55 under $300\pm100$ms. Significant differences were shown among the three ($F(2, 10) = 11.9$, $p<0.05$). Differences between the insertion points and the marked points were 1.02mm under non delay conditions, 1.38mm under delay conditions of 200ms $\pm$ 100ms, and 1.23mm under delay conditions of 300ms $\pm$ 100ms. Significant differences were not observed among those three mean distances of difference ($F(2, 10) = 2.6$, n.s.).

## 3. Experiment 2 : The evaluation of work characteristics under the zoom lens function

### 3.1. Method

The experimental system in experiment 2 was the same as that used in experiment 1. In this experiment, we compared the effects of a fixed lens and a zoom lens on the works. The viewing angle of a fixed lens was 17 degrees at the horizon. And the range of the varied angle of the zoom lens was from 9 to 24 degrees. The lens angles were changed by using the pedal system (Microsoft: SideWinder Force Feedback Wheel USB). The elevation angle of the cameras was $-47$degrees. The number of subjects in this experiment was 4. The task for the subjects was the same as that in experiment 1.

### 3.2. Experimental Procedure

The experimental procedure was the same as that used in experiment 1 except that subjects were required to control viewing angle of the cameras using the zoom lens function. The viewing angle at the beginning of the trial was 24degrees under the zooming lens conditions, and 17degrees under fixed lens condition. Subjects could adjust the viewing angles by using the pedal during the tasks performed under zoom lens conditions.

### 3.3. Results and Dissections

The mean completion times of the five needle insertions were 262.5s (SD $= 85.5$s) under fixed lens angle conditions and 389.9s (SD $= 129.3$s) under zooming lens conditions ($t(3) = 3.3$, p$<0.05$). The mean number of corrections to insertions were 0.17 times under fixed lens angle conditions, and 0.42 times under zooming lens conditions ($t(3) = 4.0$, p$<0.05$). It was suggested that these differences were caused by slow zooming speed, and that correction of the insertions was done more under zooming conditions.

## 4. Conclusion

These results lead to the conclusion that in order to do the teleoperation in shorter time it is necessary to make the operation delay less than 200 ms, and that work accuracy could be improved by using the zooming lens function.

# References

[1] Noriaki Ando, Joo-ho Lee and Hideki Hashimoto(1999). "A Study on Influence of Time Delay in Teleoperation", IEEE, pp.V-1111-1116.

[2] Katsuya Matsunaga, Kazunori Shidoji, Fumiaki Kitamura, and Joe Tabuki (1996). "The effects of the coordination of perception and movement on work performance under the virtual reality environment, The Report on the researches [256] by the Grants-in-Aid for Scientific Research from Ministry of Education of Japan, pp27-28. (in Japanese)

*Medicine Meets Virtual Reality 13*
*James D. Westwood et al. (Eds.)*
*IOS Press, 2005*

# Collaborative Biomedical Data Exploration in Distributed Virtual Environments

Falko KUESTER, Zhiyu HE, Jason KIMBALL,
Marc ANTONIJUAN TRESENS and Melvin QUINTOS
*Visualization and Interactive Systems Group*
*University of California, Irvine*

**Abstract.** Imaging techniques such as MRI, fMRI, CT and PET have provided doctors with a means to acquire high-resolution biomedical images that serve as the foundation for the diagnosis and treatment of diseases. Experts with a multitude of backgrounds, including radiologists, anatomists, psychiatrists and neuroscientists now collaboratively analyze the same images to extract a better understanding of the encoded information. Unfortunately, access to these specialists at the same physical location is not always possible and new tools and techniques are required to facilitate simultaneous and collaborative exploration of volumetric data between spatially separated domain experts. This paper presents CVMED, a collaborative visualization environment for volumetric biomedical data-sets, supporting heterogeneous hardware, rendering and display systems connected via heterogeneous networks. CVMED provides the user with the algorithms and tools for stereoscopic as well as monoscopic data visualization and annotation along with the middleware needed to exchange the resulting visuals between all participants in real-time.

## 1. Introduction

The pervasive nature of imaging techniques has provided doctors in different disciplines with a means to acquire high-resolution biomedical images. Experts with a multitude of backgrounds, including radiologists, anatomists, psychiatrists and neuroscientists, subsequently collaboratively analyze the acquired data to extract a better understanding of the encoded information. Unfortunately, access to these specialists at the same physical location is not always possible and new tools and techniques are required to facilitate simultaneous and collaborative exploration of volumetric data between spatially separated domain experts. This paper presents CVMED, a distributed visualization environment for the collaborative analysis of biomedical data, which allows researchers to virtually collaborate from any place with basic network support. All users have access to a *HybridReality* renderer [1], which offers co-located 2D and 3D views of the volumetric data and enables collaborative information exchange via sketching and annotation. The 2D view represents images slices and is suitable for precise interactions such as annotation, segmentation, and high-resolution analysis. The 3D view supports volume rendered visuals, which establishes the physical relationship between the image slices and facili-

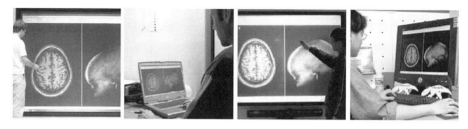

**Figure 1.** Real-time collaborative visualization utilizing 2D and 3D display technology, including a networked passive stereo display wall, laptop, digital whiteboard and desktop system (from left).

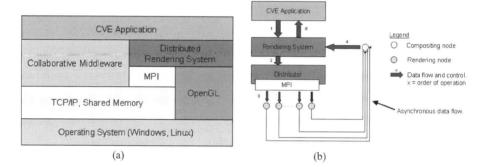

**Figure 2.** Layout of the (a) software architecture and (b) rendering system control flow.

tates navigation within the 3D space. Heterogeneous platforms, ranging from high-end graphics workstations to low performance TabletPCs, as well as heterogeneous networks ranging from wireless to dedicated gigabit links, are supported.

## 2. System Architecture

The system architecture focuses on separating the research and development paths for collaboration [2,3] and visualization algorithms, middleware and tools. An important consideration was the design of a plug-in capable harness that can support user specific visualization algorithm and communication layers without affecting other framework components. The architecture is shown in Figure 2(a), and consists of a set of discrete layers, including (1) an application layer, (2) a collaborative middleware layer and (3) a distributed rendering layer. The application layer serves as the foundation for the development of algorithms, tools and interfaces for distributed 2D/3D visuals and hides the middleware and rendering system from the user. The *Collaborative Middleware Layer* is built on TCP/IP for communications between instances of the CVMED client applications. Clients are connected through a communication server, responsible for synchronization and session management, including management of session logs that allow users to join and exit collaborative sessions at any point in time. The *Distributed Rendering System Layer* is used to distribute the rendering tasks across attached rendering nodes and to composite the final visual. In order to support multiple users that simultaneously can interact with shared data, a client-server model is supported that uses a synchronization server, responsible for managing system wide data consistency and the processing

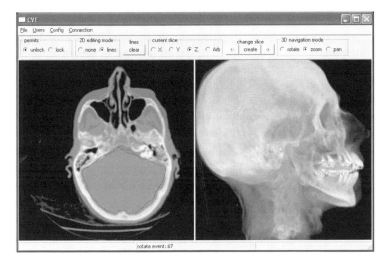

**Figure 3.** CVMED user interface combining a shared 2D view (left) and 3D view (right).

and dissemination of user events as well as the shared visual contents. The server may select to distribute rendering tasks to client nodes and to function as a compositing node, to allow the real-time processing of larger datasets. As illustrated in Figure 2(b), data can be broken up and distributed among the rendering nodes. Each rendering node loads the provided rendering algorithm as a dynamically linked library (late binding), generates an image tile and returns it to the server where the resulting image tiles are gathered and combined into the final image.

## 3. User Interface and Test Results

The CVMED GUI is shown in (Figure 3). The interface provides a side-by-side 2D as well as 3D workspace, enabling users to quickly switch between different display and interaction modes. Currently interaction modes for the 2D space include sketching, labeling and image slice selection, while the 3D space provides access to the traditional transformations, controls over transfer and opacity functions as well as slicing tools.

Tests were conducted on multiple computational platforms (Pentium4, Xeon) equipped with nVIDIA FX1000 and ATI Radeon 9700PRO graphics cards. Tests between the Brain Imaging Center (BIC) at UCI and the National Center for Microscopy and Imaging Research (NCMIR) at UCSD demonstrated that real-time collaborative work is practical. Tests for a $512^3$ MRI scan and a 512x512 final visual, in a five user distributed environment, wirelessly connected at 11Mbit/sec, showed that image generation, compression, delivery, decompression and display can be achieved at 5fps over commodity networks, with user interactions taking no more that 10msec to propagate between nodes. Stereo image pairs were locally cached to satisfy higher refresh rates.

## 4. Conclusion

The paper introduces a new distributed visualization environment for biomedical data analysis. In particular, the developed algorithms and tools provide enhanced interactivity for the collaborative analysis of biomedical image data between researchers at different physical locations. The framework implements a flexible architecture for distributed rendering that supports dynamic rendering plug-ins and on-demand distribution of rendering tasks. The architecture enables the framework to be fully functional in a wide range of hardware settings, from high-end graphics workstation with gigabit network to low-end laptop with wireless connectivity. While the current research focus is on the overall architecture, rendering as well as communication techniques, human-computer interaction challenges have been an important research component.

## References

[1]  Marc Antonijuan Tresens and Falko Kuester. Hybrid-reality: Collaborative biomedical data exploration exploiting 2-d and 3-d correspondence. In James D. Westwood et al., editor, *Medicine Meets Virtual Reality 12*, volume 98 of *Studies in Health Technology and Informatics*, pages 22–24. IOS Press, January 2004.
[2]  Vinod Anupam, Chandrajit Bajaj, Daniel Schikore, and Matthew Schikore. Distributed and collaborative visualization. IEEE *Computer*, 27(7):253–259, 549, July 1994.
[3]  Guruduth Banavar, Sri Doddapaneni, Kevan Miller, and Bodhi Mukherjee. Rapidly building synchronous collaborative applications by direct manipulation. In *Proceedings of the 1998 ACM conference on Computer supported cooperative work*, pages 139–148. ACM Press, 1998.

*Medicine Meets Virtual Reality 13*
*James D. Westwood et al. (Eds.)*
*IOS Press, 2005*

# FEM-Based Soft Tissue Destruction Model for Ablation Simulator

Naoto KUME [a], Megumi NAKAO [b], Tomohiro KURODA [b],
Hiroyuki YOSHIHARA [b] and Masaru KOMORI [c]
[a] *Graduate School of Informatics, Kyoto University, Japan*
[b] *Graduate School of Medicine, Kyoto University, Japan*
[c] *Computational Biomedicine, Shiga University of Medical Science, Japan*

**Abstract.** In surgical procedures, ablation is one of the most difficult skills to train
and acquire. For the risk of ablation failure, ablation training environments are
desired. This paper proposes FEM-based deformation and destruction soft tissue
model for ablation training simulator. The proposed model employs shearing stress
hypothesis. The result of simulation experiments shows that the model can express
different destruction progression by manipulation.

## 1. Introduction

Achievement of effective surgery support system and improving of surgical training environment is expected. VR-based training simulators [1,2] are applying to surgical planning, navigation or training. Especially, in the field of medical virtual reality, the importance for force feedback is recognized widely, and some palpation VR simulators with haptic devices are prepared [1]. Force feedback is important not only in palpation but also in ablation.

Ablation in surgery is one of the difficult and frequently used procedures. Because failure in ablation of organs causes serious damage to patients, surgeons inevitably have to learn ablation skill to be a master of surgery. Although residents have few chances to train ablation procedure repeatedly, training environment for ablation has not been provided. Therefore, development of VR-based ablation simulator is desired.

Reproducing several cases in ablation procedures, the simulator requires soft tissue destruction model. However, soft tissue destruction model considering deformation are not developed. Although FEM-based soft tissue deformation model [1] calculates accurate deformation and force feedback in real time, the model can not simulate destruction. Cutting models [2] adopt approximate algorithm that manipulation point correspond to destruction point. However, manipulation point does not correspond to destruction point in ablation. Although S. Cotin's liver tear model [2] handles deformation and destruction of soft tissue, tore position is not simulated based on deformation.

The goal of our research is to develop VR ablation simulator for training. In order to develop advanced ablation simulator that enables to provide accurate visual and force feedback, a completely physics-based destruction model is required. This paper proposes a soft tissue deformation and destruction model for ablation simulator. Effectiveness of the proposed models is examined through some tension test simulation.

## 2. Overview of ablation simulation

Ablation is a manipulation of tearing connective tissue for dividing adhesive organs. Force feedback is important for residents to learn manipulation skill in ablation. For training ablation, simulator should express success or failure of ablation caused by operator's manipulation. Therefore, tore position after expansion of soft tissue should be expressed differently by different manipulation. Ablation simulator needs to provide visual and force feedback with destruction derived from deformation of soft tissue. Consequently, ablation simulator should adopt a completely physics-based destruction model based on internal stress caused by manipulation.

This study proposes a soft tissue destruction model for ablation simulator. The proposed model needs to satisfy four functional requirements for simulation of ablation. Firstly, the proposed model should calculate accurate soft tissue deformation and internal stress for determination of destruction point. Secondly, the model decides tore position based on stress distribution. Thirdly, the model needs to represent different spread of tore position in case of different manipulation. Finally, the model calculates reaction stress at the manipulation point for haptic presentation.

## 3. FEM-based soft tissue deformation and destruction

The model should calculate accurate deformation of soft tissue. And also, the model should calculate tore position caused by stress distribution for expression of ablation instead of cutting approximation. The model is composed of the following two physical steps; deformation and destruction.

(1)  deformation step : manipulation and linear deformation of soft tissue
(2)  destruction step : destruction caused by stress distribution accompanied deformation

Figure 1 shows an image of the proposed ablation design by deformation and destruction. Both tissue A and B are soft tissue organs, and tissue C is connective tissue. While tore position appears in tissue C, manipulator succeeds in ablation. On the other hand, ablation is recognized as failure when tissue A or tissue B is destroyed.

The proposed model enhances conventional FEM based deformation model [1] for calculation of accurate deformation. The conventional FEM-based tetrahedral model has elastic physical parameter (Young's modulus and Poisson's ratio). The proposed model gives new elastic parameter that represents rupture stress to conventional FEM-based model. The rupture stress modulus provides the limit of deformation of each element. When stress of an element exceeds the set rupture stress modulus (RS), the element will be destroyed. The authors design coalescent organs as one object model because the ad-

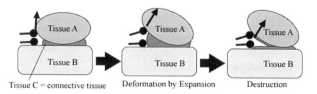

**Figure 1.** Total image of ablation of three layered organs.

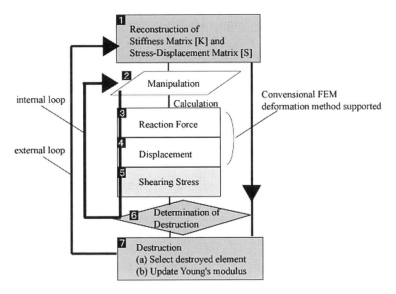

**Figure 2.** Algorithm loop for ablation simulation. This paper focuses on calculation of stress distribution and determination of destruction.

hered organs deform like as one object. Each organs region is specified with elastic and rupture stress parameters. For real time simulation of accurate deformation and force feedback, conventional FEM-based model adopts condensation technique [3] that consolidate internal elastic attribute to the surface of model. The proposed model does not adopt condensation technique for calculation internal stress. Figure 2 shows algorithm loop involving matrix construction and destruction determination online on the model.

### 3.1. Tetrahedral FEM modeling

An organ model is constructed from two dimensional images that are obtained from MRI or CT dataset. After extracted from accumulate slice images, a 3D region of target organ is divided into finite tetrahedra. The 3D region has physical parameters; Young's modulus, Poisson's ratio and rupture stress modulus. If each element size is sufficiently tiny, appropriate rupture stress modulus setting is expected to realize expression of anisotropic destruction.

Current obtaining technology of human body attributes does not support to get absolute parameter that provides a basis for rupture stress. This paper assumes that an organ has a uniform rupture stress value, doctors who recognize sensation during soft tissue ablation by empirical knowledge provide with rupture stress for the model relatively.

### 3.2. Real-time deformation with internal stress analysis

Static FEM model assumes that internal force during deformation is balanced in an object. Therefore, Hooke's law is applied to static FEM model. Conventional FEM deformation model describes stiffness matrix $[K]$ as $f = [K]u$. Where $u$ is displacement, $f$ is external force. The proposed model adopt conventional deformation model for calculation of deformation. Note that $K$ matrix cannot be reduced by condensation method at matrix reconstruction stage in Figure 2 for calculation of internal stress. The proposed model prepares stress-displacement matrix $S$ for calculating internal stress from each element displacement rapidly. $S$ matrix is provided as a parameter of each element at the matrix reconstruction stage. $S$ matrix is defined by multiplication of strain-displacement matrix and stress-strain matrix. Therefore, the proposed model fulfills the requirement for accurate deformation and calculation of reaction stress at manipulation point.

### 3.3. Destruction Model

Soft tissue destruction should be expressed based on stress distribution during deformation. The model is required to calculate destroyed element based on stress derived from deformation of it own. The proposed model adopts maximum shearing stress hypothesis [4] that defines that the maximum shearing stress distribution causes soft tissue to destroy. The hypothesis is based on empirical evidence of soft tissue tension test. During deformation stage, the model makes a comparison of the rupture stress to shearing stress all over the elements for selection of an element which should be destroyed. Because it is reasonable to suppose that the shearing stress distribution does not change abruptly between elastic and plastic deformation range, it is appropriate to adopt the approximation technique that calculate destroyed element only by maximum shearing stress distribution during elastic deformation range. In addition, the destruction is expressed only from surface element of the object because ablation is a controlled destruction manipulation.

Therefore, the proposed model enables interactive expression of destruction caused by rupture stress of each element based on distribution of maximum shear stress. After eliminating the destructed element, the model reconstructs stiffness matrix and stress-displacement matrix. This deformation and destruction of soft tissue is repeatedly simulated. Because stress distribution of the model is kept accurately, destruction is expressed by removing tetrahedral element.

## 4. Evaluation and Results

Based on the proposed model, simulation of ablation expressed by destruction of soft tissue was preliminary developed. This study prepared some experiments in order to verify certification of tore position. Following two experiments evaluate destruction distribution and reaction stress during ablation.

Accuracy of stress distribution is affected by particle size of the volumetric mesh topology. The result of a preliminary experiment showed that proper number of nodes of an organs model is over 900 nodes. The object model for the following evaluation employed 1594 nodes 3D board model consist of two elastic parameter regions that represent adhere state of organs. Figure 3 shows two regions as tissue A (Young = 5MPa, Poisson = 0.4 and RS = 2MPa) and tissue B (Young = 10MPa, Poisson = 0.4 and RS = 8MPa). The rupture stress was arbitrary set relative to Young's modulus. Visualization of destruction was expressed by destroyed element elimination method [2] that is updated Young's modulus approximate to $0$ for accurate calculation of stress distribution after destruction.

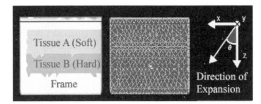

**Figure 3.** 3D board model consist of two layered soft tissue.

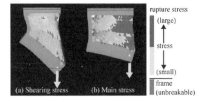

**Figure 4.** Comparison of stress distribution between shearing stress and main stress.

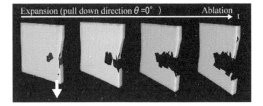

**Figure 5.** Results of tension test simulation appears ablation.

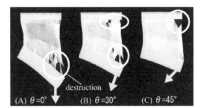

**Figure 6.** Result of tension test by three way manipulation. Different tore position appears by different manipulation.

Manipulation point was fixed on right below of the board model. Preliminary deformation experiment without destruction compared main stress distribution with shearing stress distribution. Figure 4 shows credibility of the maximum shearing stress hypothesis on the grounds of soft tissue destruction.

## 4.1. Evaluation of destruction distribution

Tore position was evaluated qualitatively with tension test on the developed system. The test was performed by three way manipulation. The results show in Figure 5 and Figure 6. As shown in Figure 5, the proposed model achieved expression of ablation. Figure 6 shows that different tore position were expressed by three way manipulation (pulling down direction $\theta = 0, 30, 45$ degree). In case of pulling down direction $\theta = 0$, tore position appeared near manipulation point approximately. On the other hand, in case of $\theta = 45$, tore position appeared near fixed above side of the object. And then, in case of $\theta = 30$, tore position appeared both sides of near manipulation point or near fixed above side unpredictably. The tests concluded that the model can express tore position appropriate for the way of different manipulation based on empirical knowledge.

## 4.2. Evaluation of reaction stress while ablation

Reaction stress while ablation is evaluated quantitatively with tension test at the same condition of the previous test. The transition of reaction stress in case of pulling down direction $\theta = 0$ are plotted in Figure 7.

During deformation, reaction stress increased sequentially. In contrast, reaction stress decreased abruptly at a point of destruction caused. The average of reaction stress effectively decreased along with progress of tore position. Decrease of reaction stress

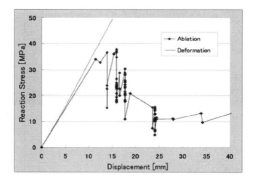

**Figure 7.** Results of reaction stress at manipulation point during ablation and only deformation.

caused by stress concentration is the same as in ablation of real tissues. This experiment confirmed that the proposed model have capability to present realistic haptic feedback through manipulators.

## 5. Discussion

This paper shows possibility that ablation simulator which adopts completely physics based model enables surgeons to feel haptic feedback at the point of soft tissue destruction based on accurate deformation while ablation. The proposed approach for destruction determination based on maximum shearing stress hypothesis performed realistic tore position spread. Accurate deformation for accuracy calculation of stress distribution has effected on accurate destruction determination directly. One of the most critical requirements is achievement of real time ablation simulation. First of all, in order to achieve real time refresh rate, the model should be improved on computational complexity at the matrix reconstruction stage. Secondly, for natural visualization of ablation instead of destroyed element elimination method, development of efficiency remeshing method is desired.

## 6. Conclusion

This study proposed physics based model that can express organs tore position caused by its own shearing stress distribution for ablation simulator. The proposed model based on FEM could calculate stress distribution and reaction stress at manipulation point. In addition, the model could appear the different destruction with different manipulation. In the future, adopting the proposed model, advanced ablation simulator achieves expression of realistic destruction progressing and force feedback.

### Acknowledgements

This research was supported by Grant-in-Aid for Scientific Research (S) (16100001) and Young Scientists (A) (16680024) from The Japanese Ministry of Education, Science, Sports and Culture.

# References

[1] M. Nakao, T. Kuroda, M. Komori and H. Oyama, "Evaluation and User Study of Haptic Simulator for Learning Palpation in Cardiovascular Surgery", International Conference of Artificial Reality and Tele-Existence (ICAT), pp. 203-208, 2003.

[2] S. Cotin, H. Delingette, and N. Ayache, "A hybrid elastic model for real-time cutting, deformations, and force feedback for surgery training and simulation", The Visual Computer, No.16, pp.437-452, 2000.

[3] M. Bro-Nielsen and S. Cotin, "Real-time volumetric deformable models for surgery simulation using finit elements and condensation", Eurographics Computer Graphics Forum, Vol.15, No.3, pp.57-66, 1996.

[4] S. Taira, "*Zairyou rikigaku* [*Strength of materials*]", Ohmsha, 1970.

*Medicine Meets Virtual Reality 13*
*James D. Westwood et al. (Eds.)*
*IOS Press, 2005*

# The VREST Learning Environment

E.E. KUNST, MSc, PhD [a],
R.H. GEELKERKEN, MD, PhD [b] and A.J.B. SANDERS, MSc [c]
[a] *Kunst & van Leerdam Medical Technology bv, Enschede, the Netherlands*
*e-mail: ekunst@kvlmt.nl*
[b] *Department of Vascular Surgery, Medisch Spectrum Twente,*
*Enschede, the Netherlands*
*e-mail: r.geelkerken@mst-ziekenhuis.nl*
[c] *Kunst & van Leerdam Medical Technology bv, Enschede, the Netherlands*
*e-mail: asanders@kvlmt.nl*

**Abstract.** The VREST learning environment is an integrated architecture to improve the education of health care professionals. It is a combination of a learning,
content and assessment management system based on virtual reality. The generic
architecture is now being build and tested around the Lichtenstein protocol for hernia inguinalis repair.

## 1. Problem

The quality of health care professionals is at stake in a number of countries in the Western
world. Due to the increase in the number of elderly people and the decrease in those potentially available to deliver care, the costliness of current master-slave training systems,
the subjectivity of the determination of the outcome of training, the quality of health care
professionals can no longer be guaranteed [1–4].

In the Netherlands in 2000 an initiative was initiated to introduce virtual reality as
a component in the training of health care professionals. Although its sope has widened
since the start, it started in the surgical environment, hence the name: Virtual Reality
Educational Surgical Tools (VREST).

## 2. Method

VREST concentrates on the development of a true learning environment in which sometimes VR-tools are necessary and sometimes they do not. VREST builds the architecture
of the virtual training house and provides the tools to build 'the walls' and the 'interior'.

To demonstrate the potential of such an environment VREST currently develops a
surgical trainer for hernia inguinalis repair according to the Lichtenstein protocol. The
prototype will be introduced into a validation setting in order to generate valuable feedback on the concept of the VREST environment and the possible role of virtual reality
tools in such an environment.

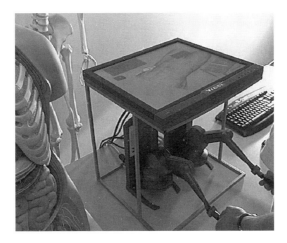

**Figure 1.** The VREST Platform for Virtual Medical Training.

Furthermore, VREST has already developed a decision support and training environment for the selection and treatment of patients with an abdominal aorta aneurysm. This EAG-tool (Effective AAA Graftmanship) is currently under validation.

## 3. Results

The prototype of the VREST learning environment for the surgical repair of a hernia inguinalis according to Lichtenstein is complete (see Figure 1). It will enter a validation research programme by the beginning of 2005.

The VREST decision support system for AAA endografts (EAG-tool) is currently under validation. The preliminary results are very promising. Submission of several scientific publication is foreseen for the end of 2004.

## 4. Conclusion

The first results with the VREST learning environment are very promising. The real strength, however, can only be presented when the basic concept is truly validated.

## 5. Discussion

The VREST learning environment provides an environment in which vr-tools and other learning gadgets are necessary and can play an important role. In the past many initiatives have mainly focussed on the technological challenges related to virtual reality tools, both visual and haptics. VREST offers a structure in which such high-tech systems need to be implemented.

Many health care professionals support the approach and the concept. A scientific validation however is necessary to come to its full potential.

# References

[1] Scott DJ, Valentine RJ, Bergen PC, Rege RV, Laycock R, Tesfay ST et al. Evaluating surgical competency with the American Board of Surgery In-Training Examination, skill testing, and intraoperative assessment. Surgery 2000; 128(4):613-622.

[2] Grantcharov TP, Kristiansen VB, Bendix J, Bardram L, Rosenberg J, Funch-Jensen P. Randomized clinical trial of virtual reality simulation for laparoscopic skills training. Br J Surg 2004; 91(2):146-150.

[3] Ahlberg G, Heikkinen T, Iselius L, Leijonmarck CE, Rutqvist J, Arvidsson D. Does training in a virtual reality simulator improve surgical performance? Surg Endosc 2002; 16(1):126-129.

[4] Bloom MB, Rawn CL, Salzberg AD, Krummel TM. Virtual reality applied to procedural testing: the next era. Ann Surg 2003; 237(3):442-448.

*Medicine Meets Virtual Reality 13*
*James D. Westwood et al. (Eds.)*
*IOS Press, 2005*

# MVL: Medical VR Simulation Library

Yoshihiro KURODA [a], Megumi NAKAO [b], Tomohiro KURODA [c],
Hiroshi OYAMA [d] and Hiroyuki YOSHIHARA [c]

[a] *Graduate School of Informatics, Kyoto University, Japan*
[b] *Graduate School of Medicine, Kyoto University, Japan*
[c] *Department of Medical Informatics, Kyoto University Hospital, Japan*
[d] *Graduate School of Medicine, University of Tokyo, Japan*

**Abstract.** In the last ten years, medical VR techniques have much progress and many simulators have been developed for education, planning, rehearsal and so on. On the other hand, developing a simulator takes much more labor and cost. In this paper, we propose MVL: Medical Virtual reality simulation Library, which supports simulation of several significant medical manipulations considering multiple organ interaction. The result of developing simulators using MVL confirmed validity about variety and developing cost.

## 1. Introduction

Virtual reality (VR) based simulation with physics-based deformation and force feedback gives much capability of medical application for education, training, planning and a lot of purposes. However, for developing simulators, much time and efforts are required for developers to learn and implement basic physics and foregoing methods. The aim of our study is to support and promote developing medical VR simulators by reducing developing burden. In this paper, we propose a simulation library *MVL: Medical Virtual reality simulation Library*, which enables easy development of simulators with several important medical manipulations considering organ-organ interaction.

## 2. MVL

The features of MVL are as follows.

1. Multiple medical manipulations and multiple organ interaction
2. High accurate and interactive deformation and force display
3. API for simulating medical manipulations

MVL supports simulations of several significant medical manipulations such as palpation, cutting, retracting, and pushing aside. Simulation of both palpation and combination of cutting, retracting, and pushing aside achieves a lot of educational and training environment in elementary diagnosis and surgical approaching procedures respectively [1,2]. Interaction model between elastic objects [1] and collision detection method for deformable model [3] enables to simulate indirect palpation and pushing aside con-

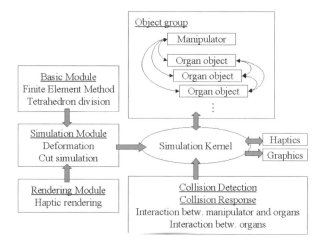

**Figure 1.** Architecture of MVL.

sidering behind objects. For high accurate deformation and force calculation, finite element method with condensation [4] and Hirota's methods [5] are implemented. API for medical manipulations is provided and enables simulation of medical manipulation with a few line coding.

Above features are achieved by *object group* based simulation architecture as shown in figure 1.

*Object group* class is an interface between users and simulation kernel. Just by adding a manipulator and organ objects into *object group* and a few line coding enables simulation of medical manipulations. All kinds of simulation modules including tetrahedron division, finite element method, haptic rendering, collision detection, organ interaction model are cooperated. Easy and flexible setting of physical parameters such as Young modulus and Poisson ratio are possible by using utility software called *Matrix Builder*, which is provided by us.

## 3. Results

Developed sample simulators using MVL and lines of coding are shown. Figure 2 and 3 show simulators of palpation and approaching thoracoabdominal aorta respectively [1,6].

The results confirm that MVL simulates various kinds of simulators and achieves reduced coding for developing simulators.

## 4. Conclusion

This paper proposes MVL, which is a supporting environment for developing force reflecting physics-based simulators. Object group based architecture manages all kinds of modules and provides API for simulating medical manipulations. The results confirmed that MVL simulates various kinds of simulators and achieves reduced coding for developing simulators. Japanese version of MVL is now available on the web site. Further development will be continued for advanced simulations.

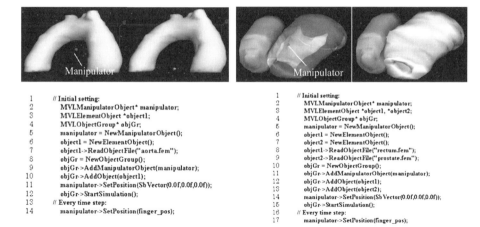

```
 1    // Initial setting:
 2       MVLManipulatorObject* manipulator;
 3       MVLElementObject *object1;
 4       MVLObjectGroup* objGr;
 5       manipulator = NewManipulatorObject();
 6       object1 = NewElementObject();
 7       object1->ReadObjectFile("aorta.fem");
 8       objGr = NewObjectGroup();
 9       objGr->AddManipulatorObject(manipulator);
10       objGr->AddObject(object1);
11       manipulator->SetPosition(SbVector(0.0f,0.0f,0.0f));
12       objGr->StartSimulation();
13    // Every time step:
14       manipulator->SetPosition(finger_pos);
```

```
 1    // Initial setting:
 2       MVLManipulatorObject* manipulator;
 3       MVLElementObject *object1, *object2;
 4       MVLObjectGroup* objGr;
 5       manipulator = NewManipulatorObject();
 6       object1 = NewElementObject();
 7       object2 = NewElementObject();
 8       object1->ReadObjectFile("rectum.fem");
 9       object2->ReadObjectFile("prostate.fem");
10       objGr = NewObjectGroup();
11       objGr->AddManipulatorObject(manipulator);
12       objGr->AddObject(object1);
13       objGr->AddObject(object2);
14       manipulator->SetPosition(SbVector(0.0f,0.0f,0.0f));
15       objGr->StartSimulation();
16    // Every time step:
17       manipulator->SetPosition(finger_pos);
```

**Figure 2.** Palpation simulators Aorta palpation simulator (Left), rectal palpation simulator (Right) Each simulator is characterized as direct and indirect palpation respectively. Haptic display considering multiple organ interaction is achieved automatically just by difference in coding of registered number of objects.

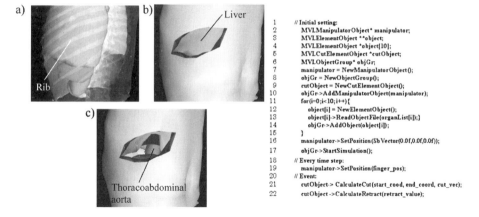

```
 1    // Initial setting:
 2       MVLManipulatorObject* manipulator;
 3       MVLElementObject **object;
 4       MVLElementObject *object[10];
 5       MVLCutElementObject *cutObject;
 6       MVLObjectGroup* objGr;
 7       manipulator = NewManipulatorObject();
 8       objGr = NewObjectGroup();
 9       cutObject = NewCutElementObject();
10       objGr->AddManipulatorObject(manipulator);
11       for(i=0;i<10;i++){
12          object[i] = NewElementObject();
13          object[i]->ReadObjectFile(organList[i]);}
14          objGr->AddObject(object[i]);
15       }
16       manipulator->SetPosition(SbVector(0.0f,0.0f,0.0f));
17       objGr->StartSimulation();
18    // Every time step:
19       manipulator->SetPosition(finger_pos);
20    // Event:
21       cutObject-> CalculateCut(start_cood, end_coord, cut_vec);
22       cutObject ->CalculateRetract(retract_value);
```

**Figure 3.** Approaching simulators Multiple surgical manipulations are conducted when approaching thoracoabdominal aorta. MVL supports development of a simulator dealing with several surgical manipulations. a) Before cutting between ribs. b) After retracting incision, liver covers a surgical field. c) Aorta is visible by pushing aside several surrounding organs.

## Acknowledgements

This research was supported by Grant-in-Aid for Scientific Research (S)(16100001) and Young Scientists (A) (16680024) from The Ministry of Education, Culture, Sports, Science and Technology, Japan.

## References

[1]  Y. Kuroda, M. Nakao, T. Kuroda, H. Oyama, M. Komori and T. Matsuda, "FEM-Based Interaction Model Between Elastic Objects for Indirect Palpation Simulator", Proceedings of 12th Medicine Meets Virtual Reality Conference, pp.183-189, 2004.

[2] M. Nakao, T. Kuroda, H. Oyama, M. Komori, T. Matsuda and T. Takahashi, "Planning and Training of Minimally Invasive Surgery by Integrating Soft Tissue Cuts with Surgical Views Reproduction", Computer Assisted Radiology and Surgery(CARS), pp. 13-18, 2002.

[3] Y. Kitamura, A. Smith, H. Takemura and F. Kishino, "A Real-Time Algorithm for Accurate Collision Detection for Deformable Polyhedral Objects", MIT PRESENCE, Vol.7, No.1, pp.36-52, 1998.

[4] M. Bro-Nielsen, "Finite element modeling in surgery simulation", Journal of the IEEE, Vol.86, No.3, pp.490-503, 1998.

[5] K. Hirota and T. Kaneko, "A method of representing soft object in virtual environment", IPSJ JOURNAL, Vol.39, No.12, pp.3261-3268, Dec. 1998

[6] M. Nakao, T. Kuroda, M. Komori and H. Oyama, "Evaluation and User Study of Haptic Simulator for Learning Palpation in Cardiovascular Surgery", International Conference of Artificial Reality and Tele-Existence, pp.203-208, 2003.

*Medicine Meets Virtual Reality 13*
*James D. Westwood et al. (Eds.)*
*IOS Press, 2005*

# Haptic Device for Colonoscopy Training Simulator

Jun Yong KWON, Hyun Soo WOO and Doo Yong LEE

*Dept. of Mechanical Engineering, Korea Advanced Institute of Science and Technology*
*e-mail: {kwonjy,lee.dooyong}@kaist.ac.kr*

**Abstract.** A new 2-DOF haptic device for colonoscopy training simulator employing flexible endoscopes, is developed. The user operates the device in translational and roll directions. The developed folding guides of the device keep the endoscope tube straight. This helps transmit large decoupled forces of the colonoscopy simulation to the user. The device also includes a mechanism to detect jiggling motion of the scopes to allow users to practice this important skill of the colonoscopy. The device includes PD controller to compensate the inertia and friction effects. This provides the users with better transparent sensation of the simulation.

## 1. Introduction

Colonoscopy requires skills in handling a long and flexible tube, and is performed mainly in translational and roll motion. The haptic device of the colonoscopy training simulator needs large workspaces in the roll and translation motions. It should also provide the reflective force and torque in these 2-DOF (degrees of freedom) independently.

The mechanism employing a rubber ball [1] cannot generate large enough forces because of slippage, and cannot completely decouple the two DOF. Körner et al. [2] developed a different 2-DOF haptic device that attached the tip of the endoscope to a carriage. This mechanism has large inertia in the translational direction, and cannot provide large torque in the roll direction. We present a new 2-DOF haptic device with large workspaces, which can generate large enough force and torque in the translational and roll directions, independently.

The jiggling motion of the endoscope tube makes the colon straight, and shortens the colon length by wrinkling its folds. It is an important skill of colonoscopy. The new device presented in this paper allows the user to practice this technique, by employing a sensor mechanism and algorithms.

## 2. Methods

Figure 1 depicts the decoupled 2-DOF haptic device for colonoscopy training simulator. Translational motion is implemented with a wire-driven mechanism. The endoscope tube, fixed on the pulley mechanism, moves along the two guiding rods in translational direction. The torque of the roll motion is transferred by a timing belt and the pulley.

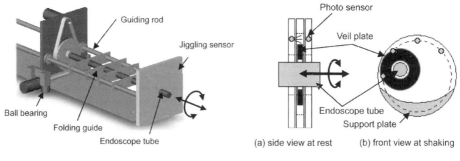

**Figure 1.** 2-DOF haptic device.

**Figure 2.** Sensor mechanism for jiggling motion.

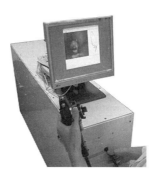

**Figure 3.** Colonoscopy simulator.

This mechanism has large friction and inertia. A closed-loop PD controller using a 6-DOF force/torque sensor is designed to reduce the friction and inertial effects. The user's maneuvering forces are measured in real-time, and compensated for including the effects of coulomb and viscous frictions.

Special guide is used to maintain the form of the tube straight as shown in Figure 1. This helps the force and torque generated by the haptic device be transmitted to the user without any loss. The guide folds and expands like a curtain. The guide panels are connected with wires so as to ease the folding motion, and endure the stretching force. The maximum distance between the guide panels is limited to about 5cm to keep the tube straight.

The sensor mechanism to detect the jiggling motion of the tube is composed of a veil plate and 4 pairs of photo sensors as shown in Figure 2. The photo sensors are placed at particular intervals to identify decoupled directions. A crescent support plate prevents the endoscope tube from drooping below the center. This mechanism is located at the entrance hole for the tube. This mechanism identifies the jiggling of 2.5Hz and above.

The developed colonoscopy simulator is shown in Figure 3. It employs specially fabricated endoscope tube and handle that share the look, feel, and functions with actual endoscopes, and the necessary electronics. The simulator also includes a virtual colon model based on real human data. The user interacts with the virtual model through the developed haptic device.

**Table 1.** Specifications of the haptic device.

|  | Max. Force | Workspace | Bandwidth |
|---|---|---|---|
| Translational Motion | 60.250 N | 980 mm | 50 Hz |
| Roll Motion | 1.028N · m | Infinite | 57 Hz |

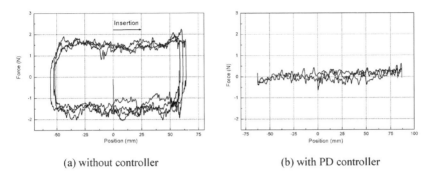

(a) without controller          (b) with PD controller

**Figure 4.** Measured maneuvering force in free motion.

## 3. Results

Table 1 shows the workspace, reflective force range, and bandwidth of the developed haptic device. It can also detect the jiggling motion at above 2.5Hz in 8 directions independently.

Figure 4 shows the measured maneuvering force in free motion when the virtual environment provides no reflective force. The user has to exert about $\pm1.314$ N to operate the haptic device forward and backward in the translational direction without a PD controller as shown in Figure 4(a). Figure 4(b) shows that the PD controller compensates the maneuvering force down to $\pm0.17$ N. The maneuvering force is also compensated by the controller when the user interacts with the virtual environment that has the stiffness K $= 750$ N/m and the damping B $= 4$ N · s/m$^2$.

## 4. Conclusion

The developed 2-DOF haptic device provides the user with decoupled active force and torque in the translational and roll directions. The included PD controller compensates 87% of the friction and inertial effects of the device so as to provide transparent sensations to the user. The new device also includes a mechanism to allow users to practice jiggling skill of colonoscopy. The developed simulator with the new haptic device and improved graphics provides more enhanced experience for the colonoscopy training.

## References

[1] K. Ikuta, K. Iritani, and J. Fukuyama, "Mobile Virtual Endoscope System with Haptic and Visual Information for Non-invasive Inspection Training," *Proceedings of the 2001 IEEE International Conference on Robotics & Automation*, Seoul, Korea, May 21-26, 2001. pp. 2037-2044.

[2] O. Körner and R. Männer, "Implementation of a Haptic Interface for a Virtual Reality Simulator for Flexible Endoscopy," *IEEE 11th Symposium on Haptic Interfaces for Virtual Environment and Teleoperator Systems*, Los Angeles, California, Mar. 2003, pp. 22-23.

*Medicine Meets Virtual Reality 13*
*James D. Westwood et al. (Eds.)*
*IOS Press, 2005*

# Developing a Simulation-Based Training Program for Medical First Responders

Fuji LAI [a], Eileen ENTIN [a], Meghan DIERKS [c],
Daniel RAEMER [d] and Robert SIMON [d]

[a] *Aptima, Inc., Woburn, MA*
*e-mail: fujilai@aptima.com*
[c] *Harvard Medical School and Beth Israel Deaconess Medical Center*
[d] *Center for Medical Simulation, Massachusetts General Hospital*

**Abstract.** A major stumbling block for widespread incorporation of simulators into
EMT training includes the limited availability of curricula infrastructure linking the
key components of skills, scenarios, and measures as well as the expertise required
to run such programs. To meet these needs we are developing a training program
for first responders that uses mannequin-based simulator technology effectively to
fill the identified training need for valid meaningful scenarios that can be integrated
into the curriculum and are applicable for a variety of EMT skill levels. The program will provide detailed scenarios, instructions for administering the program,
and measures for performance feedback. Each scenario will exercise a combination of taskwork and cognitive skills and the set of scenarios will span all of the
higher-level skills that have been identified as benefiting from targeted training.

## 1. Background

Simulation promises to provide a training solution for cognitive skills training as well as
taskwork training for Emergency Medical Technicians (EMTs). The 2001 EMS Division
of the National Highway Traffic Safety Administration (NHTSA) roundtable identified
EMS patient safety related issues including "limited access to simulation training technology" [1]. At MMVR in 2004 the call was made for educational infrastructure, curricula and validation to support the integration of simulators into actual use [2]. A major stumbling block for widespread incorporation of simulators into EMT training, especially into smaller regional EMS units, includes the limited availability of curricula infrastructure linking the key components of skills, scenarios, and measures as well as the
expertise required to run such programs. Our program is designed to meet these needs.

## 2. Training Package

Through examination of the curricula for the Army combat medic (91W) and the National Registry of Emergency Medical Technicians EMT programs, and input from an
expert advisory panel of stakeholders, we identified that training emphasis is needed on
cognitively-based skills such as situation assessment, adaptation, and decision making,

and on team-based skills such as communication and coordination at each of the stages of planning, survey, triage, treatment, and handoff. Examples include prioritizing of limited treatment resources, assessment of threats, deciding upon the need for immediate procedural intervention versus deferring intervention until arrival at a higher level care facility, and seeking direction from on-line medical direction. Furthermore, a need was identified for training under complex unusual situations where there may need to be dynamic decision making and problem solving.

Simulator-based training has the potential to enhance first responder education but its use has been hindered by cost and limited access to higher fidelity simulators, need for validation, need for simulator scenarios and curriculum, and competence in simulator use. To address these needs we are developing the First Responder Simulation-based Training (FIRST) Program. As illustrated in Figure 1 FIRST will provide all the components required to conduct a scenario-based training program using a mannequin simulator without the need for an expert trainer, and can therefore be administered as a self-contained, standalone, 'off-the-shelf' package.

There are four components to the package:

The first component is a program overview that sets forth the goals, learning objectives and course structure. This introduction will explain the links between the skills, measures, and scenarios, and lay out the support requirements for conducting the training program.

The second component is an instructor manual to guide instructors in conducting the scenarios as well as evaluating and debriefing the students. An important aspect of scenario-based training is the conduct of a post-scenario debriefing session that allows

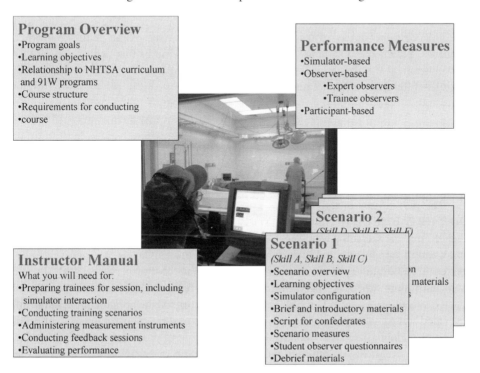

**Figure 1.** Product package.

the participants to examine and analyze their performance under the guidance of an instructor. The goal of the debriefing is not to 'score' the trainees' performance but rather to allow them to review their performance critically, but non-punitively, to see where they did well, and where they could have been more effective. The instructor's manual will include a set of guidelines and targeted questions that will support instructors in conducting the debriefing.

The third component of the package is a set of scenarios. Each scenario exercises a combination of cognitively-based skills and the set of scenarios span the domain of all the higher-level skills that have been identified as benefiting from targeted training. For each scenario, there will be a detailed outline of the scenario events, a description of the skills that are targeted and where in the scenario they are exercised, and instructions on how to set up the scenario including a list of required props, specifications on how to configure the simulator and, where necessary, scripts for confederates who are needed to play specific roles in the scenario (such as an on line medical director).

The fourth component of the package is a set of performance measures that include simulator, observer, and participant-based measures. For the observer-based measures, our objective is to develop measures that assess cognitive skills required by the scenario rather than task skills such as inserting an IV. There are many challenges in designing measures of performance. One consideration is ensuring that the response scale represents a continuum of low to high performance. Another is that the evaluation of the appropriateness or effectiveness of an action may be a function of previous actions. The underlying approach we adopted is that the measures should assess whether the actions of participants are within the bounds of what an expert would define as reasonable. Even after measurement items are developed, they need to be tried out to ensure that they accommodate the variety of responses that participants may exhibit as they perform a scenario. Yet another challenge lies in constructing measures that are appropriate for and generalizable across a range of scenarios. Finally, the measures must be sensitive to regional differences in EMT training.

## 3. Program Demonstration

We have tested the scenarios we have developed and the measures of performance for those scenarios in a simulator environment at the Center for Medical Simulation.

The participants in the scenarios ranged in skill and experience from the EMT-Basic (EMT-B) to EMT-Paramedic (EMT-P) level. Taken as a whole, the demonstrations showed that the scenarios were successful in exercising the skills they were designed to elicit and in tapping into and identifying a range of different levels of expertise and experience. For example, in one demonstration, the relatively inexperienced EMT-Bs and somewhat more experienced EMT-Intermediates performed the scenario at low to moderate levels of proficiency. The EMT-Paramedics performed the scenario well, but it still provided some challenges as was conveyed in the debrief by the participants. Our experience also emphasizes that scenario design is an iterative process and that it is vital to try out the scenarios with multiple sets as well as levels of participants in order to fine tune the scenarios to make them appropriate for various levels of expertise as well as to anticipate the spectrum of behavioral responses and decisions that may occur.

## 4. Conclusions and Future Directions

Simulators have the ability to enhance training but have not taken root because of the limited curriculum infrastructure and validation and until recently the prohibitively high cost of simulators. When completed in late 2005 the FIRST program will represent an important step towards helping the integration and incorporation of simulation-based training into medical first responder curriculum.

## Acknowledgements

This work is supported by the U.S. Army Medical Research and Materiel Command under Contract No. DAMD17-03-C-0059. The views, opinions and/or findings contained in this report are those of the author(s) and should not be construed as an official Department of the Army position.

## References

[1]  Kleiner, D.M. (2002). *Report of the NHTSA roundtable for reducing errors in EMS.*
www.saem.org/newsltr/2002/mar-apr/nhtsa.pdf.
[2]  Satava, R. (2004). From validation studies to implementation: How do we proceed? Medicine Meets Virtual Reality Conference. January 14-17, 2004.

*Medicine Meets Virtual Reality 13*
*James D. Westwood et al. (Eds.)*
*IOS Press, 2005*

# A Mechanical Contact Model for the Simulation of Obstetric Forceps Delivery in a Virtual/Augmented Environment

R.J. LAPEER

*School of Computing Sciences, University of East Anglia, Norwich, UK*
*e-mail: rjal@cmp.uea.ac.uk*

**Abstract.** During the process of human childbirth, obstetric forceps delivery can be a justified alternative to emergency Caesarean section when normal vaginal delivery proves difficult or impossible. Currently, training of forceps interventions is mainly done on real patients which poses a risk. This paper describes a pilot project on the simulation of training of obstetric forceps delivery, using Virtual Reality technology. We first give a brief historical review of the concept of 'birth simulation' and describe the current implementation of the interface. Then we report a number of experiments, conducted to test the feasibility of a real-time mechanical contact model to describe the interaction between the forceps and fetal head, eventually to be interfaced with a multi-purpose haptic feedback device. It is concluded that an explicit dynamic model to calculate the deformation of the main fetal skull bones only, or a quasi-static model to calculate the deformation of the fetal head in its entirety, can reach real-time performance.

## 1. Introduction

Human childbirth is a process that each one of us has gone through at some stage! In most cases this process runs smoothly though a certain percentage of cases (which may be well over 10% in certain western countries) will need some type of intervention: usually a Caesarean section, though often instrumental delivery using vacuum extraction or obstetric forceps. The latter is a justified alternative to emergency Caesarean section when normal vaginal delivery proves difficult or impossible. Currently, training of forceps interventions is done directly on patients due to the lack of realistic training facilities. The author has longstanding expertise in the biomechanics of human childbirth [4,5,7] and his team has recently developed an augmented environment based obstetric forceps simulation[1] which allows an obstetrician to manipulate a real forceps whilst rotating and extracting a virtual fetus from the birth canal - See Figure 1. Post-operative diagnostic assessment of the deformations of the fetal head caused by the simulated forceps movements can then be evaluated using an implicit FE-based contact model [2]. The presented

---

[1]The advantage of AR/VR based training facilities for obstetric forceps delivery, as compared to dummy models or mannequins, is their ability to regenerate different scenarios with variable parameters without the need of creating a completely new 'hardware'-based model!

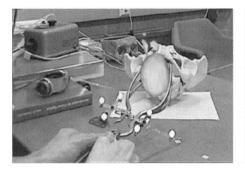 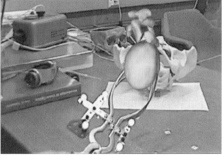

**Figure 1.** Snapshots from a simulation extracting a virtual fetus from a real pelvic model in an augmented environment. The forceps is optically tracked on both blades to allow simulation of the placement of each blade - which is a crucial part to the success of a forceps intervention.

research aims to evaluate the extension of this model to a mechanical contact model in real-time, so it can be used during the simulation in conjunction with haptic feedback.

## 2. Brief history

### 2.1. fetal head/skull deformation

In the early 1980's, a group at the Ann Arbor Institute in Michigan studied the deformation of fetal parietal bone when subjected to the pressure of the uterine cervix [8]. They derived material properties of fetal skull bone and fontanelles from six stillborn babies to perform subsequent Finite Element Analysis (FEA). This work was significantly furthered by the author in the late 1990's by analysing the deformation of the fetal skull in its entirety[2], during delivery, using a non-linear FE model [5,7].

### 2.2. Simulating birth

In the early 1990's, some researchers attempted to simulate the human birth process or in particular, the birth kinematics on computer [1,12]. Only recently, the author's research team [11] and a team at the Technical University in Münich [10] embarked on a quest to further these ideas to useful clinical applications.

## 3. Method

A Finite Element (FE) mechanical contact model adds an extra 'contact force' term - the vector $\mathbf{F}^{cont}(d(t))$ - as a function of the displacement vector $\mathbf{d}(t)$ - to the standard formulation with internal forces $\mathbf{F}^{int}(\mathbf{d}(t))$, external forces $\mathbf{F}^{ext}(\mathbf{d}(t))$, mass matrix $\mathbf{M}$ and damping matrix $\mathbf{C}$:

$$\mathbf{M\ddot{d}}(t) + \mathbf{C\dot{d}}(t) + \mathbf{F}^{int}(\mathbf{d}(t)) + \mathbf{F}^{cont}(\mathbf{d}(t)) = \mathbf{F}^{ext}(\mathbf{d}(t)) \tag{1}$$

---

[2]Including the fontanelles, which are the large soft tissue structures in between the fetal skull bones.

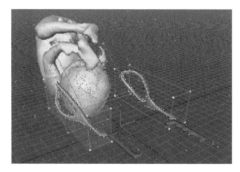
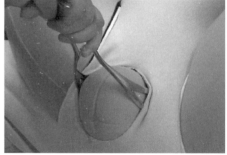

**Figure 2.** The left image shows the collision detection of the left (virtual) forceps blade - with the fetal model. The right image shows the typical 'scoop' movement as performed with the obstetric forceps to deliver the baby (shown on the Birth Training Mannequin from Southmead Hospital in Bristol, UK).

Using an explicit integration method and restricted contact at one timestep $t$, the otherwise complex problem when using implicit FEA, can be significantly reduced in time needed to calculate deformations of the fetal head in contact with the inner blades of the obstetric forceps. Restricted contact is based on efficient collision detection on sporadic contact points to avoid that large areas of the mesh, which are not in contact, are included in the calculations. The collision detection algorithm is performed in three steps. The first step uses bounding boxes (octree hierarchy) around the polygon models to establish that a forceps blade is in the vicinity of one side of the fetal head. This step delivers a selected subset of candidate polygons for contact interaction between forceps blade and fetal head model (see Figure 2a). Further refinement of the subsets is obtained by comparing the direction of surface normals. Finally, in the last step the remaining polygons for each model are pairwise checked for overclosure. For collision response, the selected polygons of the forceps mesh model are used as the master surface whilst those from the head model function as the slave surface because in contact mechanics it is a convention that the master surface can overclose (penetrate) the slave surface. Considering the fact that the forceps is in steel as compared to the bony skull/head, this choice makes sense.

## 4. Implementation and experiment

The current implementation of the simulation includes a virtual fetus model, modelled with the in-house developed volume rendering software 3DView [6][3]. The (real) forceps is tracked using an NDI Polaris optical tracking device. Fetal head deformation through forceps contact is calculated off-line using the method described in the previous section. Figure 1 shows the extraction of the virtual fetus from a real pelvic model, using the tracked forceps. Subsequent analyses based on these manipulations allow us to assess performance in time.

### 4.1. Experiment: deformation and time analysis

A typical forceps extraction movement was studied, where the baby is delivered using a 'scoop' like upwards motion, as illustrated in Figure 2b. In experiment 1, a simplified

---

[3]This software is freely available on http://www2.cmp.uea.ac.uk/~rjal/.

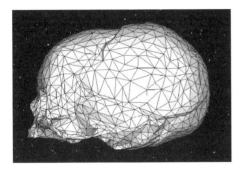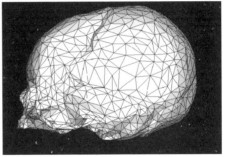

**Figure 3.** Undeformed and deformed skull model after application of a (virtual) forceps (deformation magnification = 10). Each time increment takes about 0.2s. Lifting of the frontal and parietal bones is clearly shown in the right image (deformed skull); an effect commonly observed by osbtetricians and reported in [5].

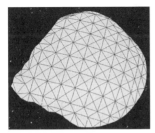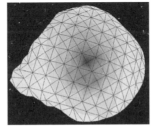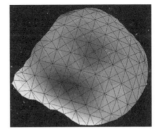

**Figure 4.** Explicit dynamic analysis of the parietal bone (complexity of 280 elements) when subjected to a forceps contact pressure of 0.027MPa and an extraction force of 15.33N in the upwards direction. Shown are contours of three timesteps showing increasing deformation throughout time (darker patches indicating larger deformations). Time increments take about 0.05s.

model of the fetal skull (complexity of about 3,000 triangular elements) was subjected to an equivalent contact pressure of a typical forceps intervention [9] of the order of 200mmHg (0.027MPa). Furthermore, the scoop motion, yields a force of 15.33N in the positive y-direction. Figure 5 shows the pressure distribution and force on the FE model of the skull. Resulting deformation animation of the fetal skull is shown in Figure 3 after FE analysis (assuming non-linear geometry) was performed using the ABAQUS FE software. This analysis took an average of 0.2s for each time increment.

In experiment 2, we tested explicit dynamic analysis. After several trials, and only when the model was simplified to calculating the deformation of parietal bones only, near real-time performance was achieved. Figure 4 shows the dynamic deformation after the same pressure/load distribution was applied as in the previous experiment. Update frequencies were around 20Hz (0.05s per time step).

## 5. Discussion

Currently a number of different analyses are at our disposal, each of which display either enhanced realism though usually at cost of real-time performance or vice-versa. Ignoring mass and damping effects (quasi-static analysis), the analysis type used in the first experiment (entire skull model), yields an update rate of 5Hz. This is not real-time

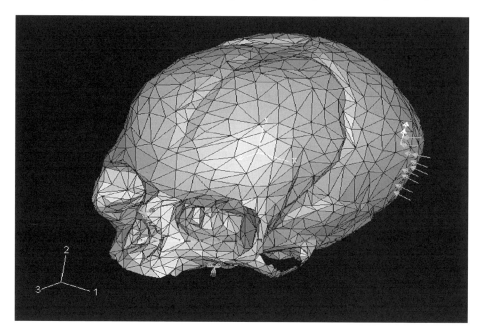

**Figure 5.** The image shows the fetal skull model (complexity of around 3,000 elements) with displayed contact pressure and upwards force (positive y-direction) to 'scoop' the baby out (arrows on left hand side).

performance though adaptive remeshing may improve this performance by reducing the complexity of the mesh where curvature is low (e.g. the skull base). Dynamic analysis (including the mass and damping matrices as shown in equation 1) is far too slow using implicit analysis and even when using explicit analysis still takes several seconds for the entire skull model with complexity of 3,000 elements. Explicit analysis was conducted in the second experiment on a simplified parietal bone model (complexity of 280 elements) which yielded results in update steps of 0.05s (20Hz). Employing such a model does ignore the fontanelle and suture structures which are crucial to realistic behaviour of the deformation of the fetal head. Opting for linear geometry analysis as opposed to non-linear geometry results in significant speed-ups (factor 5-6) but again at cost of realism and absence of incremental updates. Another problem is that mesh simplification of the fetal skull is limited as triangles need to be small to correctly capture the fontanelle and suture structures which are of the order of magnitude of millimeters. A way around this is to use adaptive remeshing though limitations do exist to the extent by which one can create triangles which differ significantly in size.

## 6. Conclusion

The implementation of a real-time mechanical contact model for obstetric forceps delivery simulation has been investigated. Collision detection between forceps and fetal head can be performed quickly using the hierarchical model as described in section 3. Collision response in the form of a mechanical surface-to-surface FE contact model poses problems when realism to the extent of accurate fetal head deformation is required. The off-line analysis, as described in this paper shows that real-time dynamic analysis is only possible on simplified structures such as the skull bones (experiment 2). Inclusion of the fontanelles and structures requires a quasi-static analysis, ignoring mass and damping effects.

The final step to provide a complete simulation to train junior obstetricians and other health professionals in the use of obstetric forceps will include the coupling of the fastest models, as described previously, to a haptic feedback device. The device of choice is the multi-purpose TELLURIS haptic feedback device [3], with a maximum force tolerance of over 200N. A further requirement is the development of an articulated interface to the feedback device, which provides the necessary degrees of freedom to simulate the traction, scoop and twist manipulations, typical for the use of obstetric forceps.

## Acknowledgments

Thanks to Mr. Tim Draycott from the Southmead Hospital in Bristol, UK for his expert advise on operating the obstetric forceps. Also thanks to Dr. Jing Deng from the Department of Medical Physics and Bio-engineering at University College London to provide the MR data of the fetus model.

## References

[1] B. Geiger. *Three-dimensional modeling of human organs and its application to diagnosis and surgical planning.* PhD thesis, Ecole des Mines de Paris, April 1993.

[2] R.J. Lapeer, M.S. Chen, and J. Villagrana. Simulating obstetric forceps delivery in an augmented environment. In *Proceedings of AMI-ARCS 2004, MICCAI Satellite Workshop*, pages 1–10, September 2004.

[3] R.J. Lapeer, P. Gasson, J-L Florens, S. Laycock, and V. Karri. Introducing a novel haptic interface for the planning and simulation of open surgery. In *in Medicine Meets Virtual Reality - MMVR12*, pages 197–199, 2003.

[4] R.J. Lapeer and R.W. Prager. Finite element model of a fetal skull subjected to labour forces. In *Medical Image Computing and Computer-Assisted Intervention - MICCAI'99*, volume 1679 of *Lecture Notes in Computer Science*, pages 1143–1155. Springer, September 1999.

[5] R.J. Lapeer and R.W. Prager. Fetal head moulding: finite element analysis of a fetal skull subjected to uterine pressures during the first stage of labour. *Journal of Biomechanics*, 34(9):1125–1133, 2001.

[6] R.J. Lapeer, R.S. Rowland, and M.S. Chen. PC-based volume rendering for medical visualisation and augmented reality based surgical navigation. In *MediViz 2004 Conference proceedings*, pages 67–72. IEEE Computer Society Press, July 2004.

[7] R.J.A. Lapeer. *A Biomechanical Model of Foetal Head Moulding.* PhD thesis, University of Cambridge - Department of Engineering, August 1999.

[8] G.K. McPherson and T.J. Kriewall. Fetal head molding : An investigation utilizing a finite element model of the fetal parietal bone. *J. Biomechanics*, 13(1):17–26, 1980.

[9] A.S. Moolgaoker. A Comparison of Different Methods of Instrumental Delivery Based on Electronic Measurements of Compression and Traction. *Obstetrics & Gynecology*, 54(3):299–309, 1979.

[10] T. Sielhorst, T. Obst, R. Burgkart, R. Riener, and N. Navab. An augmented reality delivery simulator for medical training. In *Proceedings of AMI-ARCS 2004, MICCAI Satellite Workshop*, pages 11–20, September 2004.

[11] J.G. Villagrana. Designing a 3D interface to simulate obstetric forceps. Master's thesis, School of Computing Sciences, University of East Anglia, 2003.

[12] A. Wischnik, E. Nalepa, K.J. Lehmann, K.U. Wentz, M. Georgi, and F. Melchert. Zur prävention des menschlichen geburtstraumas I. mitteilung: Die computergestützte simulation des geburtsvorganges mit hilfe der kernspintomographie und der finiten-element-analyse. *Geburtshilfe und Frauenheilkunde*, 53(1):35–41, 1993.

*Medicine Meets Virtual Reality 13*
*James D. Westwood et al. (Eds.)*
*IOS Press, 2005*

# Instant Electronic Patient Data Input During Emergency Response in Major Disaster Setting: Report on the Use of a Rugged Wearable (Handheld) Device and the Concept of Information Flow throughout the Deployment of the Disaster Response upon Hospital Admission

Christophe LAURENT M.D. [a] and Luc BEAUCOURT M.D. [b]

[a] *Monica General Hospital, Antwerp, Belgium*
[b] *University Hospital Antwerp (UZA), Antwerp, Belgium*
*e-mail: spoedman@skynet.be; Luc.Beaucourt@uza.be*

**Abstract.** A hard- and software solution has been conceived, realized, produced and used to gather clinical information about disaster victims in the field in such a way that it makes the different efforts made by mass casualty incident management managers and first responders work more efficient, ergonomic, safe and useful for further scientific and statistic analysis.

## 1. Problem

### 1.1. Introduction

Throughout the world, METTAG cards [1] are used to identify and document the state of patients in the field at smaller or major disaster events. This is an almost universally used method, which has proven to be valuable and efficient.

There are, however a number of inconveniencies, which nowadays, making use of state of the art technology [2], can be overcome. It is e.g. very hard to write on a MET-TAG card in the pouring rain. And legibility further on is still depending on the handwriting of the author of the card. Also, information is very often not structured on the card.

## 1.2. Convergence of measures

Considering the whole project, a number of factors and elements can be added, so as to augment the value and validity of the first and consecutive appreciations of the victims in the field, and so as to make it possible to use this interface to include the very first assessment of the patient in the clinical pathway of the specific patient.

This creates the possibility of acquiring not only a clear overview of the response event as a whole in retrospect, but also enhances the safety for the patients and the reliability of medical information throughout the entire process, because of the obtained clear traceability. Given the right circumstances, a genuine process control can be obtained and observed during the event itself.

We have developed, used and evaluated a device in Disaster Response Exercise Events.

## 2. Method

### 2.1. Program

Based upon the contents and possibilities of the existing disaster patient "Tags" such as METTAG, and considering the needs for a basic patient survey in the field, a model of minimum medical record has been compiled, built up in a logical order for the physician or paramedic.

The program is coded to be used in any language, as are the results and statistics. (The language is an option in the setup). Accordingly, a suited handheld device approach was chosen and the device was prepared for use in disaster response.

### 2.2. Device

The device is an ergonomic rugged light weight (single-) handheld computer, operating with DOS®. It has a full QUERTY keyboard on a limited space and an 8 line display. A barcode scanner and sticker printer are also built in. The on site printed stickers can be resistant up to 100° C and −40° C.

The use of the device has been streamlined to be as user friendly, efficient, safe and quick as possible. In fact, the use of the device may not slow down any health worker at all, but must increase the quality of the overall effort.

### 2.3. Overview

In short, the patient is assessed and the (basic) data put in the handheld device. A sticker is then printed, which contains the printed version of the information that would normally be *written* on the METTAG card, as well as a 2D and 1D barcode, which also contains some additional data.

## 2.4. "2D Bar Code" Stickers

The stickers, which are weather resistant, are attached not only to the METTAG card, but also to the patient's body. A third sticker is collected by the paramedic, in case the electronic memory of the device or the device itself should be lost or become unusable, as happens in disasters.

The barcodes can, but must not, be read by the dispatching persons, who with their device, according to the information that they have, indicate a destination for the patient (name of the hospital). A change in vital signs or symptoms can also be recorded. Then, a clearly marked second sticker can be added, stating the intended destination in text and in a 2D barcode.

This sticker and code can be read by the transporting ambulance, if they are also equipped with the device, or a similar one.

## 2.5. In the Hospital

Arrived in the hospital or final destination for extended care, the information can either be read from the printed stickers, on the person of the patient, or the barcodes can be scanned to put in the information of the original physical assessment and the additional data available in the Hospital Information Network [3], thus minimizing the administrative effort in the case of mass admission, and simplifying it to the level of a control of the information. Again, the bar code information can, but must not be used.

## 2.6. WiFi / RF

In case the handheld devices are used in a RF or WiFi environment (such as an airport, where we tested our method), the information can be processed right away. (This creates the before unseen possibility for process control in Disaster Response Interventions.) Otherwise, the read outs of the handheld devices can be collected encrypted over the internet post factum.

## 3. Results

- A user friendly method has been developed and tested to record patient data in the field in a quick, reliable and ergonomic way. The resulting information is not limited to the information put in, but permits additional statistics and other resulting information on the event.
- Processing of the data real time (when a RF or WiFi environment is available on location) or after the event permits process control and analysis, as well as appreciation of the quality and efficacy of the response event and the rescue personnel.
- Quality of information means safety of patients and better guaranties for efficient communication during and after the events.
- Efficient information flow of this nature is also beneficiary in a financial way, as it also constitutes a meticulous tracking of administrative and medical events (medication, transport, interventions, . . .)

## 4. Discussion

We know the Digital Age is moving to the battle field quickly, even in civilian environments. We should explore and use the possibilities and know how (as e.g. acquired by the industry) to improve ergonomics, safety, reliability, traceability and quality in patient care, even in the most extreme and harsh conditions. Most certainly in the most extreme and harsh conditions.

## References

[1]  www.mettag.com/mettag/.
[2]  Laurent, C. The Wireless and Paperless E.R.: an Economical and Ergonomic Approach. *Medicine Meets Virtual Reality 11*, p.181-183, J.D. Westwood et al. (ed.) IOS Press, 2003.
[3]  Laurent, C. A New Form of Application Service Provider (ASP) in the Development of Data Systems and Data Flow and Management of Data in (Multiple Campus) Health Care Instutions. *Medicine Meets Virtual Reality 12*, p.200-202, James D. Westwood et al. (ed.) IOS Press, 2004.

*Medicine Meets Virtual Reality 13*
*James D. Westwood et al. (Eds.)*
*IOS Press, 2005*

# Remote Console for Virtual Telerehabilitation

Jeffrey A. LEWIS [a,b], Rares F. BOIAN [b],
Grigore BURDEA [b] and Judith E. DEUTSCH [a]

[a] *RIVERS Lab, Program in Physical Therapy, UMDNJ*
*e-mail: lewisje@umdnj.edu*
[b] *VR LAB, CAIP Center, Rutgers University*

**Abstract.** The Remote Console (ReCon) telerehabilitation system provides a platform for therapists to guide rehabilitation sessions from a remote location. The ReCon system integrates real-time graphics, audio/video communication, private therapist chat, post-test data graphs, extendable patient and exercise performance monitoring, exercise pre-configuration and modification under a single application. These tools give therapists the ability to conduct training, monitoring/assessment, and therapeutic intervention remotely and in real-time.

## 1. Introduction

The priorities of a successful telerehabilitation system are training and counseling, monitoring and assessment, and therapeutic intervention [1] from a distance. Telerehabilitation implementations are currently being developed, providing different remote capabilities. The first Virtual Reality-based telerehabilitation system was developed by our group, in collaboration with Stanford university. It was intended for the training of musculo-skeletal patients [2] and used a server-client architecture with asynchronous patient data uploading, and an Internet video link. Subsequently researchers at the University of California – Irvine developed Java Therapy [3], in which therapists prescribe a set of exercises via the web. These exercises can then be accessed and executed by the patient through a web browser. Therapists may monitor the patient's performance on the web page and asynchronously modify the therapy, however, there is no real-time interaction or training. Another telerehabilitation application [4] uses a video conferencing link (VC) with commercial video-capture software, to provide audio/visual communication between the patient and the therapist. The same exercise environment is displayed at each site to allow for real-time monitoring and assessment. Data transfer is hindered by the fixed speed requirements of the VC link, forcing this application to reduce the rate at which remote updates are made.

Our first telerehabilitation application for the lower extremity was a real-time web based remote monitor [5], which coupled 3rd party audio and visual communication with real-time patient data, performance gauges, and simplified 3D graphics updated in real time based on the patient's exercise simulation. This monitoring system was subsequently tested for ease of use by five physical therapists [6]. While feedback was gen-

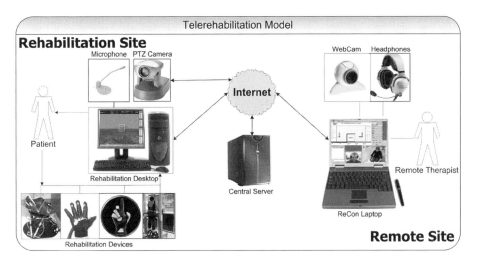

**Figure 1.** Telerehabilitation Model using the ReCon.

erally positive, the subjects raised several issues on the quality of audio communication, and the therapist's inability to make modifications of exercise parameters remotely. In response to these limitations, we have developed the "Remote Console" (ReCon), a telerehabilitation system described in this paper.

## 2. Telerehabilitation System Description

The ReCon was designed for both upper and lower extremities, as illustrated in Figure 1. The patient interacts with VR-based therapeutic exercises using custom interfaces (the Rutgers Master glove for the UE and the Rutgers Ankle and Rutgers Mega Ankle for the LE). The simulation exercises are presented to patients on one PC display, while a Pan-Tilt-Zoom (PTZ) camera captures their image. Patient video, voice and VR exercise parameters are transmitted in real-time to a remote therapist over the Internet. This information is then accessed from a PC, in this example a laptop, using the ReCon.

A remote therapist may start the ReCon application from either a desktop icon or a web link. This prompts Java Web Start to download the latest package of the application as well as the appropriate Java version. On startup, it will initiate a connection with a central server that communicates with each ReCon and rehabilitation site. The therapist may then choose to open a communication channel (audio, video, and chat) with one of the active rehabilitation sites running a copy of the media package built into the ReCon. When this connection is established with the rehabilitation site, the chat window indicates that the therapist is connected. The therapist is then able to hear the sounds at the rehabilitation site through headphones, and a small window will pop up to show the therapists face to assist in positioning the camera. In addition, a Logitech QuickCam is used for automatic face-tracking by panning and zooming in on the therapists face as it moves. This face-tracked video is received at the rehabilitation site. By opening a PTZ camera window, the therapist gains control of the camera movement at the rehabilitation site. Preset viewpoints are accessible on the bottom of the PTZ window to automatically position and zoom the camera to a specified location. For the purposes of this study the

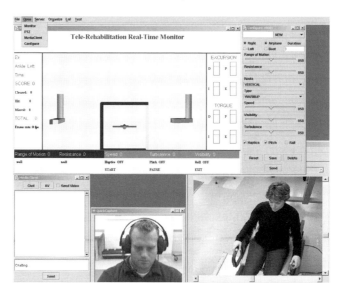

**Figure 2.** ReCon monitoring screen for LE telerehabilitation: plane exercise monitor (top left); ankle exercise configuration utility (top right); chat window (bottom left); therapist monitor (bottom middle); PTZ camera view and controls (bottom right).

PTZ camera views were preset to point to patients' upper body, or to their ankle to watch their movement during an exercise.

The ReCon desktop (shown in detail in Figure 2) incorporates patient simplified 3D exercise graphics, which are updated in real time. The same screen includes numerical exercise performance monitoring, patient video, remote configuration and modification of exercise parameters, and a private therapist chat window. The ReCon allows the therapist to remotely position the PTZ camera and to view post-test data graphs to gauge patient's performance objectively.

The ReCon is implemented using Java [7] with the Java3D API [8] for three-dimensional movement and exercise representations, Java Media Framework (JMF) [9] for audio/video communication, and Java Web Start [10] for deployment and to allow updates to be quickly propagated to users.

In our previous implementation, a remote therapist had to rely on communicating with a local therapist, who was present with the patient, to configure a new exercise or adjust an exercise in progress. The exercise had to be configured before each session by the local therapist. To make a modification, the remote therapist either contacted the local therapist using the microphone, interrupting the patient's exercise, or communicated with the local therapist over a chat mechanism, drawing their attention away from the patient. In both cases, the desired modification to the exercise would take more time than necessary and affected the efficiency of the action and the session as a whole. To remedy this situation, an additional layer of interaction has been added to ReCon, by allowing remote therapists to manipulate a rehabilitation session from their remote location. While monitoring the progress of an exercise, the therapist can create or modify an upcoming exercise using the remote configuration utility. This allows the therapist to select a pre-configured exercise from a pull-down menu. Any individual exercise can be modified or deleted before it is transmitted to the remote patient station. Before the rehabilitation site

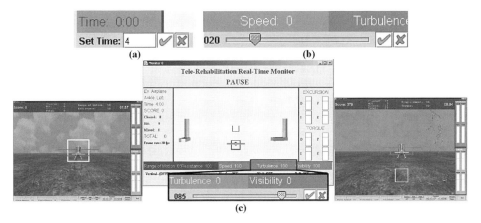

**Figure 3.** Remote real-time exercise parameter setting: a) time; b) airplane speed; c) airplane exercise; remote modification of turbulence; resulting airplane exercise.

starts the next exercise, the therapist may remotely send one of the pre-set configuration lists and start the exercise trial. Several of the simulations contain exercise configurations that can be altered while the exercise is in progress. In addition, a therapist monitoring the session can select one of these modifiable parameters and update the exercise instantly and remotely during run-time. As an example, the therapist may decide that the exercise should be shortened (Figure 3*a*) or the airplane speed should be increased (Figure 3*b*). Once the therapist clicks on the appropriate item, a modify toolbar appears underneath to accept the proper input. For time, the therapist must enter the new duration, for speed, the therapist moves the slider to the desired position and selects the green check mark to accept and transmit the new value to the running exercise. Once the value is changed at the rehabilitation site, the update will appear as the current value on the monitoring window for that exercise. Figure 3*c* shows how the remote therapist can affect an exercise in progress. After the green check mark is selected, the turbulence is increased causing a change in the virtual environment (thunder, lightning and stormy skies) and the addition of haptic perturbations of the Rutgers Ankle platform.

A training session with the RARS starts with a baseline trial where the patient's ankle range of motion and torque capabilities are measured. This stage is followed by a configuration stage where the therapist specifies the upcoming exercise parameters. Once this stage is complete the exercise is loaded on the patient's station and the exercise may begin. When monitoring a patient remotely, the therapist is involved with every step. The therapist may monitor the baseline values and instruct the remote patient in the proper ankle movements to record the data. Once therapists are satisfied with the results, they may open the configuration screen and load a configuration that was pre-set and saved. Alternatively, the local therapist may set the exercise configurations and the remote therapist may interactively make modifications to what is set. The remote therapist may then choose to start the simulation on the patient's station by selecting the "START" button on the patient monitor. During the exercise, as described above, the therapist may make any of the desired modifications, but may also pause or exit the exercise and move on to another trial. This allows the remote therapist the freedom to manipulate the exercise routines without interfering with the flow of the session..

## 3. Initial Experimental Results

During Summer 2004 the ReCon system underwent pilot clinical testing as part of a training protocol with individuals in the chronic phase post-stroke. During the first three weeks of the study, the therapist and a therapist assistant were onsite with the patient. Telerehabilitation was introduced during the last week of the four-week training regimen. The remote therapist conducted three telerehabilitation sessions for each of three subjects participating in the trails. During the remote sessions, the therapist assistant remained with the patient while the therapist interacted from a different room in the same building. This allowed the ReCon to be tested under most favorable conditions (on a single Local Area Network) without being subjected to network delays or poor quality of network service.

The remote therapist, who is considered an expert domain user, had pilot tested the original version of the tele-monitoring system in a study conducted using the same design [5]. Therefore she was able to compare the current version of the system with its earlier prototype. The improvements noted by the therapists were a decrease in communication lag (although some audio communication challenges remained), the ability to pre-configure exercises and save them, and the ability to configure and monitor exercises from the remote station. The domain expert user reported that the ReCon was much easier to use and certainly more useful than the earlier version of the software.

After the remote rehabilitation sessions, each subject was asked to fill out a questionnaire, which made several statements about the system and the interaction with the remote therapist. For each statement they rated their agreement on a scale of 1, "Strongly Disagree," to 7, "Strongly Agree". After the first session, two subjects partially agreed (5) with the statement "I felt something was missing because the therapist could not see me in person". After two complete sessions, the two subjects disagreed with this statement (2), while a third subject strongly disagreed with this statement from the first session (1). Several statements regarding their video interaction indicated that the subjects were comfortable being on camera and were not concerned that others may be watching or listening in during the session. In response to "I would feel more comfortable seeing the therapist in a face-to-face session," the responses ranged from indifferent to partial agreement (4-5). In general the patients felt that the therapist did not miss too much information from being out of the room and they still received the same advice that they would have if the therapist were in the room. Another section of the questionnaire asked the patient to order different scenarios of patient-therapist interaction during a rehabilitation session. One individual ranked "Performing exercises at home with therapist available by video connection" as most desirable. Each of the other subjects consistently chose "Performing exercises in the clinic with therapist in room" followed by "Performing exercises in the clinic with therapist available by video". While some of the subjects would prefer to have the therapist in the room, they did not object to telerehabilitation as an alternative.

## 4. Conclusions and Future Work

The Remote Console was intended to provide a larger set of telerehabilitation tools under a single application to minimize the challenges of the telerehabilitation platform. Fur-

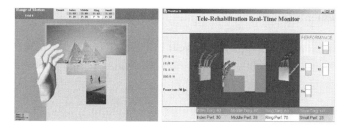

**Figure 4.** Exercise and the respective monitor displays for the upper extremity.

ther, this system incorporates therapeutic intervention by allowing a therapist to remotely access performance measures and make exercise modifications in real-time.

Patient and provider acceptance of telemedicine is integral to the future success of related technologies [11]. For this reason, we captured patient and therapist responses after using the ReCon system to remotely interact with training. After three weeks of training with the therapist and therapist assistant present, two of the patients agreed that they would prefer to have a session in a clinic with the therapist still present, while a third would have preferred to exercise at home with the therapist present only through video. Though some subjects would prefer a face-face sessions, in general, the patients did not oppose the telerehabilitation sessions and felt that the therapist was able to actively follow a session. Under our testing conditions, the subjects became comfortable with the routine of having the remote therapist training the subjects face-to-face for the first three weeks. In addition the therapist assistant was present for all four weeks, making the telerehabilitation sessions we conducted more closely resemble a clinical telerehabilitation environment than a home telerehabilitation setup. To accurately test patient acceptance, the involvement of the remote therapist in face-to-face sessions will have to be varied to determine levels of comfort with a remote provider.

The previous version of our monitoring software was only able to present data from an airplane and boat simulation for the Rutgers Ankle Rehabilitation System (RARS). The ReCon monitor package is structured to be extendable by adding new modules. Currently, the system has been extended to connect to simulations for hand exercises, using a Cyberglove and/or Rutgers Master II Haptic Glove (RMII) [12], and simulations for the Mobility Simulator currently under development [13]. For each of these simulations, the remote monitor displays a three-dimensional representation of the exercise simulation and several angles of the body part being exercised in the center of the screen, using the Java3D API. Exercise configurations, patient data, and performance gauges are shown along the sides and bottom (Figure 4). Multiplexed telerehabilitation is potentially achieved by initiating multiple monitoring windows to interact with several remote patients, each performing different exercises. Multiple monitors could be opened during the same ReCon session and may access multiple rehabilitation sites.

The development of a complete telerehabilitation system is an iterative process that will continue to require feedback from both patients and providers. A usability study will be conducted with practicing physical therapists to gain a broader sense of the ease-of-use and acceptance of ReCon. Improvements will be made to reflect the input from these therapists. The current framework that allows commands to be passed to the rehabilitation site will be extended to provide greater flexibility to the therapist.

## Acknowledgements

Research reported here was supported in part by the NSF Grant BES-0201687.

## References

[1] Rosen MJ. Telerehabilitation. Neurorehabilitation, 3:3–18, 1999.
[2] Popescu, V., G. Burdea, M. Bouzit, M. Girone, and V. Hentz, "PC-Based Telerehabilitation System With Force Feedback," *Proceedings of Medicine Meets Virtual Reality (7) Conference*, "The Convergence of Physical & Informational Technologies: Options for a New Era in Healthcare," IOS Press, Amsterdam, Vol. 62, pp. 262-267, 1999.
[3] Reinkensmeyer DJ, Pang CT, Nessler CA, Painter CC. Web-based telerehabilitation for the upper-extremity after stroke, IEEE Transactions on Neural Science and Rehabilitation Engineering, vol. 10, no. 2, 2002, pp. 102-108.
[4] Holden MK, Dyar T, Schwamm L, Bizzi E. Home based telerehabilitation using a virtual environment system. Proc. Second Int. Workshop on Virtual Rehabilitation, pp. 4-12, September 2003.
[5] Lewis JA, Boian RF, Burdea GC, Deutsch JE. "Real-time Web-based Telerehabilitation Monitoring, Proceeding of Medicine Meets Virtual Reality 11, Newport Beach, CA, January 2003, IOS Press, pp. 190-192.
[6] Deutsch JE, Lewis JA, Whitworth E, Boian RF, Burdea G, Tremaine M. Formative Evaluation and Preliminary Findings of a Virtual Reality Telerehabilitation System for the Lower Extremity, (In press) Presence Special Issue on Virtual Rehabilitation 2005.
[7] SUN Microsystems, Java API Specification for the Java 2 Platform, Standard Edition, v1.4.2, 2003.
[8] SUN Microsystems, The Java3D API Specification, Java3D v1.3.1, 2001.
[9] SUN Microsystems, The Java Media Framework API Guide, JMF v2.1.1e, 1999.
[10] SUN Microsystems, Java Web Start Guide, v1.5 2004.
[11] Collins K, Nicolson P, Bowns I. Patient satisfaction in telemedicine. Health Informatics Journal, pages 81–85, Feb 2000.
[12] Adamovich SV, et al. A Virtual Reality Based Exercise System for Hand Rehabilitation Post-Stroke, (In press) Presence, Special Issue on Virtual Rehabilitation 2005.
[13] Boian RF, Burdea GC, Deutsch JE, Winter SH. Street Crossing Using a Virtual Environment Mobility Simulator, *Proceedings of IWVR 2004*, pp. 27-33, September 2004.

*Medicine Meets Virtual Reality 13*
*James D. Westwood et al. (Eds.)*
*IOS Press, 2005*

# Improved Virtual Surgical Cutting Based on Physical Experiments

Yi-Je LIM [a], Daniel B. JONES [b] and Suvranu DE [a]

[a] *Department of Mechanical, Aerospace and Nuclear Engineering,*
*Rensselaer Polytechnic Institute, Troy, NY 12180*
[b] *Department of Surgery, Beth Israel Deaconess Medical Center, Boston, MA 02215*

**Abstract.** Simulation of surgical cutting is one of the most challenging tasks in the development of a surgery simulator. Changes in topology during simulation make any precomputed data meaningless. Moreover, the process is nonlinear and given the complexity of soft tissue mechanics, the underlying physics is not well understood. Therefore, fully realistic procedures for the simulation of surgical cutting at real time rates on single processor machines is possibly out of reach. We developed a geometry-based algorithm that is capable of simulating progressive cutting without increasing the number of primitives and have coupled it to a mesh-free physically based simulation scheme. In this paper we enhance a geometrically efficient cutting algorithm by including physical information from actual cutting experiments.

## 1. Introduction

Problems in conventional medical training have led to the development of powerful multimodal virtual surgical systems. One of the major advantages of virtual digital surgery systems is that they are more efficient than training on real patients, and eliminate the risks associated with learning a new skill. These systems can be used to objectively evaluate and measure technical competence and they are less expensive and less offensive than training on animal models. However, the complexities of developing efficient *physics-based* tool-tissue interaction algorithms that perform in *real time* have impeded the development of realistic surgery simulators that transcend the level of sophisticated computer games.

Modeling and simulation of surgical cutting is one of the most challenging tasks in the development of a surgery simulator. The process of cutting process is inherently nonlinear and given the complexity of soft tissue biomechanics, the underlying physics is far from being well understood. Therefore, fully realistic procedures for the simulation of surgical cutting at real time rates are possibly out of reach.

Mass-spring models [1,2] do not capture the underlying physics accurately and an elaborate curve-fitting process is usually required to obtain the hundreds and thousands of parameters for the individual springs and masses. The mesh-based finite elements models [3] necessitate an expensive remeshing operation after cutting and thus require nonphysical simplifications such as element removal. In our previous work [4] we presented an efficient geometry-based algorithm coupled with a physically-based numerical scheme using a ***meshfree approach*** for the simulation of surgical cutting procedure in multimodal virtual environments. Progressive cutting, without the generation of new primitives, is achieved by snapping the nearest nodes to the interaction point between the cutting tool and the underlying polygon edge. The meshfree method is used to compute the deformation fields and interaction forces.

Recently, tissue modeling has become an important research area for surgical simulation and robot-assisted surgery in order to improve realism and performance. Some authors have concentrated attention to modeling soft tissue cutting. Bielser and Gross [5] proposed a mechanical scalpel model which accounts for the interaction forces, both external and internal, between the scalpel and the tissue. They distinguish between two different forces: static and dynamic cut friction force. As long as the force applied to the scalpel is smaller then a threshold value, the scalpel will not penetrate the tissue and this is assumed to be due to the static cut friction force. If the magnitude of force exceeds the threshold, the scalpel starts to cut and the dynamic cut friction force affects this motion of the scalpel.

Mahvash and Hayward [6] introduced an energy approach inspired from fracture mechanics to evaluate the tool force given tool displacement. They observed that a deformation regime starts with a collision between the scalpel blade and the sample. The rupture occurs almost instantaneously as the release of elastic energy creates a crack. The process then switches to cutting where the work performed by the scalpel blade separates the sample. Force feedback devices have been used to display external cutting forces on a blade in surgical simulations. Recently, Chanthasopeephan et al. [7] modeled the mechanical response of pig liver during cutting. They observed the cutting process consists of a sequence of intermittent localized fracture. Cutting with scissors has been modeled by Greenish et al. [8] and Okamura et al. [9]. They collected scissors cutting data for biological tissues and tried to reproduce force profiles using haptic scissors.

For purposes of our cutting simulation, we realized the need for more realistic soft tissue behavior during cutting. In this paper we enhance a geometrically efficient cutting algorithm by including physical information from actual cutting experiments. The rest of this paper is structured as follow: in section 2 we present the experimental setup for the cutting test. In section 3 we describe the experimental results and explain the implementation from the measured data in section 4.

## 2. Experiment Setup

We have modified a Phantom Premium1.0 (Sensable Technologies) haptic interface device to perform surgical incision and cutting experiments. This device is used to deliver precise displacement stimuli and is fitted with a six-axis force sensor from ATI Industrial Automation (Nano 17) to measure reaction forces. The Phantom has a nominal position resolution of 0.03 mm, a maximum force of 8.5 N and 1 kHz sampling rate. The transducer has a force resolution of 0.781 mN along each of the three orthogonal axes and connected to a 16-bit A/D converter having a high speed sampling rate up to 7800 Hz. Blade tips are fitted to the end of the Phantom with the force transducer mounted in-between to accurately sense the reaction forces (see Figure 1).

In order to measure the cut opening distance of the soft tissue during the cutting experiments, we use a videomicroscopy system together with a high precision stimulator.

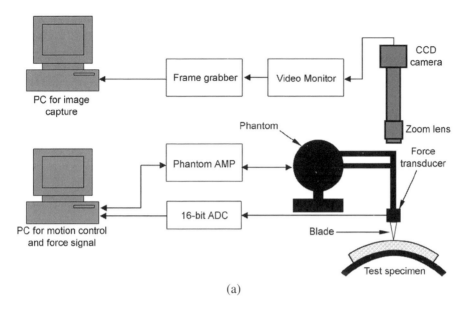

(a)

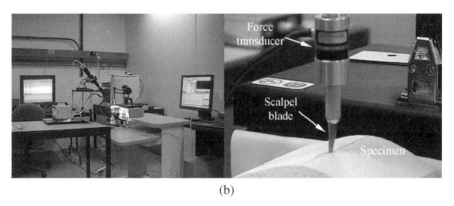

(b)

**Figure 1.** Experiment setup. (a) Schematic diagram for cutting experiments and (b) an actual experimental setup.

The videomicroscopy system is used to capture the image sequences of the soft tissue in real time (30 frames/sec) during experiment. The captured image sequences are stored for cut opening displacement analysis. The system is composed of an optical light source, a zoom lens, a CCD camera (Hitachi HV-D27) offering 800 lines of resolution, a video monitor, and a frame grabber hosted by Pentium IV PC. The zoom lens in front of the CCD camera is utilized to change the magnifications of the images. The image signals are sent to a video monitor (Sharp), through which we can observe the motion of the soft tissue in real time. The signals are then sent to the PC through a DC1000 Pinnacle video editing system. In our preliminary experiments, the specimens are attached to test plates with various radii of curvature to induce different conditions of pre-tension. It is worth mentioning that we have designed the experimental system to minimize the effect of links and flexibility.

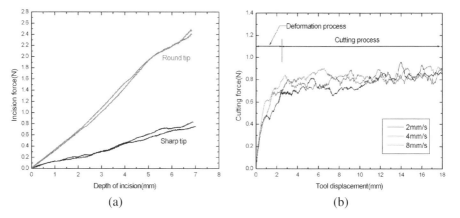

**Figure 2.** Incision and cutting force. (a) Incision force as a function of depth of incision for two different types of blades (shape and round tip) at 2 mm/s velocity. (b) Cutting force with constant velocity (2, 4, 8 mm/s).

## 3. Experimental results

In the incision and cutting tests that we describe below, abdominal pads from Limbs and Things [10] have been used as the specimen. Results on actual tissue samples will be presented at the conference.

### 3.1. Incision experiments

In the incision experiments the blade was driven into the specimen normally with velocities of 1–8 mm/s up to a depth of 7 mm and the corresponding forces required to penetrate the specimen were recorded.

The general response that we have obtained from incision tests with abdominal pad is illustrated by Figure 2a. Two different types of blades were used. The incision force is seen to increase linearly with the depth of incision without a distinct initial deformation before rupture.

### 3.2. Cutting experiments

During the cutting experiments, the specimen was cut with various velocities (1–8 mm/s), initial depths of cut, and angles of the blade. The cutting force for different lengths of cut (5–20 mm) as well as the maximum opening of the cut was recorded.

In our preliminary results using abdominal pads, we have observed that the cutting operation is essentially a two-step process. The specimen initially deforms under the action of the load applied to the blade. Rupture of the specimen occurs after some critical load is reached. Thereafter, the cutting force remains reasonably constant as the blade is translated with constant velocity (see Figure 2b). The cutting force measured is essentially invariant with the tool velocity. This is a key observation that we use in section 4 to simplify our computational process

The cut opening displacement (COD) is another important parameter that we have measured during the experiments. This is defined as the maximum opening of the cut at the midpoint (see Figure 3). Figure 4 shows that the COD is a strong function of the depth of cut, the length of cut and the pre-stress in the specimen.

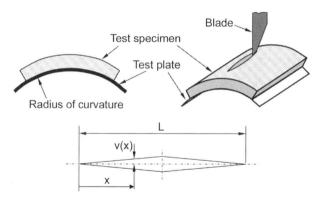

**Figure 3.** Cut opening displacement (COD) defined as the maximum opening of the cut at the midpoint, COD=2v(x=L/2).

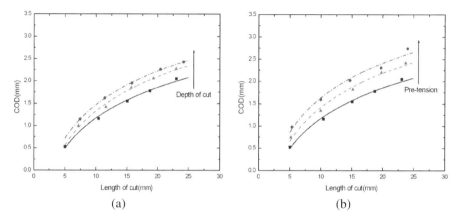

**Figure 4.** Cut opening displacement (COD) corresponding to (a) the depth of cut and (b) the pre-stress.

## 4. Implementation

We have enhanced our simulation by incorporating the information noted in section 3.2. The experimental observations have vastly simplified the simulation procedure.

The force to rupture is obtained from experiments. The physically-based meshfree method [11] is used to compute the deformation fields and reaction forces at the tool tip. When the tool tip reaction force crosses the experimentally determined threshold, rupture is assumed to have occurred. While cutting is in progress, the force on the tool tip is maintained at the value corresponding to rupture. In a practical implementation, the cutting force is calculated by subtracting the friction force determined by a second empty cut on the same spot from the total measured force. The opening of the cut is obtained from the COD measured during the experiments, which is then mapped onto the progressing cut.

In Figure 5 we present examples of our surgical cutting simulation. Figure 5a shows the cutting of a 3D inner abdominal wall while Figure 5b shows a liver model, obtained from the segmented Visible Human data set.

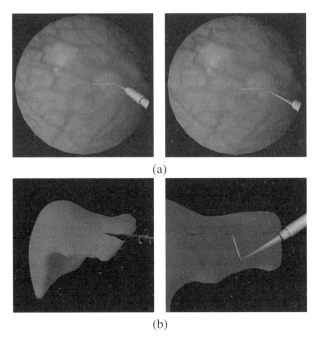

**Figure 5.** Screen shots of surgical cutting simulation of an inner abdominal wall (a) and a liver model (b).

## 5. Conclusion and future work

Accurate modeling of the physics that governs the process of cutting soft biological tissues is complex and its simulation in real time is difficult. In this paper we develop physical experimental techniques whose results are used to enhance an efficient progressive cutting algorithm using nodes snapping that we have developed earlier.

While the experiments presented in this paper have been limited to abdominal pads, results on actual soft tissues will be presented at the conference. As part of our future work we will observe and model the interactions of specific surgical blades as functions of factors such as blade type, edge sharpness, cutting depth and initial configuration of soft tissue.

## Acknowledgements

The authors would like to thank Professor X. George Xu of RPI for making available to us segmented models of the Visible Human Project and to Dr. M.A. Srinivasan of Touch Lab, MIT for loaning us the force transducer and some of the control programs. Funding has been provided by a grant from the National Institutes of Health (R21 EB003547-01).

## References

[1]  A. Mor and T. Kanade, "Modifying Soft Tissue Models: Progressive Cutting with Minimal New Element Creation", *Proceedings of MICCAI*, Vol. 1935, 2000.

[2]  C. Bruyns and K. Montgomery, "Generalized Interactions Using Virtual Tools Within the Spring Framework: Cutting", *Proceedings of MMVR 2001 Conference.*

[3]  D. Serby, M. Harders, and G. Szekely, "A new approach to cutting into finite element models", *Proceedings of MICCAI*, pp.425-433, 2001.

[4]  Y.-J. Lim and S. De, "Realistic Simulation of Surgical Cutting of Soft Tissues in Real Time with Force Feedback", *Proceedings of MMVR 2004 Conference.*

[5]  D. Bielser and M.H. Gross, "Interactive Simulation of Surgical Cuts", *Proceedings of the Eighth Pacific Conference on Computer Graphics and Applications*, China, 2000.

[6]  M. Mahvash and V. Hayward, "Haptic Rendering of Cutting: a Fracture Mechanics Approach", *Haptics-e*, Vol. 2, No. 3, 2001.

[7]  T. Chanthasopeephan, J. P. Desai, and A. Lau, "Measuring Forces in Liver Cutting for Reality-Based Haptic Display", *IEEE/RSJ International Conference on Intelligent Robots and Systems*, Las Vegas, Nevada, 2003.

[8]  S. Greenish, V. Hayward, V. Chial, A. Okamura, and T. Steffen, "Measurement, Analysis and Display of Haptic Signals During Surgical Cutting", *Teleoperators and Virtual Environments*, Vol. 6, No. 11. pp. 626-651, 2002.

[9]  A. Okamura, R. Webster, J. Nolin, K. Johnson, and H. Jafry, "The Haptic Scissors: Cutting in Virtual Environments", *IEEE International Conference on Robotics and Automation*, pp. 828-833, 2003.

[10]  Limbs and Things. Available at http:// www.limbsandthings.com.

[11]  S. De, J. Kim, and M. A. Srinivasan, "A Meshless Numerical Technique for Physically Based Real Time Medical Simulations," *Proceedings of MMVR 2001 Conference.*

308

Medicine Meets Virtual Reality 13
James D. Westwood et al. (Eds.)
IOS Press, 2005

# A Haptic-Enabled Simulator for Cricothyroidotomy

Alan LIU, Yogendra BHASIN and Mark BOWYER

*The Surgical Simulation Laboratory, National Capital Area Medical Simulation Center,*
*Uniformed Services University*
*url: http://simcen.usuhs.mil*

**Abstract.** Cricothyroidotomy is an emergency procedure that is performed when the patient's airway is blocked, and less invasive attempts to clear it have failed. Cricothyroidotomy has been identified as an essential skill for military readiness. This training is relevant to more than 40,000 U.S. military medics, and thousands of civilian health care providers. Current training methods use animals, cadavers and plastic mannequins. Animal models do not have the correct anatomy. Cadavers do not have the correct physiology. Mannequins do not adequately cover the full range of anatomical variations. In this paper, we describe our effort to build a computer-based cricothyroidotomy simulator to address these problems.

## 1. Introduction

Open cricothyroidotomy is an essential skill in emergency airway management. It is the procedure of choice when ventilation cannot be achieved by less invasive methods [1, 2]. This skill has relevance to both military and civilian medical services. For example, cricothyroidotomy is the recommended approach for the management of certain thermal or toxic gas injuries during tactical field care [3]. As another example, cricothyroidotomy may be necessary to secure the airway in gunshot wounds to the face, a situation that can be encountered both during combat and in the civilian emergency room [4,5].

In cricothyroidotomy, an incision is made in the cricothyroid membrane. A tracheostomy tube is introduced through the incision into the trachea. Air flows through the passage created, permitting the patient to breathe. When performed correctly, the procedure is safe. Current teaching methods use animals, cadavers, or mannequins. These methods have disadvantages. Animals do not have the same anatomy as humans, and their use can involve ethical issues. Cadavers cannot produce an appropriate physiological response. Mannequins and Human Patient Simulators have been used to teach cricothyroidotomy with some success [6–8]. The latter can provide some physiological response during simulation. However, they require parts that must be replaced after every exercise. They do not bleed convincingly during simulation, and different mannequins are necessary to represent patients with different injuries, body types, and age groups.

Computer-based surgical simulators using a combination of 3D graphics and haptics can provide an alternative. They can contain accurate representations of human anatomy and physiology. Different patient types can be simulated by loading the appropriate model. More importantly, computer-based simulators can incorporate metrics to measure student performance. Improvements in skill level can be quantified. They also have the potential to incorporate didactic material, and provide real-time feedback on performance. When a mistake is made, students can back up to an earlier stage in the procedure to try again.

In this paper, we describe the ongoing development of a computer-based cricothyroidotomy simulator. A mannequin model is not used. Instead, 3D computer patient models are employed. Haptic and visual feedback is provided using a hand-immersive environment similar to that described in [9]. To date, no comparable computer-based simulator for cricothyroidotomy has been developed.

## 2. Methods

This section describes the system's hardware, the software components, and our implementation of the steps in the cricothyroidotomy algorithm.

### 2.1. Hardware

The system is developed on a hand-immersive platform similar to [9]. A cathode ray tube (CRT) monitor generates a 3D frame-sequential image of the virtual patient. This image is reflected off a front-silvered mirror to the user. The user, wearing a pair of CrystalEyes shutter glasses, perceives a 3D virtual image behind the mirror. A Phantom haptic interface device [10] is positioned such that its working volume is co-registered with the visual space. An individual working in this environment can see and feel virtual objects within the working volume. Hand-eye coordination is preserved. We have chosen this configuration as the most natural interface for open cricothyroidotomy. The interface is driven by a PC with dual Pentium IV Xeon 3.02GHz processors, 2Gb of main memory, and a 3DLabs Wildcat 7110 graphics card. The system is capable of driving the visual display at better than 20 frames/sec. The haptic loop runs at 1KHz.

### 2.2. Software Components

The system was implemented using the ReachIn API [11]. The API manages visual and tactile rendering on the hand-immersive hardware. The API permits software development to focus on developing application specific 3D models and tools, and their interaction. Applications need not be explicitly involved in this aspect, but can override default actions if required. The ReachIn API uses the Virtual Reality Markup Language (VRML) [12] as the basis for its modeling language. Extensions to VRML permit additional properties, such as tissue stiffness, event triggers, and user-defined objects to be defined as nodes and connected to the VRML tree.

In our system, the software components that have been developed include: the graphical user interface, the patient model, and key surgical skill steps. We describe each in turn.

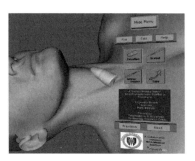
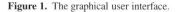
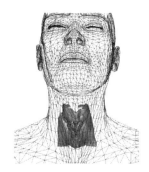

**Figure 1.** The graphical user interface.

**Figure 2.** A virtual patient model used during simulation. The skin is represented by a wire frame to highlight the thyroid model.

### 2.2.1. The Graphical User Interface

Fig. 1 illustrates the graphical user interface (GUI). The user sees a virtual patient lying supine. A palette of possible actions appears to the right. Using the Phantom stylus, the student can select from one of several possible actions, including palpation, performing an incision, widening an existing incision, and intubation. In addition, the GUI incorporates various help modes to assist the student in performing the procedure, For example, the student can toggle skin transparency in order to visually locate and study the thyroid.

### 2.2.2. The Patient Model

Patient models are developed in 3D Studio Max [13] and exported as VRML files. Additional properties, such as tissue stiffness, collision response handling, and tool interaction are incorporated in a post processing step. Since the main area of focus is the region around the thyroid, a detailed thyroid model is included. Fig. 2 illustrates.

### 2.2.3. Skill Steps

The surgical algorithm for cricothyroidotomy involves multiple steps. Each step requires a specific skill or action to be performed. Our system implements each step as a separate module. This permits additional modules to be incorporated as needed. These additioanl steps may represent common variations in performing the procedure, or additional actions that must be performed for patients with unusual injuries. For each module, the surgical instruments used as well as the expected visual and haptic feedback are encoded. Four key steps of the algorithm have been implemented. They are: identification of anatomical landmarks, performing the incision, incision enlargement, and inserting the tracheostomy tube. We describe each in turn.

**Landmark identification:** Locating the cricothyroid membrane is primarily a tactile task. The surgeon first palpates the neck anteriorly to locate the thyroid cartilage, then moves down until the space between the thyroid and cricoid cartilage is identified. The membrane is located in this space. In our system, the virtual patient model facilitates the practice of this skill. Visually, the student sees the skin on the patient's neck. Beneath the neck is a detailed model of the patient's thyroid. The skin, cartilage, and membrane have different mechanical properties. The student interacts with the model using the Phantom. As the student probes the patient's neck, different levels of stiffness are perceived, corresponding to the different cartilage structures. Once the correct location is identified, the student can mark the spot before performing the next action.

**Making the incision:** When an incision is made, the wound opens, the cut bleeds, and resistance is felt as the scalpel passes through skin. In our system, we simulate this using a novel technique described in [14]. Our approach does not require polygon subdivision [15,16]. Visually, animated textures are used to simulate the appearance of the wound opening and bleeding. The model's topology is unchanged. Haptically, a local model is used to simulate the sensation of cutting with a scalpel. For small, straight-line incisions, this can be modeled using two effects: reaction force and constrained motion. As the scalpel is pushed into tissue, it exerts a reaction force in the opposite direction. In our system we model this force as a function of scalpel depth, position, and the direction of shortest distance to the skin from the scalpel tip. During the cutting process, tissue surrounds both sides of the scalpel blade. This constrains blade motion in a plane that includes the cut. We model this as a force that is exerted whenever the scalpel drifts from the cut-plane. More details can be found in [14].

**Incision enlargement:** During an emergency cricothyroidotomy, the back of the scalpel blade is often used as an expedient to enlarge the initial incision. We model the visual and haptic effects of this step in a fashion similar to that used during incision. The appearance of the wound widening is accomplished by updating the texture map over the incision with a sequence of images. Haptic feedback is accomplished with a local model that constrains the instrument to penetrate the skin at a single point. Resistance to insertion is modeled by a reaction force, similar to that described previously.

**Intubation:** To simulate the resistance of inserting the tracheostomy tube, a simplified model of the trachea is used to provide haptic response. This model is not rendered visually. The original model could not be used because it contained too much detail for real-time collision detection and response at haptic rates. During intubation, collision with the haptic model was determined at five evenly spaced points along the tube. For each point, if a collision occurred, the reaction force was noted. The resistance on the tube was then taken as the vector sum of reaction forces.

## 3. Results

Our implementation currently permits students to practice the basic skill steps in cricothyroidotomy. In the simulation, the student, wearing CrystalEyes shutter glasses, sees a 3D rendering of a virtual patient. A menu of actions appears beside the patient. The student uses the Phantom haptic interface to interact with the environment. The student selects the appropriate action to be performed. Based on the action selected, the Phantom's stylus is replaced by various surgical instruments. For example, when making an incision, the stylus is replaced by a scalpel. As the student performs the cut, the wound opens and bleeds. The student also receives haptic feedback via the Phantom. The extent of bleeding depends on the depth of the cut. For example, if the student exerts a lot of force and creates a deep cut, the wound bleeds profusely. Figs. 3(a), 3(b), and 3(c) illustrate some other actions being performed.

Preliminary assessments by surgeons familiar with the procedure have been favorable. The evaluators commented favorably on the accuracy of tactile response during palpation, incision, and intubation, as well as the realistic bleeding.

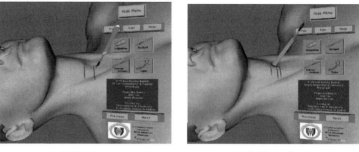

(a) Cutting                    (b) Enlarging

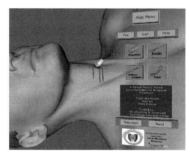

(c) Intubation

**Figure 3.** Skill Steps in the Cricothyroidotomy Simulator.

## 4. Discussion and Conclusion

In this paper, we described our cricothyroidotomy trainer currently under development. Unlike current efforts, our approach uses a hand-immersive display with both visual and tactile feedback. Our system is an improvement, as using virtual models enables students to practice on a wide range of patient types using the same hardware. Technical achievements include the use of animated textures and local haptic models for simulating incisions and instrument insertion [14]. Previous attempts have focused on incorporating the cut in the patient model. In those attempts, polygon subdivision is required, which increases model complexity. Moreover, the resulting polygons are frequently suboptimal in shape. Degradation of visual and haptic rendering performance can result. Our approach does not require polygon subdivision. The model's complexity remains constant, and visual rendering efficiency does not degrade. Using a local haptic model permits haptic feedback to be decoupled from the model's topology, and is computationally efficient.

The system is can be used as a teaching aid in its present state. However, it lacks the ability to independently instruct the student in the procedure, and metrics to measure student performance have not been incorporated. These shortcomings will be addressed in the ongoing development effort.

### Acknowledgments

This work is supported by the U.S. Army Medical Research and Materiel Command under Contract No. DAMD17-03-C-0102. The views, opinions and/or findings contained in this report are those of the author(s) and should not be construed as an official Department of the Army position, policy or decision unless so designated by other documentation.

# References

[1] American College of Surgeons Committee on Trauma. *Advanced Trauma Life Support for Doctors*, chapter Airway and Ventilatory Management, pages 59–72. Chicago: American College of Surgeons, 6th edition, 1997.

[2] Patrick Liston. Emergency awake surgical cricothyroidotomy for severe maxillofacial gunshot wounds. *ADF Health*, 5:22–24, 2004.

[3] The Committee on Tactical Combat Casualty Care. Tactical combat casualty care prehospital care in the tactical environment. Technical Report For Chapter 17: Military Medicine, in The Prehospital Trauma Life Support Manual, Fifth Edition, 21 Feb 2003 Draft, 2003.

[4] Charles W. Perry and Bradley J. Phillips. Gunshot wounds sustained injuries to the face: A university experience. *The Internet Journal of Surgery*, 5(2), 2001.

[5] Kihtir T., Ivatury RR, Simon RJ, Nassoura Z., and Leban S. Early management of civilian gunshot wounds to the face. *Journal of Trauma*, 35(4):569–75, 1994.

[6] Block E.F., Lottenberg L., Flint L., Jakobsen J., and Liebnitzky D. Use of a human patient simulator for the advanced trauma life support course. *Am Surg.*, 68(7):648–51, 2002.

[7] Gilbart M.K., Hutchinson C.R., Cusimano M.D., and Regehr G. A computer-based trauma simulator for teaching trauma management skills. *Am. J. Surg.*, 179(3):223–8, 2000.

[8] Marshall R.L., Smith J.S., Gorman P.J., Krummel T.M., Haluck R.S., and Cooney R.N. Use of a human patient simulator in the development of resident trauma management skills. *Journal of Trauma-Injury, Infection & Critical Care*, 51(1):17–21, 2001.

[9] Stevenson D.R., Smith K.A., McLaughlin J.P., Gunn C.J., Veldkamp J.P., and Dixon M.J. Haptic workbench: A multisensory virtual environment. In *Proc. SPIE: Stereoscopic Displays and Virtual Reality Systems*, volume 3639, pages 356–66, May 1999.

[10] T. Massie and K. Salisbury. The phantom haptic interface: A device for probing virtual objects. *ASME Winter Annual Meeting*, 55(1):295–300, 1994.

[11] http://www.reachin.se.

[12] Ames A.L., Nadeau D.R., Nadeau D.R., and Moreland J.L. *VRML 2.0 Sourcebook*. John Wiley & Sons Inc., 2nd edition, 1996.

[13] http://www.discreet.com.

[14] Bhasin Y., Liu A., and Bowyer M. Simulating surgical incisions without polygon subdivision. In *Medicine Meets Virtual Reality (to appear)*, 2005.

[15] Mor A. and Kanade T. Modifying soft tissue models: Progressive cutting with minimal new element creation. In *Medical Image Computing and Computer-Assisted Intervention - MICCAI 2000.*, volume 1935, pages 598–607. Springer-Verlag, 2000.

[16] Bielser Daniel., Maiwald V.A., and Gross M.H. Interactive cuts through 3-dimensional soft tissue. In *Computer Graphics Forum (Eurographics 99)*, volume 18, pages 31–38. Springer-Verlag, 1999.

*Medicine Meets Virtual Reality 13*
*James D. Westwood et al. (Eds.)*
*IOS Press, 2005*

# The Mini-Screen: An Innovative Device for Computer Assisted Surgery Systems

Benoit MANSOUX [a,b], Laurence NIGAY [a] and Jocelyne TROCCAZ [b]

[a] *CLIPS-IMAG lab., HCI group, University of Grenoble 1, France*
[b] *TIMC-IMAG lab., CAS group, University of Grenoble 1, France*

**Abstract.** In this paper we focus on the design of Computer Assisted Surgery (CAS) systems and more generally Augmented Reality (AR) systems that assist a user in performing a task on a physical object. Digital information or new actions are defined by the AR system to facilitate or to enrich the natural way the user would interact with the real environment. We focus on the outputs of such systems, so that additional digital information is smoothly integrated with the real environment of the user, by considering an innovative device for displaying guidance information: the mini-screen. We first motivate the choice of the mini-screen based on the ergonomic property of perceptual continuity and then present a design space useful to create interaction techniques based on a mini-screen. Two versions of a Computer ASsisted PERicardial (CASPER) puncture application, as well as a computer assisted renal puncture application, developed in our teams, are used to illustrate the discussion.

## 1. Introduction

The main objective of Computer Assisted Surgery (CAS) systems is to help a surgeon in defining and executing an optimal surgical strategy based on a variety of multi-modal data inputs. The key point of a CAS system is to "augment" the physical world of the surgeon: the operating theater, the patient, the surgical tools etc., by providing pre-operative information during the surgery. CAS systems are now entering many surgical specialties and such systems can take on the most varied forms. Although many CAS systems have been developed and provide real clinical improvements, their design is ad-hoc and principally driven by technologies.

In this context and as part of a multidisciplinary project that involves the (Human-Computer Interaction) HCI and the CAS research groups of the University of Grenoble, our research aims at providing elements useful for the design of usable CAS systems by focusing on the interaction between the user and the CAS system. In this paper we concentrate on interaction techniques based on a LCD mini-screen as an innovative device for displaying guidance information. In the next section, we motivate our work by presenting the existing solutions and the ergonomic issue they raise. We then present our approach based on the mini-screen: we describe a design space useful to create interaction techniques based on a mini-screen. In the final section, we present our first results drawn from our design space, namely the developed interaction techniques based on the mini-screen.

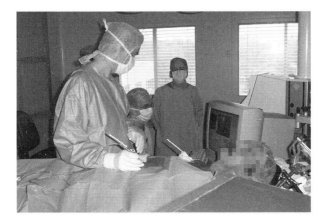

**Figure 1.** Our CASPER application in use.

## 2. Ergonomic Problem: Perceptual Discontinuity

In CAS systems, Augmented Reality (AR) interaction techniques are based on the fusion of two worlds: the digital world (e.g., MRI, scan images, computed trajectory) and the real world (e.g., the patient's body, a needle). However, there is no consensus on a definition of AR techniques highlighting the problem of delimitating the frontier between the two worlds [2,7]. As we defined in [2], the adapters are devices in charge of the fusion between the two worlds. We distinguish input adapters (inputs to the system) from output adapters (outputs from the system). The input adapters, such as an electro-magnetic localizer or a video camera, capture information from the real world that is transferred to the computing system, while the output adapters, such as a projector or a Head Mounted Display (HMD), convey information from the digital world to the real world. The results of the fusion thanks to the output adapters are either perceived in the digital world (e.g., a 3D brain model and a video of a patient merged on a screen [5]) or in the real one (e.g., a 3D model projected onto the patient's body [1,4]). For example, using CASPER, a computer-assisted pericardial puncture application, the surgeon must look at the screen to get the guidance information, as shown in Figure 1.

CASPER assists the surgeon by providing in real time the position of the puncture needle according to the planned strategy. On screen, the current position and orientation of the physical needle are represented by two mobile crosses, while a stationary cross represents the planned trajectory. When the three crosses are superimposed the executed trajectory corresponds to the planned one. A graphic gauge translates the current depth of the performed trajectory according to the pre-planned one. Ergonomic evaluations of CASPER highlighted that the required shift between looking at the graphics on screen (i.e., the crosses and the gauge) and looking at the operating field (i.e., the patient and the needle) was disturbing to the surgeon. Indeed keeping the trajectory aligned and controlling the depth of the needle by referring to the visual display was found difficult to do. The interactive system does not respect the ergonomic property of perceptual continuity. In [2] we define the perceptual continuity by having no perceptual gap between the real and the digital worlds: the user can perceive all the relevant information for her/his task within the same perceptual environment (e.g., the same visual environment).

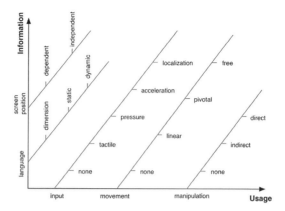

**Figure 2.** Our mini-screen design space: A 2-D space to characterize interaction techniques based on a mini-screen.

To address this problem we developed a new version of CASPER using a different output adapter: a see-through Head Mounted Display (HMD). The see-through HMD eliminates the problem of perceptual/visual discontinuity: the surgeon can see the operating field (i.e., patient and needle) through the HMD as well as the guidance data in the same location. The fusion of the digital and real worlds is then perceivable in the real world and the needle is no longer represented: only the planned trajectory as well as the depth control are displayed on the HMD. But display latency problems that can only be resolved by technical improvements as well as the HMD weight on the surgeon's head led us to set aside that second version.

## 3. Solution and Method

Different strategies for designing AR interaction techniques are defined in [6]. The target of augmentation can be the user (i.e., the surgeon), the environment (i.e., the operating theater) or the physical objects (i.e., the needle). Having already explored the possibility of augmenting the user (HMD), our solution consists of augmenting the environment or the needle. In this context, several possibilities for presenting the information from the system to the surgeon exist: some studies explore the usage of non-visual interaction techniques such as touch [9] or sound, while others explore the combination of such techniques (output multimodal interfaces). Our work focuses on visual information. Instead of techniques based on a projector such as in [1], we use mini-screens in order to augment the operating field or the needle with display capabilities.

While a mini-screen is an innovative interaction device for CAS systems, such a small device is being increasingly studied in the HCI domain and leads to the definition of new interaction paradigms like the Embodied User Interfaces defined in [3]. From those techniques, we have established a design space to characterize interaction techniques based on a mini-screen. Beyond standard technical features of a LCD screen as size, weight and resolution, our design space is based on more interaction-centered characteristics. Indeed, as shown in Figure 2, our framework is comprised of two orthogonal axes namely (i) Characterization of the displayed information (ii) Characterization of the usage of the device itself.

**Table 1.** Characterization of the two interaction techniques: Design choices for the dimension "Information".

| Information | Language | Screen position |
|---|---|---|
| | (2D, dynamic) or (3D, dynamic) | independent |

The first dimension, namely "Information", is used to describe how the device conveys information to the user. First we consider the form of the displayed information ("interaction language") that we characterize in terms of the dimension of the displayed data (1D, 2D, etc.) and of its dynamic capabilities. Secondly we consider if the displayed data is dependent on the screen's position or not. For instance, if the screen is tied to a tool handled by the surgeon, and it conveys guidance information, then the output data may be dependent on the screen's position: the displayed data change according to the screen's positions over the patient's body. Other kinds of data (e.g., blood pressure, body temperature) may be independent on the screen's position in that same case.

The second dimension, namely "Usage", characterizes the usage of the mini-screen itself by the user. Along this dimension, we identify three sets of characteristics let the designer answer three questions.

- Does the mini-screen convey information to the computer system and how (Input dimension)?
- Does the mini-screen move during the operation and how (Movement dimension)?
- Is the mini-screen manipulated by the surgeon during the operation and how (Manipulation dimension)?

## 4. Results: Developed Techniques Based on a Mini-Screen

*4.1. Developed Interaction Techniques*

We developed two techniques based on a mini-screen that have been integrated in a computer assisted renal puncture application. According to our design space, both techniques have different characteristics along the dimension "Usage" but share the same characteristics along the dimension "Information".

For both interaction techniques, the surgeon can see on the mini-screen either a pre-operative scan image of the patient's pelvis along with the planned trajectory as well as the current position of the needle, or the current position of the needle according to the planned trajectory as three 2D colored-crosses and a gauge (same representation as the one in the first version of CASPER). In Table 1 we summarize the characteristics of the two designed techniques for the dimension "Information". The surgeon can switch between the two views by a pedal command. We plan to add speech recognition to let the surgeon switch via voice commands. In addition the mini-screen size influences the displayed information. For the developed techniques, we used a 3.5 inches LCD screen. We are currently studying a new representation of the guidance information, without the graphical gauge: for example the depth information can be encoded by the size of the lines of the three crosses in order to save pixels on the mini-screen (theory of graphical excellence [8]).

Both techniques differ by their characteristics along the dimension "Usage". For the first interaction technique, the mini-screen is positioned near the operating field. This first

**Table 2.** Characterization of the first technique: Design choices for the dimension "Usage".

| Usage | Input | Movement | Manipulation |
|-------|-------|----------|--------------|
|       | none  | none     | none         |

**Table 3.** Characterization of the second technique: Design choices for the dimension "Usage".

| Usage | Input | Movement | Manipulation |
|-------|-------|----------|--------------|
|       | none  | none     | indirect     |

technique is solely a spatial improvement as compared with the first version of CASPER. We take advantage of the mini-screen small size which enables it to be closer to the operating field than a standard computer display. The mini-screen is stationary while the surgeon performs the puncture. Based on our design space, Table 2 characterizes the designed technique along the dimension "Usage".

For the second technique, the mini-screen is tied with the puncture needle, acting like a viewfinder. Such a difference in comparison with the first technique is captured within our design space by the characteristic "manipulation" that is equal to indirect for this technique. As for the previous technique and although the screen is tied with the needle, the displayed information is not dependent on the position of the screen. As a consequence the screen is not localized (Input = none). The design choices for this second technique are listed in Table 3.

So far we have developed two interaction techniques and we have characterized them within our design space. We need to develop other techniques based on different characteristics and to experimentally compare them for evaluating the ergonomic values of our characteristics.

### 4.2. Display Strategies: Standard Screen / Mini-Screen

While designing the techniques on mini-screen, we faced the problem of extending existing applications relying on a standard screen. We therefore studied the relationships that can be maintained between the information displayed on the standard screen and the one displayed on the mini-screen. We have identified three main display strategies.

The three strategies are presented in Figure 3. On the left part of Figure 3, the strategies (a) and (b) are based on the replication of information. On the right part of Figure 3, the strategy (c) is based on the distribution of information. The strategy (a) corresponds to the most generic approach. It consists of a raw copy of a part of the big screen, pixel per pixel. That strategy works without knowing what is displayed and is therefore independent of the surgical application. For defining what is displayed on the mini-screen, the user places one or several transparent windows on screen. What is visible through a transparent window is also visible on the mini-screen. The user can freely move and resize the transparent windows. Only one transparent window has the focus at a time, so only the content of that window is copied to the mini-screen. The switch between transparent windows is achieved by a pedal or voice commands. The drawback of that strategy is that the user has to place and size all the transparent windows. The strategy (b) also relies on replication but is application-dependent. It is a replication of a specific workspace of the application. The workspaces that can be replicated must be de-

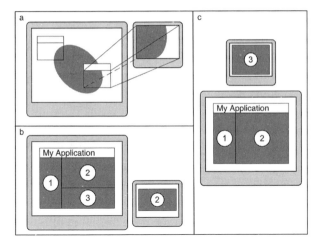

**Figure 3.** Three display strategies for two screens, a standard screen and a mini-screen.

fined by the designer. At last, in the strategy (c), a specific workspace is displayed on the mini-screen and only on it. There is no redundancy between the standard screen and the mini-screen.

For the moment, only the strategy (a) is developed and is going to be tested with our second technique (i.e., the mini-screen tied to the needle). The two other strategies must be developed.

## 5. On-Going and Future Work

As on-going work, in parallel to the software development of new techniques based on the characteristics of our design space, we need to experimentally test and compare our design solutions. Some experiments have already been made for the first technique, the mini-screen being placed near the patient's body. Such a solution clearly minimizes the perceptual discontinuity. Nevertheless we observed another ergonomic problem, related to the interpretation by the surgeon of the displayed information, namely cognitive discontinuity [2]. Indeed when the surgeon moves the physical needle, that movement has to be visualized in a coherent way on the mini-screen. Therefore, the mini-screen position according to the patient's body is important for interaction. The new solution must be developed accordingly and then experimentally tested by quantitatively comparing the technique with the first version of CASPER that relies on a standard screen.

As future work, we need to enrich our design space by considering technical issues such as connectivity and display resolution of the mini-screen: such issues also impact on the usability of the designed interaction techniques.

## Acknowledgements

Special thanks to C. Marmignon for the CASPER picture and to G. Serghiou for reviewing the paper.

# References

[1]  Blackwell, M., Nikou, C., DiGiola, A.M., and Kanade, T. An Image Overlay System for Medical Data Visualization. Proceedings of MICCAI'98, (1998), LNCS 1496, Springer-Verlag, 232-240.
[2]  Dubois, E., Nigay, L., Troccaz, J. Consistency in Augmented Reality Systems. Proceedings of EHCI'01, (2001), LNCS 2254, Springer-Verlag, 117-130.
[3]  Fishkin, K.P., Moran, T.P., Harrison, B.L. Embodied User Interfaces: Towards Invisible User Interfaces. Proceedings of EHCI'98, (1998), Kluwer Academic Publ., 1-18.
[4]  Glossop, N., Wedlake, C., Moore, J. et al. Laser Projection Augmented Reality System for Computer Assisted Surgery. Proceedings of MICCAI'03, (2003), LNCS 2879, Springer-Verlag, 239-246.
[5]  Grimson, W.E.L., Ettinger, G.J., White, S.J. et al. An Automatic Registration Method for Frameless Stereotaxy, Image Guided Surgery, and Enhanced Reality Visualization. in IEEE Transactions on Medical Imaging, 15(2), (1996), 129-140.
[6]  Mackay, W. Augmented Reality: linking real and virtual worlds. Proceedings of ACM AVI'98, (1998), ACM Press.
[7]  Milgram, P. A taxonomy of mixed reality visual displays. in IEICE Transactions on Information Systems, (1994), E77 D(12): 1321-1329.
[8]  Tufte E. The Visual Display of Quantitative Information. Graphics Press Cheshire, CT, USA, 1983, ISBN:0-9613921-0-X.
[9]  Vazquez-BuenosAires J.O., Payan Y. and Demongeot J. Evaluation of a Lingual Interface as a Passive Surgical Guiding System. Proceedings of Surgetica'2002, (2002), Sauramps medical, 232-237.

*Medicine Meets Virtual Reality 13*
*James D. Westwood et al. (Eds.)*
*IOS Press, 2005*

# Real-time Visualization of Cross-sectional Data in Three Dimensions

Terrence J. MAYES, Theodore T. FOLEY,
Joseph A. HAMILTON and Tom C. DUNCAVAGE

*Concept Exploration Laboratory, NASA-Johnson Space Center,*
*2101 NASA Road 1, Mail Code: SF12, Houston, Texas, 77058-3963*

**Abstract.** This paper describes a technique for viewing and interacting with 2-D medical data in three dimensions. The approach requires little pre-processing, runs on personal computers, and has a wide range of application. Implementation details are discussed, examples are presented, and results are summarized.

## 1. Problem

The goal of this work is to achieve real-time visualization of 2-D cross-sectional medical data as a 3-D model. These data include CT-scans and ultrasound images. User manipulation and extraction of information from the data at interactive rates is required. Another requisite is that very little pre-processing of the data is performed.

Techniques exist that create 3-D geometric models of such data, but they are often slow, expensive, and require significant data pre-processing. Visualization of cross-sectional data as geometric models also has the potential to conceal information easily gleaned from the data in image form. A software solution is desired that would run on typical, low-cost computer hardware. Ideally, images could be read directly from the scanning hardware into the software as it runs on a physician's laptop.

## 2. Method

Two assumptions were made to meet these requirements. First, maintaining original image data in memory would allow greater flexibility than 3-D geometry created from that data. Second, displaying the data as stacked slices in three dimensions would provide sufficient 3-D perception to the user. To prove these assumptions, a MS Windows-based tool has been created. Its interface is designed to be consistent with those of popular software today. The user specifies a set of 2-D cross-sectional data to be viewed. Mouse and keyboard controls allow the model to be viewed from any direction and in any scale.

Densities in the model can be selected using mouse buttons. A selected density and its 3-D position are provided to the user as feedback. Densities can be matched and regions of similar density highlighted. Size variations can be tracked by measuring the distance between any two selected points on the model. A "dissection plane" is used to

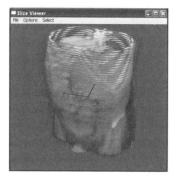

**Figure 1.**

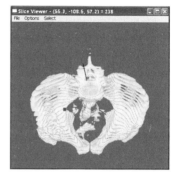

**Figure 2.**

create cut-away views. This plane provides oblique views and selection of densities in the interior model regions. The plane is parallel to the monitor screen and can be used to chip off and permanently discard regions of the image data not at interest.

Image processing operators are provided to interactively enhance the data. Image transforms can be used to repair digitization artifacts. Contrast stretching enhances dynamic range, making small magnitude densities more visible. Edge detection finds boundaries between different tissue types. Registration aids in detecting differences between two cross-sections scanned at different times. Image subtraction highlights size and shape variations between properly registered image pairs. A histogram of densities can be displayed. Comparing histograms from two sets of scans can be used to estimate changes in bone density, muscle density, etc. Finally, images refined with the tool can be saved, reloaded, and used in other medical applications.

## 3. Results

A few observations were made in the process of achieving the stated goals. The tool excelled at helping people without medical training understand the data. Bones, organs, and muscles became clearly evident to the novice when viewed with the tool. It is an effective training aid. A variety of scans can be maintained to demonstrate different medical conditions. Human or animal cadaver dissection can be performed conveniently in virtual space. It is also appropriate in cases where expensive 3-D approaches are not feasible. For example, the International Space Station has no CT-scan or MRI capability. The tool is presently being adapted to work with ultrasound at the request of NASA flight surgeons.

Figure 1 shows the tool displaying a stack of CT-scan images. Note that the rib cage, which is difficult to detect in a single slice, is now clearly visible. Figure 2 is an image of pelvic bones extracted from the stack and viewed from a different angle. Figure 3 shows slices taken from an individual at two different times. Edge detection was applied to the images and they were registered using the rib cage as a landmark. The results are presented in figure 4. The heartbeat and respiration of the subject are in different phases and spinal flexion varied between the two scans.

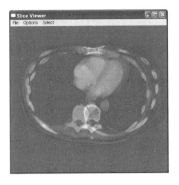

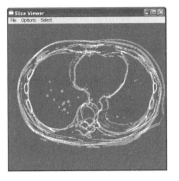

Figure 3.                                        Figure 4.

## 4. Discussion

The tool is built on the OpenGL [1] graphics library available on modern versions of Windows. Image data for test cases were originally stored in DICOM [2] format, a popular standard. At initialization, a patient is reconstructed using a set of textured, stacked planar polygons. The planes are sized and positioned using information taken from the CT data. Embedded text is removed from the scans, and density values are transformed into four component RGB-alpha textures. These textures are stored as OpenGL objects in video RAM and also as arrays of densities in processor memory for fast access.

Panning and zooming is accomplished by setting up a viewing transformation focused on the center of the polygonal slices. The dissection plane is implemented as an OpenGL clip plane perpendicular to the view plane. A half-space test determines which pixels are permanently removed when the dissection plane is used to chip off image data. Pick selection is achieved by tracing a ray from the click spot on the screen out into the field of view. The ray is intersected with polygons in the stack and the 3-D coordinates of the nearest intersection are returned.

An optimized library of image processing functions was created to support the tool's features. Popular algorithms [3] are implemented using in-line coding, pointer arithmetic, and minimal use of floating point numbers. The Sobel gradient filter is used to detect edges and show boundaries between regions of different density. Registration of two cross-sections is accomplished by transforming both into log-polar space [4] and performing cross-correlation. Lastly, the MS Windows Bitmap (BMP) file format is used for reading and writing image data to disk.

## 5. Conclusion

The software has been successfully tested on a variety of computers without special hardware. It is extensible, and several new features are currently in development. For instance, linear and cubic interpolators can be added to generate new density data in between pairs of cross-sections. Four-pixel and eight-pixel connectivity operators can organize densities into distinct classes, allowing different tissues to be segregated for individual processing. Performance can be improved by incorporating the Intel image processing library [5], which takes advantage of MMX instructions in modern processors.

The long-term goal is to turn the software into an analysis tool. Multiple sets of data could be loaded into the system and compared against each other. For example, comparing sets from the same subject taken at different times could make estimates of tumor growth possible. The potential user base is vast due to the limited resource requirements of the application. The executable is roughly 200 kilobytes in size and can readily be transported on a floppy disk or sent via e-mail. It could easily be tailored to suit the needs of users ranging from educators to battlefield medics.

## References

[1] Neider, J.; Davis, T.; Woo, M., *OpenGL Programming Guide*, Addison-Wesley, 1993.
[2] Moore, S.M.; Hoffman, S.A.; Beecher, D.E., *"DICOM shareware: A public implementation of the DICOM standard,"* in Medical Imaging 1994.
[3] Gonzales, R.C.; Woods, R., *Digital Image Processing*, Addison Wesley, 1992.
[4] Wolberg, G.; Zokai, S., *"Robust Image Registration using Log-polar Transform,"* Proceedings of the IEEE International Conference on Image Processing, September 2000.
[5] Intel Corporation, *Intel Image Processing Library Reference Manual*, 2000.

Medicine Meets Virtual Reality 13
James D. Westwood et al. (Eds.)
IOS Press, 2005

# Compressing Different Anatomical Data Types for the Virtual Soldier

Tom MENTEN, Xiao ZHANG, Lian ZHU and Marc FOOTEN
*Crowley Davis Research, 280 South Academy Ave, Eagle, ID 83616*

**Abstract.** The Virtual Soldier Project endeavors to represent the baseline physiology and anatomy of a soldier using disparate but linked digital data types (http://www.virtualsoldier.net). Processing these data for storage, transmission and encryption requires different capabilities than are typical in a single codec. These representation and coding issues are illustrated and future directions are indicated.

## 1. Challenges of Representing Disparate Data Types

The first generation of the "Virtual Soldier" makes use of multiple data components integrated by a common ontology. For example, physiological information may include electrocardiograms and other measurement data, while medical history may appear as ASCII or XML data. Computed Tomography (CT) data may be represented in DICOM format, while anatomical structures are represented by triangle mesh surface models (e.g. as VTK files.) Segmentation maps, indicating the anatomical structure of various regions of image files may be represented as PNG files. Thus the first generation of the Virtual Soldier incorporates many disparate data types that together encompass the baseline data. For machine readable data of this kind to be useful in the treatment of the individual, it must be easily and quickly accessible and interpretable by a variety of computational platforms and of immediate diagnostic use by a variety of medical personnel. No single compression method and thus no previously available codec (CODer/DECoder) can handle these various data types and requirements. A single integrated codec is being developed to more efficiently store and transmit these data components, and to respond to future more integrated data representations. We illustrate the progress of this effort with two different anatomical data types.

## 2. Coding of Whole Body Computed Tomography

A whole body CT scan of a person is represented by a series of about one thousand grey scale images that are typically stored in a DICOM, pixel based format. This representation permits direct imaging at a specified resolution, but typically these files are very large and slow to transmit. More efficient coding of these data is currently best achieved by wavelet transforms using the JPEG2000 standard [1]. Additional techniques such as Region of Interest (ROI) and scalable coding can greatly improve the storage and transmission of this kind of data.

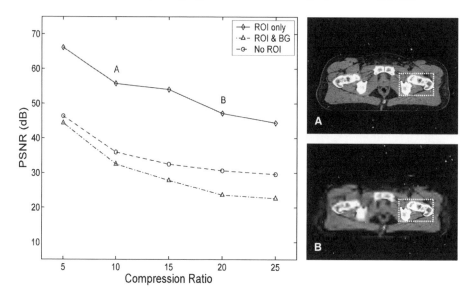

**Figure 1.** ROI Coding of Visible Human data (ROI, dashed boundary; PSNR, peak signal/noise ratio.) (A) CT scan whole body cross section, CR=10. (B) same image, CR=25. In (B) the image quality of the ROI (dashed boundary) is preserved while the surrounding area is degraded.

Region of Interest (ROI) coding [2] permits preferential allocation of storage or transmission resources to prioritized image regions. As a result, the observed image degradation is very modest in the Region of Interest, while the image quality of the non prioritized region is sacrificed. Figure 1 illustrates this benefit. 40db is widely considered to be a high fidelity representation (though this does NOT define "diagnostic image quality"). The ROI region never falls below 40db PSNR even at the high overall compression ratio (CR) of 25. In contrast, the PSNR of the non ROI coded image degrades rapidly to below 40 well before reaching a CR of 10. The ROI exhibits a gain of more than 20db from non ROI encoded format. ROI coding can be used to variously prioritize storage space or bandwidth. For example, using currently available project hardware, transmission of a whole body CT scan might require over 15 minutes. The use of ROI can facilitate the fast scan and selection of images and their subsequent transmission in less than 30 seconds.

## 3. Coding of 3D Anatomical Structures

Individualized anatomical structures derived from the computed tomography provide immediate visual and machine identification of anatomical structures [3]. For the Virtual Soldier project, the native format of these 3D triangle mesh geometry files is the VTK file. This very general data structure facilitates shape distortion, coloration and other manipulations but it is also inefficient for storage and transmission. In contrast, a much more efficient representation expands to yield the same structure [4]. Figure 2 illustrates the large reduction in file size (and correspondingly reduced transmission time) result-

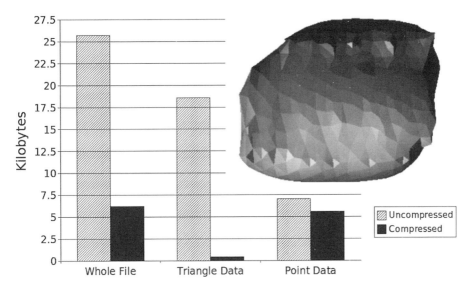

**Figure 2.** Compression of "right_nipple.vtk"; 3D model constructed from Visible Human dataset.

ing from efficient representation of the mesh geometry: the description of mesh topology was reduced losslessly by a factor of 46, leading to an overall compression ratio of 5:1. In another more extreme example, more efficient representation of a 90MB file, that would require more than 90 seconds to transmit, reduced the transmission time to less than 10 seconds.

## 4. Summary and Future Directions

We anticipate increasing complexity of data for the Virtual Soldier in terms of its anatomical and physiological scope, incorporation of encryption into the codec and an increasing level of integration of the baseline data components. While early focus has significantly emphasized the heart, we anticipate that future efforts will consider the human thorax more generally, incorporating still more data types while integrating others. Much of the value of the Virtual Soldier derives from preprocessing that identifies specific useful information in the basic data – inferred anatomical structure, for example. Future research will develop methods and tools to produce increasingly integrated and efficient representation of the basic and derived anatomical and physiological baseline information in ways that facilitate both human and automated use.

## Acknowledgements

This work was supported by contract #W81XWH-04-2-0014 (DARPA) and DAMD17-02-2-0049 (TATRC).

Data used in figures were provided by the Visible Human Project of the National Library of Medicine, and by William Lorensen, General Electric Research.

## References

[1]  Adams, M. and F.Kossentini.(2000) Jasper: A Software-Based JPEG-2000 Codec Implementation, and Proceedings of ICIP 2000.
[2]  Christopoulos,C.,Askelof,J. and M.Larsson (2000) Efficient Region of Interest Coding Techniques in the Upcoming JPEG2000 Still Image Coding Standard, Proceedings of IEEE, 2000 p41-p44.
[3]  Lorensen,W., Miller,J., Padfield,D. and J. Ross (2004) Creating Models from Segmented Medical Images. Medicine Meets Virtual Reality 13. IOS Press, Amsterdam.
[4]  Rosignac,J. (1999) Edgebreaker: Connectivity compression for triangle meshes IEEE Transactions on Visualization and Computer Graphics, Vol. 5, No. 1, pp. 47-61.

*Medicine Meets Virtual Reality 13*
*James D. Westwood et al. (Eds.)*
*IOS Press, 2005*

# A Real-Time Haptic Interface
# for Interventional Radiology Procedures

Thomas MOIX [a], Dejan ILIC [a], Blaise FRACHEBOUD [a],
Jurjen ZOETHOUT [b] and Hannes BLEULER [a]

[a] *Laboratoire de Systèmes Robotiques (LSRO), EPFL,*
*ME.B3, Station 9, 1015 Lausanne, Switzerland*
[b] *Xitact S.A.*
*Rue de Lausanne 45, 1110 Morges, Switzerland*

**Abstract.** Interventional Radiology (IR) is a minimally-invasive surgery technique (MIS) where guidewires and catheters are steered in the vascular system under X-ray imaging. In order to perform these procedures, a radiologist has to be correctly trained to master hand-eye coordination, instrument manipulation and procedure protocols. This paper proposes a computer-assisted training environment dedicated to IR. The system is composed of a virtual reality (VR) simulation of the anatomy of the patient linked to a robotic interface providing haptic force feedback.

The paper focuses on the requirements, design and prototyping of a specific part of the haptic interface dedicated to catheters. Translational tracking and force feedback on the catheter is provided by two cylinders forming a friction drive arrangement. The whole friction can be set in rotation with an additional motor providing torque feedback. A force and a torque sensor are integrated in the cylinders for direct measurement on the catheter enabling disturbance cancellation with a close-loop force control strategy.

## 1. Introduction

### 1.1. Interventional Radiology

Interventional Radiology (IR) is a minimally-invasive surgery (MIS) technique where guidewires and thin tubular instruments called catheters are navigated through the patient's vascular system. Real-time X-ray imaging (C-arm) is used for monitoring the position of the surgical tools and for controlling the ongoing intervention.

IR is an extension into therapy of the diagnostic procedures (most commonly angiographies with contrast agent injection) of vascular diseases in the peripheral, cardiac and neuro areas. Immediate treatment of various diseases is possible through techniques including local drug injection, catheter balloon inflation (angioplasty) and stent placement among others [1].

### 1.2. Training in IR

IR procedures need to be performed by well trained and experienced specialists. Difficult hand-eye coordination, complicated looping and bending of instruments, the risk of vessel injury or obstruction, and possibly lethal embolization are good reasons to provide extensive training. Some especially risky procedures, such as carotid stenting, are even expected to require specific certification and training.

Apart from traditional "see one, do one, teach one" model, radiologists have only had few mock devices for training with limitation in practical use. Training on animals is an alternative, but its use is hindered by high costs and ethical issues.

## 1.3. Computer Assisted Training System

Computer-assisted training systems are an interesting alternative for surgeons. Just as flight simulators recreate the behaviour of a plane, different weather conditions and critical situations, surgery simulators offer an environment for realistic training of medical interventions [2]. The medical procedure takes place in a virtual reality (VR) environment with the visual rendering of the imaging device used by doctors. The physical user-interface to the surgeon, the "joystick" of the simulator, consists of haptic force-feedback devices with the appearance and feel of surgical tools [3]. Several clinical studies [4–6] have already highlighted the benefits of such training systems for surgeons in different medical fields.

The existing simulation systems for IR [7–11] all have major drawbacks: the requirement to use modified instruments, high inertia of the haptic feedback that create a noticeably degraded dynamic behaviour, coupled or passive force feedback on some degrees of freedom (DOFs).

## 2. A Haptic Interface for IR

### 2.1. Requirements

The following hardware requirements have been identified. The rotation and the translation of each instrument have to be measured. Independent active force feedback must be provided for both DOFs of each instrument. The requirements for the sensors and the force feedback resolution are based on human factor studies and simple experiments: force and torque resolution shall be of 0.02 N and of 0.04 mNm respectively [12]. In IR procedures, forces and torques, estimated for a 4 French catheter (3F = 1mm), are in range of about ±2 N and ±4.5 mNm [7]. Furthermore, removing any interference from vibrations demands a high accuracy and control frequency (human hand sensitivity is of 1 μm amplitude up to 300 Hz [12]).

### 2.2. The Proposed Interface

Two measurement stations have been developed. A catheter unit, fixed at the entrance of the simulation system, measures translational and rotational movements and applies force feedback on a catheter. A mobile device tracks the motion and applies force feedback on a guidewire.

This paper focuses on the development of the unit that handles a catheter. The inserted catheter is held between two cylinders in a friction drive arrangement as illustrated in Figure 1. The first cylinder is attached to a DC torque motor in direct drive, thus applying an active force feedback for the first degree of freedom of the system, the translation

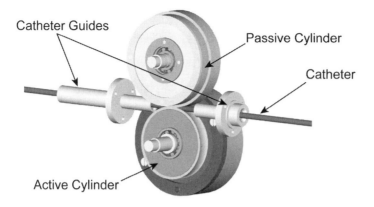

**Figure 1.** The Friction Drive Arrangement.

of the catheter. The whole cylinder system is linked with a belt to a second DC motor that provides torque feedback. Both cylinders are coated with rubber to increase friction with the catheter, hence avoiding any slippage between the catheter and the cylinders.

### 2.3. Force and Torque Sensing

In order to achieve a high-quality haptic force feedback, the inertia and the friction of the system are actively compensated. A force and a torque sensor are integrated in the friction drive enabling a close-loop control architecture. Both sensors use the same working principle. The measurand is transformed in a deformation of a mechanical structure. The deformation is measured by optical infrared reflective sensors. The mechanical structures are directly mounted in the cylinders of the friction drive, thus providing the most direct measurement possible.

The torque sensor directly forms the passive cylinder. It consists of an inner and an outer ring held with two disc springs. The stiffness of the structure is very high in all directions except the axial one. A perpendicular force (i.e. a torque applied on the catheter) applied to the outer ring induces a deflection of the disc springs that is measured by two reflective sensors. Their output signals are added to eliminate perturbations due to mechanical misalignment on the cylinder axis. The complete arrangement is presented in figure 2.

The translational force is measured on the motorized cylinder. The mechanical structure of the sensor is composed of two rings connected with four beams [13]. The inner ring is fixed to the main frame of the friction drive arrangement while the outer ring is attached to the stator of the torque motor. When a torque (i.e. a translational force applied on the catheter) is applied on one of the rings, the beams deflect. The deflection is measured by two reflective sensors as illustrated in figure 3. The outputs of the sensors are subtracted to eliminate unwanted perturbations.

The resolution of the measured force and torque of the catheter is respectively of 0.02 N over ±2 N and 0.04 mNm over ±20 mNm.

### 2.4. The Realized Prototype

Figure 4 shows the prototype of the haptic interface for catheter that has been realized and tested. The device was designed for a maximum speed of 1 m/s for translation and

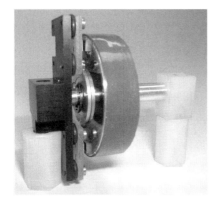

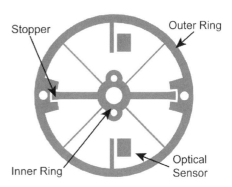

**Figure 3.** The Translational Force Sensor.

**Figure 2.** The Torque Sensor.

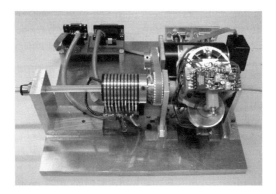

**Figure 4.** The Haptic Interface Prototype (Size: 200 x 185mm).

2 rps for rotation and a maximum acceleration of 10 m/s$^2$ and 5 rps$^2$. These values were estimated on observations of actual procedures. Emphasis has been made on the system to be light, without backlash and to display high resonance frequencies (i.e. high bandwidth).

The prototype has been integrated with the device that had previously been developed for guidewires and linked to an electronic interface thus creating a complete haptic interface for IR procedures. A communication protocol has been implemented between the electronic interface and the computer where the VR simulation is running with a *Windows®*operating system. The low-level force feedback control loop has been implemented on that same computer. The use of dedicated high priority interruptions enables a maximum force feedback sampling rate of 1 kHz.

## 2.5. Simulation Software

The software for interfacing to the hardware implements the same software interface as the commercially available Xitact CHP device, an open platform for IR simulators available from Xitact S.A. Simulation software developed in our own institution, by the Simulation group at CIMIT (Boston, USA) [14] and commercial offerings that rely on Xitact's platform are therefore compatible with our system.

## 3. Conclusions

Based on analysis of requirements and state of the art in computer-assisted training systems for IR, a new hardware haptic interface is proposed. The system offers a realistic behaviour, adapts to real or slightly modified instruments and allows their full interchangeability.

Further work includes refinement of the current prototype and experiments with different control strategies for the force feedback control loop. Testing, tuning and validation of the proposed hardware platform with a variety of simulation software will be carried out together with medical partners.

## Acknowledgement

This research is supported by the Swiss National Science Foundation within the framework NCCR CO-ME (COmputer aided and image guided MEdical interventions) and by the Swiss Innovation Promotion Agency KTI/CTI.

## References

[1] K. Valji, Vascular and Interventional Radiology. Philadelphia, PA: W.B. Saunders Company, 1999.

[2] R. Satava and S. Jones, "Current applications of virtual reality in medicine," Proc. of the IEEE, vol. 86, no. 3, pp. 484–489, Mar. 1998.

[3] E. Chen and B. Marcus, "Force feedback for surgical surgery," Proc. of the IEEE, vol. 86, no. 3, pp. 524-530, Mar. 1998.

[4] R. O'Tool, R. Playter, T. Krummel, W. Blank, N. Cornalius, W. Roberts, W. Bells and M. Raibert, "Assessing skill and learning in surgeons and medical students using a force feedback surgical simulator," in Lecture Notes in Computer Science, Medical Image Computing and Computer-Assisted Intervention (MICCAI 98), vol. 1496, pp. 899–909, 1998.

[5] P. Gorman, A. Meier and T. Krummel, "Simulation and virtual reality in surgical education," Arch. Surg., vol. 134, pp. 1203–1208, 1999.

[6] M.P. Schijven, J.J. Jakimowicz, R. Klaassen and O.T. Terpstra, "Laparoscopic skill assessment using the Xitact LS500 laparoscopy simulator," Surg Endosc, vol. 17, pp. 1978–1984, 2003.

[7] G. Aloisio, L. Barone, M. Bergamasco and al., "Computer-based simulator for catheter insertion training," in Studies in Health Technology and Informatics (MMVR 12), vol. 98, pp. 4-6, Jan. 2004.

[8] S. Z. Barnes, D. R. Morr and N. Berme, "Catheter simulation device," U.S. Patent 6 038 488, 2000.

[9] G. L. Merril, "Interventional radiology interface apparatus and method," U.S. Patent 6 106 301, 2000.

[10] B. E. Bailey, "System for training persons to perform minimally invasive surgical procedure," U.S. Patent 5 800 179, 1998.

[11] J. M. Wendlandt and F. M. Morgan, "Actuator for independent axial and rotational actuation of a catheter or similar elongated object," U.S. Patent 6 375 471, 2002.

[12] H. Tan, B. Eberman, M. Srinivasan and B. Cheng, "Human factors for the design of force-reflecting haptic interfaces," Dyn. Sys. Cont., vol. 55, no. 1, 1994.

[13] D. Vischer and O. Khatib, "Design and development of high performance torque-controlled joints," IEEE Transactions on Robotics and Automation, vol. 11, no. 4, Aug. 1995.

[14] N. Muniyandi and S. Cotin, "Real-time pc based x-ray simulation for interventional radiology training," in Studies in Health Technology and Informatics (MMVR 11), vol. 94, Jan. 2003.

*Medicine Meets Virtual Reality 13*
*James D. Westwood et al. (Eds.)*
*IOS Press, 2005*

# An Interactive Simulation Environment for Craniofacial Surgical Procedures

Dan MORRIS [a], Sabine GIROD [b], Federico BARBAGLI [a] and Kenneth SALISBURY [a]

[a] *Department of Computer Science, Stanford University*
[b] *Division of Plastic and Reconstructive Surgery, Stanford University*
*e-mail: {dmorris, barbagli, jks}@robotics.stanford.edu, sgirod@stanford.edu*

**Abstract.** Recent advances in medical imaging and surgical techniques have made possible the correction of severe facial deformities and fractures. Surgical correction techniques often involve the direct manipulation – both relocation and surgical fracture – of the underlying facial bone. The work presented here introduces an environment for interactive, visuohaptic simulation of craniofacial surgical procedures, with an emphasis on both mandibular distraction procedures and traditional orthognathic surgeries. The simulator is intended both for instruction and for procedure-specific rehearsal, and can thus load canonical training cases or patient-specific image data into the interactive environment. A network module allows remote demonstration of procedure technique, a form of 'haptic tutoring'.

This paper discusses the simulation, haptic feedback, and graphic rendering techniques used to drive the environment. Particular emphasis is placed on techniques for fracture and subsequent rigid manipulation of bone structures, a key component of the relevant procedures.

## 1. Introduction

### 1.1. Surgical Background

Incorrect alignment of the jaws – due to congenital malformation, trauma, or disease – can result in cosmetic deformation and problems with chewing and/or breathing. Orthognathic surgeries correct such problems, typically by inducing a fracture in one or both jaws (generally using a bone saw), displacing the fractured components into an anatomically preferable configuration, and installing bone screws and/or metal plates to fix the bone segments in their new positions.

This approach is often prohibited by the severity of the deformation, the size of the separation that would be required after fracture, or the sensitivity of the surrounding soft tissue. In these cases, distraction osteogenesis is often employed as an alternative. Here a similar procedure is performed, by only a minor separation is created intraoperatively. Instead of spanning the gap with a rigid plate, an adjustable distractor is fixed to the bone on both sides of the gap. The distractor can be used to gradually widen the fracture over a period of several weeks, allowing accommodation in the surrounding tissue and allowing the bone to heal naturally across the fracture.

These procedures are likely to benefit from surgical simulation for several reasons. The complex, patient-specific planning process and the significant anatomic variation from case to case suggests that an end-to-end simulator will assist physicians in preparing for specific cases. Furthermore, distraction procedures have been introduced to the craniofacial surgical community only within the last ten to fifteen years, and an effective simulator will significantly aid in the training and re-training of this new class of procedures, and with the exploration of alternative techniques for effective surgeries.

### 1.2. Previous work

Several projects [1–3] have focused on the simulation of craniofacial surgical procedures, although the focus of most previous work has been on the prediction of soft tissue movement and the prediction of post-operative facial appearance given a series of bone manipulations. The surgical procedure itself is typically represented as a series of geometric operations – defined via explicit cutting planes or analytically-specified transformations.

Other work has focused on simulation of dental [4] and otologic [5–8] procedures, which are similar to the surgeries discussed here in terms of haptic feedback and bone drilling/cutting. However, the procedures presented here additionally require the rigid manipulation of bone fragments and the attachment of rigid structures (plates, etc.) to the bone.

## 2. Methods

### 2.1. Data sources and preprocessing

Figure 1 summarizes the preprocessing stages that transform image data into the format used for interactive rendering. Isosurfaces are first generated from CT or MR data using the marching cubes method [9]; this allows us to discard regions of data that are not part of the skull. This algorithm does not generate closed meshes for all inputs, so we cap any holes in the resulting isosurfaces using the 3d Studio Max software package (Discreet Inc., Montreal, Quebec). A non-repeating set of texture coordinates is then generated on the isosurface mesh, to be used later for interactive rendering.

A flood-filling technique is then used to build a voxel grid from the isosurface data, using an AABB tree to accelerate the numerous collision tests required at this stage. For voxels situated at the boundary of the bone volume, we find the nearest triangle to the voxel center and use barycentric interpolation to assign texture coordinates and surface normals to those voxels. The resulting voxel array is exported along with density information for all voxels. This voxel array is used directly for haptic rendering, and is also retessellated into a new surface used for interactive graphic rendering (see Section 2.2). Overall preprocessing time for a typical head CT data set is on the order of fifteen to twenty minutes.

Models of bone plates have been supplied by the manufacturer, and are loaded into our environment directly as surface meshes.

### 2.2. Interactive Rendering

In order to leverage previous work in haptic rendering of volumetric data [10] while still maintaining the benefits of surface rendering in terms of hardware acceleration and visual effects, we maintain a hybrid data structure in which volumetric data are used for

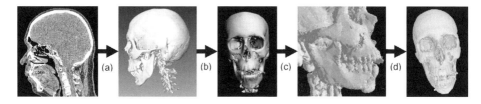

**Figure 1.** A summary of our preprocessing pipeline. CT data sets are (a) isosurfaced, (b) capped and smoothed, (c) flood-filled to generate a voxel array, and (d) re-tessellated into a final surface mesh.

haptic rendering and traditional triangle arrays are used for graphic rendering. In order to simplify and accelerate the process of updating our polygonal data when the bone is modified, we build a new surface mesh – in which vertices correspond directly to bone voxels – rather than using the original isosurface mesh.

The voxel array representing the bone model is loaded into our simulation environment, and a polygonal surface mesh is generated to enclose the voxel grid. This is accomplished by exhaustively triangulating the voxels on the surface of the bone region, i.e.:

```
for each voxel v1 that is on the bone surface
  for each of v1's neighbors v2 that is on the bone surface
    for each of v2's neighbors v3 that is on the bone surface
      generate a triangle (v1,v2,v3) oriented away from the bone surface
```

Here being 'on the bone surface' is defined as having non-zero bone density and having at least one neighbor that has no bone density. Although this generates a significant number of triangles (on the order of 200,000 for a typical CT data set), we use several techniques to minimize the number of triangles that are generated and/or rendered. To avoid generating duplicate triangles, each voxel is assigned an index before tessellation, and triangles are rejected if they do not appear in sorted order. A second pass over the mesh uses the observations presented in [11] to eliminate subsurface triangles that will not be visible from outside the mesh.

To take advantage of the fact that the user does not frequently change the simulation's perspective, we maintain two triangle arrays, one containing the complete tessellation of the current bone volume (the "complete array"), and one containing only those that are visible from positions close to the current camera position (the "visible array"). The latter array is initialized at startup and any time the camera comes to rest after a period of movement. Visible triangles are those with at least one vertex whose normal points towards (less than 90 degrees away from) the camera. Because this visibility-testing pass is time-consuming, it is performed in the background; the complete array is used for rendering the scene during periods of camera movement (when the visible array is considered 'dirty') and during the reinitialization of the 'visible' array.

As a final optimization, we use the nvtristrip library [12] to reorder our triangle and vertex arrays for optimal rendering performance. We could have further reduced rendering time by generating triangle strips from our triangle lists, but this would add significant complexity to the process of updating the surface mesh to reflect changes to the underlying voxel grid.

## 2.3. Interactive Tools

In our environment, the user makes use of one or two SensAble Phantom [13] haptic devices – providing six-degree-of-freedom control of each tool and three-degree-of-freedom haptic feedback – to control several tools that can interact with the bone data.

The primary bone modification tools are the drill/saw tools, which use the method presented in [10] to perform haptic rendering and bone removal for tools of varying size and shape. Figure 2 displays a drill tool being used to remove bone density. See [10] for a complete description of their modified Voxmap-Pointshell algorithm; only a summary will be provided here. In short, a series of sample points is distributed on the surface of the tool; at each haptic iteration, each sample is tested for immersion in the bone volume. A ray is traced from each immersed sample point toward the tool center until it reaches either the tool center or the bone surface. Bone density is removed for each voxel these rays pass through, and a haptic force is generated along each ray to push immersed points out of the bone volume.

When bone voxels are removed from our environment, our hybrid data structure requires that the area around the removed bone be retessellated. Consequently, bone voxels are queued up by our haptic rendering thread as they are removed, and the graphic rendering thread retessellates the region around each voxel pulled from this queue. That is, for each removed voxel, we see which of his neighbors have been "revealed" and create triangles that contain the centers of these new voxels as vertices. Specifically, for each removed voxel v, we perform the following steps:

```
for each voxel v' that is adjacent to v and on the bone surface
  if a vertex has not already been created to represented v'
    create a vertex representing v' and compute the surface gradient at v'
    queue v' for triangle creation
for each voxel v' that is "queued for triangle creation"
  generate triangles adjacent to v' (see below)
```

Once again, a voxel that is "on the bone surface" has a non-zero bone density and has at least one neighboring voxel that contains no bone density. When all local voxels have been tested for visibility (i.e. when the first loop is complete in the above pseudocode), all new vertices are fed to a triangle generation routine. This routine finds new triangles that can be constructed from new vertices and their neighbors, orients those triangles to match the vertices' surface normals, and copies *visible* triangles to the "visible triangle array" (see Section 2.2). The reason for "queuing triangles for triangle creation" is that the generation of triangles – performed in the second loop above – depends on knowing which local voxels are visible, which is only known after the completion of the first loop.

An additional bone modification tool allows the introduction of large bone cuts via a planar cut tool (see Figure 4). This tool generates no haptic feedback and is not intended to replicate a physical tool. Rather, it addresses the need of advanced users to make rapid cuts for demonstration or for the creation of training scenarios. Bone removal with this tool is implemented by discretizing the planar area – controlled in six degrees of freedom – into voxel-sized sample areas, and tracing a ray a small distance from each sample along the normal to the plane. This ray is identical to the rays traced from the surface of a drill-type tool, discussed in more detail above. No haptic feedback is generated, and each ray is given infinite "drilling power", i.e. all density is removed from any voxels through which each ray passes. The distance traced along each ray is controlled by the user. This

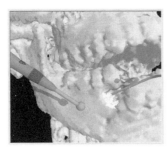

**Figure 2.** Using the drill tool to interactively modify bone volume.

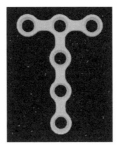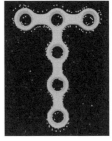

**Figure 3.** Sampling and extrusion of the surface of a bone plate for collision detection with bone.

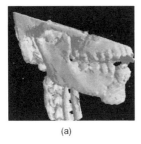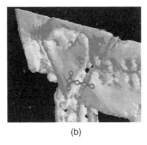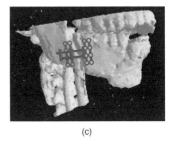

(a)                              (b)                              (c)

**Figure 4.** Binding of bone plates to a bone model. (a) Bone model before fracture (a planar cut has been applied to simplify the image for demonstration). (b) A standard bone plate fixed across a fracture. (c) A distractor fixed on both sides of a fracture.

allows the user to remove a planar or box-shaped region of bone density, demonstrated in Figure 4.

A final set of tools allows the user to manipulate models of several distractors and/or Synthes bone plates. The inclusion of these plate models allows users to plan and practice plate-insertion operations interactively, using industry-standard plates. Collision detection for haptic feedback is also performed using a set of sample points; in this case, the sample points are generated by sampling 100 vertices of each model and extruding them slightly along their normals (because these models tend to be very thin relative to our voxel dimensions) (Figure 3). Since there is no well-defined tool center toward which we can trace rays for penetration calculation, rays are traced along the model's surface normal at each sample point. At any time, the user can rigidly affix a plate tool to a bone object with which it is in contact. Future work will include a simulation of the bone-screw-insertion process.

## 2.4. Continuity detection

A critical step in simulating craniofacial procedures is the detection of cuts in the bone volume that separate one region of bone from another, thus allowing independent rigid transformations to be applied to the isolated bone segments.

In our environment, a background thread performs a repeated flood-filling operation on each bone structure. A random voxel is selected as a seed point for each bone object, and flood-filling proceeds through all voxel neighbors that currently contain bone density. Each voxel maintains a flag indicating whether or not it has been reached by the flood-

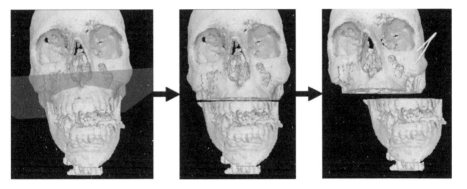

**Figure 5.** The use of the cut-plane tool and the independent manipulation of discontinuous bone regions. (a) The cut-plane tool is used to geometrically specify a set of voxels to remove. (b) The volume after voxel removal. (c) The flood-filling thread has recognized the discontinuity, and the bone segments can now be manipulated independently.

filling operation; at the end of a filling pass, all unmarked voxels (which must have become separated from the seed point) are collected and moved into a new bone object, along with their corresponding data in the vertex and triangle arrays.

Figure 5 displays a bone object that has been cut and the subsequent independent movement of the two resulting structures. Here – for demonstration – the cut-plane tool is used to create the fracture; during simulated procedures, most fractures will likely be created by the drilling/sawing tools.

## 2.5. Network Training

Surgical training is typically focused on visual observation of experienced surgeons and verbal descriptions of proper technique; it is impossible for a surgeon to physically demonstrate the correct 'feel' of bone manipulation with physical tools. With that in mind, we have incorporated a 'haptic tutoring' module into our environment, allowing a trainee to experience forces that are the result of a *remote* user's interaction with the bone model.

Ideally, the trainee would experience both the movements of the instructor's tool and the force applied to/by the instructor, but it is difficult to control both the position and the force at a haptic end-effector without any control of the compliance of the user's hand. To address this issue, we bind the position of the trainee's tool to that of the instructor's tool via a low-gain spring, and add the resulting forces to a 'playback' of the forces generated at the instructor's tool. I.e.:

$$F_{trainee} = K_p(P_{trainee} - P_{instructor}) + F_{instructor}$$

...where $F_{instructor}$ and $F_{trainee}$ are the forces applied to the instructor's and trainee's tools, and $P_{instructor}$ and $P_{trainee}$ are the position of the instructor's and trainee's tools. $K_p$ is small enough that it does not interfere significantly with the perception of the high-frequency components transferred from the instructor's tool to the trainee's tool, but large enough that the trainee's tool stays in the vicinity of the instructor's tool. In practice, the error in this low-gain position controller is still within reasonable visual bounds, and the trainee perceives that he is experiencing the same force *and* position trajectory as the instructor.

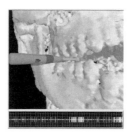

**Figure 6.** Interactive monitoring of virtual nerves. When the virtual tool makes contact with the bone in the vicinity of the virtual nerve bundle (highlighted here in blue), a series of neural pulses is presented via graphic and auditory monitoring tools. Several such bursts are displayed in this clip, captured from the graphic monitor.

## 2.6. Neurophysiology simulation

Another goal of our simulation environment is to train the surgical skills required to avoid critical and/or sensitive structures when using potentially dangerous tools. The inferior alveolar nerve is at particular risk during most of the procedures this environment is targeting. We thus incorporate a virtual nerve monitor that presents the user with a representation of the activity of nerve bundles in the vicinity of the procedure (Figure 6). Nerves are currently placed explicitly for training scenarios; future work will include automatic segmentation of large nerves from image data.

## 3. Discussion and Conclusion

Initial work with surgeons indicates that the haptic feedback associated with bone manipulation is quite realistic. Future work on this environment will thus focus on the incorporation of soft tissue data into the simulation. Online soft tissue representations will be critical for the simulation of constraints imposed on bone movements, and for the training of complete procedures including incisions and soft tissue displacement. Offline soft tissue simulation will allow us to incorporate previous work on the prediction of soft-tissue appearance following craniofacial surgery (e.g. [1–3]). Furthermore, we hope to extend our training of sensitive structure avoidance; a representation of potentially sensitive blood vessels will be valuable, as will the automated or semi-automated extraction of such structures directly from image data.

## Acknowledgements

We thank Doug Wilson for his implementation of shadowing and bone dust, Nik Blevins for his drill models, and Synthes for providing plate models. Support for this work was provided by NIH grant LM07295, the AO Foundation, and the NDSEG fellowship.

## References

[1] Keeve E, Girod S, Kikinis R, Girod B. Deformable modeling of facial tissue for craniofacial surgery simulation. Computer Aided Surgery, 1998, 3:228–38.
[2] Schmidt JG, Berti G, Fingberg J, Cao J, Wollny G. A Finite Element Based Tool Chain for the Planning and Simulation of Maxillo-Facial Surgery. Proceedings of the fourth ECCOMAS, Jyvaskyla, Finland, 2004.

[3] Koch RM, Roth SHM, Gross MH, A. Zimmermann P, Sailer HF. A Framework for Facial Surgery Simulation. Proc of the 18th Spring Conference on Computer Graphics, p33–42, 2002.

[4] Thomas G, Johnson L, Dow S, Stanford C. The design and testing of a force feedback dental simulator. Computer Methods and Programs in Biomedicine. 2001 Jan;64(1):53-64.

[5] Morris D, Sewell C, Blevins N, Barbagli F, Salisbury K. A Collaborative Virtual Environment for the Simulation of Temporal Bone Surgery. Proceedings of MICCAI 2004, v. II pp. 319-327.

[6] Agus M, Giachetti A, Gobbetti E, Zanetti G, John NW, Stone RJ: Mastoidectomy simulation with combined visual and haptic feedback. Proceedings of MMVR 2002.

[7] Bryan J, Stredney D, Wiet G, Sessanna D. Virtual Temporal Bone Dissection: A Case Study. Proceedings of IEEE Visualization 2001, Ertl et. Al., (Eds): 497-500, October 2001.

[8] Pflesser B, Petersik A, Tiede U, Hohne KH, Leuwer R Volume cutting for virtual petrous bone surgery. Computer Aided Surgery 2002;7(2):74-83.

[9] Lorensen WE, Cline HE. Marching Cubes: A high resolution 3D surface construction algorithm. ACM Computer Graphics 1987, 21:163–169.

[10] Renz M, Preusche C, Potke M, Kriegel HP, Hirzinger G. Stable haptic interaction with virtual environments using an adapted voxmap-pointshell algorithm. Proc Eurohaptics, p149-154, 2001.

[11] Bouvier, D.J. Double-Time Cubes: A Fast 3D Surface Construction Algorithm for Volume Visualization. Int'l Conf on Imaging Science, Systems, and Technology, June 1997.

[12] NVIDIA Corporation. nvtristrip library. February 2004. http://developer.nvidia.com/.

[13] Massie TH, Salisbury JK. The PHANTOM Haptic Interface: A Device for Probing Virtual Objects. Symposium on Haptic Interfaces for Virtual Environments, Chicago, IL, Nov 1994.

*Medicine Meets Virtual Reality 13*
*James D. Westwood et al. (Eds.)*
*IOS Press, 2005*

# A GPU Accelerated Spring Mass System for Surgical Simulation

Jesper MOSEGAARD [a,b], Peder HERBORG [b] and Thomas Sangild SØRENSEN [b]

[a] *Department of Computer Science, University of Aarhus, Denmark*
[b] *Centre for Advanced Visualization and Interaction, University of Aarhus, Denmark*

**Abstract.** There is a growing demand for surgical simulators to do fast and precise calculations of tissue deformation to simulate increasingly complex morphology in real-time. Unfortunately, even fast spring-mass based systems have slow convergence rates for large models. This paper presents a method to accelerate computation of a spring-mass system in order to simulate a complex organ such as the heart. This acceleration is achieved by taking advantage of modern graphics processing units (GPU).

## 1. Problem

In recent years simulators have been introduced in the surgical curriculum in several fields [1]. Many surgical simulators used in practice are based on spring-mass deformable models [2] due to performance reasons. The spring-mass model is considered physically based and achieves real-time visualization and fast convergence for geometry of moderate size.

In surgical simulation in general, there is a tradeoff between the costs of calculations, how realistic the tissue-deformation is reproduced, and how detailed the morphology being simulated appears. It is the goal of this paper to simulate a very high degree of morphological detail in real-time. As an example, the cardiac morphology is complex and requires a high degree of geometric detail to be modeled accurately.

We present a surgical simulator based on a spring-mass system accelerated by an implementation on the graphics processing unit (GPU). The purpose is to achieve a considerable speedup due to the parallel processing capabilities of the GPU [3]. This acceleration could be used to increase the accuracy and convergence of the numerical calculations and to increase the complexity of the simulated morphology. Previously, simple spring-mass systems have been implemented on the GPU (e.g. [4]). However, they were limited to simple shapes. Slow data transfer from the GPU to the CPU has been an additional bottleneck when handling interaction and visualization. With the recent generation of GPUs (Geforce 6800, Nvidia, USA) simulation, interaction, and visualization of a spring-mass based surgical simulator can be accelerated on the GPU. To our knowledge we present the first implementation of a fully GPU-based surgical simulator. The driving force behind the current research is the development of a virtual training system for complex interventions in congenitally malformed hearts [5,2], see Figure 1. The approach however, is general and can be applied to other organs directly.

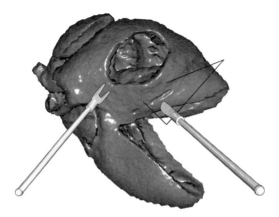

**Figure 1.** The Cardiac Surgery Simulator on a pig heart.

## 2. Methodology

### 2.1. Spring-Mass System

The GPU spring-mass implementation is based on the basic linear spring-mass formulation where each particle $x_i$ with mass $m_i$ is given by the following 2nd order differential equation:

$$m_i \ddot{x}_i = -y_i \dot{x}_i + \sum_j g_{ij} + f_i$$

where $y_i$ is the damping factor and $f_i$ is the external forces. $g_{ij}$ is the force vector defined by spring stiffness $k_{ij}$, spring rest length $l_{ij}$ and particle positions $x_i$ and $x_j$ as:

$$g_{ij} = \frac{1}{2} k_{ij} \left( l_{ij} - \|x_i - x_j\| \right) \frac{x_i - x_j}{\|x_i - x_j\|}$$

The differential equation can be solved with standard numerical methods, such as the verlet integration [6]:

$$x(t + h) = 2x(t) - x(t - h) + \ddot{x}(t)h^2$$

### 2.2. GPU Pipeline

The focus of this paper is to express the calculation of the spring-mass system effectively in terms of the hardware accelerated features of the GPU. Recently, the vertex processor and fragment processor have become programmable. Both processors are parallel processors with a number of pipelines working simultaneously. Vertex and fragment computation can depend on previous iterations through texture lookups and render-to-texture functionality exposed through Pixel Buffers (PBuffers). The PBuffer can be bound as the rendering target and as a texture. Throughout this paper we will refer to the PBuffer as a texture or as the rendering target interchangeably depending on the context. Using floating point texture extensions we can do computation on IEEE 32 bit floating point numbers. These features enable general purpose computation on the GPU.

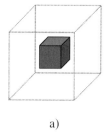
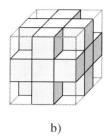

a)                                          b)

**Figure 2.** Particle connectivity in a 3D grid. Each particle a) is connected to 18 neighbors b) (blocking the black particle).

### 2.3. A Spring-Mass System with Implicit Connections

To calculate spring forces and perform verlet integration a fragment program was developed. The fragment processor was chosen as there are generally more fragment pipelines available than vertex pipelines. Equally important, texture lookups are more efficient in fragment programs. We associate the position of each particle with a single fragment in a PBuffer. The PBuffer is referred to as the *position-texture*. The fragment program is responsible for calculating forces affecting each particle, doing verlet integration, and outputting the calculated position to the associated fragment in the position-texture. Each fragment receives a texture coordinate as input, which gives the position of the associated particle through a texture lookup.

To calculate the forces affecting particles we need to fetch the position of neighboring particles connected through springs. The most important choice in our implementation and the major source of the performance we achieve is that we use only one texture lookup to obtain the position of each neighbor particle. The texture coordinates needed to lookup neighboring particles is given directly as input to the fragment program from the output of the vertex program. To avoid that the vertex processor becomes a bottleneck by rendering individual fragments as geometry, we conceptually invoke the fragment computation with a single quad covering the position-texture. Texture coordinates are specified for each vertex and interpolated automatically by the rasterizer before being received as input in the fragment programs. This means that particles must be connected in such a way that their neighbors can be fetched from per vertex interpolated texture-coordinates. That is, particles should be connected in a fixed pattern. We use a 3D grid as depicted in Figure 2 to construct a spring-mass system with eighteen springs constraining axis aligned changes as well as shearing.

The grid must be mapped to the two-dimensional position-texture to use the proposed approach. This is achieved through a derivation of the flat 3d-texture approach [7], see Figure 3. Each vertex rendered to invoke fragment computation will be given eighteen texture coordinates offset a fixed amount from the texture coordinates identifying the particle, see Figure 4. Instead of the conceptual model of rendering only one quad to invoke full fragment computation, it is necessary to render five quads with texture-coordinates constructed to take into account the border-cases of the flat 3d-texture approach.

After each iteration, the PBuffer that was rendered to is bound as a texture and used for input to subsequent iterations. The verlet integration depends on the previous two

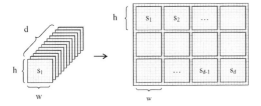

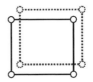

**Figure 3.** The flat 3d-texture approach. The 3D volume of voxels is mapped to a 2d texture by laying out each of the $d$ slices of size $h \cdot w$ in the 2d texture one after another. The slices are padded with elements containing unique alpha values of zero to detect the volume borders.

**Figure 4.** The solid box represents the quad drawn to invoke fragment processing. Solid spheres represent texture coordinates to the particles themselves. The dotted box and spheres represent one of the eighteen neighbors; the top left neighbor offset with texture coordinate $(1,-1)$ in comparison to the solid box.

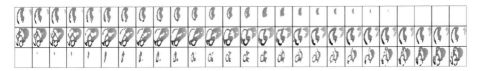

**Figure 5.** The position-texture of a 42.745 particle pig heart. White areas are grid points not associated with particles.

calculated positions; consequently we cycle three PBuffers containing the old, current and new positions.

As in [4] the geometry is connected in a regular grid. Unlike [4] however, we operate on a 3D grid. The grid must furthermore approximate an arbitrary geometry. Hence, it is necessary to exclude some of the particles in the grid. Conceptually we carve out the morphology in the grid of particles. Grid points are active particles in the simulation if inside the myocardium or a vessel wall and otherwise discarded with a depth-buffer based cull. See Figure 5 for an example.

## 2.4. Visualization and Interaction

To visualize the calculated positions we need to define vertex positions of a surface based on position-texture values. Since a large amount of grid-points are not associated to particles, a visualization based on vertex texture fetches is advantageous compared to a transfer of the entire position-texture to either the CPU or directly to a vertex buffer. Through vertex texture fetches we transfer only particles that are part of the surface of the mesh. The geometry specified to the 3D API to visualize the current simulation-step is a static mesh where each vertex is associated to a particle through a per vertex specified texture coordinate. Through texture lookups in the vertex program we can fetch the current position of the particle. We hereby defined a mapping from one surface vertex of the visualization to one particle on the surface of the spring-mass system.

The vertex-normal (indicating the curvature of the surface) to be used for shading is approximated by the normalized sum of all normalized vectors from particle neighbors to the particle in question. This value is already calculated as part of the force computation, packed into the position-texture as the alpha component.

To handle grabbing, the collision detection is done on the CPU based on a single read-back of the position-texture when grabbing is initiated. Subsequently we render the position of grabbed particles, based on the interaction device, as geometric primitives directly into the fragments corresponding to the grabbed particles. We hereby override the simulation results.

The collision detection for cutting is also done on the CPU based on a single read-back of the position-texture. As a result of cutting, we furthermore need to change the static mesh rendered for visualization. Because the connectivity between particles is implicitly based on their location in the position texture, the smallest incision possible in the proposed model is two springs wide – by removing a particle. To support incisions as small as a single spring, we extend the proposed model. If a spring is erased, we will setup the invocation of fragment computation so that the connected particles receive invalid texture coordinates for that spring whereby the spring is considered non-existing in the fragment program doing the spring-mass computations. This means that we need to render additional geometric primitives for each particle that is missing springs. The added granularity comes at the cost of performance because additional vertex processing and fragment processing is necessary – this approach is advantageous when we only make small cuts in the morphology.

## 2.5. Hardware and Test-case

A Gainward CoolFX Ultra/2600 graphics card in a Pentium 4 3 GHz was used for the presented simulation and visualization. A detailed (630.000 faces) model of a pig heart was reconstructed from a CT dataset using the marching cubes algorithm [8]. Additionally, a model with lower resolution (42.745 grid points) was obtained. The spring-mass simulation was performed on the latter which was normal-mapped to visually appear as detailed as the higher resolution model (Melody, Nvidia, USA).

## 3. Results

The GPU spring-mass system was implemented in OpenGL, C++, Cg, NV_fragment_program2and NV_vertex_program3 and compiled with Visual Studio C++. As a comparison for the GPU implementation a CPU implementation was implemented in C++ and compiled in Visual Studio C++. The CPU spring-mass system is a port of the GPU implementation. The resulting performances can be seen in Table 1.

We have extended the Cardiac Surgical Simulator [2] to support GPU based spring-mass systems. A real-time system simulating and visualizing the deformable heart was implemented. Screenshots are seen in Figure 6. In a setup where we do six iterations before visualizing, the simulation runs at 192 iterations per second and 32 frames visualized per second. The simulation step alone could be run at 219 iterations per second.

## 4. Discussion and Conclusion

We successfully expressed the spring-mass model in terms of the GPU. This is seen from Table 1 as a noticeable speedup compared to a similar CPU implementation. This speedup can be used to model and simulate morphology with a larger number of primitives than previously seen as well as faster numerical calculations. An added geometrical detail is expected to more accurately simulate complex organs such as the heart.

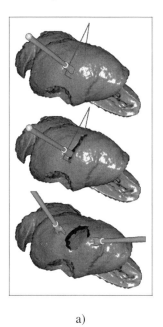
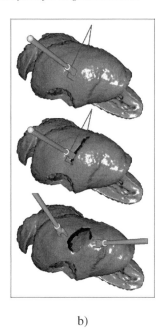

a)                                                          b)

**Figure 6.** A pig heart consisting of 42.745 particles in a regular grid reconstructed from a CT data set. We illustrate a) cutting and b) deformation by grabbing.

**Table 1.** Iterations per second (excluding visualization) with the CPU spring-mass and GPU spring-mass implementations.

| Nodes \ Method | CPU | GPU | GPU / CPU speedup |
|---|---|---|---|
| 10.000 | 45,8 | 839,8 | 18,7 |
| 20.000 | 20,2 | 476,9 | 23,6 |
| 40.000 | 9,9 | 264,6 | 26,9 |
| 50.000 | 7,8 | 218,0 | 28,1 |
| 100.000 | 3,3 | 104,1 | 31,4 |

In the past decade, GPU performance growth has exceeded that of the CPU [9]. This is expected to extrapolate well into the future. Hence the acceleration factor is expected to grow correspondingly.

With a CPU based simulation it is a potential bottleneck to visualize particle-positions since this requires a transfer of vertex attributes each frame. Visualization of the GPU based solution has the advantage that the surface-mesh is cached in video memory since there are no CPU based changes.

If we consider a standard spring-mass implementation, there are many improvements that can accelerate the simulation on the CPU. These might, however, not be easily ported to the GPU. Hence, the presented speedup is not to be interpreted as a speedup compared to the fastest CPU implementation available.

In cases where the spring-mass model is not considered adequate, other physically based models of deformation could be ported to the GPU following the principles of this paper.

## 5. Future Work

The current visualization is based on a mapping from one surface particle of the simulation to one surface vertex of the visualization. A more flexible mapping would enable us to decouple the details of visualization and simulation. This would enable a smoother appearance of the proposed spring mass implementation.

Future work should also include studies on how the GPU and CPU can work more closely together. In the presented solution, the CPU is not utilized efficiently because the transfer of data from the GPU to the CPU becomes a bottleneck. When this communication becomes faster (i.e. through PCI-express), we must consider what kind of processing is suitable for the GPU and CPU.

The clinical significance of the added morphological detail as well as clinical use of the Cardiac Surgery Simulator will be examined.

## Acknowledgements

We acknowledge pediatric heart surgeons Vibeke Hjortdal and Ole Kromann Hansen for their clinical feedback. For the data acquisition we acknowledge the contributions of Dr. Gerald Greil and Dr. Axel Kuettner, University of Tübingen, Germany as well as Dr. T. Flohr and Dr. I. Wolf.

## References

[1] Richard M. Satava. *Accomplishments and challenges of surgical simulation*. Surg Endosc;, 15(3), pp 232-41, 2001.

[2] Jesper Mosegaard. *LR-spring-mass model for cardiac surgical simulation*. Medicine Meets Virtual Reality 12, pp 256-258, 2003.

[3] Chris J. Thompson, Sahngyun Hahn and Mark Oskin. *Using modern graphics architectures for general-purpose computing: a framework and analysis*. Proceedings of the 35th annual ACM/IEEE international symposium on Microarchitecture., pp 306—317, 2002.

[4] Simon Green. *OpenGL Shader Tricks*. Game Developers Conference, 2003.

[5] Thomas S. Sørensen, Erik M. Pedersen, Ole K. Hansen, Keld Sørensen. *Visualization of morphological details in congenitally malformed hearts*. Cardiol Young; 13(5), pp 451-60, 2003.

[6] Loup Verlet. *Computer Experiments on Classical Fluids. I. Thermodynamical. Properties of Lennard-Jones Molecules*. Physical Review, Vol. 159, pp 98–103, 1967.

[7] Mark J. Harris, William V. Baxter III, Thorsten Scheuermann and Anselmo Lastra. *Simulation of Cloud Dynamics on Graphics Hardware*. Proceedings of Graphics Hardware, pp 92-101, 2003.

[8] William E. Lorensen and Harvey E. Cline. *Marching Cubes: A High Resolution 3D Surface Construction Algorithm*, Computer Graphics (Proceedings of SIGGRAPH '87), Vol. 21, No. 4, pp. 163-169, 1987.

[9] Buck I, Purcell T. A toolkit for computation on GPUs. GPU Gems. Addison Wesley 2004.

*Medicine Meets Virtual Reality 13*
*James D. Westwood et al. (Eds.)*
*IOS Press, 2005*

# Interactive 3D Region Extraction of Volume Data Using Deformable Boundary Object

Megumi NAKAO [a], Takakazu WATANABE [b], Tomohiro KURODA [a]
and Hiroyuki YOSHIHARA [a]

[a] *Dept. of Medical Informatics, Kyoto University Hospital, Japan*
[b] *Graduate School of Informatics, Kyoto University, Japan*

**Abstract.** This study aims to establish an interactive and intuitive region extraction environment for volume data. A volume clipping method using deformable boundary object is proposed to support 3D region extraction task. Slice-based volume rendering of boundary elements enables to visualize clipped results in real time. Geometrical transformation and physic-based deformation support intuitive modification of 3D region of interest. Some extraction tasks are tested using CT dataset on the developed system. All tests confirmed real-time visualization of clipped results is effective for interactive 3D region extraction in volume visualization and virtual object modeling.

## 1. Introduction

3D region extraction or clipping [1] is frequently utilized for volume visualization and anatomical model construction. For computer aided diagnosis and virtual object modeling in surgical simulation, medical doctors and researchers eager to extract 3D region of interest flexibly and interactively. In order to extract anatomical structure of organs, a large number of algorithmic approaches [2] have been proposed. However, the foregoing approaches cannot always work properly (e.g. anomalous organs). Interactive modification of 3D region may increase applicability of conventional volume visualization and algorithmic segmentation. To support interactive edit of voxels, advanced interaction interface 3D with volume visualization is indispensable.

This study aims to establish interactive extraction environment of arbitrary 3D region for volume data. A novel volume clipping method using 3D geometry data is proposed. This paper reports outline of the proposed methods and extraction results from several medical images measured from CT.

## 2. 3D Interactive Extraction for Volume Data

The proposed environment supports users (1) to extract while checking extracted results and (2) to set and modify free 3D extracted region interactively. 3D definite closed re-

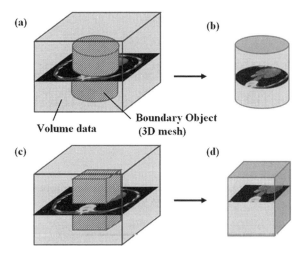

**Figure 1.** Outline of interactive extraction: (a) cylinder-shaped boundary object defined on volume data, (b) extracted volume, (c) the shape of boundary object is changed and (d) different extracted result is immediately visualized.

gion is formed using a volumetric 3D boundary object. Interactive manipulation of the geometrical object enables to set or modify visible area while observing extracted region of interest. Labeling all voxels inside the assigned 3D region performs region extraction or segmentation of anatomical organs from medical images.

General geometry format like tetrahedral grid is available as the boundary. Extracted results are visualized in real time by slice-based volume rendering with volume clipping method. Also, the environment enables users to set and modify 3D position and shape of the object through graphical and haptic interface.

Fig. 1 shows outline of the proposed interactive extraction method. Firstly, volumetric dataset of human body is visualized. (Fig. 1 (a)) A boundary object which consists of tetrahedral grid extracts 3D region from volume data, and extracted area is visualized by volume clipping and rendering (Fig 1. (b)). Then, the user can modify the boundary by changing 3D shape and size of the grid. (Fig 1. (c) (d))

In order to realize this concept on standard PCs, the following requirements are to be satisfied. This study developed some key techniques to solve these issues.

### 1) Real-time voxel clipping and volume visualization

The proposed method enables flexible clip using 3D boundary object. Because general volumetric mesh (e.g. tetrahedra) is available as the boundary, voxel data can be extracted by any 3D shape. Although the number of available clip planes has been limited for achieving real-time performance, our new approach combining 3D texture and geometry performs high speed visualization on standard PC while handling complex boundaries.

### 2) Interactive adaptation of the boundary object

For modifying extracted region, an interface to manipulate the boundary is provided. Geometrical transformation and physic-based deformation algorithms support intuitive

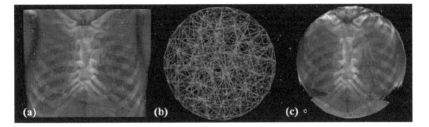

**Figure 2.** Volume clipping using sphere-shaped boundary object: (a) full volume, (b) spehere-shaped boundary and (c) extracted volume.

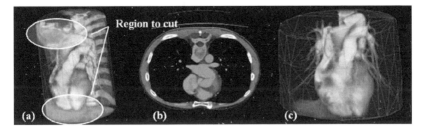

**Figure 3.** Fitting visible region by scaling and deforming cylinder-shaped boundary: (a) extracted volume by cylinder-shaped boundary, (b) selected region on 2D image and (c) interactive modification of 3D visible region.

manipulation of the grids. Specifically, curved surface based grid control method is developed for fitting the boundary into 3D shapes of organs.

## 3. Results

$256 \times 256 \times 256$ CT dataset were applied to the developed system. Fig 2 shows real-time visualization result of the extracted area clipped by spherical mesh. Fig 3 demonstrates interactive adaptation of the boundary. The initial cylindrical boundary in Fig 3 (a) covers surrounded voxels which are to be eliminated in observing or modeling heart. Changing scale and FEM-based deformation of the boundary efficiently eliminates such needless voxels. (Fig 3 (c)) This extraction task was achieved within 10 seconds. Real-time visual feedback of the extracted results efficiently supported fitting operation.

## 4. Conclusion

The proposed real-time voxel clipping method using deformable boundary mesh efficiently supports interactive region extraction while observing extracted results. All results confirmed real-time visualization of clipped results is effective for interactive 3D region extraction in volume visualization and virtual object modeling.

## Acknowledgements

This research is supported by Grant-in-Aid for Scientific Research (S)(16100001) and Young Scientists (A) (16680024) from The Ministry of Education, Culture, Sports, Science and Technology, Japan. This study is also supported by COE (Center of Excellence) program of JSPS (Japan Society for the Promotion of Science) "Establishment of International COE for Integration of Transplantation Therapy and Regenerative Medicine".

## References

[1]  D. Weiskopf, K. Engel and T. Ertl, "Interactive Clipping Techniques for Texture-Based Volume Visualization and Volume Shading", IEEE Trans. on Visualization and Computer Graphics, Vol. 9, No. 3, pp. 298-312, 2003.
[2]  Advanced Algorithmic Approaches to Medical Image Segmentation, Suri, Jasjit S., Kamaledin Setarehdan, S., Singh, Sameer (Eds.), ISBN: 1-85233-389-8, 2002

*Medicine Meets Virtual Reality 13*
*James D. Westwood et al. (Eds.)*
*IOS Press, 2005*

# Virtual Surgical Telesimulations in Otolaryngology

Andrés A. NAVARRO NEWBALL, MSc [a,b], Carlos J. HERNÁNDEZ C, BEng [c],
Jorge A. VELEZ B, MD [d], Luis E. MUNERA S, PhD [e], Gregorio B. GARCÍA, PhD [f],
Carlos A. GAMBOA, MD [g] and Antonio J. REYES, MD [h]

[a] *Pontificia Universidad Javeriana,Cll 18 # 118 -250, Cali, Colombia*
[b] *Colombian Telemedicine Center, Cr 103 #12C 50, I3, Cali, Colombia*
[c] *Pontificia Universidad Javeriana, Cali, Colombia*
[d] *Colombian Telemedicine Center, Cali, Colombia*
[e] *Universidad Icesi, Cali, Colombia*
[f] *DITEC, Universidad de Murcia, Spain*
[g] *Colombian Telemedicine Center, Cali, Colombia*
[h] *Colombian Telemedicina Center, Cali, Colombia*

**Abstract.** Distance learning can be enhanced with the use of virtual reality; this paper describes the design and initial validation of a Web Environment for Surgery Skills Training on Otolaryngology (WESST-OT). WESST-OT was created aimed to help trainees to gain the skills required in order to perform the Functional Endoscopic Sinus Surgery procedure (FESS), since training centers and specialist in this knowledge are scarce in Colombia; also, it is part of a web based educational cycle which simulates the stages of a real procedure. WESST-OT is one from the WESST family of telesimulators which started to be developed from an architecture proposed at the Medicine Meets Virtual Reality conference 2002; also, it is a step towards the use of virtual reality technologies in Latin America.

## 1. Introduction

During the last two decades the usefulness of virtual reality in medicine has been evidenced [1]; actually, many simulators successfully run and help in surgery training, some of these are aimed to train particular skills [2], others, are aimed to simulate a whole surgical process [3]; however, most of the developments are still costly, run on a stand alone computer and do not serve the Latin American region; in contrast, some groups have developed simulators which are capable to run on communication networks [4].

The Colombian Telemedicine Center is the first group that has developed a set of prototype telesimulators aimed to serve Latin America via Internet [5,6]; here, inspired on experiences on virtual reality and medicine at the University of Hull in 1997 [7] and on the need of medical knowledge diffusion with telemedicine technologies, an architecture was proposed at the Medicine Meets Virtual Reality Conference 2002 [8]; later, this architecture was evolved and tested with a prototype telesimulator on ophthalmology (WESST-OP) [6] and WESST-OT was created aimed to help trainees to gain the skills required in order to perform the FESS procedure [9].

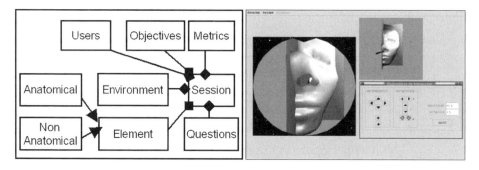

**Figure 1.** Left. WESST-OT's Architecture. Right. WESST-OT's Environment.

## 2. Method

WESST-OT was developed by an interdisciplinary team following an object oriented software development methodology; here, otolaryngologists helped to define the most important skills to be represented and the information to be presented to the trainees; meanwhile, computer scientists abstracted and implemented WESST-OT in the JAVA programming language; also, the development of the project required a close interaction with research groups at the universities Javeriana and Icesi in Colombia and Murcia in Spain. At the end, a testing plan aimed to validate the system and measure its performance was developed and executed. Today, a validation process in a Latin American network is about to start [10].

## 3. Results

For the fist version of WESST-OT, the orientation skill was chosen for implementation, since it was considered the basic one. Figure 1 shows the WESST-OT's architecture to the left; here, the session class abstracts a real practice session; the environment class abstracts a real practice environment and it is related to anatomical and non anatomical elements, which are part of the FESS surgical procedure and are also abstracted as classes; the metrics class represents the measurement of the practitioner's performance; additionally, the users class allows administrative and trainee users, the questions class displays questions inside the simulation and, the objectives class abstracts the objectives of the practice.

The WESST-OT's environment is shown in figure 1 to the right; it consists of two views, an anatomical view serves as an educational aid and an endoscopic view simulates the real procedure; also, it counts with two levels, the beginners' level allows training and the advanced level provides objective evaluation for the trainee. Complementarily, an educational cycle has been implemented; it starts confronting the practitioner with a web expert decision support system which suggests the need for surgery; if surgery is required a surgical planning instrument is presented; then, a video about the procedure is transmitted and finally, the telesimulator runs.

The performance measures of WESST-OT give average times of 10 minutes in order to download the simulator from the Internet connected at 56 kilobits per second; also, the number of frames per second using a 1.6 GHZ Pentium IV with 256 RAM using LINUX

**Table 1.** WESST-OT's preliminary validation.

| Factor | Easy to access | Performance | Realism | Friendly | Potential | **Average** |
|--------|---------------|-------------|---------|----------|-----------|-------------|
| **Degree** | 5 | 4,3 | 3,7 | 4,7 | 5 | **4,54** |

is 8,972 and using Windows XP is 38,841. The table 1 shows the qualifications obtained during the initial validation among a group of ten medical doctors; here, 1 is the lowest degree and 5 is the highest.

## 4. Discussion

Surgical telesimulation is possible and it can be part of a whole educational cycle. WESST-OT is one of the first telesimulators in Latin America and, it may help to make specialized medical knowledge more accessible. Actually, a preliminary validation of WESST-OT shows a high level of acceptance by specialists and good performance of the system was evident from the performance tests.

In contrast, the implemented skill (orientation) is good, but not enough for a FESS procedure; actually, skills like coordination and spatial location are under construction and, the degree of realism of WESST-OT is being improved; at the same time, the telesimulator is being complemented by the use of 2D scanographic images which will enhance learning

Finally, the successful deployment of telesimulation in the Latin American region requires continuing interdisciplinary and interinstitutional work; also, a Latin American network of telemedicine teams can help to promote distance learning in the field and to validate telesimulators.

## References

[1] Robb RA. The virtualization of medicine: a decade of pitfalls and progress. *Studies in health technology and informatics* **2002**;85:1–7.

[2] Payandeh S, Lomax AJ, Dill J, Mackenzie CL, Cao CGL. On defining metrics for assessing laparoscopic surgical skills in a virtual training environment. *Studies in health technology and informatics* **2002**;85:334–340.

[3] Wills DPM, Abblard E, Sherman KP. A generic arthroscopy simulator architecture. *Studies in health technology and informatics* **2002**;85:573–579.

[4] Alverson D, Kalishman S, Jacobs J, Saland L, Caudell T, Saiki S. Interactive virtual reality in distance medical education. *Telemedicine journal and ehealth* **2004**;10: S43.

[5] Navarro Newball AA, Hernández CJ, Vélez JA, Múnera LE, García GB. A virtual telesimulation scenario for otolaryngologic surgery skills training. *Telemedicine journal and ehealth* **2004**;10: S71.

[6] Navarro Newball AA, Vélez JA, Satizabal JE, Múnera LE, Bernabé G. Virtual surgical telesimulations in ophtalmology. *International congress series* **2003**;1256:145–150.

[7] Navarro Newball AA. *The implementation of a windows 95 based virtual environments knee arthroscopy training system (PC VEKATS)*, MSc dissertation, University of Hull, **1997**.

[8] Navarro Newball AA, Vélez B JA, Múnera LE. A software architecture for virtual simulation of endoscopic surgery in a web based scenario. *The 10th annual Medicine Meets Virtual Reality Conference. Course Syllabus* **2002**; 116–117.

[9] Hernández CJ. *Análisis, diseño e implementación del prototipo de un entorno de práctica de habilidades quirúrgicas en otorrinolaringología.* Undergraduate dissertation, Pontificia Universidad Javeriana, **2003**.

[10] Vélez JA, Navarro Newball AA, Múnera LE, Kopec A, García GB. Methodological basis for distributed web testing of surgical simulators prototypes in a telemedicine Latin America Network (TLAN). *Telemedicine journal and ehealth* **2004**;10: S116.

*Medicine Meets Virtual Reality 13*
*James D. Westwood et al. (Eds.)*
*IOS Press, 2005*

# Emerging Technologies for Bioweapons Defense

Sinh NGUYEN, Joseph M. ROSEN M.D. and C. EVERETT KOOP M.D.

**Abstract.** The Global War on Terrorism (GWOT) has changed the way we think about national security. The tragic events of Sept.11 have shown us that world of the 21$^{st}$ century is clearly a dangerous place. Terrorism, more than ever, affects the very lives of each and every citizens of our country Al Qaida has proven that it is able to use simple rudimentary methods to invoke strategic economic losses to our society with our own domestic resources as its weapons. The dawn of the new century has brought forth a new kind of asymmetric war where guerilla fighters are armed not with rifles but with technology at the touch of a keyboard. Warfare as we know it has changed and just as the military has its "transformation", medicine so too must have its own transformation in order to protect our citizen against the ever changing threat of bioterrorism. Virtual Reality and its applications can play a vital role in developing new countermeasures to minimize the catastrophic effects of a potential bioterror attack.

## Background

The collapse of the Soviet system in 1991 left the United States as the only superpower and it unfortunately also created a huge power vacuum in many areas of the world especially the Middle East were Islamic fundamentalism is now taking hold. It is ironic to note that we helped foster these sentiments in the 80's a bulwark against the leftist socialism engendered by the Soviet in the region. In our common struggle against the Soviet aggression in Afghanistan, we have trained the freedom fighters that fought a guerrilla war against the Soviets until their withdrawal in 1989. The enemy of my enemy is my friend indeed. Fueled by the riches of oil and freed of the iron shackles of the Soviet menace, the Islamic fundamentalist sought recognition for their cause and has now focused these actions against the US hegemony, the only superpower left. Moreover, emboldened by there success against Soviet and armed in the latest technology taught to them by our advisors, they seek to fight a net-centric guerrilla war against the very United States of America that helped train and armed them. They are no doubt highly successful as seen with their success in the 9/11 attack. The Global War on Terrorism is not a different type of war. Rather, it is a natural evolution of conflict in the 21$^{st}$ century. Our adversaries understanding full well that they cannot do battle with us vis a vis choose to strike at us strategically using the element of surprise to do the utmost damage to our economic and social wellbeing. Terrorism imposes to strike fear in the civilian masses hoping to change the political climate from within the enemy. The war of the future will not be won on the battlefield but in the hearts and minds of the people. A clear example of this is the collapse of the Soviet Empire. It broke up from within not because in defect in ideology but because it could no longer sustain the economic stress to its system inflicted upon itself from the intense competition during with the Reagan Era military buildup [1]. Lest we forget our lessons of history, the TET offensive in 1968 during the Vietnam War although a tactical failure on the battlefield was hugely successful strategically as it solidified the anti-war movement domestically forcing Kissinger initiate talks with North Vietnam which eventually led to the withdrawal of US forces from the Vietnam in 1972. The planners of the 9/11 attack having learned their history sought emulate these practices to force the withdrawal of US troops from the Middle East theatre.

## Biothreat

The CDC has classified Anthrax, Botulinium Toxin, Plague, Small Pox, Tularemia, and hemorrhagic fever as potential bioweapons that could be used against the Continental United States (CONUS). This is in part due because of our past experiences with these agents as part of our biological weapons program at Ft. Detrick, Maryland. We discontinued our research and stockpiling of these weapons after signing the Biological Weapons Convention in 1972 [2]. These agents were also developed by our counterparts the Soviet Union during the Cold War mainly to potentially serve as tactical weapons on the conventional battlefield because as a weapon, they were cheap to manufacture and could inflict heavy casualty upon opposing forces with minimal losses on friendly forces because of prior vaccination. The Anthrax scare in October 2001 shortly after 9/11 in which Senator Daschle and other prominent figures were targeted caused renewed fear among the populace of a possible bioterror attack in CONUS. In the general media hysteria following the scare, the mindset of the CDC as well as the general population has focused more intensely on these agents as possible weapons of choice for a future bioattack and they have directed viable resources to develop countermeasures against them. The focus on these agents is perhaps to narrow of a view for any future bioattack. Our prospective must be broadened less we forget the lessons learned from our "failure of imagination" in of the attacks of 9/11 for we might repeat them [3]. Keep in mind that terrorist groups such as Al-Qaida act strategically and the weapon of choice is terror. They want to possess the means to serve a political end. Thus our paradigm of potential bioweapons should be redefined and we should think more non-linearly and asymmetrically as to others agents that could be possibly used as bioweapons.

    The SARS pandemic in 2003 is an example a virus that could possibly used as a future bioweapon. The epidemic initially began in early November 2002 in southern China and by July 31, 2003, it was spread to 29 countries with a total of 8096 confirm cases resulting in 774 total deaths [4]. The negative economic impact felt by the countries affected were devastating as quarantine procedure and travel restrictions were put in place to limit the spread of the infection. The World Bank even lowered the GDP growth rate of East Asia by O.5% bringing the estimated economic loss to about 20-30 billion USD [5]. In dealing with the virus, the fragile healthcare systems of the countries affected were inundated with people seeking medical attention some real others imagined stretching the limits of the public health system. In Toronto alone, the healthcare infrastructure was overwhelmed with 251 cases, 43 deaths with 27,000 healthcare workers needing quarantine [6]. The SARS outbreak has taught us that public health is a now a global concern with economic effects ever far reaching as the world is more interconnected by globalization. Clearly the SARS epidemic has tested our paradigm of a potential bioweapon.

## Emergency Medical Response

The Presidential Directive 39 set forth guidelines under the Federal Response Plan for dealing with emergency response in the case of an act of bioterrorism. In such an event, the FBI is designated the federal lead agency in charged of crisis management and FEMA will act as the consequence management. The medical response is directed under the Emergency Support Function #8 of the Federal Response Plan which assigns the National Disaster Medical System in coordinating the relief effort under the management of FEMA [7]. NDMS was created in the mid 80's to serve the purpose of supplementing the state and local relief effort during natural disaster and major emergency. Its also serves as a dual purpose as a DOD/VA backup in case of an overseas emergency where mass casualties has overwhelmed the federal system. The currently system has not really been tested for a major medical response to a bioterror attack and if recent mock exercises of TOPOFF and Dark Winter are any indication, the system as it stands now is inadequate to respond to major medical disaster presented by a bioterror attack [8].

Post 9/11, the President on February 28, 2003 issued the Homeland security presidential directive HSPD-5 which directs the Secretary of Homeland Security to administer a National Incident Management System to streamline the response system to better coordinate the relief effort in case of a national disaster learning from the mistakes of 9/11 [9]. However the medical response under NDMS has remained relatively unchanged.

## Revolution

Now more than ever, the healthcare infrastructure needs to change in order to meet the challenges for the medical disasters of the future, be it natural or man made. Our current healthcare system is geared more towards treating chronic diseases of the elderly and is not well equipped to deal with natural disaster especially the one involving biological weapons. There needs to be a transformation in the medical infrastructure similar to the Revolution in Military Affairs by the Department of Defense [10]. There is a need to incorporate the latest technology using net-centric platforms to revolutionize the way we administer care in times of peace as well as in times of war. The NDMS needs to shifts it paradigm from a pyramidal centralized command and control structure to one that is more net-centric and decentralized one in order to respond to emerging medical threats of the 21$^{st}$ century. Information should be made on demand and pertinent distributed seamlessly in real time through secure networks. Clearly current technologies exist to leverage this transformation to create the National Disaster Response system of the future.

## Biosurveillance

Monitoring the health of the population is a critical public health activity to ensure awareness of emerging threats. There are number of current projects underway that are collecting data for detection of potential biological attacks. The CDC is developing a program called BioSense to serve as a "syndromic" surveillance model monitoring CD9 diagnosis, OTC sales of health remedies, lab test order and nurse's calls and analyze them with complex algorithms for early detection. DARPA has a similar syndromic project code named BioALIRT that possesses similar attributes [11]. These data could in turned be further analyzed using Virtual Reality Geographical Imaging Systems (VRGIS) to better visualize patterns of infection. One such effort is project BioSTORM of Stanford University [12]. They are developing computer models using spatial interpolation, data fusion, and cluster detection to better understand illness behaviors and epidemics. This would enable epidemiologist to see patterns using 3-D visualization of 2D data to better develop plans for effective countermeasures. In addition to clinical "syndromic" data, the ideal surveillance system would also integrate data from autonomous biosensors placed at strategic site for detection of biological vectors. The Department of Homeland Security (DHS) project BIOWATCH, collaboration between the EPA and CDC, has environmental biosensors that are strategically placed in over 30 cities monitor chemical and biological threats [13]. MIT Lincoln Labs is aiding such efforts with the development a genetically engineered biosensor called CANARY (Cellular Analysis and Notification of Risks and Yields) that could possibly be used to detect emerging infectious pathogens such as West Nile Virus, BSE and SARS [14]. Effective biosurveillance is definitely possible with current technology but what is more important is what we do with the information once collected.

## Clinical Assessment, Mitigation, Classification

Real time clinical assessment of ongoing infections in the field is essential to developing an effective response to a biological threat. First responders could be equipped wireless portable analyzer with DNA chip technology (Nanogen Inc.) to screen out affected population quickly and transmit such information to a central location for analysis [15]. Another prospective technology for field assessment is the use of Laser Induce Breakdown Spectroscopy (LIBS) technology to non-invasively scan for biomarkers of infectious disease [16]. These clinical assessment technologies could be incorporated on to handheld devices connected to wireless networks for real time data distribution and retrieval. These handhelds (PDAs) could be loaded with decision aid software to help the first responder deal with the emergency systematically. For example, ADASHI first responder system provides an ideal software aid for rapid identification of biological agents, on demand operation procedures and checklist, action documentation, and incidents mapping [17]. Such systems will help responders be more efficient in disaster setting providing guidance when time is of the essence.

## Quarantine and crowd controls

In the event of a bioterror attack, the setup of quarantine is necessary to isolate the disaster site in order to effectively administer support to those affect and to mitigate the spread of the agents and to establish some means of control in an otherwise disorderly chaotic situation. Radio Frequency ID (RFIDs) a popular technology with retailers such as Walmart is ideal for helping in such an environment. These tags could be place on the medical responders and affected individuals to monitor their location and track their movements. Pinpoint locations of each person could be map on a VRGIS system in order to set limits to quarantine. Audible sensors could be place on the perimeters to notify any unidentified person infringing on or out of the quarantine area. RFID technology could also track "super spreader" to ensure that they are isolated from the rest of the population and led towards to special de-containment if necessary. RFID tags could also store personal biometric, procedure, treatment for later analysis at the Incident Command (IC).

## Command and Control

Managing disaster caused by bioweapons require the manager to process complex information simultaneously in order to make effective decision at the IC. DARPA has developed ENCOMPASS (Enhanced Consequence Management Planning and Support System) as a web based software tool for effective medical surveillance for medical disaster and crisis event [18]. It has two subsystem 1) Incident Command Management System (ICMS) which function as incident commander 2) DARPA syndromic surveillance system (D-S3) that offer biosurveillance and tracks patients signs and symptoms. DARPA is leveraging it military technology in its Command Post of the Future creating an integrated biodefense system for homeland security.

## Emergency Planning and Training

Preparation and training for a future biological event is vital to mitigating its effects. This is where the application of Virtual Reality has the most immediate and potential benefits. Virtual Reality simulation and training allows medical responders to learn procedural skills necessary to treat mass casualties. One such system is BiosimMer developed by Sandia National Labs [19]. It provides first responder an opportunity to hone there skills in treating virtual patients of biological disaster allowing them to make better decision if ever needed in a real attack. Eon Reality Inc., a developer of virtual reality systems, is teaming up with 10 universities to develop Virtual Homeland Defense Center Networks to provide web base Virtual Reality training on a wide variety of CBRNE events across multiple locations [20]. Another system, Virtual Emergency Training System (VERTS) developed by Unitech allows for crisis management simulation in its Emergency Operation Command Center so that first responders can have ability to manage an EOC and see how their decision affects the final outcome of the disaster [21]. Virtual Reality is an emerging technology and its application to homeland defense is relatively new but it has great potential as a low cost method of training medical responder to bioterror threat.

## Conclusion

The Global War on Terrorism has forced us to reconsider and reassess our current medical response system in order to be more prepared for an uncertain future. The potential for a major medical disaster is no longer unthinkable but a reality that must be dealt with immediately if we are going to be successful in mitigating the effects of a major bioterror attack from an asymmetric enemy. We must change or face the possibility of another attack like 9/11 and live to regret the fact that we did not fully prepare given our awareness of the threat. Let us not have another "failure of imagination".

# References

[1]  Lefcowitz, M. Homeland Defense: Avoiding the Bear Trap, Journal of Homeland Security, June 2002.
[2]  U.S. Congress, Office of Technology Assessment, Proliferation of Weapons of Mass Destruction: Assessing the Risk, OTA-ISC-559, U.S. Government Printing Office, August 1993.
[3]  The National Commission on Terrorist Attacks Upon the United States, The 9/11 Report, St. Martin Press, New York, 2004.
[4]  WHO SARS probable case report November 1, 2002-July 31 2003
      http://www.who.int/csr/sars/country/table2004_04_21/en/.
[5]  "World Bank Responds to SARS" June 4, 2003 http://web.worldbank.org/WBSITE/EXTERNAL/NEWS.
[6]  Svoboda T, Henry B. Shulman et al, Public health measures to control the spread of severe acute respiratory disease syndrome in Toronto, NEJM, 2004:350:2352-2361.
[7]  PPD-39, Http://www.fas.ort/irp/offdocs/pdd/index.html.
[8]  Thomas Inglesby, et al, A plague on our City: Observation from TOPOFF, Clinical Infectious Disease, 2001:32; 436-435.
[9]  Department of Homeland Security, NIMS, March 1, 2004.
[10] Office of Force Transformation, http://oft.osd.mil.
[11] Henry R. Rolka, Overview of Syndromic Surveillance presentation, CDC Feb. 19, 2004
      http://dimacs.rutgers.edu/Workshops/AdverseEvent2/slides/rolka.ppt.
[12] BIOSTORM project, http://smi-web.stanford.edu/projects/biostorm/index.htm.
[13] BioWatch powerpoint presentation, http://www.health.ri.gov/disease/communicable/epi/256,1,BioWatch.
[14] Innovative Biosensors Inc company profile, www.bio.org/midamerica/present/pdfs/Innovative.pdf.
[15] Nanogen Inc., www.nanogen.com.
[16] David W. Hahn et al, Laser Induced Breakdown Spectroscopy: An introduction to the feature issue, Applied Optics, 42:30:5937.
[17] ADASHI : automated decision aids, www.adashi.org.
[18] Advanced Consequence Management, http://www.darpa.mil/dso/trans/acm.htm.
[19] John German, "Virtual Reality training tool pits rescue against computerized terrorist attacks", http://www.sandia.gov/LabNews/LN07-30-99/vr_story.html.
[20] EON Security Solutions, http://www.eonreality.com/industry/defense/homeland_security_solution.htm.
[21] Sandra Erwin, "Virtual Metropolis Underpins Emergency Response Trainer", November 2001, http://nationaldefense.ndia.org/article.cfm?Id=639.

*Medicine Meets Virtual Reality 13*
*James D. Westwood et al. (Eds.)*
*IOS Press, 2005*

# Assessment of Brain Activities in Immersive Environments

Max M. NORTH Ph.D., Sarah M. NORTH Ed.D., John CRUNK, S.E.
and Jeff SINGLETON, R.A.

*Virtual Reality Technology Laboratory, Computer Science and Information Systems,*
*Kennesaw State University*
*e-mail: Max@acm.org; url: www.vrt1.com*

**Abstract.** The primary goal of this study was to establish an objective baseline for subjects who participated in a study in an immersed environment created for the virtual reality therapy (VRT) situation. Since the effects of VRT on the subjects treated for neurosis have traditionally been measured by subjective measurements, there is a need to include objective measures. This will improve and validate the effectiveness of VRT. Fifteen college students participated in this study. Specifically, the researchers measured the activity of the subjects' brainwaves in response to the VRT using EEG technology. The preliminary data indicated that, in most cases, subjects had a decline in brain wave activity between what is deemed a normal / baseline brain activity and the brainwave activity recorded when they were when they were connected to the virtual reality equipment and under influence of an immersive scene. In rare instances, there were some subjects that showed extreme increases in brain activities. In addition, the data indicated that, in most cases, subjects are more relaxed while under the immersive influence with respect to brain activities than those that are not.

## 1. Introduction

Some type of phobia is reported in most people to some extent today. These phobias range from manageable to extreme and in most cases only cause mild discomfort. Some though experience more severe often uncontrollable fears that must be treated in some form. The most common form of treatment is the confrontation of these fears in some form either by imagination or in real life situations [4]. Treatment of phobias can take on many forms, but using one that the subject is comfortable with particularly in an uncomfortable situation already is often difficult. Where it possible to put someone in a situation they were comfortable with and at the same time treat their psychosis in a measurable fashion, this would present real possibilities [1–3].

Virtual reality (VR) promises to extend the realm of possible treatments of phobias. The use of electroencephalography (EEG) offers the ability to measure success in treatment [5,6]. The establishment of a baseline reading and subsequent reading of subjects experiencing true phobias will determine the effectiveness of VR therapy on those experiencing problems in this area.

The primary goal of this study was to establish an objective baseline for subjects who participated in the study in an immersed environment created for the virtual reality therapy (VRT) situation. Since the effects of VRT on the subjects treated for neurosis have traditionally been measured by subjective measurements, there is a need to include objective measures. This will improve and validate the effectiveness of VRT. Subjects who participated in this study were selected because they exhibited no visible or admit able signs of fear of the simulated environments. Specifically, the researchers measured the activity of the subjects' brainwaves in response to the VRT using EEG technology.

## 2. Methodology

Fifteen college students were chosen at random to participate in the study. There was no preference in the selection of subjects regarding gender, age, race, or any other character-istic. With no outside stimuli, the study used an EEG to measure the brain waves of the subjects. Four sessions were conducted consecutively in 5 minute intervals, the sessions where to include reading as follows:

1. *Without VR equipment and quite*
2. *Without VR equipment and with interaction*
3. *With VR equipment and quite*
4. *With VR equipment and interacting with program*

The selection of the program to be used was random as well as the order in which the sessions were given. All sessions where given in one sitting. This was done to get a normal base brain activity measurement with and without movement. Next, the same session was recorded while the subjects were in an immersed environment. While the sessions were being conducted, measurements using an EEG were collected to determine what if any effect the VR equipment would have on a normal subject with no admit able phobias.

## 3. Preliminary Results

Several different statistical mathematical expressions were conducted on the collected data. The min, peak, and mean were evaluated, also the standard deviation and coefficient of V. From this, we also arrive at an average min, peak and mean for each area in which the data was collected (Table 1).

Results from the data collected on the subjects indicate that the subject has less measured brain activity in the VR and no movement experiment (Table 1). In all but one case subjects were actually more relaxed while on the VR equipment than just normal. In addition, the Standard Deviation (Std. Dev.) and Coefficient (Coeff) V are also lower on the trials where VR experience was presented.

**Table 1.** Averages reported (Alpha 8 – 13 Hz) for four experiments.

| Experiments | Min. | Peak | Mean |
|---|---|---|---|
| With VR and Without Movement – Alpha 8 – 13 Hz | 0.803333 | 51.93167 | 6.295 |
| With VR and With Movement – Alpha 8 – 13 Hz | 1.070833 | 73.59 | 9.221667 |
| Without VR and Without Movement – Alpha 8 – 13 Hz | 1.136667 | 90.61417 | 11.82417 |
| Without VR and With Movement – Alpha 8 – 13 Hz | 1.34 | 158.7158 | 21.16917 |

## 4. Conclusions and Discussions

With the limited data collected, the results indicated that, in most cases, subjects are more relaxed while under the immersive influence with respect to brain activities than those that are not. Since this is a small random sampling, future study is under way to investigate a larger group and determine what causes some people to experience increased activities as a result of being under the VR influence, while others show a decrease in brain activities.

It is widely believed that VRT is a viable solution for treating varieties of fears. It is well documented that the best way of treating most fears is to put them in a situation where they have to face those fears. This requires many years of working the individual up to being able to face phobia with a manageable amount of anxiety. VRT is an alternative that can be used at an earlier stage in treatment since it can be brought to the patient and then be used to put the patient in the situation needed. For instance, this arrangements will make it possible for people who suffer from agoraphobia (fear of crowds) be able to face their fear in the comfort of their own home and without putting them at risk of anxiety attacks or any unnecessary discomforts.

## References

[1] Ashcraft, M. H. & Kirk, E. P. (2001). The relationships among working memory, math anxiety, and performance. *Journal of Experimental Psychology* 130(2), 224-237.
[2] North, M.M, North, S.M., and Coble, J.R. (1996). *Virtual reality therapy, An innovative paradigm*. CO: IPI Press.
[3] Wiederhold, B.K. & Wiederhold, M.D. 1998. A review of virtual reality as a psychotherapeutic tool, *CyberPsychology & Behavior*, 1(1), 45-52.
[4] http://www.saviodsilva.net/ph/2.htm
[5] Pugnetti, L., Mendozzi, L., Barberi, E., Rose, F.D., and Attree, E. A. (1996). Nervous system correlates of virtual reality experience, *Proceedings of European Conference Disability & Association Technology*, UK. 239-246.
[6] Slater, M. and Steed, A. (2000). A virtual presence counter (PDF), *Presence: Teleoperators and Virtual Environments*, 9(5), 413-434.

Medicine Meets Virtual Reality 13
James D. Westwood et al. (Eds.)
IOS Press, 2005

# Evaluation of 3D Airway Imaging of Obstructive Sleep Apnea with Cone-beam Computed Tomography

Takumi OGAWA [a], Reyes ENCISO [b], Ahmed MEMON [b],
James K. MAH [b] and Glenn T. CLARK [a]

[a] *Orofacial Pain/Oral Medicine Center, Division of Diagnostic Sciences*
[b] *Division of Craniofacial Sciences and Therapeutics*
*School of Dentistry, University of Southern California Los Angeles, CA 90089-0641*
*e-mail: ogawa-t@tsurumi-u.ac.jp*

**Abstract.** This study evaluates the use of cone-beam Computer Tomography (CT) for imaging the upper airway structure of Obstructive Sleep Apnea (OSA) patients. The total airway volume and the anteroposterior dimension of oropharyngeal airway showed significant group differences between OSA and gender-matched controls, so if we increase sample size these measurements may distinguish the two groups. We demonstrate the utility of diagnosis of anatomy with the 3D airway imaging with cone-beam Computed Tomography.

## 1. Introduction

The most recognized risk factor for obstructive sleep apnea is an anatomical narrowing of the upper airway [1]. In particular, the locus is in the oropharyngeal area. Identifying the exact location of the obstruction is important and upper airway imaging techniques can help with this question.

This study used cone-beam CT to image the airway. This method offers 3D imaging with reduced radiation exposure [2]. From the original CT images we reconstructed 3D surfaces and computed the oropharyngeal volume. In this study we performed a comparison of the anatomy of upper airway in the OSA patients and a gender matched control group. Our null hypothesis was that there would be no difference in the airways of these two groups.

## 2. Materials and Methods

This prospective study included six OSA subjects and 6 gender matched controls. All patients were seen at the Orofacial Pain/Oral Medicine at the Division of Diagnostic Sciences, School of Dentistry, University of Southern California. The control subjects were six healthy volunteers who were imaged for non-OSA related purposes. Age, gen-

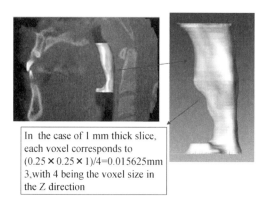

In the case of 1 mm thick slice, each voxel corresponds to $(0.25 \times 0.25 \times 1)/4 = 0.015625$ mm 3, with 4 being the voxel size in the Z direction

**Figure 1.** The total airway volume of oropharyngeal region.

der and body mass index (BMI) were recorded. The subjects were evaluated using three-dimensional cone-beam CT during awake periods.

The cone-beam volumetric tomography Newtom QR-DVT 9000 (QA sri, Via Silvestrini 20,37135 Verona, Italy) is a dental maxillofacial, volumetric imaging system. The device acquires 360 images at 1-degree intervals, with a resolution of 512*512 pixels and 8 bits per pixel (256 grey scale). The reconstruction volume size is 150*150 mm and the imaging takes 75–77 seconds. The reconstruction matrix voxel is 0.25*0.25*1 mm.

Patients were imaged using the Newtom. The reconstructed axial images were exported to Amira software (Mercury Computer Systems / 3D Viz group, San Diego, CA). First, the volume region of interest was selected by the operator between the most proximal edge of the hard palate defined in a sagittal image, and a line extending from the most anterior-inferior point of C2 and perpendicular to the most posterior wall of the airway space. In addition, the lateral extend of the analysis area was selected arbitrarily such that the airway was completely included in an axial image. Next, the upper airway cross-sectional area on each slice was automatically segmented using a threshold grayscale value of 71. In order to know the location of the minimum airway locus, our program identifies the slice with the smallest computed cross-section. With these data we were able to calculate: 1) the total airway volume of oropharyngeal region (Fig 1). 2) Smallest cross-section area (Fig 2). 3) The smallest anteroposterior and lateral dimensions of smallest cross-section area (Fig 2). We then compared the control group data with the apnea group. Descriptive results are expressed as mean ± one standard deviation; differences between two groups were compared by non-parametric Mann-Whitney U test, using SPSS software.

## 3. Results

In Figure 3 comparison of OSA vs. non-OSA is shown, including gender, age and BMI (body-mass index). We computed total airway volume ($mm^3$), smallest cross-section area ($mm^2$), and the anteroposterior (AP) and lateral (L) dimensions of the smallest cross-section area.Our case-control study consisted of 6 patients with apnea and 6 non-apnea subjects matched by gender. While they are not matched perfectly, these two groups did not have significant differences in age. BMI was significant in this study sample, with

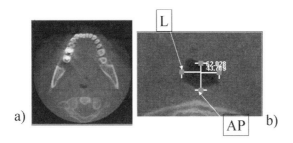

**Figure 2.** a) The smallest cross section area b) The measurements included the anteroposterior (AP) and lateral (L) dimension of the smallest cross-section area (Using Amira 3.1): This study calculates the smallest cross-section area by MATLAB software.

| | OSA AVE. | SD | non-OSA AVE. | SD | P value |
|---|---|---|---|---|---|
| Gender | F=2, M=3 | | F=3, M=3 | | ---- |
| BMI(kg/M2) | 29.8 | ±0.35 | 21.3 | ±1.74 | 0.028 |
| Age | 46.4 | ±6.56 | 34.3 | ±18.3 | 0.429 |
| Volume(mm3) | 3705.6 | ±545.7 | 6217.0 | ±2377.6 | 0.023 |
| Smallest Area (mm²) | 41.4 | ±17.1 | 99.6 | ±82.3 | 0.082 |
| AP(mm) | 15.3 | ±4.6 | 31.2 | ±8.7 | 0.006 |
| L(mm) | 45.1 | ±20.2 | 64.6 | ±35.6 | 0.273 |

**Figure 3.** Comparison Between OSA and Control. BMI=body mass index = wt(kg)/sq(ht(m)); Volume= total Pharyngeal Volume; Smallest area= smallest cross-section area; AP=anteriopesterior diameter of smallest cross-section area; L=lateral diameter of smallest cross-section area.

the OSA patients having a BMI near the obesity standard definition ($29.8 \pm 0.35$), and the controls having a lower BMI ($21.3 \pm 1.74$).

The total airway volume and the AP dimension showed significant group differences. On the other hand, the smallest cross-section area and the L dimension did not show significant group differences.

## 4. Discussion

The primary focus of this investigation was to identify anatomic risk factors for obstructive sleep apnea, using volumetric cone-beam CT. In this study we demonstrate that the AP dimension of the airway of the obstructive sleep apnea patients and its total oropharyngeal volume were smaller in OSA subjects. Based on these results we can reject our null hypothesis that there is no difference in shape or size of the airways for these two groups. Our results agree with data reported by cephalometric based studies, fluoroscopy imaging study, as well as other CT and MR imaging studies [3,4]. These other studies speculated that the airway collapse is caused by hypertrophy by inflammation of pharynx, uvula and tongue, narrowing of airway by enhancement of the lateral wall and emphasis of airway by mandible retrusion [1,3,4]. We can not confirm or refute these theories since this would require a longitudinal based study where multiple images over time were taken. One other possibility is that the airway of OSA patients is abnormal or different in size or shape before they develop apnea and it is the loss of pharyngeal muscle tone or fascial rigidity that shifts a subject from non-snoring to snoring to OSA. If so then there is a possibility that abnormal airway form and shape may be a risk factor for OSA that is evident in younger non-OSA patients. Finally, while the cone-beam CT is not the highest resolution or more sophisticated airway imaging method it has value in that the radiation dosage is relatively low and data is being routinely taken on a young cohort (orthodontics, TMJ and dental patients). In the future we will explore this application and test our concept.

## 5. Conclusion

The following conclusions were provided about the OSA patients: (1) we demonstrate the utility of diagnosis of anatomy with the 3D airway imaging with cone-beam Computed Tomography; (2) we show the characteristics of OSA airway that may distinguish OSA cases from non-OSA cases.

## References

[1] Masumi S, Clark G.; Effect of jaw position and Posture On forced Inspiration Airflow. Chart 109:1477-1483, 1996.
[2] Mah J, Danforth RA, Bumann A, Hatcher D.: Radiation absorbed in maxillofacial imaging with a new dental CT. Oral Surgery, Oral Medicine, Oral Pathology, Oral Radiology and Endodontics 96:508-513, 2003.
[3] Schwab J. R., Pasirstein M., Pierson R.: Identification of upper airway anatomic risk factors for obstructive sleep apnea with volumetric magnetic resonance imaging.: Am J Respir Crit Care Med 168: 522-530, 2003.
[4] Rama N A,Tekwani HS, Kushda AC: Site of obstruction in Obstructive Sleep Apnea. Chest 122(4):1139-1147, 2002.

*Medicine Meets Virtual Reality 13*
*James D. Westwood et al. (Eds.)*
*IOS Press, 2005*

# Multi-Sensory Surgical Support System Incorporating, Tactile, Visual and Auditory Perception Modalities

Sadao OMATA [a], Yoshinobu MURAYAMA [a] and Christos E. CONSTANTINOU [b]

[a] *College of Engineering, Nihon University, Koriyama, Fukushima, Japan*
[b] *Department of Urology, Stanford University Medical School, Stanford, California, USA*

**Abstract.** The incorporation of novel broad band sensory modalities, integrating tactile technology, with visual and auditory signals into the evolution of the next generation of surgical robotic is likely to significantly enhance their utility and safety. In this paper considerations are made of a system, where tactile information together with visual and audio feedback are integrated into a multisensory surgical support platform. The tactile sensor system uses a piezoelectric transducer (PZT) system to evaluate the haptic properties of tissues. The spatial position of the sensor is tracked by a video camera, visualizing the location of the marker. Tactile information is additionally converted to an audio signal, to represent tissue properties in terms of a frequency/amplitude modulated signal. Representative data were obtained from biological tissues demonstrating that the technology developed has potential applications in virtual systems or robotic tele-medical care. In view of these technical developments, consideration is made as to whether visual audio and tactile modalities act as independent sources of information.

## 1. Introduction

The role of integration of multi-sensory inputs by the human brain is currently under consideration by psycho-physiological investigators [1]. The importance of these consideration is based on the need to identify whether multimodal sensory perception is done independently or can be integrated. To examine the role of multi-sensory perception we constructed a prototype system suitable for the evaluation of the elastic properties of biological tissues [2,3].

This system's principal specifications are to measure in vivo the tactile characteristics of a variety of organs. Particular emphasis was placed in presenting the user with spatial map of the organ under evaluation referenced to haptic tissue characteristics. In addition we transformed haptic characteristics to auditory signals as an additional enhancement of presenting data to the users.

## 2. Perception of Multi-sensory information

In practice discrimination between healthy and pathological tissues is potentially perceived from simultaneous information available from many of our senses. For example tactile exploration done by palpation is accompanied by visual and depending on the anatomical structures from other sensory inputs. In this context, an important psycho-physiological question is whether there is evidence that using multiple senses simultaneously improves discrimination of tissue characteristics. The answer to this question is particularly important when considerations are made of employing remote monitoring devices such as robotic systems in comparison to direct clinical observations. Indeed available evidence suggests that tactile and visual cues act as independent sources of characterizing tissues in general and texture in particular. Clearly it is not apparent whether this type of psycho-physiological evidence applies in the interpretation of data from robotic sensors and systems. It is therefore important to identify whether use of multiple sources of signals can be used as independent sources of information or can be integrated within the data presentation and display format. This is particularly important when the desired functions are translated to robots systems that are required to be capable of performing tele-medical care or surgical operations. As with humans these system are required to have safety control systems as well as functional qualities comparable to identify tissue pathology.

## 3. Requirements for tissue characterization

Currently in the development of robotic systems focus is placed on image recognition, control systems, and sensors and actuators. More advanced and intelligent robots are none the less required to collect and act upon the demands of the environment. In such systems it is important to know whether visual information using a CCD camera and computer programs, to recognize the surrounding conditions and autonomously control their own direction of movement, can be processed independently of each other or require integration.

In this context it is useful to consider that for the next generation of robots to function appropriately, the need to have sensor elements abilities that are analogous to a human's five senses and are optimized to use these senses effectively for the task intended. Image recognition technologies have qualities similar to human visual function, and some voice recognition technologies that surpass human hearing function. However, the control systems of robots currently in use are primarily based on image processing or voice recognition technologies, but not tactile, taste, or olfactory sensing.

In this paper, we discuss a sensor system possessing individual tactile sensory components configured to transform tissue properties to modulated sound. This sensor system is made of PZT transducer and a phase shift circuit. The spatial position of the sensor is visually mapped using a video camera. This system can be used in studies relating to multi-sensory integration to identify the extend to which information to be used remotely can be used independently or in combination. Resolution of this question would ultimately facilitate the application of this class of sensors for effective use as a surgical instrument suitable for virtual reality representations and robotic interventions

## 4. Basic principle of a tactile sensor

The tactile sensor system, must approach hand-like abilities to sense the properties of the tissue, recognizing its dynamic properties qualitatively, by changing contact pressure and gauging the response. Using the sense of touch or contact pressure, tissue properties can be estimated with a series of movements of the finger. Perceived tissue hardness is closely related not only on physical properties, but also to contact area, pressure, thickness and size. The performance of a finger pressed against the surface of the tissue, yields a sense of touch for a given force applied. The characteristics considered in this study have already been described [3–5]. Construction of sensor probe showing: marker for video localization, pressure sensor for the measurement of contact pressure, and PZT transducer for stiffness. Sensor probe, having a 5mm diameter nylon sensing hemisphere, mounted on handle. Orientation is made possible by focusing on marker placed on top and is monitored by a video camera.

## 5. Conclusion and future work

Real time tactile data from probe were transformed to an audio signal and combined with a the visual information provided by a video camera and. It is expected that the combination of the tactile technology developed in this study with the visual and auditory integration may be applicable for use in virtual systems or tele-medical involving robotic systems. With continued enhancement of the system, the spatial position of the probe may be detected using a magnetic location system, where the 3D position of the sensor can be identified. Ultimately it is expected that this navigation system will find practical clinical application as well as an aid for training and improving the surgical skills of the physician.

## References

[1] Guest S, Spence C: What role does multisensory integration play in the visoactive perception of texture? Int J Phychophysiology 50 63-80 2003.
[2] Omata S. and Terunuma Y., "New tactile sensor like the human hand and its applications," *Sensors and Actuators A*, vol.3, pp.9-15, 1992.
[3] Omata S, Murayama S, Constantinou CE. Real time tactile sensor for the determination of the physical properties of biomaterials. Sensors and Actuators A (112), 278-285, 2004.
[4] Omata S, Murayama S, Constantinou CE Development of a novel surgical support system and virtual system incorporating a new tactile sensor technology. MMVR (12): 288-290, 2004.
[5] Murayama Y, Constantinou CE.& Omata S. Micro mechanical sensing platform for the characterization of the elastic properties of the ovum via un axial measurement. J of Biomechanics (37), 67-72, 2004.

*Medicine Meets Virtual Reality 13*
*James D. Westwood et al. (Eds.)*
*IOS Press, 2005*

# Estimation of Dislocation after Total Hip Arthroplasty by 4-Dimensional

Yoshito OTAKE [a], Naoki SUZUKI [a], Asaki HATTORI [a], Hidenobu MIKI [b],
Mitsuyoshi YAMAMURA [c], Nobuo NAKAMURA [c], Nobuhiko SUGANO [b],
Kazuo YONENOBU [d] and Takahiro OCHI [e]

[a] *Institute for High Dimensional Medical Imaging, Jikei University School of Medicine*
*4-11-1, Izumi Honcho, Komae-shi, Tokyo, Japan*
[b] *Department of Orthopaedic Surgery, Osaka Univ. Grad. Sch. of Med.*
*2-2 Yamadaoka, Suita 565-0871, Osaka, Japan*
[c] *Kyowa-kai Hospital 1-24-1 Kishibe-kita, Suita 564-0001, Osaka, Japan*
[d] *Department of Orthopaedic Surgery, Osaka Minami National Hospital*
*2-1 Kidohigasi-machi, Kawachinagano 586-0008, Osaka, Japan*
[e] *Department of Computer Integrated Orthopaedics, Osaka Univ. Grad. Sch. of Med.*
*2-2 Yamadaoka, Suita 565-0871, Osaka, Japan*

**Abstract.** We constructed a 4-dimensional musculoskeletal model for patients who have undergone total hip arthroplasty (THA), which aimed to simulate the movement of the patient's inner body structure and estimate the complications that can arise with THA. The model reflects patient-specific characteristics of the bone geometry, implant alignment and hip movement. In order to estimate the direction of the muscle force and the length of the muscles, we developed a string-type muscle model that represents the route of the muscles. The strings expand and contract according to the movement of the origin and insertion location of the muscle. We developed models for the seven muscles related to movement of the hip joint. By using this model, clinicians will be able to predict the possibility of dislocation or recognize the actual causes of dislocation, as well as any possible influences the muscle may have on dislocation.

## 1. Introduction

Dislocation is a major postoperative complication for patients who undergo total hip arthroplasty (THA), and hence the daily activity of patients is generally restricted to some extent. However, prediction of the actual possibility for dislocation, based on patient-specific data that reflect the geometry of the bones or the characteristics of the movement of each patient, has proved to be particularly difficult. Although various causes of dislocation can be considered, Bartz et al. [1] found through cadaveric studies that the primary mechanisms of dislocation could be classified into 3 main groups, namely impingement of the femoral neck on the cup liner, impingement of the femur on the pelvis and spontaneous dislocation due to excessive external force against the muscle force. Although several previous systems for predicting dislocation have been developed [2–4] and each has been utilized to provide data for preoperative planning, these systems only considered the geometry of an artificial joint or were based on the assumption that patients have the same standardized bone geometry. Consequently, differences in the skeletal or muscle structure between patients have not yet been addressed.

## 2. Purpose

In this study, we added a 4-dimensional (4-D) muscle model to our system, which was originally developed for motion analysis after total hip arthroplasty (THA) and designated the patient-specific lower extremity model [5–7]. From this muscle model, we can calculate the tension generated by the muscles surrounding the hip or estimate the possibility of dislocation during movement by analyzing the muscle tension data in concert with the collision of the bones. As a result, this system allows clinicians to give precise guidance to each patient for how to prevent dislocation after surgery.

## 3. Methods

We constructed a skeletal model of a THA patient using CT data (HiSpeed CT; GE Medical Systems, Milwaukee, WI). Since we planned to use this system routinely for clinical use, we tried to reduce the amount of exposure while maintaining the accuracy of the model. Therefore, we scanned the peripheral parts of the joint at fine intervals and other parts at rough intervals. The parameters of the helical scanner around each part were as follows: joint periphery (including implants): 2 mm slices and 1 mm pitch (120 kV, 150 mA); skin markers for motion capturing: 5 mm slices and 1 mm pitch (120 kV, 50 mA); all other areas: 10 mm slices and 3 mm pitch (120 kV, 30 mA). In order to accurately estimate the movement of implants, an estimation of the implant alignment after surgery is essential. However, due to the metal artifact we cannot construct an accurate model from CT data. Hence, we reconstructed a rough-shaped model of the implants from the CT data and then registered the CAD model to the rough model.

Next, we added muscle models to the skeletal model. These models represent each muscle as a cylindrical shape that expands and contracts according to the movement of the origin and insertion location of the muscle. In the present study, we modeled the following 7 muscles or muscle groups related to movement of the hip joint; gluteus medius, gluteus maximus, iliopsoas, rectus femoris, adductor magnus, hamstrings and short lateral rotator. We portrayed the muscles that have multiple directions of tension via the use of multiple muscle models. Next, the transition of the muscle path during hip joint motion was estimated from the movement of the attached bones. When the muscle penetrated the bone or artificial joint, we calculated the collision between the muscle path and the hard tissue and estimated the path avoiding the hard tissue.

From the skeletal movement and estimated muscle path, we then analyzed the risk of dislocation for each patient. Two analysis tools were developed for this purpose.

The first tool is for static analysis and uses the information from the range of hip motion, which can then be used to estimate the dislocation due to impingement of the hard tissue around the hip. From the length of the muscles and the length-tension relationship data [8], we calculated the intensity of the muscle force in each hip position. Since estimation of the force induced by surrounding muscles was also available, we could pre-

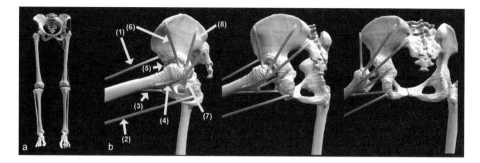

**Figure 1.** Musculoskeletal model of the patient's lower extremity. a: whole model; b: close-up of the hip joint with the hip flexed at 90 degrees. (1:rectus femoris, 2:hamstrings, 3:adductor magnus, 4:gluteus maximus, 5:iliopsoas, 6:gluteus medius, 7:short lateral rotator, 8:gluteus medius).

dict the dislocation due to excessive external force against the muscular force. In order to observe the direction of the muscle tension relative to the acetabular cup, we added a new function to the system that represents the direction via a 3-dimensional (3-D) vector on the cup.

The second tool is for 4-D dynamic motion analysis and uses both the musculoskeletal structure data and the motion capture data. The motion capture was conducted using an optical motion capture system (VICON; VICON Motion Systems, UK) via 15 infrared markers attached to the patient's lower extremity. By combining the 3-D skeletal structure and the marker motion data, we computed the 4-D movement of the skeletal structure

## 4. Result

We constructed 9 muscle models representing 7 muscles and muscle groups related to movement of the hip joint (Fig. 1a). Regarding the gluteus medius and hamstrings, 2 muscle models were created to represent each muscle structure as the effective muscle force direction is divided into two directions. An example of the estimation of the muscle path at 90 degrees flexion and 20 degrees internal rotation is shown in Fig. 1b. The estimation of the muscle path was conducted around 15 fps and the length and force direction of the muscles was calculated from the estimated path. The results were represented in the display by differentiation in color. The muscles extracted 1.5 times were rendered in purple and those contracted 0.5 times were rendered in yellow, while the muscles in between were rendered in a color according to the length of the muscle. By using this method we can figure out the extraction and contraction of the muscle groups intuitively. By conducting 4-D musculoskeletal movement simulations, we could predict the risk of dislocation during daily activities, such as walking (Fig. 2), sitting down on a chair or picking something up from the floor.

And further more, from analysis of the muscle force direction in each posture (Fig. 3), we calculated the sum force generated by these muscles at the hip joint. This vector came to represent the muscle force direction at the hip joint relative to the bone geometry. The number displayed at the tip of the vector indicates the strength of the force. Subsequently, we could also predict dislocation due to impingement between hard tissues, such as bones or implants, by using a collision detection algorithm [9].

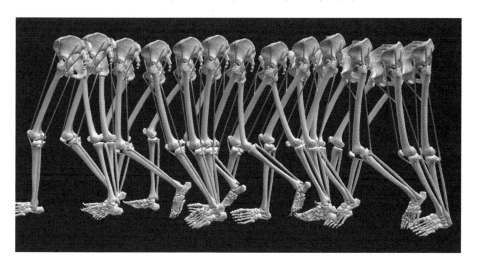

**Figure 2.** Time-sequential images of the patient's lower extremity model while walking. The muscle color indicates the ratio of the muscle length relative to the length at the neutral hip position.

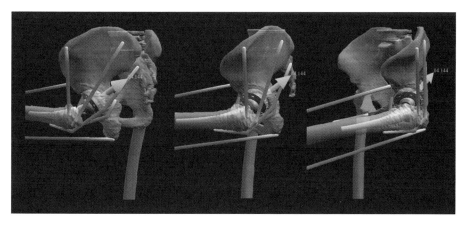

**Figure 3.** Estimated muscle force. The vector represents the muscle force direction relative to the bone geometry. The number displayed at the tip of the vector indicates the strength of the force.

## 5. Conclusion

Preoperative planning and postoperative guidance in daily activities should be individualized to address each patient's risk of complications, since the component design, component alignment and skeletal structure can vary among patients after THA. Although several recent studies have focused on preoperative planning and intraoperative image guided navigation systems, and these systems have enabled the performance of accurately planned surgeries, the planning was based on data acquired in the static position, which does not account for individual differences in dynamic motion during the activities of daily life. Thus, the same limited guidance for postoperative daily motion (e.g., prohibiting hip flexion greater than 90 degrees or encouraging the use of aids) is frequently applied to all patients regardless of the individual differences in component alignment, skeletal structure and characteristics of daily motion. Obviously, the effects of muscle force are not considered in the current systems.

Our new muscle model can reveal which muscle is the main contributor to dislocation, even if the analyzable parameters are limited. Although there are several previous studies that have created muscle models and estimated the muscle path [10–12], the bone geometry in these models was assumed to be a simple geometric shape, such as a sphere or cylinder, and the models did not reflect patient-specific differences in the bone structure or implant alignment. In our system, we detected the collision between muscles and each patient's bone geometry, such that the contraction patterns can be calculated based on patient-specific data. In addition, this system revealed the movement of the patient's skeletal structures and muscle contraction patterns during various types of motion by integrating the patient-specific 3-D model from CT data and the patient's motion capture data. From this model, we can recognize the movement of the components both intuitively and quantitatively. Furthermore, by comparing graphs representing the muscle contraction pattern among two or more patients, we can acquire the characteristics of the movement as the difference between the muscle contraction patterns, and provide guidance reflecting these patient-specific characteristics. By using these novel tools, clinicians will be able to predict the potential for dislocation for each patient and recognize the causes or mechanisms of dislocation, including the influence of the muscles. Our next step will be validation of the estimated muscle force. In this study, we used muscle length-tension relationship data from the literature [8] acquired on the basis of electromyograms. However, the error factor for electromyogram data due to cross-talk between neighboring muscles is widely known, and in order to validate the accuracy of the muscle force estimated by our model, we plan to conduct experiments that measure the real contact force at the hip joint using a pressure sensor installed with the implants. Hence, we will be able to modify the parameters of the muscle model to match the real muscle features.

## References

[1] Bartz, R.L., Noble, P.C., Kadakia, N.R., Tullos, H.S.: The Effect of Femoral Component Head Size on Posterior Dislocation of the Artificial Hip Joint, J Bone Joint Surg 82-A(9), pp.1300-1307, 2000.

[2] D'lima D.D., Urquhart A.G., Buehler K.O., Walker R.H., Colwell C.W.: The Effect of the Orientation of the Acetabular and Femoral Components on the Range of Motion of the Hip Different Head-Neck Ratios. J Bone Joint Surg, 82-A(3), pp.315-321, 2000.

[3] Delp S.L., Komattu A.V., Wixson R.L. Superior Displacement of the Hip in Total Joint Replacement: Effects of Prosthetic Neck Length, Neck-Stem Angle, and Anteversion Angle on the Moment-Generating Capacity of the Muscles. J Orthop Res, 12(6), pp.860-870, 1994.

[4] Seki M., Yuasa N., Ohkumi K. Analysis of Optimal Range of Socket Orientations in Total Hip Arthroplasty with Use of Computer-Aided Design Simulation. J Orthop Res, 16, pp.513-517, 1998.

[5] Otake Y., Hagio K., Suzuki N., Hattori A., Sugano N., Yonenobu K., Ochi T.: Development of 4-Dimensional Human Model System for the Patient after Total Hip Arthroplasty, MICCAI2002, pp.241-247, 2002.

[6] Hagio K., Sugano N., Nishii T., Miki H., Otake Y., Hattori A., Suzuki N.: A novel system of 4-dimensional motion analysis after total hip arthroplasty, CARS 2002, pp.1059, 2002.

[7] OtakeY., Hagio K., Suzuki N., Hattori A., Sugano N., Yonenobu K., Ochi T.: 4-dimensional Computer-based Motion Simulation after Total Hip Arthroplasty, MMVR11, pp.251-256, 2003.

[8] Zajac F.E.: Muscle and tendon: properties, models, scaling, and application to biomechanics and motor control, Crit Rev Biomed Eng, 17(4), pp.359-411, 1989.

[9]  S. Gottschalk, M. C. Lin, D. Manocha.: OBBTree: a hierarchical structure for rapid interference detection, Proc. SIGGRAPH '96, pp.171-180, 1996.

[10] Scott L. Delp, J. Peter Loan, Melissa G. Hoy, Felix E. Zajac, Eric L. Topp, Joseph M. Rosen. An Interactive Graphics-Based Model of the Lower Extremity to Study Orthopaedic Surgical Procedures, IEEE Trans Biomed Eng, 37(8), pp.757-767, 1990.

[11] Iain W. Charlton, Garth R. Johnson. Application of spherical and cylindrical wrapping algorithms in a musculoskeletal model of the upper limb, J Biomech, 34, pp. 1209-1216, 2001.

[12] Allison S. Arnold, Silvia Salinas, Deanna J. Asakawa, Scott L. Delp. Accuracy of Muscle Moment Arms Estimated from MRI-Based Musculoskeletal Models of the Lower Extremity, Comput Aided Surg , 5, pp.108-119, 2000.

*Medicine Meets Virtual Reality 13*
*James D. Westwood et al. (Eds.)*
*IOS Press, 2005*

# BrainTrain: Brain Simulator for Medical VR Application

Bundit PANCHAPHONGSAPHAK [a], Rainer BURGKART [b] and Robert RIENER [a,c]

[a] *Automatic Control Laboratory,*
*Swiss Federal Institute of Technology (ETH), Switzerland*
[b] *Clinic for Orthopaedics and Sport-Orthopaedics, Klinikum Rechts der Isar,*
*Technical University of Munich, Germany*
[c] *Spinal Cord Injury Center, Balgist University Hospital, Switzerland*

**Abstract.** The brain is known as the most complex organ in the human body. Due to its complexity, learning and understanding the anatomy and functions of the cerebral cortex without effective learning assistance is rather difficult for medical novices and students in health and biological sciences.

In this paper, we present a new virtual reality (VR) simulator for neurological education and neurosurgery. The system is based on a new three-dimensional (3D) user-computer interface design with a tangible object and a force-torque sensor. The system is combined with highly interactive computer-generated graphics and acoustics to provide multi-modal interactions through the user's sensory channels (vision, tactile, haptic and auditory).

The system allows the user to feel the simulated object from its physical model that formed the interface device, while exploring or interacting with the mimicked computer-generated object in the virtual environment (VE). Unlike other passive interface devices, our system can detect the position and orientation of the interacting force in real-time, based on the system's set-up and a force-torque data acquisition technique. As long as the user is touching the model, the positions of the user's fingertip in the VE can be determined and is synchronized with the finger's motion in the physical world without requirement of an additional six-degree-of-freedom tracking device.

The prior works have shown the use of the system set-up in medical applications. We demonstrate the system for neurological education and neurosurgery as a recent application. The main functions of the simulator contribute to education in neuroanatomy and visualization for diagnostic and pre-surgery planning. Once the user has touched the model, the system will mark the associated anatomy region and will provide the information of the region in terms of text note and/or sound. The user can switch from anatomy to the brain's function module, which will give details of motor, sensory or other cortical functions associated to the touch areas. In addition, the user can generate and visualize arbitrary cross-sectional images from corresponding to the magnetic resonance imaging (MRI) datasets either for training or for diagnostic purpose. The user can manipulate the cross-section image interactively and intuitively by moving the finger on the interface device.

## 1. Introduction

The brain is known as the most complex organ in the human body in terms of appearance, topography, structure, and function of the nervous system etc. Due to its complexity, learning and studying the anatomy and function of the brain without effective learning assistance is rather difficult and personnel-intensive for medical novices and students in health and biological sciences who just enter the field of human neuroanatomy. Conventional learning materials for neuroanatomy in medical schools are ranged from a low fidelity such as books or pictures to a higher fidelity such as anatomical plastic model ("phantoms"), interactive software, and VR technology, which has gained increased attention over the last decade.

In this paper, we will present a new VR simulator for neuroanatomy training called "BrainTrain" system. The main objective of the system is to provide an assistant tool for helping young medical students to learn and to recognize brain anatomy, cerebral cortex's functions and to visualize the brain's cross sectional image with VR technology. The system combined a tangible interface, highly interactive computer graphic and acoustic displays to provide multi-modal interactions to the user and to increase a realism of the system.

## 2. The BrainTrain Simulator

### 2.1. Related Works

The prior use of tangible objects as an interface device for VR has been presented by [2]. The authors have introduced "passive physical props" as two-handed interaction devices for bimanual manipulation and visualization of neurosurgical data in pre-operation planning process. A doll's head represents the "head prop" held in the user's non-dominant hand, providing tactile cues that allow the user to manipulate the virtual model of the patient's brain comfortably. A piece of rectangular plate or a stylus tool, held in the dominant hand, acts as an interacting tool. It allows the users to visualize the MRI dataset or specify a trajectory for surgical target easily and intuitively with human's skill in bimanual action.

Our BrainTrain system is developed based on the concept presented by [1]. The authors have integrated a six-degrees-of-freedom (6 dof) force-torque sensor into the tangible object in order to detect a contact position when the user touches on the anatomy model. The system allows the user to touch the model at any surface location and to display the name of each organ, which is being touched by the user. In addition, the system can animate the movement of the organ when removing the organ.

However, the system suffered from using a soft object, which introduced large error in contact location computation, and the relationship between a surface region and information is a *one-to-one* database, which only allows the system to display single information per object or region. These drawbacks have been improved in our system and additional interaction modules have been implemented, which will be explained in detailed in the following sections.

### 2.2. System Overview

Our system consists of a stereolithograph model of the brain (plastic model) obtained from processing of the brain MRI data, a 6 dof force-torque sensor (90M31A-I50, JR3. Inc.), a Pentium-4 2.8 GHz PC, speakers and an LCD display (see Figure 1). The

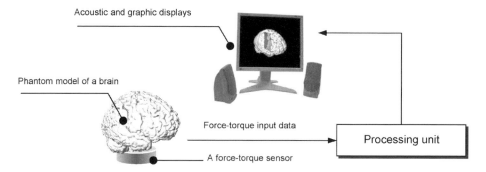

**Figure 1.** The BrainTrain simulator set-up (graphic and acoustic display and a tangible interface device).

Virtual Environment (VE) and the graphical interactions have been written with Open Inventor$^{TM}$ toolkit [5]. The brain model is used as a user interface allowing the user to interact with VE by touching on its geometry.

The 6 dof force-torque sensor is connecting the brain model with the fundament, sensing the exerted force and torque information at each time step. As the plastic brain model is rigid enough, it can prevent the sensor to send an incorrect force-torque data due to dynamic effects resulting from object's deformation. The sensing data is processed and then a contact or touch location is computed. The system and a graphical display updates at a rate of 50 frames/second. The user can touch directly on the brain model and feel tactile feedback without additional haptic interface device. In addition, As long as the user is touching the model, the determined touch location can be synchronized with the finger's motion in the actual world without any additional tracking system required.

### 2.3. Touch Location Computation

The six-degrees of freedom force-torque sensor is capable of sensing vector components of the applied force and moment based on three-dimensional orthogonal coordinate system. We assume that an external force $\vec{F}$ and an external moment $\vec{M}$ are exerted on the object at a contact point $P$. A vector $\vec{r}$ represents the vector pointing from the sensor's origin $O$ to the contact point $P$. The sensor detects the magnitude and direction of the exerted force and moment and gives the outputs in terms of a force vector $\vec{F}_s$ and a moment vector $\vec{M}_s$.

During the simulation, we assume that there is only a pure force applied to the object at the contact point without torque ($\vec{M} = \vec{0}$). Such condition exists when a point load or a contact load that is applied on a relatively small area is exerted on the object either with or without friction such as pointing with a pen or a stylus. This type of contact is known as the "hard finger contact" [4].

In any static condition, we obtain:

$$\vec{M}_s = \vec{r} \times \vec{F}_s$$

However, we cannot solve the solution of the location $\vec{r}$ with this technique because the system of equation is underdetermined. Therefore, we must consider a line of action *l*, which passes through the contact point *P* and parallel to the force $\vec{F}$. The mathematical decription of the line *l* is given in a parametric form as:

$$\vec{r}(\lambda) \equiv \vec{r}^* + \lambda\vec{F} = \vec{r}^* + \lambda\vec{F}_s$$

where $\lambda$ is scalar parameter and

$$\vec{r}^* = (\vec{F}_s \times \vec{M}_s)/|\vec{F}_s|^2$$

The $\vec{r}^*$ is the vector that is orthogonal to $\vec{F}_s$ and $\vec{M}_s$, pointing from the sensor's origin *O* and intersecting the line *l* at a point *P\**. From a physical viewpoint, the solution is laying somewhere along the line *l* and can be determined if we know parameter $\lambda$ at the location where the intersection occurs. Therefore, we have to test intersections between the geometry's surface and the force vector. In our approach, the geometrical information of the object is described by a polyhedral surface. In other words, the object's surface contains a set of triangles that forms its shape. Thus, we can find the intersection point by testing ray-triangle intersections through the whole set of the surface's triangles. The whole computation is repeated at each time step and the solution can be recorded. Therefore, we know not only the position of the touch location at a particular time, but also the force direction and magnitude as well as motion of the touch location from the history.

To guarantee the uniqueness of the solution, the following propositions must be satisfied:

- The shape the object or, at least, the interacting region must be convex.
- Only the compression forces (pushing against the model rather than pulling) are allowed to apply on the object

## 3. User Interactions

### 3.1. Information Feedback

This interaction mode aims to provide anatomical information, cortex's name and function of the brain surface where the user touches. As soon as the contact position is known, the position will then be compared with the regions, that are predefined, in our database to display the associated information. The relationship between a surface region and information is in a form of *one-to-many*. Therefore, for a surface region, information can be selected and displayed according to the user's choice i.e. cortex's name or function's name. The information is displayed by text, color highlight and an audio cue (see Figure 2).

### 3.2. Cross-Sectional Image Visualization

In this interaction module, the system will display a cross-sectional image of the brain, which corresponds to the contact location and force information. The user can define the location where to display the cross sectional images by just touching on the brain model. The cross-sectional image is reconstructed from the volumetric dataset of medical data such as MRI data (with a resolution of $256 \times 256$ pixels per slide). The image is then mapped onto the plane, which is moved and controlled by the user. The following subsections present three methods used to control the cross sectional plane.

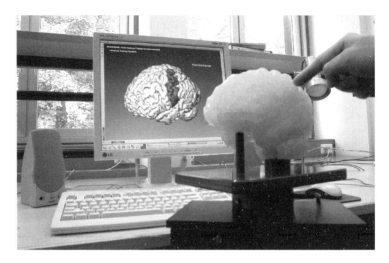

**Figure 2.** A view from the system when a user interacts with the system in the anatomy and brain's cortical functions training.

### 3.2.1. Control by Contact Location

In this method, the cross-sectional plane is controlled by the location of the contact point. The user can move the cross-sectional plane back and forward or up and down by only changing the touch location on the brain model. The orientation of the plane can be set to be parallel to one of the principal views, i.e. coronal, sagittal or axial, during the simulation. This is similar to a conventional way to visualize the medical dataset (see Figure 3a).

### 3.2.2. Control by Contact Location and Force Direction

In this method, we can control the cross sectional plane by using a contact point and the direction of the exerted force. However, only one point and one direction vector is not enough to define a plane because one direction vector is missing. Therefore, we must assume a dummy vector, which is picked from one of the principal axes. The orientation of the cross sectional plane is described by the cross product of the force vector and the dummy vector. Moreover, the user is allowed to select the preferred dummy vector during the simulation (see Figure 3b).

### 3.2.3. Control by Force Vector

In the last method, the cross sectional plane is fully controlled by a contact force vector. The plane is always normal to the force direction and it can be pushed into the brain model when the amount of exerted force is larger then a threshold value. The plane will travel along the direction of the exerted force vector. The moving distance is related to the amount of force applied. The movement will stop as soon as the user retracts his/her finger from the model (see Figure 3c).

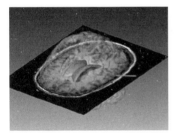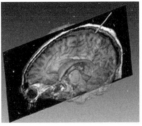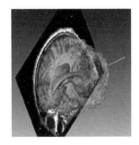

**Figure 3.** Views of the interactive visualization of the brain's cross-section from three different control methods: a) with contact location b) with contact location and force direction and c) with force vector.

## 4. Discussion

We have performed qualitative evaluations of the system. The subjects are students and visitors in our laboratory. We let the subjects test our system with their finger or with stylus tool and the touch location error was observed. The error of touch location computation is a function of the force magnitude, angle between a touched plane and the force direction, and the distance of the plane from the sensor's origin. From theory, when a 5 N force is applied on a plane, which locates 20 cm away from the sensor's origin and normal to the force direction, the maximum location error that can be presented is 0.88 mm. The maximum error will decrease if the applied force increases. However, in our experiment, the user was pointing the model with a force approximately 5 N, using a sharp-pointed tool and applying in the direction normal to the surface. We observed that the contact point error was about 2~3 mm which is about 3 to 4 times higher than the theoretical value.

We believe that the increased error comes from the noise of the sensor. We can reduce the error if we use a stronger filter. However, a strong filter could lead to a longer delay time and could limit our system from real-time capable. In addition, since the force-torque sensor is sensitive to force, it is possible that, in an uncontrolled room, the surrounding environments may affect to the outputs of the sensor.

The limitation of our simulation system results from the computing method of the touch location. As we mentioned earlier, this technique is applicable for a single touch point and a rigid object. We have tried to test our technique by replacing the rigid body object with a soft object. The error of the contact point computation was highly increased due to the dynamic effects of the object's deformation. Therefore, it is challenging to apply this method to a soft object such as a human brain.

## 5. Conclusion

We have developed a new VR simulation system for training neuroanatomy and brain function. Medical students can experience a new way of interactive interface based on a real physical object and VR technology. Once the user touches the model, the system can react to the touch region and provide the region-related information in terms of text and/or sound. The user can switch from anatomy mode to the brain function mode, which will give region-related details of motor, sensory or other cortical functions. These could help the medical students to understand complex anatomy and functions of the brain effectively.

In addition, the user can generate and visualize arbitrary cross-sectional images from corresponding magnetic resonance imaging (MRI) datasets interactively by touching and moving the finger on the interface device. The application is either for educational training or for diagnostic visualization of brain tumors or lesions.

## Acknowledgements

The authors would like to thank Dr. Spyros Kollias, Dr. Paul Summers, and Marion Funk from the University Hospital Zurich for providing the magnetic resonance images data and giving suggestions for the brain image segmentation. This project is partly supported by 3B Scientific GmbH, Hamburg.

## References

[1] Riener, R., Sae-Kee, B., Frey, M., Burgkart, R.: A Sensorized Human Torso Phantom. Proceeding of MMVR 12, Vol. 98. IOS Press (2004) pp. 323-326.
[2] Hinckley, K., Pausch, R, Goble, J., Kassell, N.: Passive Real-World Interface Props for Neurosurgical Visualization, ACM CHI'94 Conference on Human Factors in Computing Systems (1994) pp. 452-458.
[3] Sae-Kee, B., Riener, R., Frey, M., Pröll, T., Burgkart, R.: Phantom-based Interactive Simulation System for Dental Treatment Training. Proceeding of MMVR 12, Vol. 98. IOS Press (2004) pp. 327-332.
[4] Bicchi, A.: Intrinsic contact sensing for soft fingers. Proc. IEEE Int. Conf. Robotics Automation, Vol. 2 (1990) pp. 968-973.
[5] Wernecke, J.: The Inventor Mentor: Programming Object-Oriented 3D Graphics with Open Inventor$^{TM}$, *Release 2*. Addison-Wesley (1994).

*Medicine Meets Virtual Reality 13*
*James D. Westwood et al. (Eds.)*
*IOS Press, 2005*

# Smart Tutor: A Pilot Study of a Novel Adaptive Simulation Environment

Thai PHAM MD [a], Lincoln ROLAND MD [b],
K. Aaron BENSON BS [c], Roger W. WEBSTER PhD [c,d],
Anthony G. GALLAGHER PhD [e] and Randy S. HALUCK MD FACS [a,c]

[a] *Penn State University College of Medicine,*
*Department of Surgery Hershey, PA USA 17033*
[b] *Soundshore Medical Center, New Rochelle, NY USA*
[c] *Verefi Technologies, Hershey, PA USA*
[d] *Millersville University, Department of Computer Science, Millersville, PA USA*
[e] *Emory University, Atlanta, GA, USA*

**Abstract.** Computer-based learning environments create the possibility of dynamic adaptation to address learner capabilities and user performance. Software algorithms, code-named Smart Tutor, for motor skill learning were developed and applied to an abstract environment for laparoscopic surgery (RapidFire). Smart Tutor dynamically adjusts the environment to minimize frustration and optimize learning conditions for all learners.

This study compared the first generation RapidFire / Smart Tutor (RF / ST) to the Minimal Invasive Surgery Trainer Virtual Reality (MIST VR) system for laparoscopic performance improvement and level of frustration. Two groups of novice laparoscopic learners were assessed by pre- and post- training paper cutting exercise and subjective surveys.

Users of both systems showed improvement of laparoscopic skills as measured by the paper cutting exercises. No differences were shown between groups for level of improvement. However, a significant difference was seen in the subjective ratings on the post-training survey with less frustration for the RF / ST training group. Important information was acquired for refinements of the Smart Tutor algorithms.

## 1. Introduction

A major challenge to training, especially for complex tasks and medical procedures, is illustrated by the Yerkes-Dodson Principal, also known as the inverted "U" principal [1]. This principal states that in situations of high or low stress, learning and performance are compromised. This was confirmed by Moorthy et al for high stress and laparoscopic task performance [2]. The Yerkes-Dodson Law further states that optimal learning and performance occurs in a situation of moderate stress. Simulators designed for one level of difficulty will not be optimal for some users by virtue of a standard bell curve. For some users the preset level will be optimal for learning, but low performers may be frustrated or overwhelmed and high performers may become bored or not progress further.

Computer-based simulators create the possibility of performance recognition and can adapt a learning environment to the user in real time. Until recently, stimulators

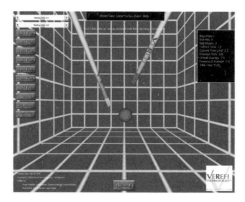

**Figure 1A.** RapidFire task involves the user touching spheres while alternating laparoscopic gaspers.

were designed with discrete difficulty levels that were selected by the user or administrator. A Smart Tutor Computing Algorithm (Verefi Technologies, Inc. Hershey, PA, patent pending) has been developed and integrated into RapidFire Simulation Trainer (Verefi Technologies, Inc. Hershey, PA) tasks to create real-time adjustments in the environment based on the user's performance. The Smart Tutor algorithm was designed to keep all learners in an optimal learning "zone" and to allow users of varying levels of abilities to start training without frustration or boredom. Smart Tutor increases difficulty in tasks automatically without discrete levels. To our knowledge, this is the first adaptive learning environment applied to surgical skill simulation. The aim of this pilot study was to compare RapidFire / Smart Tutor (RF / ST) to the Minimally Invasive Surgery Trainer Virtual Reality (MIST VR, Mentice AB, Sweden) system which has been shown to be an effective trainer of laparoscopic skills [3]. This pilot study was done to examine levels of frustration in training of novices, differences in pre-and post-training assessment between the two systems, and to acquire data for improvements of the Smart Tutor algorithm.

## 2. Methods

RapidFire is a PC-based laparoscopic motor skill trainer using the Immersion Virtual Laparoscopic Interface (Immersion Corporation, San Jose, CA). Three tasks from Rapid-Fire were modified with two different Smart Tutor algorithms (one emphasizing speed and one emphasizing accuracy) to create six tasks. The three RapidFire tasks were: 1. touching a virtual sphere with a virtual laparoscopic instrument (Figure 1A); 2. touching a sphere simultaneous with both virtual laparoscopic instrument tips (Figure 1B); and 3. grasping of one sphere and transfer to the other grasper (Figure 1C).

The Smart Tutor software is a layer of control over all key parameters of the Rapid-Fire environment including number of trials, left versus right handed tasks, time parameters, and target sizes. Smart Tutor does not alter the physical functionality of the environment such as the physics of the instruments. Smart Tutor records performance and makes adjustments in the task environment parameters.

Expert performance criteria (EPC) were established on the RF / ST, the MIST VR medium (MIST VR factory preset) and MIST VR master levels (Settings courtesy of Dr. Gallagher). This was done using the performance of two attending laparoscopic sur-

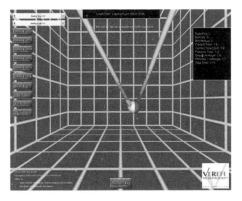

**Figure 1B.** RapidFire task involves user touching spheres with both laparoscopic graspers simultaneously.

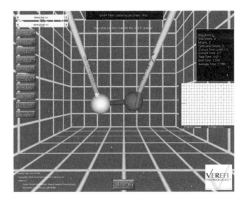

**Figure 1C.** RapidFire task involves user transferring objects from one laparoscopic gasper to another gasper.

geons, a laparoscopic surgery fellow, and two general surgery chief residents. Twenty medical students (year 1 thru 4) were randomized to either the RF / ST or MIST VR simulator. During the training sessions, the medical students were not permitted to train more than 45 minutes in a 24 hour period.

In the RF / ST group, training was completed when subjects achieved EPC in four of the six tasks in two consecutive trials. In the MIST VR group, only the Acquire Place, Transfer Place, and Traversal tasks were used and subjects were advanced from medium to master level when EPC were achieved in two of the three MIST VR tasks for two consecutive trials. In addition, for the MIST VR group, subjects' training was complete once they were able to achieve EPC at master level on two of the three tasks on two consecutive trials. The novice users were assessed by a standard pre- and post-training laparoscopic paper cutting task [4]. Post training, the subjects completed a questionnaire regarding levels of frustration on a five point Likert scale. Data were compared using a standard t-test.

**Table 1.** Summary of scores and number of trials.

|  | RF / ST ($n = 10$) | MIST VR ($n = 10$) |
|---|---|---|
| Average Pre-Cutting Score | $15 \pm 8.5$ | $17 \pm 8.3$ |
| Average Post-Cutting Score | $21 \pm 7.7$ | $28 \pm 13$ |
| Average Number of Trials to Achieve EPC | $10.5 \pm 3.4$ | $15.4 \pm 4.6$ |

EPC = Expert Performance Criteria
RF / ST: Rapid Fire / Smart Tutor

**Table 2.** Summary of Post-training Survey.

| | Post Training Survey Questions | RF / ST | MIST VR | p Value |
|---|---|---|---|---|
| 1. | I found training on the simulator to be difficult and frustrating. | $2.0 \pm 0.8$ | $3.2 \pm 1.1$ | 0.014 |
| 2. | I thought the training on the simulator was frustrating / difficult / or challenging at first, but then became easier. | $3.8 \pm 1.0$ | $3.6 \pm 1.2$ | 0.69 |
| 3. | I was frustrated with the simulator training at one point that I wanted to give-up. | $1.6 \pm 0.5$ | $2.4 \pm 1.0$ | 0.032 |
| 4. | I found training on the simulator to be boring or tedious. | $1.9 \pm 0.9$ | $2.3 \pm 0.5$ | 0.22 |
| 5. | I was bored by the simulation trainer at one point and wanted to quit. | $1.6 \pm 0.7$ | $1.8 \pm 0.4$ | 0.44 |

## 3. Results

Novice users acquired laparoscopic motor skills on both the RF / ST and MIST VR systems. There was no statistical difference in the medical student school year and the length of time needed to complete training between the two groups. The average percent increase in paper-cutting scores was 14% for RF / ST ($p = 0.05$) and 23% for MIST VR ($p = 0.001$). The improvement in paper-cutting scores were not significant between RF / ST and MIST VR ($p = 0.09$). The average number of training trails required to achieve EPC on RF / ST and MIST VR environments were $10\pm3$ and $15\pm4$ respectively ($p = 0.13$).

The subjects post training survey questions and mean responses $+/-$ standard deviation are outlined in Table 2. A difference in subjective frustration ratings was noted between RF / ST and MIST VR on questions 1 and 3. As demonstrated by questions 4 and 5, no differences were noted when subjects were asked about level of boredom.

## 4. Discussion

With the Smart Tutor Computing Algorithm applied to the RapidFire simulation environment, we have demonstrated that novices do learn laparoscopic motor skills with less stress. Though not statistically significant, users of the RF / ST simulators did show a trend towards more rapid acquisition of laparoscopic motor skills than users of he standard MIST VR simulator. Failure to achieve statistical significance is likely attributable to the small test groups. A study with larger groups is planned following refinements to the Smart Tutor Computing Algorithm.

We were encouraged that subjects felt less frustration in training with our adaptive system than the MIST VR system with non-adaptive levels. To establish EPC, two of our five experts were chief residents and we feel that more stringent EPC would have yielded better training, a higher percentage increase from pre- to post paper-cutting scores, less variability in post-training scores within groups, and a better comparison between systems. We expect that considerable refinement of the adaptive algorithms will be necessary to optimize the systems and that process is underway.

## 5. Conclusion

Novices can acquire laparoscopic skill as assessed on their paper cutting scores before and after training with RF / ST. Although not statistically significant, our pilot data show a trend of novice users are achieving EPC with less number of trails with RF / ST. While we were optimistic, we expect that further refinements of the Smart Tutor algorithms will be necessary. Of importance is that the RapidFire with Smart Tutor adaptive environment is providing a less frustrating learning environment, which may enhance acquisition of laparoscopic skills for novice users.

## References

[1] Whitman N. Student stress, effects and solutions. Assoc for Study of Higher Education, Washington, D.C., 1984.
[2] Moorthy K, Munz Y, Dosis A, Bann S, Darzi A. The effect of stress-inducing conditions on the performance of a laparoscopic task. Surg Endosc 2003;179:1481-4.
[3] Seymour NE, Gallagher AG, Roman SA, O'Brien MK, Bansal VK, Andersen DK, Satava RM. Virtual reality training improves operating room performance: results of randomized, double blinded study. Ann Surg. 2002;236(4):458-63.
[4] Gallagher AG, McClure N, McGuigan J, Ritchie K, Sheehy NP. An ergonomic analysis of the fulcrum effect in the acquisition of endoscopic skills. Endoscopy 1998;30:617-620.

*Medicine Meets Virtual Reality 13*
*James D. Westwood et al. (Eds.)*
*IOS Press, 2005*

# Immersive Visualization Training of Radiotherapy Treatment

Roger PHILLIPS [a], James W. WARD [a] and Andy W. BEAVIS [b]

[a] *Department of Computer Science, University of Hull, HU6 7RX, Hull, UK*
[b] *Department of Radiation Physics, Princess Royal Hospital, Hull, UK*

**Abstract.** External radiation beam treatment of cancer tumours involves delivery of invisible radiation beams through the body where internal structures can not be seen. Beam targeting of patient anatomy has to very accurate to achieve the desired therapeutic result. Good understanding of radiotherapy treatment (RT) concepts is essential to training. This paper presents a virtual environment simulator developed by the authors for training and education of intensity modulated radiotherapy (IMRT) treatment of cancer. This simulator employs immersive visualization to provide a high fidelity spatial awareness of the complex relationships between tumour, organs at risk, treatment beam and radiation dose. All these visualization are provided by a 3D virtual environment based on the patient in a RT treatment room. Immersive visualization using this simulator is being used to train radiation oncologist and radiation physicists about radiotherapy treatment.

## 1. Introduction

External radiation beam treatment of cancer tumours involves the delivery of invisible radiation waves through the body where internal structures can not be seen. Furthermore beam targeting of patient anatomy has to be accurate to achieve the desired therapeutic result.

This paper presents a virtual environment (VE) simulator developed by the authors for intensity modulated radiotherapy (IMRT) [1,2] treatment of cancer. For IMRT the therapeutic radiation fields are matched to the 3D profile of a tumour using a computer controlled delivery system. IMRT plans are typically created from a CT/MRI scan of a patient and a computerised optimisation algorithm guided by constraints based on patient volumes (tumour, organs at risk) and dose constraints for these volumes. The patient is irradiated using a linear accelerator with multiple shaped beams over a number of treatment sessions.

Immersive visualization has the potential to provide high fidelity spatial awareness of complex relationships between patient anatomy, treatment beam, radiation dose and equipment in the treatment room. This is helpful because IMRT delivers a complex 4D (i.e. 3D plus varying fluence) radiation dose on geometrically complex 3D anatomy. This is further complicated by issues such as patient set-up error [3], patient motion, etc.

This paper first presents the various visualizations of the VE simulator for radiotherapy treatment (RT) and then discusses uses of the VE simulator for training radiation oncologist and radiation physicists about the logistics of radiotherapy treatment.

## 2. Visualization Facilities of the Radiotherapy Treatment VE Simulator

The authors have developed a generic virtual environment (VE) simulator for radiotherapy treatment rooms. The simulator is intended for training and education of medical physicists, radiotherapy treatment planners, radiation oncologists, etc. This VE simulator provides a range of visualizations that are patient centric. This simulator provides visualization for the following:

1. A radiotherapy linear accelerator that delivers the therapeutic radiation beams.
2. Anatomy of patient and segmented anatomical structures relevant to the treatment plan.
3. Therapeutic radiation beams and representations showing the planned radiation dose to be delivered.

### 2.1. Visualization of the Linear Accelerator and the Treatment Room

The VE simulator provides a virtual world of a radiotherapy treatment room at the Princess Royal Hospital in Hull (UK) that has a Varian 600CD linear accelerator with a 160 leaved multi-leaf collimator (MLC). This initial model was constructed from measurements and photographs taken in the treatment room, and from CAD drawings available on the web. We intend to extend the simulator to cater for a range of linear accelerators from various manufacturers and to create virtual worlds based on actual treatment rooms associated with the training context. To build these new virtual worlds, the treatment rooms and the linear accelerators will be laser scanned using a Leica CDS 3000. This will provide accurate surface geometry and true colour for the captured scene. This scanning approach provides a rapid means to produce highly accurate models of linear accelerators and room layouts.

The virtual linear accelerator has the full articulation of a real accelerator. Thus the gantry and the delivery head rotate. Similarly, the virtual couch has a full range of articulation. The linear accelerator has manual virtual controls (see Fig. 1(a)), which is useful for training purposes. We are currently integrating an existing control handset (see Fig. 1(b)) so that trainees can move the VE linear accelerator and the couch using an actual handset.

The treatment room has three orthogonal lasers which intersect at the treatment isocentre. These are used to help position the patient on the couch during treatment. These lasers are provided in the VE model (see Fig 1(a)).

### 2.2. Visualization of Patient Anatomy

From the training perspective, an important feature of the VE simulator is that treatment plans of actual patients' IMRT treatment can be loaded into the virtual world. This flexibility provides the trainee with experience of the treatment of various cancer sites and it allows experience of complications that may arise during various treatment delivery situations. Being patient specific also means that it is easy to tailor the VE training session to match the needs of the curriculum. Currently, the plan is loaded from a native format of the commercial CMS (Computerised Medical Systems) RT planning system. This was chosen as it was the format used at the Princess Royal Hospital. We intend to extend this to cater for DICOM RT so that patient specificity is independent of treatment planning

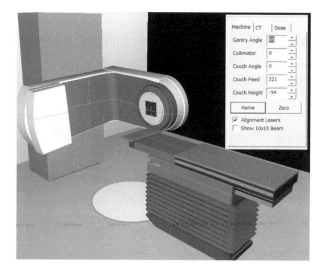
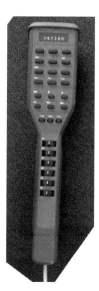

**Figure 1.** (a) Virtual linear accelerator, couch and alignment lasers (used for positioning the patient). Inset is the dialogue box for manual manipulation of the gantry and couch of the VE linear accelerator. Actual handset (b) that is being adapted for control of the VE linear accelerator.

system suppliers. The following information is extracted from the CMS treatment plan for patient visualization.

1) Anatomy as defined by a CT and / or MRI slice stack.
2) Contours and 3D surfaces delineating the treatment volumes of interest. Such volumes include the tumour, gross tumour and planned tumour volume [4], and functional anatomy that is particularly sensitive to radiation such as kidneys, spinal cord, pituary glands, etc, which need to be taken account of specifically when designing the treatment plan for the patient. The latter are known as organs at risk (OARs). These volumes and their associated radiation dose constraints, along with the number and direction of the treatment beams, provide the inputs to an inverse planning optimisation algorithm. This algorithm computes both the shape and intensity distribution of each radiation treatment beam.

The VE simulator provides various immersive facilities for anatomy visualization, all of which are displayed in 3D and registered to the patient space in the treatment room. The tumour and OAR volumes, and the patient's skin surface, can be visualized selectively either as contours or as surfaces. Colour and transparency of these volumes can be selected interactively to provide the best visualization for training purposes. The usual controls for viewing CT/MRI slices are provided in the VE simulator. To help trainees understand relationships between anatomy and treatment volumes, the displayed CT/MRI slice is registered to the patient space in the treatment room and displayed in 3D. In addition the slice can be clipped to the patient skin surface. Fig. 2 illustrates the 3D visualization of anatomy and planning volumes for a patient.

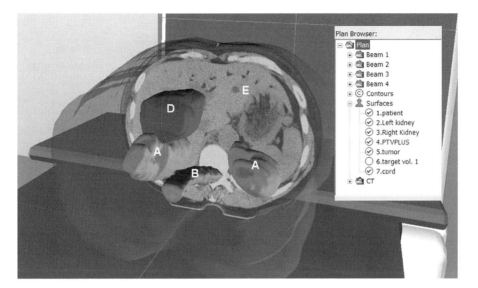

**Figure 2.** Visualization showing patient anatomy on couch of radiotherapy treatment room. View shows tumour (D) being treated, organs at risks (A – kidneys, B – spinal cord) where dose must be below a specified level, (E) CT slice clipped to patient's skin surface. Inset is the dialogue box showing elements of the treatment plan.

## 2.3. Visualization of Radiation Treatment Plans

An intensity modulated radiotherapy (IMRT) treatment plan comprises a set of therapeutic radiation beams each delivered from a different direction. Using a technique known as 'step and shoot' [5] each beam is delivered as a sequence of beam segments. Each segment is shaped individually using a multi-leaf collimator (MLC) inside the gantry head of the linear accelerator. The radiation time for each segment may also vary; this allows the intensity of the dose to be modulated over the beam's cross section.

In order to visualize treatment delivery the following information is extracted from the patient's treatment plan.

1) Details of each radiation beam.
2) Details of all segments that make up each beam.
3) The planned volumetric distribution of dose for the patient's anatomy.

To visualize a treatment beam, the simulator first moves the gantry and its head to the correct position. The beam is then visualized as a semi-transparent green projection (see Fig 3.) registered with the patient space. This visualization in fact represents the accumulation of all segments that comprise this beam. This allows the trainee to appreciate the margins between OARs and the treatment beams, and to appreciate why a particular configuration of beams is used. Individual segments of a beam can also be visualized as a green projection. The MLC leaf settings for a segment can be displayed as an inset in the 3D view (see Fig 3.).

Visualization of dose distribution is also provided. A dose intensity map can be displayed that shows the intensity of dose delivered over the cross section of a beam (see

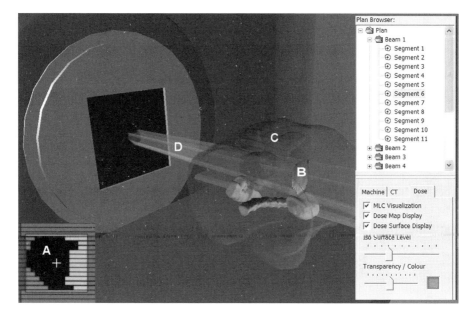

**Figure 3.** Visualization of the radiation treatment. (D) visualization of segment 6 of treatment beam 1. The segment is shaped using a MLC inside the gantry head. (A) shows the leaf positions of this MLC. (B) dose map of the radiation intensity for beam 1. (C) dose isosurface showing the tissue volume that receives at least 30% of the maximum dose level. Inset is a dialogue box of dose visualization options.

Fig. 3). A very important issue in treatment planning (and thus knowledge to impart to trainees) is the coverage of the tumour with the prescribed dose and the distribution of dose to OARs. Visualization of planned dose distribution is provided by displaying a dose isosurface (see Fig 3.). By choosing a high dose setting for the isosurface the trainee can see how well the plan produces a dose that conforms to the planned tumour volume. By choosing a low dose setting for the isosurface the trainee can check the proximity of a harmful dose level to OARs.

## 3. Training Use of the VE Simulator for Radiotherapy Treatment

### 3.1. Modes of Training

The Hull Immersive Visualization Environment HIVE (www.hive.hull.ac.uk) at the University of Hull has an immersive visualization auditorium. This auditorium features an immersive work wall that has a display area of 5.3 × 2.4 metres. The workwall is back projected by 2 triple DLP projectors (each 2000 lumen) that together provide a display resolution of 2048 * 1024 pixels. The workwall supports stereoscopic 3D display using active shutter glasses. The workwall also supports head tracked stereoscopic display that provides motion parallax effects for a user's head movements. For tracking the user's viewpoint a real time optical motion tracking system with 7 cameras is used. These facilities allow a RT treatment room to be displayed in real size, and larger if needed. Users navigate around the room via a remote gamepad or simply by walking around the room using the head tracked stereo facility.

The VE simulator presented in this paper was developed specifically to exploit the capabilities of workwalls such as the one in HIVE. There are two main modes of using the VE simulator and the workwall. The first is where a small group of trainees view the workwall a distance of 2 to 3 metres. In this setting the tutor would typically demonstrate various treatment plans and demonstrate various operational scenarios in the treatment room. In this mode the screen more or less covers the trainees' field of view with a stereoscopic 3D scene. This creates an excellent sense of being present in the treatment room. Combined with the rich set of facilities for visualizing the treatment plan and the patient, this creates a very compelling environment which seems to greatly enhance the learning experience for trainees.

The other mode is where a trainee would be given a task to perform within the treatment room. The trainee would use head tracked stereo and the trainee would have direct control of the virtual equipment and patient to complete the task. Again the sense of presence, now even greater through motion parallax, reinforces learning and assists the trainee in developing manipulation skills for positioning the patient and equipment. Our experience so far of using the VE simulator is limited. A number of classes are planned for the current academic session.

The VE simulator also runs on a range of other stereoscopic display technologies. These include a passive stereo projection system with a 2.4 × 1.8 metres screen, a Sharp auto-stereo LCD laptop computer and a PC with active stereo glasses. We have found the latter very useful for trainee education on a one to one basis.

The VE simulator has been widely used for lectures (in Hull and Sheffield) on RT treatment in a classroom setting. Here the simulator is often run during the lecture using normal mono projection facilities to demonstrate RT concepts. Alternatively, prior to the lecture, patient plans of interest can be loaded into the simulator and relevant screen grabs and animations output by the simulator for presentation in the lecture. Our experience indicates that by using the simulator's facilities, the difficult spatial concepts of RT treatment can be taught more quickly, and it also results in better understanding by the trainees.

## 3.2. Training of Patient Set-up Errors

It is important that the patient's anatomy be in the correct position prior to and during RT treatment. Positioning errors can arise due to mal alignment of the lasers with the isocentre, sag in the gantry of the linear accelerator, incorrect positioning of the patient on the couch, internal organs being in a different position from that defined by the planning CT/MRI, breathing motion, tumour reduction after a number of treatment sessions, etc. The impact of poor patient positioning can be demonstrated using the VE simulator.

In the simulator the patient anatomy is attached to the couch and the radiation beams and dose distribution are attached to the gantry head of the linear accelerator. Thus the couch of the simulator can be moved manually to mimic errors in patient position and anatomy. By then visualizing the beams and dose distribution of the treatment plan, the trainee can observe whether the positioning error is significant in terms of the tumour being under dosed or the OARs being overdosed. Similarly, some errors in equipment set up can be mimicked by manually moving the linear accelerator and observing the consequences.

## 4. Conclusions

Immersive visualization aids the understanding of complex spatial relationships of anatomy and radiation beam therapies such as IMRT. Stereoscopic views, large displays, immersion and motion parallax greatly aid the assimilation of these relationships. A key benefit of the VE simulator presented is its patient-specific approach. This allows trainees to experience a range of patient treatments selected to improve the skills and understanding of the trainees. Another key feature of the simulator is the close integration between the visualizations of patient anatomy, the treatment plan and the treatment room. We believe immersive visualization provides a cost effective training solution as it reduces learning time, improves trainee understanding and reduces the need for training in real linear accelerator treatment rooms.

Plans are well advanced to set up radiotherapy training centres (in UK and USA) based on the VE simulator presented in this paper and using immersive visualization facilities similar to that provided by HIVE. We are also investigating the use of the VE simulator for informing patients and relatives about their treatment.

## References

[1] Intensity Modulated Radiation Therapy Collaborative Working Group, *Intensity-modulated Radiotherapy: current status and issues of interest*, Int. J. Radiation Oncology Biol. Phys, Vol. 51, No. 4, pp 880-914, 2001.

[2] Webb S, *Intensity-modulated radiation therapy*, Institute of Physics Publishing, Bristol, 2000.

[3] Samuelssom, Mercke C, Johansson K-A, Systematic set-up errors for IMRT in the head and neck region: effect on dose distribution, Radiotherapy and Oncology, Vol 66, pp 303-311, 2003.

[4] International Commission on Radiation Units and Measurements (ICRU), *Prescribing, Recording and Reporting Photon Beam Therapy (supplement to ICRU Report 50)*, Report 62, Nuclear Technology Publishing, 1999.

[5] Beavis AW, Ganney P, Whitton VJ and Xing L, *Optimisation of the step-and-shoot leaf sequence for delivery of intensity modulated radiation therapy using a variable division scheme*, Phys Med Biol, Vol 46, pp 2457-2465, 2001.

Medicine Meets Virtual Reality 13
James D. Westwood et al. (Eds.)
IOS Press, 2005

# Toward *In Vivo* Mobility

Mark E. RENTSCHLER [a], Jason DUMPERT [a], Stephen R. PLATT [a],
Shane M. FARRITOR [a] and Dmitry OLEYNIKOV [b]

[a] *Department of Mechanical Engineering, University of Nebraska-Lincoln*
[b] *Department of Surgery, University of Nebraska Medical Center*

**Abstract.** Today's laparoscopic tools impose severe ergonomic limitations and are constrained to only four degrees of freedom. These constraints limit the surgeon's ability to orient the tool tips arbitrarily, and can contribute to a variety of complications. Robots external to the patient have been used to aid in the manipulation of the tools and improve dexterity. However, these robots are expensive, bulky, and are used for only select procedures. *In vivo* robotic assistants have the potential to enhance the capabilities of the surgeon, reduce costs, and reduce patient trauma. The motion of these *in vivo* robots will not be constrained by the insertion incisions. Such assistants will need to attain optimal viewing angles by traversing the abdominal organs without causing trauma. This paper presents an experimental analysis of miniature *in vivo* robot wheels.

## 1. Background

In minimally invasive surgery, the small incisions are the advantage and the limitation. These small holes reduce patient trauma, but do not allow the surgeon to directly view or touch the surgical environment, and they constrain the motion of the endpoint of the tools and cameras to arcs of a sphere whose center is the insertion point. Vision limitations are significant [1,2] because the current field of view cannot encompass the frequent changes of instruments as they pass through the abdominal cavity. This has led to accidental injury to organs and vascular structures [3,4]. Additional viewpoints—showing the entire body cavity—would be very helpful [5]. Such limitations have slowed the expanded use of laparoscopic techniques. Within about a decade of the first laparoscopic cholecystectomy, 85% of all gall bladder excisions were performed laparoscopically [6], suggesting a rapid conversion of many other conventional procedures to less invasive approaches. The reality is that laparoscopic surgery has not realized this potential. In 2000, less than 3% of colon resections [7] and only 17% of cardiothoracic surgeries [6] were performed laparoscopically.

Robots have been used to increase the surgeon's dexterity. The robots can filter the natural tremor present in the human hand, correct for the effects of motion reversal, and/or perform motion scaling to provide greater control of instrument movements in the surgical field. In such systems the robots are implemented from outside the body and are therefore still fundamentally constrained by the small access ports. Moreover, each of the robotic arms is necessarily long and bulky to accommodate the range of motion required to maneuver the long instruments attached to each arm. Large excursion arcs of the arms lead to collisions outside the patient, and improper placement of the access

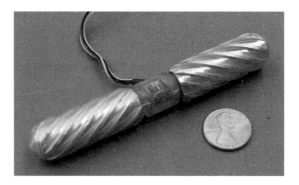

**Figure 1.** *In vivo* mobile robot prototype.

ports leads to collisions inside the patient [8]. Each arm requires a separate access port into the abdominal cavity; hence the number of incisions is not reduced compared to conventional laparoscopy. Tool changes still require the removal of the existing tool and the reinsertion of the new one, adding to the overall surgical time and adversely affecting the efficiency of the operation [9,10].

Use of miniature *in vivo* robotic assistants offers a new approach to laparoscopy. Robotic assistants placed inside the abdominal cavity during surgery have the potential to enhance the capabilities of the surgeon, reduce costs, and improve patient care. Several prototype *in vivo* camera robots have been used during porcine cholecystectomies to provide the surgeon with additional visual feedback [11]. In addition, image quality from these robot cameras has been found to be comparable to current laparoscopic systems [12].

## 2. Methods

### 2.1. Mobile Robot

An *in vivo* mobile robot prototype has been developed [13]. This robot is 15 mm in diameter, 85 mm long and weighs 0.3 N (Fig.1). It has two wheels that are independently driven, and a small tail (not shown) to prevent the body from spinning. It has a center space that is sized to hold a small camera. The robot has been tethered in these early tests. The addition of a tail will increase frictional resistance and may provide small changes to the robot's normal force. However, testing of the tethered robot shows that the tether does not significantly obstruct steering, nor significantly affects motion resistance.

### 2.2. Wheel/Tissue Modeling

Wheel-terrain interaction has been studied extensively for passenger vehicle applications. However, the environment inside the abdomen is much different than any of the studies done on wheel and soil interaction. For *in vivo* applications, the wheel interacts with organs that are highly deformable and very slick, and the constitutive relations describing wheel-organ interaction generally do not resemble those of soils.

The mobility of a wheeled robot can be characterized by the drawbar force produced. This force is a strong function of the normal force between the wheel and the surface, the

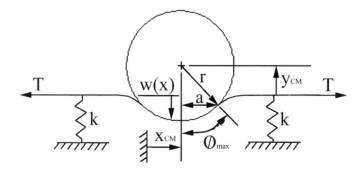

**Figure 2.** Wheel/tissue interaction analytical model.

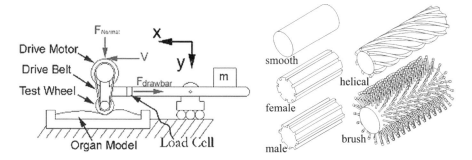

**Figure 3.** Bench top platform and wheel profiles.

effective coefficient of friction between the wheel and the surface, and wheel torque [14]. The surface mobility of *in vivo* robots has been modeled using the surface interaction model of Filonenko-Borodich [15] for a membrane on an elastic foundation [16]. The model represents the load distribution for an elastic material covered by a surface membrane in tension (Fig. 2). The fundamental issue affecting mobility is the contact angle, which is essentially a measure of vertical wheel displacement. The trends established by this model have been used to help design the wheel diameter.

## 2.3. Drawbar Force

Ultimately a wheel that produces the most drawbar force, without damaging the abdominal organs, is desirable. Current work has focused on designing and testing the crawler's wheels. This has been done by testing wheels on both a bench top platform, and on the mobile robot itself (*ex vivo* and *in vivo*).

### 2.3.1. Bench Top Platform

A laboratory system was created to test wheel performance (Fig 3, left). This system consists of a linear slide that moves a wheel similar in size, shape, and material to the proposed robot, across a model of an organ. The wheel is independently driven by a motor attached with a drive belt. The wheel assembly is mounted to a lever that is used to dictate the wheel/organ normal force. A load cell is used to measure the drawbar force and an inclinometer on the lever is used to determine surface deflections.

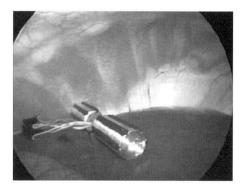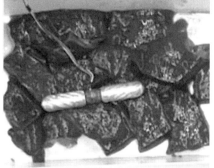

**Figure 4.** *In vivo* and *ex vivo* mobile robot performance.

Excised, previously frozen, bovine liver was used to replicate the characteristics of internal organs. A set of experiments was performed to determine the performance of several different wheel profiles (Fig. 3, right) on bovine liver. In each experiment the wheel assembly was driven across the organ model at a fixed linear velocity of 1.0 cm/s while the angular velocity of the wheel was independently controlled at various slip ratios. The slip ratio is defined as

$$SR = \text{slip ratio} = \frac{r\dot{\theta}_{cm}}{\dot{x}_{cm}},$$

where $\dot{x}_{cm}$ is the linear forward velocity of the center of mass of the wheel, $\dot{\theta}_{cm}$ is the angular velocity of the wheel, and $r$ is the wheel radius.

### 2.3.2. Mobile Robot Drawbar Force

A helical wheel was implemented on the mobile robot (Fig. 1). A load cell was attached to the base of the mobile robot body. The other end of the load cell was rigidly clamped using a standard laparoscopic grasper tool. The grasper was then fixed using an arm clamp affixed to the surgical table.

The robot wheels were then rotated at various speeds, while the drawbar force was measured with the load cell. These tests were done *ex vivo* on excised, previously frozen, bovine liver; and *in vivo* on porcine liver, bowel, and spleen.

## 3. Results

### 3.1. Traversing Abdominal Organs

The mobile robot has demonstrated the capability to traverse *in vivo* porcine liver (Fig. 4, left). However, this wheel design proved ineffective on the bowel. A helical wheel design has been tested in a laboratory (Fig. 4, right). This design has the ability to traverse uneven surfaces and can turn easily. This design will be tested *in vivo* in the near future.

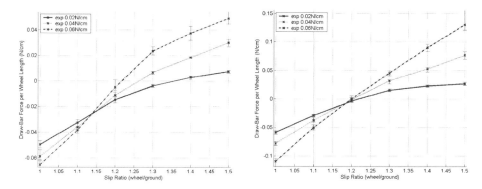

**Figure 5.** Helical and brush wheel performance.

## 3.2. Drawbar Force

### 3.2.1. Bench Top Platform

The drawbar force was measured and averaged over a set of five tests for each slip ratio and applied normal force. Positive drawbar force indicates tension in the load cell (the wheel is pulling), while negative force indicates the load cell is in compression. Several different wheel designs were tested: smooth, female, male, helical, brush (Fig. 3, right). The helical wheel and brush wheel showed superior performance (Fig. 5).

The left plot in Figure 5 shows experimental drawbar force measurements for the 15mm diameter, helical wheel on bovine liver. This wheel generated positive drawbar force for slip ratios greater than 1.2. For low slip ratios, the wheel was not able to overcome the drag associated with the wheel sinkage and bow effect of the liver in front of the wheel.

The 30mm diameter, brush wheel was designed so that it can be pushed through a smaller diameter trocar for surgical applications, while maintaining a larger diameter for functionality. This wheel's performance (Fig. 5, right) is a scaled version of the helical wheel's performance. At a slip ratio of 1.3, the brush wheel produces similar drawbar forces as the helical wheel at a slip ratio of 1.5. The brush wheel shows the best performance. On the surface of the liver, the brush wheel produces the highest drawbar force by a factor of three. This is not unexpected as this design has many channels allowing fluid flow, and low ground pressure that avoids sinkage.

### 3.2.2. Mobile Robot Drawbar Force

The 15mm diameter helical wheel design was tested in the laboratory (Fig. 6, left) to quantify drawbar force production on bovine liver. The mobile robot was tethered to a load cell to measure the force generation at various wheel speeds (Fig. 6, right). The results show that the robot is capable of producing drawbar forces nearly equal to the weight of the robot (0.3N).

Similar tests were performed *in vivo* on porcine small bowel (Fig. 7), liver and spleen. The results, from both the *ex vivo* and *in vivo* tests, suggest that sufficient drawbar forces exist to maneuver within the abdominal environment. Future tests with this wheel design, and others, *in vivo* will help quantify an appropriate wheel design for traversing the abdominal organs without causing trauma.

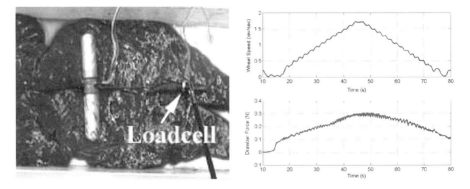

**Figure 6.** *Ex vivo* wheel drawbar force production on beef liver.

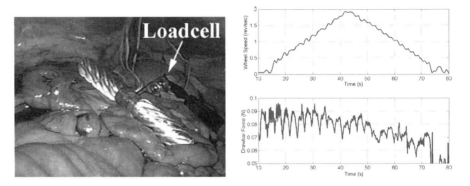

**Figure 7.** *In vivo* wheel drawbar force production on porcine bowel.

## 4. Conclusions

Experiment results have been shown to help develop wheels that are capable of traversing the abdominal environment. Currently, different wheel materials and tread designs are being explored, in addition to porcine *in vivo* testing of several additional wheel designs. These tests will aid in the design of wheels that will not damage tissue. Preliminary tests suggest that it is possible to generate sufficient drawbar forces to maneuver within the abdominal cavity with negligible tissue damage.

An optimized wheel design will be implemented into a mobile robot camera system for porcine *in vivo* exploration and experimental laparoscopic surgeries (e.g. cholecystectomy). Ultimately, the goal is to provide mobile robotic *in vivo* assistance to laparoscopic surgeons. Such robotic assistants will eliminate the port used for the laparoscope, therefore reducing patient trauma.

## References

[1] Treat, M., 1996, "A Surgeon's Perspective on the Difficulties of Laparoscopic Surgery," Computer Integrated Surgery.
[2] Tendick, F., Jennings, R., Tharp, G., and Stark, L., 1996, "Perception and Manipulation Problems in Endoscope Surgery," Computer Integrated Surgery: Technology and Clinical Applications.

[3] Wolfe, B., Gardiner, B., and Leary, B., et al, 1991, "Endoscopic Cholecystectomy: Analysis of Complications," Arch Surg **126**.

[4] Southern Surgeons Club, 1991, "A Pospective Aalysis of 1518 Lparoscopic Colecystectomies," New England Journal of Medicine, **324**, pp. 1073-1078.

[5] Schippers, E., and Schumpelick, V., 1996, "Requirements and Possibilities of Computer-Assisted Endoscope Surgery," Computer Integrated Surgery: Technology and Clinical Applications.

[6] Medtech Insight, 2000, Mission Viejo, CA.

[7] Lo, P., et. al., 2001, "Which Laparoscopic Operations Are the Fastest Growing in Residency Programs?," Surgical Endoscopy, **15**, pp. S145.

[8] Ballantyne, G.H., 2002, "Robotic Surgery, Telerobotic Surgery, Telepresence, and Telementoring," Surgical Endoscopy, **16**, pp. 1389-1402.

[9] Kim, V.B., Chapman, W.H.H., Albrecht, R.J., Bailey, B.M., Young, J.A., Nifong, L.W., and Chitwood, W.R., 2002, "Early Experience With Telemanipulative Robot-Assisted Laparoscopic Cholecystectomy Using da Vinci," Surgical Laparoscopy, Endoscopy & Percutaneous Techniques, **12-1**, pp. 33-44.

[10] Kang, H. and Wen, J.T., 2001, "Robotic Assistants Aid Surgeons During Minimally Invasive Procedures," IEEE Engineering in Medicine and Biology, pp. 94-104.

[11] Oleynikov, D., Rentschler, M., Hadzialic, A., Dumpert, J., Platt, S., Farritor, S., 2004, "Miniature Robots Can Assist in Laparoscopic Cholecystectomy." SAGES.

[12] Rentschler, M., Oleynikov, D., Hadzialic, A., Dumpert, J., Platt, S., Farritor, S., 2004, "In Vivo Camera Robots Provide Improved Vision for Laparoscopic Surgery." Computer Assisted Radiology and Surgery Conference.

[13] Rentschler, M., Hadzialic, A., Dumpert, J., Platt, S., Farritor, S., Oleynikov, D., 2004, "In Vivo Robots for Laparoscopic Surgery." Studies in Health Technology and Informatics – Medicine Meets Virtual Reality, **98**, pp. 316-322.

[14] Jo-Yung Wong and A..R.. Reece, 1967, "Prediction of Rigid Wheel Performance Based on the Analysis of Soil-Wheel Stresses, Part I. Performance of Driven Rigid Wheels", Journal of Terramechanics, **4-1**, pp. 81-98.

[15] Selvadurai, A.P.S., 1979, *Elastic Analysis of Soil-Foundation Interaction,* Elsevier Scientific Publishing Company.

[16] Rentschler, M., Dumpert, J., Hadzialic, A., Platt, S., Oleynikov, D., Iagnemma, K., Farritor, S., 2004, "Theoretical and Experimental Analysis of In Vivo Wheeled Mobility." ASME 28th Biennial Mechanisms and Robotics Conference.

*Medicine Meets Virtual Reality 13*
*James D. Westwood et al. (Eds.)*
*IOS Press, 2005*

# E-Learning Experience: A Teaching Model with Undergraduate Surgery Students in a Developing Country

Rafael E. RIVEROS, M.D [a], Andres ESPINOSA, M.D [b], Pablo JIMENEZ, M.D [c]
and Luis MARTINEZ, MS VI

[a] *Chairman Department of Surgery, School of Medicine, Universidad Colegio Mayor de Nuestra Señora del Rosario Bogota, Colombia*
[b] *Medical Informatics Unit Coordinator, School of Medicine, Universidad Colegio Mayor de Nuestra Señora del Rosario Bogota, Colombia*
[c] *Undergraduate Program Coordinator Department of Surgery, School of Medicine, Universidad Colegio Mayor de Nuestra Señora del Rosario Bogota, Colombia*

**Abstract.** Colombian medical students do not have an effective approach to electronic facilities *in situ* or at home, in contrast with most of American and European medical programs. Our aim is to help medical students to handle current biomedical data, specifically surgical information, in the benefit of patients, themselves and the community via ICT. The model implemented as a pilot study had a good acceptance amongst undergraduate surgery students and faculty.

## 1. Problem

The increasing use of information technology (ICT) in common medical life has led recent generations of students and teachers to realize that informatics are vital in the construction of the medical doctor [1]. There have been sporadic efforts in our country to approach the use of ICT in higher education although, unfortunately, the general trend is still in germinal status [2].

In general, our medical students (MS) do not have an effective approach to electronic facilities *in situ* or at home, in contrast with most of American and European medical programs [3]. Our main objective is to help MS to handle current biomedical data, specifically surgical information, in the benefit of patients, themselves and the community via ICT [4].

## 2. Methods

Through our medical school website (http://medicina.urosario.edu.co) we link an e-learning platform with our virtual course in Surgery and related specialties (including Anesthesia, Ophthalmology, Othorynolaryngology, Orthopedic surgery, Pediatric surgery and Plastic surgery).

The surgery undergraduate program coordination and the medical informatics unit administer the course. Only MS who are at 4th and 6th year of medicine can access to the course.

This course has been organized in the following modules:

- Course contents: Academic syllabus, Calendar, Finder, Glossary and Academic contents.
- Communication tools: e-mail, chat and forums.
- Other tools: My progress and Personal websites.

4th year MS receive 83 theoretical classes in surgical sciences through the academic semester and they visit our virtual course in the e-learning platform finding relevant information of every topic.

We realized a pilot study with 6th year MS during 2 months to evaluate this model. They received 20 theoretical classes about general topics in surgical sciences and they could review related information in the virtual course. In addition, 4 chat sessions with teachers were carried out to solve questions.

## 3. Results

128 MS are being evaluated (30 MS at 4th year and 98 MS at 6th year). In the pilot study, 98 MS during 2 months using the virtual course in Surgery and related sciences were evaluated. 64% were women, age among 21 to 25 years old. 559 visits to the system were registered: 358 (64%) to the course contents, 163 (29%) to the communication tools and 38 (7%) to other tools.

The percentage of students that visited the platform was 82,7% (81 students) with an average of 6,9 visits/student (range: from 1 to 122 visits). Final results of 4th year MS will be obtained and analyzed in January 2005.

## 4. Discussion

Virtual courses at Universidad del Rosario School of Medicine are a novel experience in Colombian medical education. The model implemented with theoretical classes with virtual resources had good results with the students, much more than it was supposed to be expected.

Department directors and faculty in general had shown intermediate enthusiasm to cooperate with similar projects in other biomedical areas. Cooperative meetings with faculty of the Basic Sciences, Clinical, Public Health and Research Departments are in progress with positive results.

Follow up papers with final reports will be published to share this experience with the informatics and academic communities.

## 5. Conclusions

E-learning as a teaching model in this undergraduate surgery program has been a grateful and successful experience.

The model implemented as a pilot study had a good acceptance amongst 6<sup>th</sup> year MS and faculty. Currently, we are working to achieve results with 4<sup>th</sup> year MS.

Faculty and MS teamwork, in search to reach the use of ICT in our medical school, is a challenging scenario today at germinal state but initial results are demanding.

We will compare in 2005 the results obtained from 4<sup>th</sup> and 6<sup>th</sup> year MS with coming undergraduate surgery students of first and second semester of 2005. We want to assess relevance, advantages and disadvantages of this model for educational and learning processes of our students.

## References

[1] Carothers R. Classism and Quality. In: Pursuit of Quality in Higher Education: Case Studies in Total Quality Management. L.G. Teeter D. San Francisco, Jossey-Bass Publishers: 133;1993.
[2] Unigarro M. Educacion Virtual, encuentro formativo en el ciberespacio. Bucaramanga, Editorial Universidad Autonoma de Bucaramanga: 92;2001.
[3] Wilson A. Moving Beyond Performance Paradigms in Human Resource Development. In: Handbook of adult and continuing education. San Francisco, Jossey-Bass Inc: 735;2001.
[4] Riveros R, Isaza A, Espinosa A, Lobelo F, Pacheco S, Younes R. A program for electronic medical education in Colombia: Educacion Electronica Estructurada (E3). A successful experience. Journal of Systemics, Cybernetic and Informatics [serial online] 2004 May; 2(1): [2 screens]. At: URL: http://www.iiisci.org/Journal/SCI/Home.asp.

*Medicine Meets Virtual Reality 13*
*James D. Westwood et al. (Eds.)*
*IOS Press, 2005*

# Development of a VR Therapy Application for Iraq War Military Personnel with PTSD

Albert RIZZO, Jarrell PAIR, Peter J. MCNERNEY, Ernie EASTLUND,
Brian MANSON, Jon GRATCH, Randy HILL and Bill SWARTOUT
*University of Southern California Institute for Creative Technologies*
*13274 Fiji Way, Marina del Rey, CA. 90292*

**Abstract.** Post Traumatic Stress Disorder (PTSD) is reported to be caused by traumatic events that are outside the range of usual human experiences including (but not limited to) military combat, violent personal assault, being kidnapped or taken hostage and terrorist attacks. Initial data suggests that 1 out of 6 returning Iraq War military personnel are exhibiting symptoms of depression, anxiety and PTSD. Virtual Reality (VR) exposure therapy has been used in previous treatments of PTSD patients with reports of positive outcomes. The aim of the current paper is to specify the rationale, design and development of an Iraq War PTSD VR application that is being created from the virtual assets that were initially developed for the X-Box game entitled *Full Spectrum Warrior* which was inspired by a combat tactical training simulation, *Full Spectrum Command*.

## 1. Introduction

In 1997, researchers at Georgia Tech released the first version of the Virtual Vietnam VR scenario for use as a graduated exposure therapy treatment for Post Traumatic Stress Disorder with Vietnam veterans. This occurred over 20 years following the end of the Vietnam War. During that interval, in spite of valiant efforts to develop and apply traditional psychotherapeutic approaches to PTSD, the progression of the disorder in some veterans severely impaired their functional abilities and quality of life, as well as that of their family members and friends. The tragic nature of this disorder also had significant ramifications for the U.S. Veteran's Administration healthcare delivery system often leading to designations of lifelong service connected disability status. Just recently, the first systematic study of mental health problems due to the Iraq conflict revealed that *"... The percentage of study subjects whose responses met the screening criteria for major depression, generalized anxiety, or PTSD was significantly higher after duty in Iraq (15.6 to 17.1 percent) than after duty in Afghanistan (11.2 percent) or before deployment to Iraq (9.3 percent)"* [1]. With this history in mind, the USC Institute for Creative Technologies (ICT) has initiated a project that is creating an immersive virtual environment system for the treatment of Iraq War veterans diagnosed with combat-related PTSD. The proposed treatment environment is based on a creative approach to recycling virtual assets that were initially built for a combat tactical simulation scenario entitled

*Full Spectrum Command*, which later inspired the creation of the commercially available X-Box game, *Full Spectrum Warrior*. This paper will briefly present the vision, rationale, technical specifications, clinical interface design and development status of the Full Spectrum PTSD treatment system that is currently in progress at the USC ICT.

## 2. Post Traumatic Stress Disorder

According to the DSM-IV [2], PTSD is caused by traumatic events that are outside the range of usual human experiences such as military combat, violent personal assault, being kidnapped or taken hostage, terrorist attack, torture, incarceration as a prisoner of war, natural or man-made disasters, automobile accidents, or being diagnosed with a life-threatening illness. The disorder also appears to be more severe and longer lasting when the event is caused by human means and design (bombings, shootings, combat, etc.). Such incidents would be distressing to almost anyone, and is usually experienced with intense fear, terror, and helplessness. Typically, the initiating event involves actual or threatened death or serious injury, or other threat to one's physical integrity; or witnessing an event that involves death, injury, or a threat to the physical integrity of another person. Symptoms of PTSD are often intensified when the person is exposed to stimulus cues that resemble or symbolize the original trauma in a *non-therapeutic* setting. Such *uncontrolled* cue exposure may lead the person to react with a survival mentality and mode of response that could put the patient and others at considerable risk.

Prior to the availability of VR therapy applications, the existing standard of care for PTSD was *imaginal* exposure therapy. Such treatment typically involves the graded and repeated imaginal reliving of the traumatic event within the therapeutic setting. This approach is believed to provide a low-threat context where the patient can begin to therapeutically process the emotions that are relevant to the traumatic event as well as decondition the learning cycle of the disorder via a habituation/extinction process. While the efficacy of imaginal exposure has been established in multiple studies with diverse trauma populations [3,4], many patients are unwilling or unable to effectively visualize the traumatic event. In fact, avoidance of reminders of the trauma is inherent in PTSD, and is one of the defining symptoms of the disorder. It is often reported that, *". . . some patients refuse to engage in the treatment, and others, though they express willingness, are unable to engage their emotions or senses."* [5]. Research on this aspect of PTSD treatment suggests that the inability to emotionally engage (*in imagination*) is a predictor for negative treatment outcomes [6].

The use and value of Virtual Reality for the treatment of cognitive, emotional, psychological and physical disorders has been well specified [7,8]. The first use of VR for a Vietnam veteran with PTSD was reported in a case study of a 50-year-old, Caucasian male veteran meeting DSM-IV criteria for PTSD [9]. Results indicated post-treatment improvement on all measures of PTSD and maintenance of these gains at a 6-month follow-up. This case study was followed by an open clinical trial of VR for Vietnam veterans [10]. In this study, 16 male PTSD patients were exposed to two HMD-delivered virtual environments, a virtual clearing surrounded by jungle scenery and a virtual Huey helicopter, in which the therapist controlled various visual and auditory effects (e.g. rockets, explosions, day/night, yelling). After an average of 13 exposure therapy sessions over 5-7 weeks, there was a significant reduction in PTSD and related symptoms. Similar positive results have also recently been reported for VR applied to PTSD resulting from the attack on the World Trade Center [5]. In this report, a case study was presented using VR to provide re-exposure to the trauma with a patient who had failed to improve with traditional exposure therapy. The authors reported significant reduction of PTSD symptoms by exposing the patient to explosions, sound effects, virtual people jumping from the burning buildings, towers collapsing, and dust clouds and attributed this success partly due to the increased realism of the VR images as compared to the mental images the patient could generate in imagination. Such early results suggest that VR may be a valuable technology to apply as a component within a comprehensive treatment approach for persons with combat-related PTSD.

## 3. Full Spectrum Warrior Background and Development History

The primary aim of the current project is to use the already existing ICT Full Spectrum Warrior graphic assets (go to: http://www.ict.usc.edu/disp.php?bd=proj_games_fsw for video demo) as the basis for creating a clinical VR application. The ICT games project has created two training tools for the U.S. Army to teach leadership and decision making skills. Full Spectrum Command (FSC) is a PC application that simulates the experience of commanding a light infantry company. FSC teaches resource management, adaptive thinking, and tactical decision-making. Full Spectrum Warrior, developed for the Xbox game console, puts the trainee in command of a nine person squad. Trainees learn small unit tactics as they direct fire teams through a variety of immersive urban combat scenarios. These tools were developed through collaboration between ICT, entertainment software companies, the U.S. Army Training and Doctrine Command (TRADOC), and the Research, Development, and Engineering Command, Simulation Technology Center (RDECOM STC). Additionally, Subject Matter Experts from the Army's Infantry School contributed to the design of these training tools. The current VR PTSD application is designed to run on two Pentium 4 notebook computers each with 1 GB RAM, and a 128 MB DirectX 9 compatible graphics cards. The two computers are linked using a null Ethernet cable. One notebook runs the therapist's control application while the second notebook drives the user's head mounted display (HMD), orientation tracker and navigation controls. The application is built on ICT's FlatWorld Simulation Control Architecture (FSCA). The FSCA enables a network-centric system of client displays driven by a single controller application. The controller application broadcasts user triggered or scripted event data to the display client. The client's real-time 3D scenes are presented using Numerical Design Limited's (NDL) Gamebryo graphics engine.

## 4. Full Spectrum Warrior PTSD VR System Features

We have created a prototype virtual environment designed to resemble a middle-eastern city (see Figures 1-3). This VE was designed as a proof of concept demonstrator and as a tool for initial user testing to gather feedback from both Iraq War military personnel and clinical professionals in order to refine the city scenario and to seek guidance regarding the future expansion of the system to include other relevant scenario settings. The vision for the project includes, not only the design of a series of diverse scenario settings

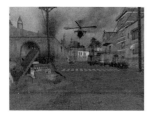

**Figure 1.** City View.

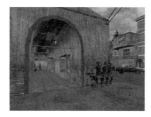

**Figure 2.** "Flocking" Patrol.

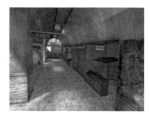

**Figure 3.** Interior View.

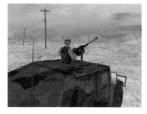

**Figure 4.** Desert Road View.

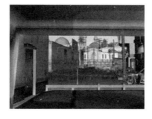

**Figure 5.** HUMVEE View.

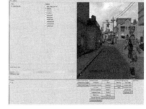

**Figure 6.** Clinical Interface.

(e.g. outlying village and desert scenes), but as well, the creation of options for providing the user with different first person perspectives. These choice options when combined with real time clinician input via the "Wizard of Oz" clinical interface is envisioned to allow for the creation of a user experience that is specifically customized to the needs of the patient participating in treatment. The software is being designed such that clinical users can be teleported to specific scenario settings based on a determination as to which environment most closely matches the patient's needs, relevant to their individual combat related experiences. These settings include:

1. **City Scenes** – In this setting, we are creating two variations. The first city setting (similar to what we have in our prototype) will have the appearance of a desolate set of low populated streets comprising of old buildings, ramshackle apartments, a mosque, factories and junkyards (see Figures 1-2). The second city setting will have similar street characteristics and buildings, but will be more highly populated and have more traffic activity, marketplace scenes and monuments.

2. **Checkpoint** – This area of the City Scenario will be constructed to resemble a traffic checkpoint with a variety of moving vehicles arriving, stopping and then moving onward.

3. **City Building Interiors** – Some of the City Scenario buildings will have interiors modeled that will allow the user to navigate through them. These interiors will have the option of being vacant (see Figure 3) or have various levels of populated virtual characters inhabiting them.

4. **Small Rural Village** – This setting will consist of a more spread out rural area containing ramshackle structures, a village center and much decay in the form of garbage, junk and wrecked or battle-damaged vehicles. It will also contain more vegetation and have a view of a desert landscape in the distance that is visible as the user passes by gaps between structures near the periphery of the village.

5. **Desert Base** – This scenario will be designed to appear as a desert military base of operations consisting of tents, soldiers and an array of military hardware.

6. **Desert Road** – This will consist of both paved and dirt roadway which will connect the City scenario with the Village scenario. The view from the road will
mainly consist of desert scenery and sand dunes (see Figure 4) with occasional
areas of vegetation, ramshackle structures and battle wreckage.

Once the scenario setting is selected, it will be possible to select from a variety
of user perspective and navigation options. These are being designed in order to again
provide flexibility in how the interaction in the scenario settings can be customized to
suit the clinical user's needs. These options will include:

1. User walking alone on patrol from a first person perspective (Figure 1).
2. User walking with one soldier companion on patrol. The accompanying soldier
   will be animated with a "flocking" algorithm that will place them always within
   a 5-meter radius of the user and will adjust position based on collision detection
   with objects and structures to support a perception of realistic movement.
3. User walking with a patrol consisting of a number of companion soldiers using a
   similar "flocking" approach as in #2 above (Figure 2).
4. User view from the perspective of being in a HUMVEE or other moving vehicle
   as it automatically travels through the various setting scenarios (Figure 5). The
   interior view can have options for other occupant passengers that will have ambient movement. The view will also be adjustable to support the perception of
   travel within a convoy or as a lone vehicle.
5. User view from the perspective of being in a helicopter hovering above the scenarios.

In each of these user perspective options, the user may or may not possess a weapon,
and in some cases the weapon will be usable to return fire when it is determined by the
clinician that this would be a relevant component for the therapeutic process. We have
also created an initial version of a "Wizard of Oz" type clinical interface (Figure 6). This
interface is a key element in the application, as it needs to provide a clinician with a
usable tool for placing the user in VE locations that resemble the setting and context in
which the traumatic events initially occurred. As important, the clinical interface must
also allow the clinician to further customize the therapy experience to the patient's individual needs via the systematic real-time delivery and control of "trigger" stimuli in the
environment. This is essential for fostering the anxiety modulation needed for therapeutic habituation. In our initial configuration, the clinician has a separate computer monitor
that displays the clinical interface controls. While the results from planned user studies
will ultimately guide the interface design process, one possible candidate setup is to provide four quadrants in which the clinician can monitor ongoing user status information,
while simultaneously directing trigger stimulus delivery. The upper left quadrant will
contain basic interface menu keys used for placement of the patient (and immediate removal if needed) in the appropriate scenario setting and user perspective. This quadrant
will also contain menu keys for the control of time of day or night, atmospheric illumination, weather conditions and initial ambient sound characteristics. The lower left quadrant will provide space for real-time display of the patients' heartrate and GSR readings
for monitoring of physiological status. The upper right quadrant will contain a window
that displays the imagery that is present in the user's field of view in real-time. And the
lower right quadrant contains the control panel for the real-time delivery of specific trig-

ger stimuli that are actuated by the clinician in an effort to modulate appropriate levels of anxiety as required by the theory and methodology of exposure-based therapy.

The specification and creation of such trigger stimuli is an evolving process that has begun with our intuitive efforts to include options that have been reported to be relevant by returning soldiers and combat environment experts. For example, Hoge et al., [1], present a useful listing of combat related events that were commonly experienced in their sample of returning Iraq War military personnel. These events provide a useful starting point for conceptualizing how relevant trigger stimuli could be presented in a VE, including: "*Being attacked or ambushed, Receiving incoming artillery, rocket, or mortar fire, Being shot at or receiving small-arms fire, Shooting or directing fire at the enemy, Being responsible for the death of an enemy combatant. . .* " (p. 18). From this and other sources, we have begun our initial effort to conceptualize what is both functionally relevant and pragmatically possible to include as trigger stimuli in our current clinical interface.

## 5. Conclusion

War is perhaps one of the most challenging situations that a human being can experience. The physical, emotional, cognitive and psychological demands of a combat environment place enormous stress on even the best-prepared military personnel. One of the more foreboding findings in the recent Hoge et al., [1] report, was the observation that among Iraq War veterans, "*. . . those whose responses were positive for a mental disorder, only 23 to 40 percent sought mental health care. Those whose responses were positive for a mental disorder were twice as likely as those whose responses were negative to report concern about possible stigmatization and other barriers to seeking mental health care.*" (p. 13). While military training methodology has better prepared soldiers for combat in recent years, such hesitancy to seek treatment upon return from combat, especially by those who may need it most, suggests an area of military mental healthcare that is in need of attention. In this regard, perhaps a VR system for PTSD treatment could serve as a component within a reconceptualized approach to how treatment is accessed by veterans returning from combat. One option would be to integrate VR combat exposure as part of a comprehensive "assessment" program administered upon return from a tour of duty. Since past research is suggestive of differential patterns of physiological reactivity in soldiers with PTSD when exposed to combat-related stimuli [11,12], an initial procedure that integrates our VR PTSD application with physiological recording could be of value. If indicators of such physiological reactivity are present during an initial VR exposure, a referral for continued care could be negotiated and/or prescribed. Finally, one of the guiding principles in our development work concerns how VR can *extend* the skills of a well-trained clinician. This VR approach is not intended to be an automated treatment protocol that could be administered in a "self-help" format. The presentation of such emotionally evocative VR combat-related scenarios, while providing treatment options not possible until recently, will most likely produce therapeutic benefits when administered within the context of appropriate care via a thoughtful professional appreciation of the complexity and impact of this disorder.

## Acknowledgement

This paper was developed with funds of the Department of the Army under contract number DAAD 19-99-D-0046. Any opinions, findings and conclusions or recommendations expressed in this paper are those of the authors and do not necessarily reflect the views of the Department of the Army.

## References

[1] Hoge, C.W., Castro, C.A., Messer, S.C., McGurk, D., Cotting, D.I. and Koffman, R.L. (2004). Combat Duty in Iraq and Afghanistan, Mental Health Problems, and Barriers to Care. *NE Jour of Med*, 351:13-22.

[2] DSM-IV. (1994). American Psychiatric Association, Washington, D.C.

[3] Rothbaum, B.O., Meadows, E.A., Resick, P., et al. (2000). Cognitive-behavioral therapy. In: Foa, E.B., Keane, T.M., Friedman, M.J. (eds.), *Effective treatments for PTSD*. New York: Guilford, pp. 60–83.

[4] Rothbaum, B.O., & Schwartz, A.C. (2002). Exposure therapy for posttraumatic stress disorder. American Journal of Psychotherapy 56:59–75.

[5] Difede, J. & Hoffman, H. (2002). Virtual reality exposure therapy for World Trade Center Post Traumatic Stress Disorder. *Cyberpsychology and Behavior,*5:6, 529-535.

[6] Jaycox, L.H., Foa, E.B., & Morral, A.R. (1998). Influence of emotional engagement and habituation on exposure therapy for PTSD. *Journal of Consulting and Clinical Psychology* 66, 186–192.

[7] Glantz, K., Rizzo, A.A. & Graap, K. (2003). Virtual Reality for Psychotherapy: Current Reality and Future Possibilities. *Psychotherapy: Theory, Research, Practice, Training*, 40, 1/2, 55–67.

[8] Rizzo, A.A., Schultheis, M.T., Kerns, K. & Mateer, C. (2004). Analysis of Assets for Virtual Reality Applications in Neuropsychology. *Neuropsychological Rehabilitation*. 14(1) 207-239.

[9] Rothbaum B., Hodges, L., Alarcon, R., Ready, D., Shahar, F., Graap, K., Pair, J., Hebert, P., Gotz, D., Wills, B., & Baltzell, D. (1999). Virtual reality exposure therapy for PTSD Vietnam veterans: A case study. *Journal of Traumatic Stress* 12, 263-271.

[10] Rothbaum, B., Hodges, L., Ready, D., Graap, K. & Alarcon, R. (2001) Virtual reality exposure therapy for Vietnam veterans with posttraumatic stress disorder. *Journal of Clinical Psychiatry* 62, 617-622.

[11] Laor, N., Wolmer, L., Wiener, Z., Reiss, A., Muller, U., Weizman, R. & Ron, S. (1998). The function of image control in the psychophysiology of PTSD. *Jour of Traumatic Stress*, 11, 679-696.

[12] Keane, T. M., Kaloupek, D., Blanchard, E., Hsieh, F., Kolb, L. C., Orr, S. P., Thomas, R. G. & Lavori, P.W. (1998). Utility of psychophysiological measurement in the diagnosis of posttraumatic stress disorder: Results from a Department of veterans affairs cooperative study. *Jour of Consulting & Clin Psy.* 66, 914-923.

*Medicine Meets Virtual Reality 13*
*James D. Westwood et al. (Eds.)*
*IOS Press, 2005*

# The LapSim: A Learning Environment for Both Experts and Novices

Charles Y. RO [a], Ioannis K. TOUMPOULIS [a], Robert C. ASHTON Jr. [a],
Tony JEBARA [b], Caroline SCHULMAN [a], George J. TODD [a],
Joseph J. DEROSE Jr. [a] and James J. McGINTY [a]

[a] *Department of Surgery, St. Luke's-Roosevelt Hospital Center, New York,
New York, U.S.A.*
[b] *Columbia University, New York, New York, U.S.A.*

**Abstract.**

*Background*: Simulated environments present challenges to both clinical experts and novices in laparoscopic surgery. Experts and novices may have different expectations when confronted with a novel simulated environment. The LapSim is a computer-based virtual reality laparoscopic trainer. Our aim was to analyze the performance of experienced basic laparoscopists and novices during their first exposure to the LapSim Basic Skill set and Dissection module.

*Methods*: Experienced basic laparoscopists (n = 16) were defined as attending surgeons and chief residents who performed >30 laparoscopic cholecystectomies. Novices (n = 13) were surgical residents with minimal laparoscopic experience. None of the subjects had used a computer-based laparoscopic simulator in the past. Subjects were given one practice session on the LapSim tutorial and dissection module and were supervised throughout the testing. Instrument motion, completion time, and errors were recorded by the LapSim. A Performance Score (PS) was calculated using the sum of total errors and time to task completion. A Relative Efficiency Score (RES) was calculated using the sum of the path lengths and angular path lengths for each hand expressed as a ratio of the subject's score to the worst score achieved among the subjects. All groups were compared using the Kruskal-Wallis and Mann-Whitney U-test.

*Results*: Novices achieved better PS and/or RES in Instrument Navigation, Suturing, and Dissection ($p<0.05$). There was no difference in the PS and RES between experts and novices in the remaining skills.

*Conclusion*: Novices tended to have better performance compared to the experienced basic laparoscopists during their first exposure to the LapSim Basic Skill set and Dissection module.

Training novices in minimally invasive techniques has moved from the operating room to the classroom due to issues such as patient safety, quality control, work hour restrictions, and cost-effectiveness [1–4]. Methods devised to improve laparoscopic skills include cadaveric human models, live animal models, and video box trainers. A new technology to train and assess the laparoscopic skills of surgeons is the virtual reality simulator. The LapSim (Surgical Science, Göteborg, Sweden) is a computer-based application designed to simulate laparoscopic conditions. Students are able to practice basic and complex skills with immediate feedback on performance variables including completion time, errors, and instrument motion without extra equipment or supervision as would be needed with conventional training methods.

Virtual reality simulators provide objective evaluation of performance and have been validated to distinguish novices from advanced laparoscopic experts [5–7]. The performance of a less advanced laparoscopist, referred to in this study as a 'basic' laparoscopist, on the LapSim has not been well defined. Whereas an advanced expert has been shown to perform better than a novice on a simulator, possibly due to superior familiarity with visual-spatial challenges required, the performance of a basic laparoscopist compared to that of a novice remains to be determined. Our goal was to analyze the performance of experienced basic laparoscopists and novices on their first encounter with the Basic Skill set and Dissection module.

## Material and Methods

Basic laparoscopists (n = 16) were defined as attending surgeons and chief residents who performed >30 laparoscopic cholecystectomies, yet who do not have advanced skill training. Novices (n = 13) were surgical residents with minimal laparoscopic experience. None of the subjects had used a computer-based laparoscopic simulator in the past.

Subjects were given one practice session on the LapSim and were supervised throughout the testing. The skills tested were Instrument Navigation, Coordination, Grasping, Lifting & Grasping, Cutting, Clip Applying, Suturing, and the cholecystectomy Dissection module. Instrument motion, completion time, and errors were recorded by the LapSim.

A Performance Score (PS) was calculated using the sum of total errors and time to task completion. A Relative Efficiency Score (RES) was calculated using the sum of the path lengths and angular path lengths for each hand expressed as a ratio of the subject's score to the worst score achieved among the subjects. Higher scores indicated worse performance. All groups were compared using the Kruskal-Wallis and Mann-Whitney U-test.

## Results

All 29 subjects completed each task. Analysis of the data revealed no statistical difference between basic laparoscopists and novices in the PS for 6 of 8 skills (Table 1) and in the RES for 6 of 8 skills (Table 2).

Novices achieved significantly better PS in Instrument Navigation and Suturing (p<0.05). Novices also achieved significantly better RES in Suturing and Dissection (p<0.05). Furthermore, novices tended to perform better (lower PS and RES) for each task, except for Clip Applying.

## Discussion

Our study demonstrated that subjects with basic laparoscopy experience performed worse than novices, specifically when confronted with advanced tasks such as Suturing and Dissection. This is in contrast to what may be expected, given that basic laparoscopists have more experience in performing laparoscopic tasks in general.

**Table 1.** Mean Performance Scores (PS).

| Subject | Instrument Navigation | Coordination | Grasping | Lifting & Grasping | Cutting | Clip Applying | Suturing | Dissection |
|---------|-----------------------|--------------|----------|--------------------|---------|---------------|----------|------------|
| Basic   | **35.8**              | 76.0         | **83.7** | 184.0              | **192.3** | 198.4       | **3100.2** | 553.1    |
| Novices | **24.4**              | 54.7         | **51.8** | 147.3              | **138.3** | 216.4       | **995.5**  | 397.9    |
| p-value | **0.018**             | 0.189        | **0.148**| 0.125              | **0.293** | 1.000       | **0.001**  | 0.293    |

**Table 2.** Mean Relative Efficiency Scores (RES).

| Subject | Instrument Navigation | Coordination | Grasping | Lifting & Grasping | Cutting | Clip Applying | Suturing | Dissection |
|---------|-----------------------|--------------|----------|--------------------|---------|---------------|----------|------------|
| Basic   | **2.67**              | 1.99         | **2.54** | 3.19               | **2.27** | 1.44        | **2.46**   | 1.72     |
| Novices | **2.44**              | 1.69         | **2.26** | 2.94               | **1.90** | 1.10        | **1.58**   | 1.09     |
| p-value | **0.293**             | 0.160        | **0.236**| 0.066              | **0.188** | 0.273      | **0.009**  | 0.039    |

Surgical simulators were developed to help students overcome the learning curve of laparoscopy in an environment safe for patients and without the need for direct supervision or additional supplies. A major drawback to current systems, including the LapSim, is the lack of realistic tactile feedback. We believe that the basic laparoscopists' expectations and reliance on haptic feedback from their prior clinical laparoscopic experience may have a negative effect on their first attempt with the system. Interestingly, this effect has not been shown in studies investigating the more advanced experts. It is possible that the need for haptic feedback is negated by the advanced visual-spatial abilities acquired by the experts. Furthermore, novices, who have not honed any laparoscopic skills and may rely primarily on visual cues, approach this novel simulated environment without any preconceived tactile sensory feedback. We anticipate that the difference found in our study would be minimized with repeated attempts as basic laparoscopists learn to use visual cues as opposed to haptic feedback. In addition, the use of models with haptic feedback may also reduce this effect. Finally, our LapSim scoring system may not be the appropriate measure to determine construct validity in this study.

Previous studies have demonstrated that novices benefit from virtual reality training. At minimum, they are able to familiarize themselves with laparoscopic instrumentation and video assisted tasks. Experienced basic laparoscopists may benefit by improving their reliance on visual cues. Whether improving these skills leads to improved performance in the operating room or assists in learning advanced laparoscopic techniques is unknown. Further studies will be required to determine the educational benefit of the LapSim to both novices and experienced basic laparoscopists.

## References

[1]  Villegas L, Schneider E, Callery MP, Jones DB. Laparoscopic skills training. Surgical Endoscopy 2003; 17:1879-1888.
[2]  Munz Y, Kumar BD, Moorthy K, Bann S, Darzi A. Laparoscopic virtual reality and box trainers: is one superior to the other? Surgical Endoscopy 2004; 18:485-494.
[3]  Bridges M, Diamond DL. The financial impact of teaching surgical residents in the operating room. The American Journal of Surgery 1999; 177:28-32.

[4]  Scott DJ, Bergen PC, Rege RV, Laycock R, Tesfay ST, Valentine RJ, Euhus DM, Jeyarajah DR, Thompson WM, Jones DB. Laparoscopic training on bench models: better and more cost effective than operating room experience? Journal of the American College of Surgeons 2000; 191:272-283.

[5]  McNatt SS, Smith CD. A computer-based laparoscopic skills assessment device differentiates experienced from novice laparoscopic surgeons. Surgical Endoscopy 2001; 15:1085-1089.

[6]  Taffinder N, Sutton C, Fishwick RJ, McManus IC, Darzi A. Validation of virtual reality to teach and assess psychomotor skills in laparoscopic surgery: results from randomized controlled studies using the MIST VR laparoscopic simulator. Studies in Health Technology and Informatics 1998; 50:124-130.

[7]  Gallagher AG, Richie K, McClure N, McGuigan J. Objective psychomotor skills assessment of experienced, junior, and novice laparoscopists with virtual reality. World Journal of Surgery 2001; 25:1478-1483.

*Medicine Meets Virtual Reality 13*
*James D. Westwood et al. (Eds.)*
*IOS Press, 2005*

# A Novel Drill Set for the Enhancement and Assessment of Robotic Surgical Performance

Charles Y. RO [a], Ioannis K. TOUMPOULIS [a], Robert C. ASHTON Jr. [a],
Celina IMIELINSKA [b], Tony JEBARA [b], Seung H. SHIN [a], J.D. ZIPKIN [a],
James J. McGINTY [a], George J. TODD [a] and Joseph J. DEROSE Jr. [a]

[a] *Department of Surgery, St. Luke's-Roosevelt Hospital Center, New York,
New York, USA*
[b] *Columbia University, New York, New York, USA*

**Abstract.** *Background*: There currently exist several training modules to improve performance during video-assisted surgery. The unique characteristics of robotic surgery make these platforms an inadequate environment for the development and assessment of robotic surgical performance.

*Methods*: Expert surgeons ($n = 4$) ($>50$ clinical robotic procedures and $>2$ years of clinical robotic experience) were compared to novice surgeons ($n = 17$) ($<5$ clinical cases and limited laboratory experience) using the da Vinci Surgical System. Seven drills were designed to simulate clinical robotic surgical tasks. Performance score was calculated by the equation Time to Completion + (minor error) $\times 5$ + (major error) $\times 10$. The Robotic Learning Curve (RLC) was expressed as a trend line of the performance scores corresponding to each repeated drill.

*Results*: Performance scores for experts were better than novices in all 7 drills ($p<0.05$). The RLC for novices reflected an improvement in scores ($p<0.05$). In contrast, experts demonstrated a flat RLC for 6 drills and an improvement in one drill ($p = 0.027$).

*Conclusion*: This new drill set provides a framework for performance assessment during robotic surgery. The inclusion of particular drills and their role in training robotic surgeons of the future awaits larger validation studies.

Robotics facilitates video-assisted surgery by offering a 3-D imaging system, camera stability, wrist-like instrument navigation, motion scaling, and improved ergonomics [1,2].

These characteristics improve operator performance on standard laparoscopic bench models and also allow for steeper learning curves among novice surgeons [3–6].

Nonetheless, the robotic surgery environment requires familiarity with the device's innate lack of haptic feedback and altered grip strength control. Smooth coordination of the camera with the arms via seamless manipulation of the masters and the foot pedals must also be learned. These unique characteristics of robotic surgery demand novel drills in order to train surgeons and to appropriately assess their robotic surgical performance.

**Table 1.** Mean Performance Scores

| Groups | Drill 1 Precision Beads | Drill 2 Simple Rope Pass | Drill 3 Russian Roulette | Drill 4 Mobile Mobile Precision Beads | Drill 5 Beaded String Pass | Minefield | Suturing |
|---|---|---|---|---|---|---|---|
| Novices | 59.9 | 90.4 | 112.6 | 177.0 | 167.1 | 214.4 | 95.9 |
| Experts | 40.2 | 49.5 | 75.0 | 143.6 | 143.7 | 144.6 | 61.7 |
| p-value | <0.001 | <0.001 | <0.001 | 0.017 | 0.036 | <0.001 | <0.001 |

## 1. Methods

Expert surgeons ($n = 2$, total 4 sets of drills) (>50 clinical robotic procedures and >2 years of clinical robotic experience) were compared to novice surgeons ($n = 17$) (<5 clinical cases and limited laboratory experience) using the da Vinci Surgical System (Intuitive Surgical, Mountain View, CA, USA). Seven drills were designed to simulate clinical robotic surgical tasks in a box trainer using instruments specific for each drill. After an introduction to the robot, each subject was allowed to practice each drill once. Each drill was repeated 5–6 times depending on the specific drill. Time to completion, minor errors and major errors were recorded. Performance score was calculated by the equation Time to Completion + (minor error) × 5 + (major error) × 10. Larger scores corresponded to worse performance. The Robotic Learning Curve (RLC) consisted of a trend line of the performance scores corresponding to each repeated drill. Data was analyzed with the Friedman Test and Mann-Whitney U Test.

### 1.1. Drills

Drill 1: Precision Beads – Large beads are transferred between two cups alternating hands.
Drill 2: Simple Rope Pass – Rope made of large beads is passed from nondominant to dominant hand grasping at pre-determined beads.
Drill 3: Russian Roulette – Pins are transferred from an outer to inner circle alternating hands. The camera must be adjusted for adequate visualization.
Drill 4: Mobile Precision Beads – Small beads are dropped through a hole in a mobile disk.
Drill 5: Beaded String Pass – Similar to Drill 2 but with small beads.
Drill 6: Minefield – Needle from a 6-0 Prolene suture is passed through loops in a pre-arranged pattern. The camera must be adjusted for adequate visualization.
Drill 7: Suturing – 2-0 Vicryl suture is placed within a target area. One surgeon's knot and 3 square knots are tied.

## 2. Results

Performance scores for experts were better than novices in all 7 drills (Table 1, $p<0.05$).
The RLC for novices reflected an improvement in scores ($p<0.05$), but did not reach statistical significance in Drills 6 & 7 (Figures 1–5). In contrast, experts demonstrated a flat RLC for 6 drills and an improvement in Drill 3 ($p = 0.027$).

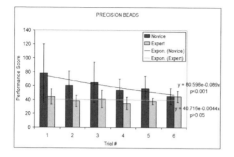

**Figure 1.** Precision Beads.

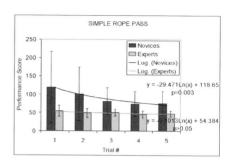

**Figure 2.** Simple Rope Pass.

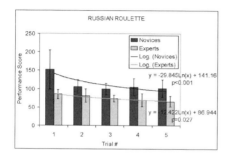

**Figure 3.** Russian Roulette.

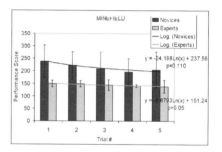

**Figure 4.** Minefield.

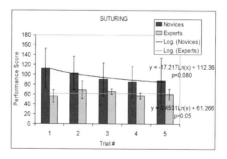

**Figure 5.** Suturing.

## 3. Discussion

This new drill set provides a framework for performance assessment during robotic surgery. Experts performed better at each drill, but novices approached their scores at the end of the drill set indicating a relatively steep learning curve. Drills will be evaluated in future studies using video-linked time and motion analysis through da Vinci system's API (Application Programming Interface). The inclusion of particular drills and their role in training robotic surgeons of the future awaits larger validation studies.

# References

[1] Ballantyne GH. Robotic surgery, telerobotic surgery, telepresence, and telementoring: review of early clinical results. Surgical Endoscopy 2002; 16:1389-1402.

[2] Ballantyne GH, Moll F. The da Vinci telerobotic surgical system: the virtual operative field and telepresence surgery. Surgical Clinics of North America 2003; 83:1293-1304.

[3] Moorthy K, Munz Y, Dosis A, Hernandez J, Martin S, Bello F, Rockall T, Darzi A. Dexterity enhancement with robotic surgery. Surgical Endoscopy 2004; 18:790-795.

[4] Hubens G, Coveliers H, Balliu L, Ruppert M, Vaneerdeweg W. A performance study comparing manual and robotically assisted laparoscopic surgery using the da Vinci system. Surgical Endoscopy 2003; 17:1595-1599.

[5] Sarle R, Tewari A, Shrivastava A, Peabody J, Menon M. Surgical Robotics and Laparoscopic Training Drills. Journal of Endourology 2004; 18:63-67.

[6] Hernandez JD, Bann SD, Munz Y, Moorthy K, Datta V, Martin S, Dosis A, Bello F, Darzi A, Rockall T. Qualitative and quantitative analysis of the learning curve of a simulated surgical task on the da Vinci system. Surgical Endoscopy 2004; 18:372-378.

*Medicine Meets Virtual Reality 13*
*James D. Westwood et al. (Eds.)*
*IOS Press, 2005*

# Spherical Mechanism Analysis of a Surgical Robot for Minimally Invasive Surgery – Analytical and Experimental Approaches

Jacob ROSEN, Ph.D. [a,b], Mitch LUM, BSEE. [a], Denny TRIMBLE, BSME [c],
Blake HANNAFORD, Ph.D. [a,b] and Mika SINANAN M.D., Ph.D. [a,b]

[a] *Department of Electrical Engineering, University of Washington, Seattle, WA, USA*
[b] *Department of Surgery, University of Washington, Seattle, WA, USA*
[c] *Department of Mechanical Engineering, University of Washington, Seattle, WA, USA*
*e-mail: {rosen,mitchlum,mssurg,blake}@u.washington.edu*
*Biorobotics Lab: http://brl.ee.washington.edu*
*Center of Videoendoscopic Surgery: http://depts.washington.edu/cves/*

**Abstract.** Recent advances in technology have led to the fusion of MIS techniques and robot devices. However, current systems are large and cumbersome. Optimizing the surgical robot mechanism will eventually lead to its integration into the operating room (OR) of the future becoming the extended presence of the surgeon and nurses in a room occupied by the patient alone. By optimizing a spherical mechanism using data collected *in-vivo* during MIS procedures, this study is focused on a bottom-up approach to developing a new class of surgical robotic arms while maximizing their performance and minimizing their size. The spherical mechanism is a rotational manipulator with all axes intersecting at the center of the sphere. Locating the rotation center of the mechanism at the MIS port makes this class of mechanism a suitable candidate for the first two links of a surgical robot for MIS. The required dexterous workspace (DWS) is defined as the region in which 95% of the tool motions are contained based on *in-vivo* measurements. The extended dexterous workspace (EDWS) is defined as the entire abdominal cavity reachable by a MIS instruments. The DWS is defined by a right circular cone with a vertex angle of 60° and the EDWS is defined by a cone with an elliptical cross section created by two orthogonal vertex angles of 60° and 90°. A compound function based on the mechanism's isotropy and the mechanism stiffness was considered as the performance metric cost function. Optimization across both the DWS and the EDWS lead to a serial mechanism configuration with link length angles of 74° and 60° for a serial configuration This mechanism configuration maximized the kinematic performance in the DWS while keeping the EDWS as its reachable workspace. Surgeons, using a mockup of two mechanisms in a MIS setup, validated these results experimentally. From these experiments the serial configuration was deemed most applicable for MIS robotic applications compared to a parallel mechanism configuration. The mechanical design of a cable actuated surgical robot was based on optimized link length angles. The system is currently being integrated into a fully operated two-arm system. Small form-factor surgical robotic arms with optimized dexterous workspaces will facilitate the integration of multiple arms while avoiding self-collision in the OR of the future.

# 1. Introduction

The OR of the future has been envisioned as a space that will contain only one human being - the patient [1] the presence of surgeons and nurses will be replaced by enabling technologies such as surgical robots, tool changers, equipment dispensers and imaging modalities. Pioneering work in the field of surgical robotics demonstrates that the surgeon can be safely removed from the immediate surgical scene and maintain interaction with the patient in a teleoperational mode [2–5], for review see [6,7]. Duplicating the presence of two surgeons would require at least four highly dexterous surgical robotic arms. Using four robotic arms will clutter the limited space above the patient, while exposing the arms to possible self-collision and limit access to internal anatomy. The scope of this study is to optimize the mechanism of a spherical serial mechanism based on a measured workspace database acquired during MIS setup [8] and to assess its performance.

# 2. Tools and Methods

## 2.1. Spherical Serial Mechanism - Analytical Analysis

The mechanism under study is a member of a class of spherical mechanisms in which all the links' rotation axes intersect in a signal point located at the center of the mechanism. Aligning this point with the location of the port through which tools are inserted into the body in MIS eliminates any tool translation along the orthogonal axes of the tool's shaft. The center of the sphere is the origin for all reference frames of the mechanism. Thus, each link frame is a pure rotation from one to the next.

The coordinate frames are assigned such that the Z-axis of the $n$th frame points outward along the $n$th joint [19]. The numbering scheme for the frames has odd numbers (Frames $0'$, 1, 3 and 5). The end-effector frame is Frame 5. Frame $0'$ is oriented such that the z-axis points along joint 1 and the y-axis points to the apex of the sphere. The link angle, $\alpha_{i+1}$ expresses the angle between the $i$th and $(i+1)$th axis. These are fixed parameters defined by the mechanism geometry. The rotation angle $\theta_i$ defines the angle as a function of time between the rotation axis $i-1$ and $i$. When all joint angles are set to 0 ($\theta_1 = \theta_3 = 0$), link 13 lies in a plane defined by $Z_{0'}$ and $Y_{0'}$, link 35 is folded back on link 13.

Analyzing a database collected by the Blue DRAGON [8] of generic surgical tasks including tissue handling/examination, tissue dissection, and suturing performed on an animal model in-vivo by 30 surgeons in a MIS environment indicates that 95% of the time the positions of the surgical tools encompass in a cone with a vertex angle of 60° with a tip located at the port. In addition, measuring the reachable workspace of an endoscopic tool performed on a human model showed that in order to reach any organ in the abdomen the tool needed to move 90° in the lateral/medial direction (left to right) and 60° in the superior/inferior (foot to head) direction (Fig. 1c).

The reachable workspace of the spherical manipulator is a sector of a sphere. The size and the shape of this sector are determined by the mechanism joint lengths ($\alpha_{13}, \alpha_{35}$), and joint limits. Based on the in-vivo measurements, the dexterous workspace (DWS) for the surgical robot was defined as the area on the sphere bounded by the closed

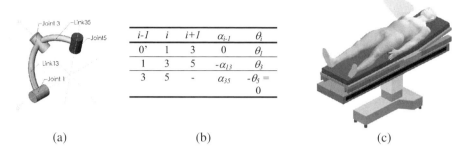

|        | (a) |        |        | (b)    |        |        | (c) |        |

| $i-1$ | $i$ | $i+1$ | $\alpha_{i-1}$ | $\theta_i$ |
| --- | --- | --- | --- | --- |
| 0' | 1 | 3 | 0 | $\theta_1$ |
| 1 | 3 | 5 | $-\alpha_{13}$ | $\theta_3$ |
| 3 | 5 | - | $\alpha_{35}$ | $-\theta_5 = 0$ |

**Figure 1.** Spherical serial two link mechanism (a) link and joint assignment based on the Denavit-Hartenberg (DH) notation (b) the mechanism DH parameter notation summary where link number is denoted by $i$ the link length denoted by $\alpha_{i-1}$, and the joint angles denoted by $\theta_i$ (c) Workspace in Minimally invasive surgery: An elliptical cone with a vertex angle of 60-90 degrees represents the reachable workspace such that any organ in the abdomen can be reached by the endoscopic tool. Note that the azimuth and elevation angles of the cone are free parameters that are determined by the relation between the port location and the targeted organ, (c) The EDWS plotted in one pose with respect to the human body.

line created when a right circular cone with a circular cross section and a vertex angel of 60° located at the center of the sphere intersected the sphere. The extended dexterous workspace (EDWS) of the surgical robot was defined in a similar fashion; however, the 'cone' had an elliptical cross section created by two orthogonal vertex angels of 60° and 90°. The optimization process aimed to define the mechanism parameters (link lengths) allowing it to reach any point the EDWS and provide high dexterity in the DWS. Based on the mechanical design limits of the mechanism, the range of motion of the first joint angle is 180° ($0° < \theta_1 < 180°$) and the range of motion of the second joint angle is 160° ($20° < \theta_3 < 180°$). These constrains were further used to limit the design space from which an optimal solution was searched.

The forward and inverse kinematics of the serial spherical mechanism were developed in [9]. The Jacobian matrix ($J$) relates joint velocities ($\dot{\theta}_i$) to end-effector angular velocities ($\omega_i$) where $^{i+1}_iR$ is the rotation matrix expressing the origin of frame $i + 1$ in frame $i$, and $\hat{z}_{i+1}$ is a unit vector along the Z-axis of the $i + 1$ frame aligned along the rotational axis. Utilizing the recursive expression for the Jacobian matrix (Eq. 1) [10] along with DH transformation matrices of the mechanism Jacobian can be explicitly expressed in Eq. 2. The eigenvalue corresponding to the angular velocity of Frame 5 has a value of 1 for all poses and joint velocities when the Jacobian matrix is expressed in Frame 5. This allows for the reduction of the Jacobian dimension. The upper $2 \times 2$ submatrix of the $3 \times 3$ Jacobian matrix is thus used. This truncated version of the Jacobian relates the two controlled joint velocities, 1 and 3 to end-effector velocity. The current analysis uses mechanism isotropy (*ISO*) as the performance metric, defined in Eq. 3 as the ratio between the lowest eigenvalue ($\lambda_{min}$) and the highest eigenvalue ($\lambda_{max}$) of the Jacobian matrix. For a given a design candidate ($\alpha_{13}, \alpha_{35}$), the mechanism isotropy is a function of the joint angles ($\theta_1, \theta_2$) and has a value in the range of 0 to 1. An isotropy measure of 0 means the mechanism is in a singular configuration and has lost a degree of freedom. A typical singular configurations of the mechanism under study is obtained when the to links are fully stretched. An isotropy measure of 1 means that the eigenvalues of the Jacobian are all equal and the mechanism can move equally well in all directions.

$$\left[ {}^{i+1}\omega_{i+1} \right] = \left[ {}^{i+1}_iR \right]\left[ {}^i\omega_i \right] + \dot{\theta}^{i+1}_{i+1}\hat{z}_{i+1} \qquad (1)$$

$$\begin{bmatrix} ^5\omega_{5x} \\ ^5\omega_{5y} \end{bmatrix} = [J_5] \begin{bmatrix} \dot{\theta}_1 \\ \dot{\theta}_3 \end{bmatrix} = \begin{bmatrix} -\text{Sin}\theta_3 \, \text{Sin}\alpha_{35} & 0 \\ -\text{Cos}\theta_3 \, \text{Sin}\alpha_{13} \, \text{Cos}\alpha_{35} + \text{Cos}\alpha_{13} \, \text{Sin}\alpha_{35} & \text{Sin}\alpha_{35} \end{bmatrix} \begin{bmatrix} \dot{\theta}_1 \\ \dot{\theta}_3 \end{bmatrix}$$

(2)

$$ISO(\theta_1, \theta_3) = \frac{\lambda_{\min}}{\lambda_{\max}} \quad ISO \in \langle 0, 1 \rangle$$

(3)

A scoring function defined in Eq. 4, that is later used as the cost function of the mechanism optimization process, is a compound function that utilizes isotropy measure (Eq. 3) for quantitatively assessing the mechanism performance over its entire designated workspace. The scoring function is a synthesis of three individual elements including (1) an integrated average isotropy measure over the mechanism workspace, (2) a minimal isotropy measure score in the mechanism workspace and (3) the cube of the angular length of the links

$$\phi\,(\alpha_{13}, \alpha_{35}) = \frac{S_{\text{sum}} \cdot S_{\min}}{(\alpha_{13} + \alpha_{35})^3}$$

(4)

In order to analyze the mechanism performance, the hemisphere is discretized into points distributed equally in azimuth and elevation. Given the ranges of the azimuth angle $\sigma$ and the elevation angle $\zeta$, defining the intersection area between a right circular cross section cone (DWS and EDWS) with a vertex angle of 60° or 90° and located at the center of the sphere and the sphere itself, the set of all possible intersection areas on the hemisphere is $K = \{k\,(\sigma, \zeta) : 0 < \sigma < 2\pi, \ 0 < \zeta < \pi/4\}$. The set of all the discrete points contained in the intersection area is $k_{\sigma,\zeta}^p \subset k_{\sigma,\zeta}$. Due to the discrete nature of the computation, each point included in the intersection area has an associated isotropy value $ISO$ and sector area $A$. Thus the components of the scoring function (Eq. 4) are defined as follows

$$S_{\text{sum}} = \underset{K}{MAX} \left\{ \sum_{k_{\sigma,\zeta}^p} ISO\,(\theta_1, \theta_3)\, A\,(\sigma, \zeta) \right\} \qquad \text{(a)}$$

(5)

$$S_{\min} = \underset{K}{MAX} \left\{ \underset{k_{\sigma,\zeta}^p}{MIN}\,\left(ISO\,(\theta_1, \theta_3)\,\right) \right\} \qquad \text{(b)}$$

A requirement of the optimization is that over the DWS or EDWS, the mechanism does not encounter any singularities or workspace boundaries. By multiplying the summed isotropy by the minimum isotropy (Eq. 4), candidates that fail to meet this requirement have a score of zero. By dividing by the cube of the sum of the link angles the score reflects proportionality to the mechanisms stiffness or mass. Thus, over a scan of the potential design space, the peak composite score represents a design with maximum average performance, a guaranteed minimum performance, and maximized stiffness.

The optimization considered all combinations of $\alpha_{13}$, and $\alpha_{35}$ from 16° to 90° in 2° increments for a total of 1444 design candidates. The hemisphere was discretized into 3600 points, distributed evenly in azimuth and elevation.

$$max\,\phi(\alpha_{13}, \alpha_{35}) \quad \begin{cases} 16° < \alpha_{13} < 90° \\ 16° < \alpha_{35} < 90° \end{cases}$$

(6)

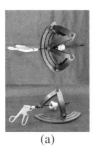 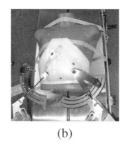 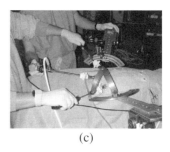

(a)                          (b)                          (c)

**Figure 2.** Experimental setups of the spherical mechanism mock-ups with adjustable link length and base length. The surgical endoscopic tool is inserted into a guide located at mechanism apex in a configuration that allow to test different design candidates in a real MIS setup. (a) Parallel configuration – (top) and serial configuration- (bottom) (b) Two serial configurations tested in a MIS setup with a human torso (c) Two serial configurations tested with an animal model.

## 2.2. Spherical Mechanism - Experimental Evaluation

Two re-configurable mockups of both serial and parallel versions of the spherical mechanism were design and fabricated with adjustable link lengths. The human torso was used to assess potential collisions between two surgical arms with different combinations. In addition, the selected configurations were tested in a real MIS setup in which surgical tools were inserted through the apex of the spherical mechanisms. Using real surgical tools, gross tasks such as tissue manipulation as well as high dexterous tasks such as suturing were performed by surgeons while the spherical mechanism following passively the motion of the tools. Qualitative assessment of range of motion and potential collisions were performed.

## 3. Results

Optimizing for the DWS, the best design was achieved with link angles of $\alpha_{13} = 52°$ and $\alpha_{35} = 40°$ (Fig. 2a). In contrast, running the same optimization but requiring a cone with a vertex angle of 90° indicated that the optimal mechanism design has link angles $\alpha_{13} = 90°$ and $\alpha_{35} = 72°$ (Fig. 2b). The difference in the results is not un-expected but it does pose an interesting dilemma. If one chooses the design that optimizes on a cone with a vertex angle of 90°, the resulting design should be more likely to reach all the poses that manipulator would be asked to reach. However, this design has lower overall performance than the design optimized on for the DWS and larger links, which may increase the likelihood for problems of collisions between two manipulators.

One interesting consideration is to take the best design that is optimized for the DWS that also has the ability to reach a cone with a vertex angle of 90°. This is done by eliminating all the solutions representing mechanism candidates that that cannot reach a cone with a vertex angle of 90°. This optimal design has link angles with $\alpha_{13} = 72°$ and $\alpha_{35} = 60°$ (Fig. 2c).

Assessing the different combinations of two arms (serial and parallel) in the same surgical scene indicated that two serial mechanisms could be integrated into a MIS sur-

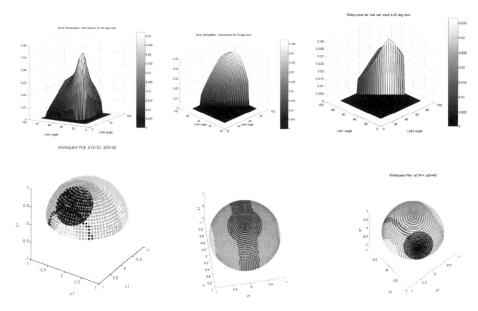

**Figure 3.** The composite score $\phi$ of a serial mechanism as a function of the link length angles Link1 ($\alpha_{13}$), Link2 ($\alpha_{35}$) along with the workspace of the mechanism with the best performance for each design criterion (peak of a) DWS, a cone with a vertex angle of 60° (b) Workspace plot for optimal mechanism (a) with link angles $\alpha_{13} = 52°$ and $\alpha_{35} = 40°$ (c) EDWS, a cone with a vertex angle of 90° (d) Workspace plot for optimal mechanism (peak of c) with link angles $\alpha_{13} = 90°$ and $\alpha_{35} = 72°$, (e) subset of (a) which can reach a cone with a vertex angle of 90°. (f) Workspace plot for optimal mechanism (peak of e) with link angles $\alpha_{13} = 74°$ and $\alpha_{35} = 60°$. For subplots c,d,f, the workspace plots show the hemisphere in green, the reachable workspace in purple, and the orientation of the best cone in black, with the strip of maximum isotropy also in black.

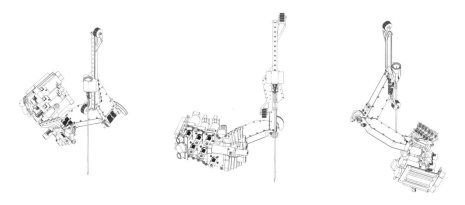

**Figure 4.** CAD rendering of a serial spherical surgical robotic arm design that was based on link length angles obtained as part of the optimization process under study.

gical scene with minimal potential of self-collision. Setting the adjustable link length angles of the two mockups while manipulating MIS tools through the apex of the mockups indicated that they provided the required workspace needed to complete the surgical tasks under study.

## 4. Discussion

Robotic arms that replace the presence of the surgeon and nurses in the operating room occupy both the space above and inside the patient during both open and MIS setups. These spaces are strictly dictated by the human anatomy. This study provides an optimization methodology for minimizing the size of a spherical surgical robotic arm in order to avoid potential collisions when more than one arm is introduced into the surgical scene. The optimization balanced a guaranteed minimum and integrated isotropy over the DWS as well as total link length in order to yield a very compact, high-dexterity mechanism. The definitions of the DWS and EDWS were derived based on an experimental database of the kinematics of surgical tools in MIS as collected by the Blue DRAGON system. The optimization results were translated into an actual mechanical design. A further system optimization could include placement of two or more manipulators over a patient while optimizing the individual sub system position and orientations to avoid robot-patient collisions as well as robot-robot collisions and self-collision.

## References

[1]  Satava, R. Disruptive visions: the operating room of the future, Surgical Endoscopy, 2003, 17(1), 104-107.

[2]  Taylor, R.; Lavallee, S.; Burdea, G.; Mosges, R. Computer-Integrated Surgery, MIT Press: Cambridge, MA, 1996.

[3]  M.C. Cavusoglu, F. Tendick, M. Cohn, and S.S. Sastry, ``A Laparoscopic Telesurgical Workstation,'' IEEE Trans. Robotics and Automation, vol 15, no. 4, pages 728-739, August 1999.

[4]  Madhani, A.; Niemeyer, G.; Salisbury, K. The Black Falcon: A Teleoperated Surgical Instrument for Minimally Invasive Surgery. IEEE/RSJ Int. Conf. on Intelligent Robots and Systems (IROS), Victoria B.C., Canada, October, 1998.

[5]  Marescaux, J.; Leroy, J.; Gagner, M.; Rubino, F.; Mutter, D.; Vix, M.; Butner, S.; Smith, M.K. Transatlantic Robot-Assisted Telesurgery, Nature Magazine, 2001, 413, 379-380.

[6]  Howe, R.; Matsuoka, Y. Robotics for Surgery. In Annual Review of Biomedical Engineering, 1999, 1, 211 - 240.

[7]  J. E. Speich and J. Rosen, Medical Robotics, In Encyclopedia of Biomaterials and Biomedical Engineering, Gary Wnek and Gary Bowlin (Editors), pp. 983-993, Marcel Dekker, Inc, NY, 2004.

[8]  Rosen, J.; Brown, J.; Chang, L.; Barreca, M.; Sinanan, M.; Hannaford, B. The Blue DRAGON - A System for Measuring the Kinematics and the Dynamics of Minimally Invasive Surgical Tools In–Vivo, Proceedings of the 2002 IEEE International Conference on Robotics & Automation, Washington DC, USA, May 11-15, 2002.

[9]  M.J.H. Lum, J. Rosen, M. N. Sinanan, B. Hannaford, Kinematic Optimization of a Spherical Mechanism for a Minimally Invasive Surgical Robot, 2004 IEEE International Conference on Robotics & Automation, pp. 829-834, New-Orleans, USA, April 26-30, 2004.

[10]  Craig J., Introduction to Robotics Mechanics and Control, Addison, Wesley Logmen, Second Edition, 1989.

*Medicine Meets Virtual Reality 13*
*James D. Westwood et al. (Eds.)*
*IOS Press, 2005*

# Using an Ontology of Human Anatomy to Inform Reasoning with Geometric Models

Daniel L. RUBIN, Yasser BASHIR, David GROSSMAN,
Parvati DEV and Mark A. MUSEN

*Stanford Medical Informatics, Stanford, California 94305-5479 USA*
*e-mail: rubin@smi.stanford.edu*

**Abstract.** The Virtual Soldier project is a large effort on the part of the U.S. Defense Advanced Research Projects agency to explore using both general anatomical knowledge and specific computed tomographic (CT) images of individual soldiers to aid the rapid diagnosis and treatment of penetrating injuries. Our goal is to develop intelligent computer applications that use this knowledge to reason about the anatomic structures that are directly injured and to predict propagation of injuries secondary to primary organ damage. To accomplish this, we needed to develop an architecture to combine geometric data with anatomic knowledge and reasoning services that use this information to predict the consequences of injuries.

## 1. Introduction

Medical assessment of penetrating injuries is a knowledge-intensive task. Rapid and effective medical intervention in response to civil and military-related injuries is crucial for saving lives and limiting disability [1]. Accurate assessment of penetrating injures is challenging because the spatial relationships among anatomic regions can be complex, and potential damage to some vital structures may not be recognized. Intelligent tools that can integrate patient-specific geometric data and anatomic knowledge to inform care providers about internal injuries could improve patient care and outcomes.

Dramatic advances have occurred in recent years in the quality and resolution of cross sectional imaging modalities such as computed tomography (CT), which now serve a critical role in evaluating an injured subject [2]. While these images contain detailed spatial information, they lack any knowledge of anatomy, such as the identity of anatomic structures and relationships among anatomic structures. To develop computerized tools to support diagnosis of traumatic injury, these tools need to be provided both with patient-specific geometric data and anatomic knowledge. Anatomic knowledge adds meaning to geometric data, labeling regions in space with particular organs, relating organ parts and subparts to other anatomic structures, and identifying critical structures that may affect patient prognosis and management.

The Virtual Soldier project is being undertaken by the U.S. Defense Advanced Research Projects agency to use both geometric data derived from images and canonical anatomic knowledge to aid the rapid diagnosis of penetrating injury [3]. The vision for the project is that each soldier would carry pre-injury CT images and other relevant base-

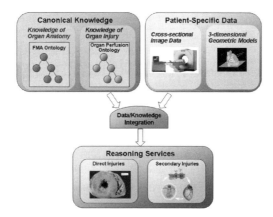

**Figure 1.** Architecture for integrating patient-specific data and canonical knowledge to reason about penetrating injury.

line clinical data on a small memory card. At the time of an injury, an information system would read the baseline data and offer advice about the nature of the wound, the patient's prognosis, and requirements for therapy.

Our goal is to develop a methodology to automate reasoning about penetrating injuries using canonical knowledge combined with specific subject image data. Our approach is to build three dimensional geometric models of subjects from segmented images. We link regions in this model to concepts in two knowledge sources: (1) a comprehensive ontology of anatomy containing organ identities, adjacencies, and other information useful for anatomic reasoning, and (2) an ontology of regional perfusion containing formal definitions of arterial anatomy and corresponding regions of perfusion. We are developing computerized reasoning services that can determine the organs that are injured given particular trajectories of projectiles, whether vital structures—such as a coronary artery—are injured, and can predict the propagation of injury ensuing after a vital structure is injured. This methodology may improve the speed and accuracy of rapid assessment of penetrating injury.

## 2. Methods

The architecture of our system to integrate patient-specific geometric data with anatomic knowledge in ontologies is shown in Figure 1. Canonical knowledge sources are ontologies containing detailed knowledge of organ anatomy as well as knowledge about structural anatomic dependencies that are important for predicting secondary injuries. Patient-specific data consist of cross-sectional imaging data and three dimensional geometric models that are built from these data. Data structures in our software architecture integrate the canonical knowledge and patient-specific geometric data, making both available to applications (reasoning services) that can perform intelligent tasks such as predicting direct and secondary injuries (Figure 1).

### 2.1. Knowledge of Anatomy

We use the Digital Anatomist Foundational Model of Anatomy (FMA) as our knowledge source of anatomy [4]. The FMA is a comprehensive ontology of human anatomy, containing more than 70,000 concepts that describe the elements of canonical human morphology in a clear and consistent manner. It provides declarative descriptions of detailed anatomic structures in a computationally accessible format; it is modeled using the Protégé ontology-management environment (http://protege.stanford.edu), and it adheres to the conventions of the OKBC frame language [5].

Intelligent applications can be developed that use this representation to reason about anatomic relationships, such as inferring organ injuries related to a projectile trajectory. This is accomplished by reading anatomic concepts ("classes" in the ontology), and their attributes ("slots" on the class). Slots can be atomic types (such as integers, strings, etc.) or other classes (e.g., the "part-of" slot contains classes that have a partonomic relationship with the given class). Components in the FMA that we use in this project include organ names, compositionality (partonomy relationships), organ adjacencies, containment, and continuities. The FMA is particularly useful because it contains anatomic structures that may be too small to be visible on images, and thus may not be present in geometric models. This knowledge is useful for a reasoning service to deduce possible injury to small but vital structures that are adjacent to visible structures.

### 2.1.1. Knowledge of Organ Injury

While the FMA is an excellent knowledge source describing morphology and composition of anatomic structures, it lacks physiological knowledge. For example, it does not describe the regions of myocardium supplied by branches of the coronary arteries. Such knowledge is needed to reason about secondary organ damage—injury that occurs to particular anatomic structures as a result of damage to other structures.

We built an ontology of coronary artery anatomy and regional myocardial perfusion (Figure 2) using the Web Ontology Language (OWL) [6]. The OWL classes contain formal definitions, represented using logical statements, specifying the necessary and sufficient conditions ("assertions") for class inclusion. For example, the definition of the lateral wall of the left ventricle includes assertions specifying all of the branches of the coronary arteries that ordinarily supply it (Figure 2). This ontology specifies the segments and continuities in coronary arteries, the composition of myocardial regions (e.g., the left ventricle has anterior, lateral, posterior, apical, and septal parts), and it describes the myocardial regions supplied by particular coronary arterial branches. This ontology also defines the coronary arteries as being "critical" structures—anatomic structures that result in damage to other structures if they are injured.

The class definitions contained in the OWL ontology allow reasoning services to deduce important physiological consequences of arterial injury. First, the ontology encodes the knowledge that arterial branches downstream from an injured branch will be functionally impaired. Second, the ontology contains knowledge of all arterial branches feeding a myocardial region. There are also definitions about when a region is totally or partially ischemic (a region is totally ischemic if all arteries supplying it are impaired, and is partially ischemic if one ore more arteries are not impaired).

### 2.2. Geometric data sources and model

We obtained segmented images from the Visible Human project [7]. These comprise serial cross-sectional images from a cadaver, and they are analogous to reconstructed images available from CT on live patients. Each organ in these images was labeled,

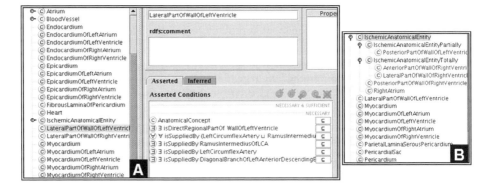

**Figure 2.** A) Ontology (in OWL) of coronary anatomy and regional myocardial perfusion. Classes of anatomic structures are shown on the left panel, and formal definitions of the concepts are shown on the right. The class "Lateral part of wall of left ventricle" is seen to be defined by six assertions, all necessary conditions for this class. Some of these assertions specify the coronary arterial branches that supply this structure. B) OWL ontology updated with the knowledge that the second segment of the right coronary artery has been injured. After automatic classification, new classes (light color) appear, suggesting the ischemic regions of myocardium that occur as a consequence of the right coronary artery injury.

and these labels were used to map these anatomic structures to corresponding anatomic classes in our ontologies.

The segmented two-dimensional images cannot be used directly for spatial anatomical reasoning; a three-dimensional representation of patient anatomy must be built from these images to reason with a three-dimensional projectile trajectory. We used the Insight Toolkit (ITK; http://itk.org) to build solid three-dimensional tetrahedral mesh models from the serial segmented images of the chest (Figure 3). These geometric mesh models created from the imaging data represented the three-dimensional coordinates of anatomic structures in space. Collections of vertices in the mesh model were labeled with FMA class names to identify the anatomic structures that they represent. Thus, the mesh model of patient-specific geometry is linked to canonical anatomic structures in the FMA (as well as the OWL ontology of myocardial perfusion). This provides a software architecture that makes patient-specific geometric data and canonical anatomic knowledge accessible to intelligent applications such as reasoning services.

We created a graphical visualization application that displays patient-specific geometric data models (Figure 3). Spatial objects comprising sets of tetrahedrons that represent particular organs or organ parts are displayed in different colors. A specified trajectory of penetrating injury can be incorporated into the geometric model as an additional spatial object. Rendering methods are applied to highlight the surface regions and internal volume of organs affected by the penetrating injury and area surrounding it.

## 2.3. Reasoning services

We have initially implemented two applications that use patient-specific geometric data and anatomic knowledge sources to perform useful reasoning capabilities: (1) a tool to determine which organs are injured by a penetrating injury ("Direct Injury Reasoner"), and (2) a tool that determines whether any vital structures are injured and the consequences of such injury ("Secondary Injury Reasoner").

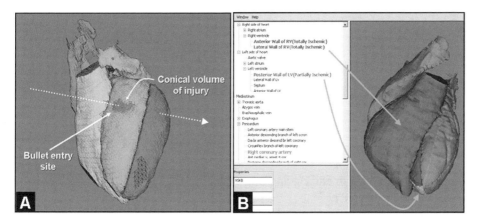

**Figure 3.** Three dimensional geometric model of the heart linked to FMA ontology of anatomy. A) A bullet path was described to traverse the patient, and predicted primary injuries are displayed (shaded conical region). B) Reasoning about secondary injury in graphical user interface display of patient anatomy and geometry. Shaded volumes in the geometric model (right) correspond to anatomic structure classes in the FMA ontology (left). An OWL reasoning service deduces parts of the myocardium that are injured consequent to a coronary artery injury, shown as highlighted structures in the FMA (left) and shaded parts of heart (right).

The Direct Injury Reasoner takes as input an entry wound and an exit wound on the patient, and it deduces the anatomic structures that have been injured by direct impact by the penetrating injury (or from shock waves in close proximity to the trajectory of injury). To accomplish this task, the Direct Injury Reasoner defines a parametric trajectory path of the penetrating injury using the observed wounds and three-dimensional tetrahedral mesh model of the patient derived from the image data. This trajectory is used to infer the organs that are injured by the projectile. The Secondary Injury Reasoner takes as input a list of anatomic structures that have been injured by the penetrating injury (deduced by the Direct Injury Reasoner) and it deduces additional tissue injury that are occurring or will occur as a consequence of the primary injuries. To accomplish this task, the Secondary Injury Reasoner uses the OWL ontology of anatomic knowledge to assert primary injuries and deduce secondary injuries by applying an automatic classifier to the ontology.

If any critical structures have been injured, the OWL ontology is updated with this information by creating new assertions (new subclasses indicating the structures that have been injured). For example, if the second segment of the right coronary artery (RCA) is injured, then a new subclass of the ontology class "functionally impaired blood vessel" would be created by the Secondary Injury Reasoner.

After the Secondary Injury Reasoner asserts the damaged critical structures, it calls a classification engine that updates the OWL ontology, inferring new classes and relationships given the asserted knowledge and pre-existing class definitions. In the case of the RCA injury above, new subclasses of the injury classes "IschemicAnatomicEntity-Totally" and "IschemicAnatomicEntityPartially" would be created, indicating that regions of myocardium are ischemic secondary to the RCA injury (Figure 2B). These secondary injuries would be deduced by the Secondary Injury Reasoner, and are used to update the graphical display of patient geometry (Figure 3B). In our example, the Secondary Injury Reasoner would deduce that most of the right ventricle and portions of the left ventricle and right atrium were ischemic as a result of the injury to the second segment of the right coronary artery.

By combining the Direct and Secondary Injury Reasoners in series, we can begin with baseline patient imaging data and patient wounds and rapidly deduce the anticipated extent of direct and secondary injuries.

## 3. Discussion

Our goal is to develop intelligent applications to improve the ability of practitioners to assess and triage injured patients. Creating geometric models of internal anatomic structures alone is not adequate to solve this task. Images of patient anatomy may contain labels, but there is little knowledge in those labels beyond a name. By enhancing geometric models with anatomic knowledge, it is possible to build reasoning services that can predict the primary and secondary injures caused by a trajectory of injury that crosses different parts of the geometry. In the future we plan to add physiological knowledge to these models so that our reasoning services can inform practitioners about the physiological significance of injuries. Such information could be useful in developing decision support tools that assist practitioners prioritize treatment options for patients at the scene of injury.

Previous work on assessing penetrating injury focused on developing simulation environments and teaching aids to assist in assessing penetrating injuries [8]. Such teaching activity is valuable to give practitioners general experience managing trauma cases, but this differs from our approach which provides patient-specific information. Ogunyemi and colleagues developed a system that calculates the probabilities of organ injuries using a canonical geometric model of human anatomy [9]. This can be a helpful guide to typical injuries, but the geometric models are not specific to a particular patient. Our reasoning services operate on patient-specific representations of knowledge, an approach we believe is advantageous since there can be considerable variation in anatomy among people.

A limitation of our current approach is that it does not incorporate uncertainty relating to injuries. We are currently extending our representation to represent different possible trajectories, from which probabilities of organ injury can be calculated. Another limitation is that we have not yet performed a formal evaluation of our approach. We are now planning these evaluation studies.

## Acknowledgments

This work was supported by a contract from DARPA, executed by the U.S. Army Medical Research and Materiel Command/TATRC Cooperative Agreement, Contract W81XWH-04-2-0012. We are grateful to Cornelius Rosse for many years of exciting discussion and collaboration. This work was also supported by the Protégé resource, under grant LM007885 from the U.S. National Library of Medicine.

# References

[1] West JG, Trunkey DD, Lim RC. Systems of trauma care. A study of two counties. Arch Surg 1979;114(4):455-60.

[2] Alkadhi H, Wildermuth S, Desbiolles L, Schertler T, Crook D, Marincek B, et al. Vascular emergencies of the thorax after blunt and iatrogenic trauma: multi-detector row CT and three-dimensional imaging. Radiographics 2004;24(5):1239-55.

[3] Virtual Soldier Project. http://www.virtualsoldier.net/summary.htm. 2004.

[4] Rosse C, Mejino JL, Jr. A reference ontology for biomedical informatics: the Foundational Model of Anatomy. J Biomed Inform 2003;36(6):478-500.

[5] Noy NF, Musen MA, Mejino JLV, Rosse C. Pushing the envelope: challenges in a frame-based representation of human anatomy. Data & Knowledge Engineering 2004;48(3):335-359.

[6] Smith MK, Welty C, McGuinness D. OWL Web Ontology Language Guide, http://www.w3.org/TR/owl-guide/. 2004.

[7] Ackerman MJ, Yoo TS. The Visible Human Data Sets (VHD) and Insight Toolkit (ITk): Experiments in Open Source Software. Proc AMIA Symp 2003:773.

[8] Freeman KM, Thompson SF, Allely EB, Sobel AL, Stansfield SA, Pugh WM. A virtual reality patient simulation system for teaching emergency response skills to U.S. Navy medical providers. Prehospital Disaster Med 2001;16(1):3-8.

[9] Ogunyemi OI, Clarke JR, Ash N, Webber BL. Combining geometric and probabilistic reasoning for computer-based penetrating-trauma assessment. J Am Med Inform Assoc 2002;9(3):273-82.

436

*Medicine Meets Virtual Reality 13*
*James D. Westwood et al. (Eds.)*
*IOS Press, 2005*

# Assessing Surgical Skill Training Under Hazardous Conditions in a Virtual Environment

Mark W. SCERBO [a], James P. BLISS [a], Elizabeth A. SCHMIDT [a],
Hope S. HANNER-BAILEY [a] and Leonard J. WEIRETER [b]

[a] *Old Dominion University*
[b] *Eastern Virginia Medical School*

**Abstract.** The present study examined the performance of a surgical procedure under simulated combat conditions. Eleven residents performed a cricothyroidotomy on a mannequin-based simulator in a fully immersive virtual environment running a combat simulation with a virtual sniper under both day and night time lighting conditions. The results showed that completion times improved between the first and second attempt and that differences between day and night time conditions were minimal. However, three participants were killed by the virtual sniper before completing the procedure. These results suggest that some participants' ability to allocate attention to the task and their surroundings was inappropriate even under simulated hazardous conditions. Further, this study shows that virtual environments offer the chance to study a wider variety of medical procedures performed under an unlimited number of conditions.

## 1. Background

Simulators have been a standard component of military training for many years in a variety of contexts including aviation, dismounted infantry operations, weapons training, and command and control operations. By contrast, using simulation technology for medical procedures is relatively new [1]. In the last five years, however, there has been a dramatic increase in the number and variety of medical simulation systems commercially available [2,3]. Further, medical schools are now incorporating this technology into training curricula due to increased pressure to train physicians and surgeons to higher levels of competency, in less time, while simultaneously improving safety [4].

At present, most current medical simulators are designed to train basic skills or specific procedures. However, another important advantage of simulation technology is that it enables one to train under conditions that would be too dangerous in actual operational settings. Although this represents a standard use of simulation for training many different skills in military contexts, it has been largely overlooked in medicine.

Accordingly, the goal of the present study was to examine the performance of surgical skills in a virtual environment (VE) in which the operational context was simulated. Military medical personnel who have been in war have commented that traditional medical school training and practice in standard hospital settings do not always transfer to combat situations [5]. Thus, the specific purpose of this study was to determine whether surgical skills acquired in a traditional medical school and practiced in a standard hospital environment might be compromised in a simulated combat scenario.

The procedure selected for investigation in the present study was cricothyroidotomy, used when endotracheal intubation is not possible. It requires the use of one hand to lock thyroid cartilage in place and the other to make an incision in the cricoid membrane and insert tubing into the airway. The procedure was performed on a mannequin-based simulator in a VE under simulated combat conditions including visual and auditory depictions of munitions fire, gunfire, and a virtual sniper who would shoot at the participants if they did not take proper cover. The battle scenario was designed to provide a heightened sense of realism in which to examine performance. Further, the procedure was performed under two different lighting conditions: daytime and nighttime. The two lighting conditions were included to create different levels of workload and stress within the combat scenario. In particular, the nighttime condition was included because military medical personnel might not always have control over the visibility conditions in which they must perform. It was expected that if performance were compromised under the simulated combat scenario, it would suffer more under the nighttime visibility conditions.

## 2. Methodology

### 2.1. Participants

Participants were 11 surgical residents (4 PGY-3, 3 PGY-4, 2 PGY-5, and 2 PGY-6) from Eastern Virginia Medical School in Norfolk, VA. They ranged in age from 21 to 38 years ($M = 30.9$, $SD = 1.8$). All participants had experience with cricothyroidotomy, tracheostomy, or percutaneous tracheostomy procedures. The mean reported frequency of having performed one or more of these procedures was 9 ($SD = 3$) and 87% of the participants indicated that they had performed one of these procedures within the last 6 months. The residents were paid $15 for their participation.

### 2.2. Procedural training simulator

The procedure was performed on the Simulab® Inc., TraumaMan® System. This is a mannequin-based simulator used throughout the world for surgery education and is the only simulator approved for the ATLS® Surgical Skills Practicum by the American College of Surgeons. The simulator includes a realistic anatomical model of the neck, chest, and abdomen with replaceable tissue components and fluid reservoirs that permit instruction on six surgical procedures including cricothyroidotomy.

### 2.3. Virtual Environment Implementation

A CAVE Automatic Virtual Environment was used to present the combat scenario. The system consisted of two main computers connected through a 100-mbps network switch. An SGI® ONYX® 2 computer was used to display the application in the CAVE, provide the sound playback, and read the information from the tracking device. This computer used MultiGen-Paradigm's Vega software running on the IRIX® 6.5 operating system. An SGI® O2 computer served as the main console and was used to launch the application and issue command overrides controls during the simulation. Images were presented on three 10x10 ft walls of the CAVE with a resolution of 1024x768. In addition, a Radio Shack electronic beam was fixed to the top of the boxes (approximately 3 ft. above the ground) to engage the virtual sniper (see below).

## 2.4. Combat Simulation

The combat simulation depicted a small town under fire. Combat was simulated using the Vega special effects module to trigger visual and auditory explosion events as well as background gunfire at specific times. The events were timed to repeat at specific intervals. The scenario was run in a continuous loop until the participant was finished.

Day and nighttime conditions were created by adjusting the luminance intensity of the image with the time-of-day feature in the Vega software. Under the daytime conditions, there was enough ambient illumination emanating from the walls of the CAVE to make the barricade, mannequin, and instruments easily visible. Under the nighttime conditions, however, there was very little illumination provided by the CAVE walls. Thus, the participants performed the procedure in near total darkness except for the occasional explosions that provided temporary increases in illumination.

The audio track was created using sound samples from unrestricted sources on the Internet. They were downloaded and filtered. Voice samples were saved in monophonic format at a 22.1 kHz sampling rate. Background and other supplemental audio sounds included gunfire, explosions, machine gun fire, and some M1 tank fire. The audio files were presented over two channels. The left and right speakers were placed at approximately 225 and 315 degrees from center, respectively. The speakers were mounted on speaker stands at an elevation of approximately five feet. None of the audio sounds exceeded 90dB during the session.

A virtual sniper was included in the combat scenario as well. If the participant disrupted the electronic beam, an audio file would be played that provided either a warning or informed the participant that they had been killed.

## 2.5. General Procedure

All participants had formal training and experience with airway management; therefore, they were given no additional information or training for the procedure prior to the experimental session. The participants were tested individually and told they were going to play the role of an Army medic with a team of soldiers under fire. A member of the team had been injured and required a cricothyroidotomy. (The participants actually performed a cricothyroidotomy and a chest tube thoracostomy; however, only the cricothyroidotomy procedure is presented here.) Their goal was to get to the patient and perform the procedure to save his life. They were given a standard Special Operations medic kit that contained a knife and cric tube and were escorted into the CAVE. They were told that they would perform the procedure twice: once under daylight and once under nighttime conditions. Each attempt began with the participant standing at a starting point marked with tape on the floor. They were instructed to listen for a call for a medic. As soon as they heard the call, they were to get to the patient and perform the procedure as quickly as possible. They were not required to assess the need for the procedure. Further, they were not required to anesthetize the patient or secure the tube after placing it in the neck.

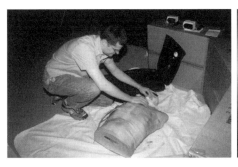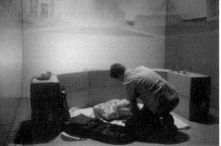

**Figure 1.** Participant performing the procedure under daylight combat conditions.

When they finished, they were told to return to the starting mark on the floor. Figure 1 shows the configuration of the CAVE facility and a participant performing the procedure.

The participants were also told that there was a sniper in one of the nearby buildings and that they had to take cover behind the barricade. Further, if the sniper acquired a clear line of sight he would shoot to kill and they would hear a loud rifle shot. If the sniper missed, they would hear someone tell them to "Get down." If they were hit, they would hear the phrase, "Hasta la vista, baby." At that point, they were considered dead; however, they were instructed to continue and finish the procedure. They were not fired upon again. In actuality, all participants received one warning shot if they disrupted the electronic beam. If they disrupted the beam a second time, they were killed.

The order of day and nighttime conditions was counterbalanced across participants. After the first attempt, the simulation was stopped, a second mannequin was placed in the CAVE, and the participant performed the procedure again. After their second attempt, the participants were escorted out of the CAVE and asked to complete a brief survey. During this interval, a surgeon qualified to teach ATLS® examined the mannequin and determined whether the cric tube had been placed correctly.

*2.6. Dependent Measures*

There were two dependent measures: completion time and performance ratings. The total time to complete the procedure was recorded from the initial call for the medic until the participant returned to the starting mark. The performance rating was based on correct placement of the tube in the trachea.

## 3. Results

Only one participant placed the tube incorrectly. This occurred on the first attempt under daylight conditions. Thus, completion time was the more sensitive measure.

The mean completion times for each attempt and the day and nighttime conditions are shown in Table 1. A comparison of the means showed a decrease in completion time from the first to the second attempt and this difference was statistically significant, $t(10) = 2.4$, $p < .025$. Also, although the procedure took longer to perform under night as compared to day conditions, this difference did not reach significance ($p > .05$).

The completion time analyses included data from all participants; however, there were several instances in which participants were "killed" by the virtual sniper (see Ta-

**Table 1.** Mean Completion Times (in seconds) for Attempts and Day/Night Conditions (standard deviations in parentheses).

|            | All Participants (n = 11) | Surviving Participants (n = 8) |
|------------|:-------------------------:|:-----------------------------:|
| Attempt 1  | 64.9 (34.5)               | 60.5 (30.1)                   |
| Attempt 2  | 37.0 (11.2)               | 40.4 (10.4)                   |
| Day        | 48.2 (29.3)               | 40.2 (9.2)                    |
| Night      | 53.7 (28.8)               | 60.6 (30.4)                   |

**Table 2.** Participants "Killed" by Sniper.

|           | Condition |
|-----------|:---------:|
| *Order*   |           |
| Attempt 1 | 3         |
| Attempt 2 | 1         |
| *Lighting*|           |
| Day       | 3         |
| Night     | 1         |

ble 2). As can be seen in the table, most of the participants who were killed were shot during their first attempt. Although participants who were killed were allowed to complete the procedure, one could argue that these data should not be included in the overall means. Thus, the mean completion times were recalculated excluding data from participants who were killed. The means for the 8 "surviving" participants are also presented in Table 1. The overall pattern for attempts and lighting conditions remained the same; however, the difference between day and night conditions was more pronounced and approached significance ($p < .08$).

## 4. Discussion

The primary goal of the present study was to examine the performance of a surgical procedure under simulated combat conditions. Overall, the results were encouraging. Only one tube placement was judged unsatisfactory. The completion time data showed that on average, participants were able to get to the patient and perform the procedure in under a minute. Completion times were only slightly longer under the nighttime conditions, but this difference was not statistically significant. Thus, impoverished lighting conditions did not hamper performance. This finding was contrary to initial expectations, but may be due to studying a procedure that draws so heavily on the sense of touch.

The results also showed that completion times became approximately 40% quicker from the first to the second attempt irrespective of lighting conditions. This improvement in performance likely reflects increased familiarity with the testing conditions and efforts by the participants to adjust their actions to meet the task requirements. For example, in the post-experimental surveys, most participants indicated that they made a concerted effort to better organize their equipment in the medic kit so that they did not waste time fumbling around on their second attempt.

On the surface, these results seem encouraging; however, they may paint an overly optimistic picture of performance. First, there were 3 instances in which participants failed to heed the warning shot and were "killed" before they could complete the procedure. Anecdotal comments offered by some of the residents indicated that they saw little difference between the "chaos" in an Emergency Room and the "chaos" in our combat simulation and that they were able to "tune out" the noise and focus on the procedure. A finding such as this is troubling because it suggests the presence of *attentional narrowing*. Research has shown that under stressful conditions, even well trained individuals can fixate on a particular stimulus or strategy to the exclusion of other potentially relevant information [6]. Thus, even with the levels of stress created by our *simulated* combat conditions, some participants exhibited inappropriate and potentially dangerous behavior that would likely be exacerbated under genuine combat conditions.

One criticism of the present study may lie with the basic scenario. One could argue that it is unlikely this procedure would be performed under the conditions we created in our simulation. That is, the injured patient normally would be moved to a safer location before performing the procedure. Although that may be true, our primary goal was to examine how skills practiced in standard hospital settings would hold up under stressful conditions simulated in a VE. Further, even though standard practice might dictate moving the patient to a safer environment before performing the procedure, it does not preclude the possibility that transporting the patient would be unfeasible in some situations. Thus, emergency medical personnel might be called upon to perform such a procedure to prolong a patient's life until he or she could be moved at later time.

## 5. Conclusion

From a general perspective, the present study shows that VEs can be a valuable tool for medical training because they provide a rich context under which performance can be examined. They also provide a safe environment for training medical personnel on a wide range of scenarios under a variety of stressful conditions. The context chosen for the present study was a combat environment; however, other scenarios could also be developed addressing emergency response to natural or man made disasters or even performance within a standard hospital emergency room.

Second, VEs extend the range of applications for current medical simulators. For example, the TraumaMan®system used in this study was designed primarily as an emergency medicine training device. Obviously, other mannequin-based or even VR simulators can be used in a similar fashion. Thus, we have shown that the ability to combine varieties of simulation technology can broaden the scope of applications for medical simulation well beyond classroom instruction. Most important, however, they offer a laboratory in which to study new training techniques and countermeasures for medical personnel who must perform in dangerous situations.

## Acknowledgements

This study was a collaborative project between the Virginia Modeling, Analysis and Simulation Center (VMASC) at Old Dominion University and the Eastern Virginia Medical School. Funding for this study was provided in part by the Naval Health Research Center through NAVAIR Orlando TSD under contract N61339-03-C-0157, entitled "The National Center for Collaboration in Medical Modeling and Simulation". The ideas and opinions presented in this paper represent the views of the authors and do not necessarily represent the views of the Department of Defense.

## References

[1] Satava, R. M. (1993). Virtual reality surgical simulator: The first steps. *Surgical Endoscopy, 7*, 203-205.
[2] Satava, R. M. (2001). Accomplishments and challenges of surgical simulation: Dawning of the next-generation surgical education. *Surgical Endoscopy, 15*, 232-241.
[3] Dawson, S. L. (2002). A critical approach to medical simulation. *Bulletin of the American College of Surgeons, 87*(11), 12-18.
[4] Healy, G. B. (2002). The College should be instrumental in adapting simulators to education. *Bulletin of the American College of Surgeons, 87*(11), 10-11.
[5] Miller, R. (2003, Aug.). 75th Ranger: Casualty response lessons learned. Paper presented at the Advanced Technology Applications for Combat Casualty Care Annual Meeting, St. Pete Beach, FL.
[6] Wickens, C.D., & Hollands, J.G. (2000). *Engineering psychology and human performance, 3rd Ed.*, Upper Saddle River, NJ: Prentice Hall.

*Medicine Meets Virtual Reality 13*
*James D. Westwood et al. (Eds.)*
*IOS Press, 2005*

# An Automatic Robust Meshing Algorithm for Soft Tissue Modeling

Sascha SEIFERT, Sandro BOEHLER, Gunther SUDRA and Rüdiger DILLMANN
*Institut für Rechnerentwurf und Fehlertoleranz, Fakultät für Informatik,*
*Universität Karlsruhe (TH), Haid-und-Neu-Straße 7, 76128 Karlsruhe, Germany*

**Abstract.** Soft tissue simulation with the finite element method is based on discretizations of anatomical objects. The structure of organs is mostly heterogeneous. To compute the deformation of composite materials correctly borders between adjacent tissues must be preserved. In this paper a new meshing algorithm is presented that fulfill this requirement. Additionally it works automatically in a straight forward manner to produce high quality 3d meshes from input triangle surfaces. The algorithm shows robust behavior and allows even to generate mesh from the most complex geometries. The processing time depends directly on the size of the input mesh and not on topology. This makes this algorithm calculable hence useful for time dependant cases, for example to adapt intraoperatively to modified operation status.

## 1. Introduction

The quality of soft tissue simulation for surgery planning depends strongly on geometrical modeling of human anatomy. For biomechanical modeling, the finite element method (FEM) has established as "Gold-Standard". FEM is an important technique to solve differential equations from continuum mechanics which govern the formulation of soft tissue deformation behavior. Calculations with FEM rely on a discretization of the domain in simple elements, mostly in tetrahedra, that as a whole approximate the complexity of the domain. However, in practice, the level of automation of mesh generation becomes a significant, if not controlling factor. Existing automatic meshing tools are often not robust enough to mesh very complex geometries and terminate prematurely without returning a suitable mesh. This algorithm has been developed for use in spine surgery. Here meshing of vertebrae with its complex geometry is still a challenge. Even in this case our algorithm has proven robust. Other approaches need to modify the triangle input mesh before the algorithm can start. But this is a critical factor especially for heterogeneous organs. Additionally, for intraoperative use our meshing algorithm fulfills time requirements.

## 2. Methods

Our algorithm is implemented as a part of our simulation framework MEDIFRAME [1]. The overall structure can be seen in Fig. 1. Meshing consists of three steps:

- Move a sweep line to generate a lattice of equidistant points in the inner

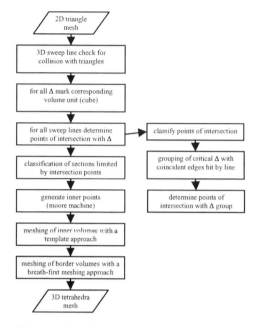

**Figure 1.** Overall structure of the meshing algorithm.

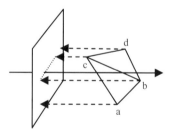

**Figure 2.** Back projection.

- Tetrahedronize inner points
- Connect inner mesh with triangle surface

Using a closed 2d mesh consisting of triangles, the algorithm starts scanning triangles with a sweep line which checks for collisions. This triangle intersection test uses tolerances because of the finite precision of the computer. However, all doubtful cases are resolved by looking at the group of neighboring triangles at the intersection. For example if the sweep line intersects two triangles on their sharing edge a projection backwards allows classifying these triangles correctly (Fig. 2). Sections limited by intersection points are then classified by their continuation (Fig. 3), which allows us to use a *Moore Machine* to generate mesh nodes in the inner of the object. Afterwards every eight inner neighbor points are meshed with tetrahedra by alternating use of templates which subdivide a hexagonal region into five regular tetrahedra. The banded region between the

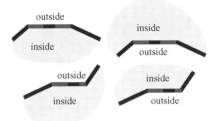

**Figure 3.** Intersection cases.

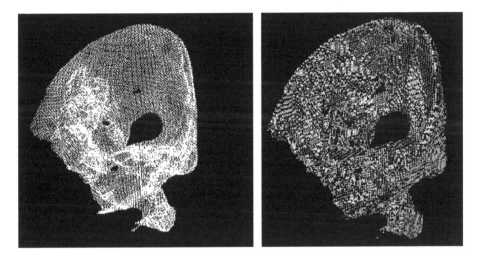

**Figure 4.** Human skull base portion; (left) lattice of inner points (right) inner mesh.

inner mesh and the triangle surface are filled by the use of a *breadth-first approach*. Starting with a tetrahedron from the inner mesh an adequate point on the surface is searched. Then neighboring tetrahedra are generated by recursively searching adequate points on the triangle surface and the new border of the inner mesh to completely fill the banded region. Finally, all tetrahedra are collected and renumbered to get the entire mesh . For an example of a human skull base portion see Fig. 4 and 5.

## 3. Conclusion

The algorithm shows a robust behavior in experiments with different anatomical objects, especially for vertebrae. The maximum processing time correlates with the input size of the problem and can be determined in advance. The average complexity is $O(n^{3/2})$ in worst case it is $O(n^2)$. Therefore the algorithm is also suitable for intraoperative use to adapt the mesh to the current operation state. Since we use a template approach for the inner meshing, high quality tetrahedra are guaranteed. For the banded region the only new tetrahedra are generated which fulfil the delaunay criterion and have good shape. In future we want to improve our algorithm with hp-adaptiveness.

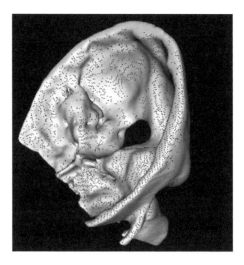

**Figure 5.** Resulting mesh of a human skull base.

## References

[1] S. Seifert, R. Kussaether, W. Henrich, N. Voelzow, R. Dillmann, "Integrating Simulation Framework MEDIFRAME", IEEE EMBC 2003, Cancun, September 2003.

*Medicine Meets Virtual Reality 13*
*James D. Westwood et al. (Eds.)*
*IOS Press, 2005*

# Visualizing Volumetric Data Sets Using a Wireless Handheld Computer

Steven SENGER

*Dept. of Computer Science, University of Wisconsin – La Crosse*

**Abstract.** We describe two extensions to the Nomadic Anatomy Viewer application that both make use of a statistical clustering analysis. In the first case the results of clustering are used to identify the geometry of the local neighborhood and provide for automated navigation along structures. In the second case the analysis is used to support a pen-based interface for interactively rendering selected portions of a volumetric data set.

## 1. Introduction

Wireless handheld pen-based computers provide a ubiquitous and intuitive technology for accessing remote data and computational resources. The Nomadic Anatomy Viewer (NAV) application was developed, as part of a Next Generation Internet project, to interactively explore volumetric data sets, such as CT or the Visible Human cryosection data, in cross section from an iPaq Pocket PC (Figure 1). Utilizing a client/server design, the client tracks user input by rotating and translating the user's frame of reference. The server uses this frame of reference to compute and return to the client the appropriate cross-section image. In addition to the basic client/server functionality, the application can form multicast connections among peers, allowing users to collaborate.

We describe two extensions to the NAV application. Both make use of statistical clustering applied to a local neighborhood of the data set. In the first case, clustering analysis together with principle component analysis is used to determine the geometry of local structures. Information on the local geometry is used to automate navigation through the data set. This navigational assistance appears to the user as a collaborating partner that offers to navigate along the local geometry. For example, if the local geometry is an axial structure, the navigating partner will follow the structure, keeping the structure centered and perpendicular to the image plane. If the local geometry is a boundary surface, the navigating partner will move in the principle direction of the surface.

In the second version, the cross-sectional view of the data set is replaced with a volume rendered reconstruction. In this version, the user's pen position is interpreted as a location on the visible surface of the data set. Local cluster analysis determines a primary voxel category that includes the visible voxels at the pen position. Pen movements are then interpreted as requests to "dissect" away visible structures composed of voxels in the primary category.

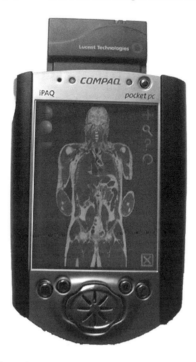

**Figure 1.** Nomadic Anatomy Viewer application.

## 2. Cross-Section Navigation

This version is implemented through a separate server process independent of the client and cross-section server. The navigation server monitors for the existence of multicast channels used by collaborating clients. When it finds a collaborating client, the server continuously monitors the frame of reference exchanged over the collaboration channel.

The coordinate frame determines the voxel at the center of the corresponding cross-section image and this voxel is used as the center of a spherical neighborhood. Voxels within this neighborhood are sampled and a cluster analysis is performed.

The result of the cluster analysis is an assignment of voxel types into categories based upon their similarity. The primary category is that category with majority representation at the center of the neighborhood. A principle component analysis of the spatial distribution of voxels in the primary category is used to identify geometric characteristics of the neighborhood. A single strong eigenvector indicates an axial geometry while two strong eigenvectors indicate a planar or boundary structure (Figure 2).

When the navigation server is able to determine a clear local geometry, it uses that information to determine a direction of movement and communicates that change in position over the collaboration channel. Consequently, to the user it appears that they are collaborating with a remote partner who is able to accurately control navigation along identifiable structures.

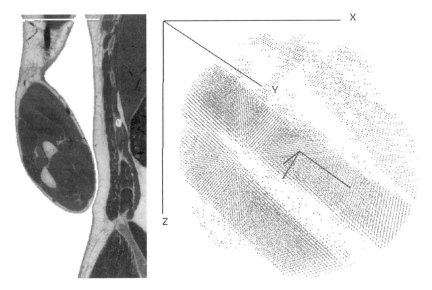

**Figure 2.** Cross-section of Visible Male centered on radius of the right arm and the corresponding spherical neighborhood with bone voxels rendered as a point cloud. The coordinate frame at the center of the neighborhood consists of the eigenvectors resulting from the principle component analysis.

## 3. Volume Dissection

In this version, the client manages a user frame of reference that is used by the server to compute a ray-cast reconstruction of the data volume. The client application allows the user to transform this coordinate frame to rotate and translate the viewing position for the data volume.

Pen strokes are interpreted as actions on the visible surface. During a pen stroke the 2D coordinates of the pen are continuously streamed to the server. The initial point of contact is projected by the server onto the visible surface of the volume and determines the center of a spherical neighborhood. The server performs a cluster analysis within the neighborhood. The primary category is taken to be the category that contains the visible voxels at the point of contact. The server sets all primary category voxels within the neighborhood to be transparent. Subsequent points on the pen stroke are similarly projected to points on the visible surface, and using the primary category of the initial cluster analysis, voxels in the neighborhood of these points are also set to be transparent. This is similar to one of the techniques used in the Immersive Segmentation system [1].

The effect is that as the user moves the pen over the displayed image, the voxels under the pen in the primary category become transparent, or are "dissected away" and expose underlying and dissimilar structures composed of voxels belonging to other categories. Inverting the interpretation of the primary category allows the user to reverse the process and selectively re-visualize structures by rendering them opaque. Figure 3 shows the Visible Human male data set after several actions have progressively exposed the musculature of the chest and ribs.

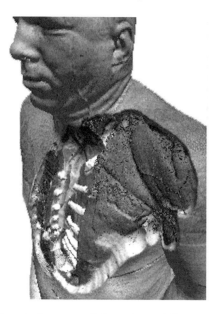

**Figure 3.** Ray-cast rendering with partial dissection.

## 4. Discussion

The cluster analysis technique operates on raw data values in rgb space. It can be extended to voxel value spaces containing an arbitrary number of dimensions. No pre-classification or segmentation of structures is presumed. Consequently it is limited by the quality of the data set and the ability to identify distinct voxel categories. The determination of categories is effected by the relative representation of voxels in the chosen neighborhood. The user can however exploit this property to bias the cluster results in a favorable way by appropriately controlling the position of the center voxel.

Both versions of this application support a high degree of user involvement. Used in an educational setting they would support an active learning style, where users must make choices about how to navigate through the data set or visualize structures of interest. The ability to do this from a wireless handheld device means that access to the data can be taken virtually anywhere and used in a spontaneous manner to support other activities.

## Acknowledgements

This work was partly supported by the NLM (NO1-LM-3506, Dr. Parvati Dev P.I., SUMMIT, Stanford University) and the NSF (ACR 0222519 Dr. Steven Senger P.I.).

## References

[1]  Senger, S. Visualizing and Segmenting Large Volumetric Data Sets. IEEE Computer Graphics and Applications, Vol. 19, No. 3, pp. 32-37, 1999.

*Medicine Meets Virtual Reality 13*
*James D. Westwood et al. (Eds.)*
*IOS Press, 2005*

# Quantifying Risky Behavior
# in Surgical Simulation

Christopher SEWELL [a], Dan MORRIS [a], Nikolas BLEVINS [b],
Federico BARBAGLI [a] and Kenneth SALISBURY [a]

[a] *Departments of Computer Science, Stanford University*
[b] *Departments of Otolaryngology, Stanford University*

**Abstract.** Evaluating a trainee's performance on a simulated procedure involves determining whether a specified objective was met while avoiding certain "injurous" actions that damage vulnerable structures. However, it is also important to teach the stylistic behaviors that minimize overall risk to the patient, even though these criteria may be more difficult to explicitly specify and detect. In this paper, we address the development of metrics that evaluate the risk in a trainee's behavior while performing a simulated mastoidectomy. Specifically, we measure the trainee's ability to maintain an appropriate field of view so as to avoid drilling bone that is hidden from view, as well as to consistently apply appropriate forces and velocities. Models of the maximum safe force and velocity magnitudes as functions of distances from key vulnerable structures are learned from model procedures performed by an expert surgeon on the simulator. In addition to quantitatively scoring the trainee's performance, these metrics allow for interactive 3D visualization of the performance by distinctive coloring of regions in which excessive forces or velocities were applied or insufficient visibility was maintained, enabling the trainee to pinpoint his/her mistakes and how to correct them. Although these risky behaviors relate to a mastoidectomy simulator, the objectives of maintaining visibility and applying safe forces and velocities are common in surgery, so it may be possible to extend much of this methodology to other procedures.

## 1. Introduction

The education of a surgeon-in-training involves the acquisition of the sensorimotor skills necessary for performing surgical tasks as well as the refinement of the cognitive processes involved in performing a full procedure. While a number of existing surgical simulators have been developed to train specific skills, there is also substantial benefit to providing trainees with increased experience through simulation in dealing with the wide range of potential scenarios that can arise in the course of performing a full procedure. Ideally, such a simulator should allow the trainee to interact with the virtual environment in a free-form manner, while evaluating his/her performance according to criteria devised and tuned by the instructing surgeon. It should also provide the user with feedback, both in the form of quantitative metrics and constructive criticism, detailing the trainee's weaknesses and how they can be improved.

At a basic level, the trainee's performance can be critiqued according to whether he/she achieved an objective (such as exposing a lesion; see Figure 1A) while avoiding

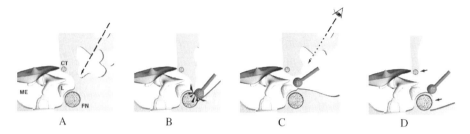

A    B    C    D

**Figure 1.** A) Schematic cross-sectional view of the temporal bone illustrating a lesion (L) within the middle ear (ME) cavity. The goal of this simulation is to access this lesion, in the direction shown by the arrow. The chorda tympani (CT) and the facial nerve (FN) are shown. B) An "injurious" action has occurred, with the burr contacting the facial nerve. C) A "dangerous" action has occurred, when the surgeon has drilled away bone without first establishing clear exposure of the region. D) Correct bone removal has occurred. The nerves have been avoided, and adequate exposure has been established. When the drill is in close proximity to a vulnerable structure, as shown here, applied force and velocity magnitudes should be sufficiently small.

"injurous" actions (such as cutting a nerve; see Figure 1B). We have previously proposed an event based framework that allows for the development of such simulations, and have illustrated the feasibility of the methodology in a simulation of a mastoidectomy procedure [1]. However, a more thorough simulator should also be able to assess the trainee's adherence to stylistic guidelines specified by the instructing surgeon. While there may be multiple techniques that a trainee, with a little luck, may be able to use to perform a procedure while avoiding injurous actions, it would be far better for him/her to learn the specific technique developed over many years by expert surgeons that minimizes the overall risk to the patient. Nevertheless, such criteria are significantly more difficult to specify and to quantify.

## 2. Types of Risky Surgical Behaviors in a Mastoidectomy

In this paper, we consider three types of risky behavior in a mastoidectomy procedure: removing bone outside the current field of view (see Figure 1C); moving the drill too quickly, especially when in close proximity to vulnerable structures (such as the facial nerve or the sigmoid sinus); and applying excessive force, again especially when operating near vulnerable structures (see Figure 1D).

Recognizing the need for customizable surgical simulators, we have previously developed a graphical scripting environment in which the instructing surgeon can design specific training scenarios using finite state machines. However, it would be much more difficult to attempt to encode stylistic guidelines in this way. Also, explicitly segmenting the bone and assigning the appropriate velocities and forces in each region would be very tedious, error-prone, subjective, and applicable only to one specific model. Substantial research has been conducted both in the fields of non-explicit encoding of procedures [2] and of applying probabilistic and machine learning techniques to the evaluation of surgical skill [3,4]. The paradigm of "programming by demonstration" can enable the simulator to develop an internal model of "good style" for a procedure by learning from exemplary runs of the simulation by expert surgeons.

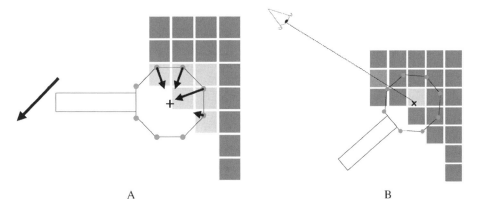

A                                                                    B

**Figure 2.** A) Algorithm for generating forces when the drill contacts bone. The bone is represented as voxels (shown here in 2D as squares), and the drill as a cloud of points (the dots along the perimeter of the circular drilling surface). Each drill point is tested for intersection with the voxel mesh (using direct indexing based on location). The generated force vector is the sum of the vectors from each intersected voxel to the drill center. The density of each voxel along these vectors (here shown with light-colored squares) is decreased, eventually causing them to be removed and turn into bone dust (rendered graphically with a simple particle simulator). B) Algorithm for visibility testing. In order to determine whether bone being removed is within the current field of view, a line is simply traced from the voxel (here shown as the light-colored square) to the view point (the OpenGL camera position). Points at discrete intervals along this line are tested for intersection with the voxel mesh. If any voxels (besides those covered by the drill) are intersected (such as the one on the middle far left highlighted here), they obstruct the view and the removed voxel is determined to not be visible. Otherwise, the voxel is visible.

## 2.1. Drill Force

One of the primary components of good technique in a mastoidectomy is applying appropriate forces with the drill when removing bone. The maximum "safe" force is some function primarily dependent on the distance of the current drilling location from key vulnerable anatomic structures. In our simulator, the bone is represented haptically as a collection of voxels (although a hybrid data structure is used to graphically render a triangulated mesh [5]), and the drill is modeled haptically as a cloud of points, as in the method described by Petersik et. al. [6]. Forces are generated by testing the drill points for intersection with bone voxels (via direct indexing), and summing the vectors from each intersected voxel to the drill center (see Figure 2A).

We want to develop a function that, given a trainee's drill location, returns the maximum force magnitude that can safely be applied there. In order to learn the appropriate force profile, we record the location and force magnitude for each voxel as it is drilled by the training surgeon (or another expert surgeon). Instead of defining locations with respect to a fixed coordinate system, location is specified in terms of distance from key vulnerable structures, allowing use of the function in any bone model (including patient-specific models) in which the locations of these structures are known.

To determine the appropriate type of function to use, we performed a trial run in which an expert otolaryngologist performed a mastoidectomy on our simulator. Distances from each voxel to six key structures (the sigmoid sinus, facial nerve, dura, incus, chorda tympani nerve, and inner ear) were pre-computed (using a brute-force method, finding, for each voxel and each key structure mesh, the minimum distance between the

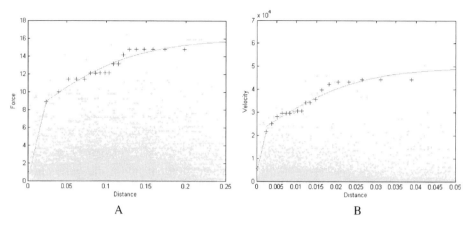

A                                    B

**Figure 3.** A) A plot of applied force magnitudes for voxels as a function of the distance from the voxel to a key structure, in this case the chorda tympani nerve. The raw data points for the 12,573 voxels removed during a mastoidectomy performed on the simulator by an expert surgeon are shown as light dots. Averaged upper bound sample points, shown as crosses, are calculated at regular distance intervals as the average of the five largest force magnitudes at any equal or smaller distance. The initial, steeply sloping region was fitted using linear regression and the region that gradually ascends to a plateau using logistic regression, both shown as solid lines. At somewhat larger distances (off the scale as shown here), the upper hull of the force magnitudes of the raw data starts to decrease again, probably a result of the drill approaching other key structures. B) A plot of instantaneous drill velocity magnitudes for voxels as a function of the distance from the voxel to a key structure, in this case the sigmoid sinus. The raw data points for the 12,573 voxels removed during a mastoidectomy performed on the simulator by an expert surgeon are shown as light dots. Averaged upper bound sample points, shown as crosses, are calculated at regular distance intervals as the average of the five largest velocity magnitudes at any equal or smaller distance. The initial, steeply sloping region was fitted using linear regression and the region that gradually ascends to a plateau using logistic regression, both shown as solid lines. At larger distances, the upper hull of the velocity magnitudes of the raw data starts to decrease again, probably a result of the drill approaching other key structures.

voxel center and a vertex of the mesh), and then recorded along with applied force magnitude when drilled by the expert.

Distance versus force magnitude plots were constructed for each key structure. An example, for the chorda tympani nerve, is shown in Figure 3A. Examining the upper hull of the plotted raw data for each key structure, there appeared to be a steep, roughly linear increase in maximum forces for small distances from the structure, and then a gradual ascent to a plateau as distance from the structure increased further. For many of the plots, maximum forces then began to decrease again at even further distances, presumably as the drill began to approach other key structures.

Rather than attempt to develop a single, complex, global function for maximum safe force magnitudes, separate functions were constructed for each key structure. Also, since we were primarily concerned with the upper hull of maximum safe forces, sample points were created by calculating, at regular distance intervals, the averages of the five maximum forces at any equal or smaller distance. These sample points were then fitted using linear regression for the initial, steeply sloping region, and logistic regression for the region ascending to a plateau.

When the trainee then performs a mastoidectomy on the simulator, the force magnitude applied at each drilled voxel can be compared to the safe force function for each of the key structures, evaluated at the voxel's distance from the structure. The trainee's performance can be evaluated quantitatively by summing, for all voxels for which the applied force magnitude exceeds the maximum of the safe force functions at that location, the amount by which the maximum safe force is exceeded. Perhaps more importantly, upon request, the removed voxels can be re-rendered green if removed with a safe force and red if removed at an unsafe force (with darkness shading according to the amount by which the safe force was exceeded), providing the trainee with constructive graphical criticism, clearly showing where he/she should be observing greater caution.

## 2.2. Drill Velocity

In addition to refraining from applying excessive forces, caution should also be exercised when in proximity to vulnerable structures by maintaining drill velocities at sufficiently small magnitudes. As for the drill forces, we want to develop a function that, given a trainee's drill location (in terms of its distance from key structures), returns the maximum velocity magnitude that can safely be applied there, and to learn this function by recording the location and velocity magnitude for each voxel as it is drilled by an expert surgeon. Velocities are obtained directly from the haptic device's API.

During the trial run described in the previous subsection in which an expert otolaryngologist performed a mastoidectomy on our simulator, we also recorded velocities for each removed voxel. Distance versus velocity magnitude plots were constructed for each key structure. An example, for the sigmoid sinus, is shown in Figure 3B. Examining the upper hull of the plotted raw data for each key structure, the behavior appeared similar to that for force magnitude data, exhibiting a steep, roughly linear increase for small distances, tapering off into a plateau at further distances, and often decreasing again at even further distances. Thus, as before, these regions were fitted with linear and logistic regression, respectively. Quantitative and graphical feedback can then be provided to the trainee based on drill velocities as well as applied forces, showing regions in which he/she should drill more slowly and carefully.

## 2.3. Visibility

Another type of dangerous behavior in performing a mastoidectomy is drilling bone that is hidden from view, usually by other bone. An otolaryngologist is trained to recognize a variety of subtle but important visual cues that indicate the proximity of vulnerable structures just below the surface of the bone, but these cues cannot be heeded if they cannot be seen.

When the trainee removes a voxel, its visibility is tested using a simple algorithm that traces a line from the voxel to the view point (i.e., the OpenGL camera position). Points along this line are tested for intersection with the bone voxel mesh; if any voxel between the drill and the viewpoint is intersected, the removed voxel must have been hidden. See Figure 2B. As for the other risky behaviors, the trainee's performance can be both scored, according to the percentage of removed voxels that were hidden, and visualized, showing voxels that were visible when removed in green and those that were not in red, as shown in Figure 4. Optionally, selected structures can be prevented from being rendered, and the scene can be rotated, allowing unobstructed visualization of the locations of the removed voxels and their proximities to other structures.

Although ideally no invisible voxels should be removed, the severity of the consequences of removing invisible voxels can vary depending on location. Thus, rather than

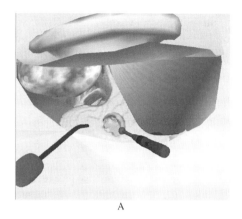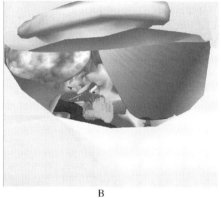

A                                    B

**Figure 4.** A) A trainee drills the temporal bone while performing a mastoidectomy on the simulator. In this example, the trainee "saucerized" on the right side, removing only visible bone, while he "undercut" on the left side, removing bone that was hidden by other bone. B) On the final report, it was noted that 33% of voxels were hidden when removed. Here the trainee can visualize where he performed well (visible voxels in green) and where he did not (invisible voxels in red), and realize that undercutting in close proximity to the sigmoid sinus (in blue) was dangerous as he could not see the visual cues indicating the vein's location below the bone surface.

a binary visible/invisible rating for each voxel, scoring and shading could be graded depending upon distances to key structures, although we have not implemented this.

## 3. Future Work and Conclusions

In this paper we have introduced a methodology for training stylistic surgical techniques that avoid risky behavior. In the context of a mastoidectomy procedure, we evaluated a trainee's ability to maintain an appropriate field of view, as well as to apply forces and velocities consistent with those implicitly defined by an expert surgeon by performing model procedures on the simulator. Although these risky behaviors were identified by an otolaryngologist as among the most important for training specifically in a mastoidectomy simulator, the goals of maintaining visibility in the operating region and of recognizing crucial structures and exercising appropriate caution around them are common in surgery, so many of these ideas may be generalized and applied to other procedures.

The performance of anyone using the simulator is highly dependent upon the quality of the simulator. Thus, as we continue to improve the visual and haptic realism of the simulator, new expert force and velocity profiles will need to be recorded, and will more closely approximate the forces and velocities actually used in the operating room. Other additions to the simulator, such as more realistic stereo rendering and a viewpoint positioning device that mimics the microscope used in the operating room, will also affect the ways in which users can maintain visibility and avoid removing hidden bone. We also hope to employ more sophisticated learning algorithms to better model expert force and velocity profiles, as well as to explore other risky surgical behaviors, perhaps even in the context of other procedures.

# References

[1] Christopher Sewell, Dan Morris, Nikolas Blevins, Federico Barbagli, and Kenneth Salisbury: An Event-Driven Framework for the Simulation of Complex Surgical Procedures. Proceedings of the International Conference on Medical Imaging Computing and Computer Assisted Intervention (MICCAI), St. Malo, France, September 2004, Springer Lecture Notes in Comptuer Science, Vol. II, pp. 346-354.

[2] David Canfield Smith: Kidsim: Programming Agents Without a Programming Language. Communications of the ACM, July 1994, Vol. 37, No. 7.

[3] Jacob Rosen, Massimiliano Solazzo, Blake Hannaford, and Mika Sinanan: Objective Laparoscopic Skills Assessments of Surgical Residents Using Hidden Markov Models Based on Haptic Information and Tool/Tissue Interactions. Medicine Meets Virtual Reality, Newport Beach, CA, January 2001.

[4] Louai Adhami. An Architecture for Computer Integrated Mini-Invasive Robotic Surgery: Focus on Optimal Planning. PhD Thesis, Ecole des Mines de Paris, 2002.

[5] Dan Morris, Christopher Sewell, Nikolas Blevins, Federico Barbagli, and Kenneth Salisbury: A Collaborative Virtual Environment for the Simulation of Temporal Bone Surgery. Proceedings of the International Conference on Medical Imaging Computing and Computer Assisted Intervention (MICCAI), St. Malo, France, September 2004, Springer Lecture Notes in Comptuer Science, Vol. II, pp. 319-327.

[6] A. Petersik, B. Pflesser, U. Tiede, K.H. Hohne, and R. Leuwer: Haptic Volume Interaction with Anatomic Models at Sub-Voxel Resolution. Proceedings of the IEEE Virtual Reality, Orlando, FL, March 2002, pp. 66-72.

*Medicine Meets Virtual Reality 13*
*James D. Westwood et al. (Eds.)*
*IOS Press, 2005*

# Haptic Herniorrhaphy Simulation with Robust and Fast Collision Detection Algorithm

Yunhe SHEN [a], Venkat DEVARAJAN [b] and Robert EBERHART [a]

[a] *Joint BME Program in the University of Texas at Arlington and University of Texas Southwestern Medical Center at Dallas*
[b] *Department of Electrical Engineering, University of Texas at Arlington*

**Abstract.** Collision detection and soft tissue deformation are two major research challenges in real time VR based simulation, especially when haptic feedback is required. We have developed a real time collision detection algorithm for a prototype laparoscopic surgery trainer. However, this algorithm makes no assumptions about its applications and thus can be a generic solution to complicated collision detection problems. For soft tissue modeling, we use the mass-spring model enhanced with volume constraint and, stability control methods. We use both the new collision detection and tissue modeling algorithms in a bimanual hernia repair simulator which performs a mesh prosthesis stapling operation in real time.

## 1. Introduction

### 1.1. Inguinal herniorrhaphy

There are about 500,000 new inguinal hernia incidences each year in the United States, according to NIH [1]. Indirect inguinal hernias pass from the deep/internal inguinal ring, protruding along with the spermatic cord. Direct inguinal hernias pass directly through the abdominal wall leaving the abdominal cavity medial to the inferior epigastric vessels. Indirect inguinal hernias are more common than direct cases. The sacs of inguinal hernias contain some abdominal viscera, commonly part of the small intestine.

During laparoscopic hernia repair, a mesh prosthesis is stapled on the inner side inguinal floor to prevent early recurrence of herniation. Compared with open surgery, laparoscopic herniorrhaphy causes less pain, bleeding, faster recovery and improved cosmesis to the patients [2].

### 1.2. Simulation of laparoscopic stapling operation

To setup a virtual environment for the training of hernia repair procedures, 18 deformable or rigid tissues and instruments are considered necessary objects by the surgeons in the Center of Minimally Invasive Surgery (SCMIS) at UTSWMC. The modeled and simulated human tissues are (in figure 1): left and right rectus abdominis muscles, transver-

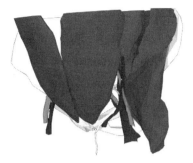

**Figure 1.** Polygonal models for the simulation of inguinal hernia repair.

sus abdominis muscles, iliopsoas muscles, external iliac artery and vein, inferior epigastric artery and vein, spermatic artery and vein, vas deferens, peritoneum, iliopubic tract, cooper's ligament, pelvic bones and pubic symphysis.

Our modeling of human tissues is based on 3D visualization of their anatomical data defined in 2D slices from the Visible Human Project [3].

For real time collision detection, we design a new data structure and an algorithm that performs non-pairwise processing in the broad-phase collision detection at sub-object level. For real time soft tissue modeling, we choose a mass-spring model and enhance it with volume or area constraints, and stability control methods. This fast algorithm simulates tissue deformation at close to haptic rates.

## 2. Method

### 2.1. Collision detection

The fundamental processing of collision detection can be classified as distance calculation, overlapping prune (Z-buffer / Occlusion tests on graphics hardware, for example), or Spatial Occupancy Test (SOT). Introductions of different kinds of collision detection problems and their solutions can be found in [4–6].

To overcome their computation load in real time, algorithms developed for specific applications generally exploit certain features of these applications; for example, the closest features among objects, spatial and temporal coherence etc. Assumptions made on convex, rigid, and static objects substantially simplify the geometric computation required for collision detection. However, these algorithms encounter difficulties when their assumptions are invalidated by some complex issues in the collision detection context:

- Highly deformable objects which violate the convex assumption and make it hard to find the closest features.
- Objects with topological complexity, such as clustered, bundled, concave or sponge structures, voxel objects, particles or polygon soup. Construction of bounding hierarchies of these objects is expensive or inefficient.
- Dynamic updating problem: topology changes due to cutting or suturing operations, adding or removing objects in scenarios, etc.
- Large number of moving objects. This is fatal to pairwise processing.

- Large scale environment or high subdivision resolution. For non-pairwise algorithms performing spatial tessellation, these two factors cause problems in data
storage and access.

Algorithms resolving the above complexity would be robust and generic. Possible
solutions could be hybrid methods, which integrate different kinds of detection modules,
classify and forward the detection tasks to their corresponding algorithms.

Other than combining algorithms, the so called "occupancy test based, spatial tessellation" method, is also a candidate for such a task, if we design a data structure and
an algorithm that is efficient for the uniform tessellation - a non-pairwise processing that
is independent of the complexities of the objects in collision detection applications.

We propose a new *Occupancy* test based algorithm, with a new *Hashing* and *Cascaded* structure (OHC), which deals with the above complex factors in the detection
context without introducing excessive complexity to the detection scenario itself.

The concept of inspecting spatial occupancy for collision detection has been implemented since 1980's [7]. Gibson implemented a SOT based algorithm to detect collisions
between two voxel objects - a deformable sphere and a rigid probe [9], whose occupancy
data was maintained in an array, a static structure that is not efficient for storage or access.
Hash table has been proposed as an optimization for indexing the occupied space containing a given set of coordinates [8]. However, the storage limitation remained in the implementation [10] of the SOT; and the resolution of tessellation is at only object level and not
at sub-object level. Another occupancy test [11] created a hash table indexing the occupied space (buckets) that contains a given node on a liver model. This structure contains
tessellated cell level and primitive level information, and is capable of node-based collision detection between a pair of objects. Note that when we apply an occupancy test for
more than one pair of objects, the structure should support object level indexing as well.

The pruning efficiency of an occupancy test is determined by the resolution of spatial
tessellation, as well as the pruning level. A broad phase detection with primitive level
pruning sends primitives to further primitive-to-primitive (narrow phase) detection, while
object level pruning passes entire objects to its subsequent process.

We resolve the above collision detection complexities with the OHC method that
uses condensed memory allocation supported by hashing plus cascaded data structure
design, which is different from generally used hierarchical trees. Comparison among the
different approaches is briefly shown in table 1.

To perform the non-pairwise processing beyond object level, we need an occupancy
data structure containing both object level information and primitive level information.
Instead of using tree structure, OHC cascades its data into three levels: spatial cells,
objects and primitives. Below is an example of the 3-level structure with 2 cascaded
hashing:

```
Cell set typedefine:
    tOMap: H₁ <cell I.D. type, tObjSet>;
        objSet = h₁(cell I.D.);
Objects set typedefine:
    tObjSet: H₂ <obj I.D. type, tPrimSet>;
        primSet = h₂(obj I.D.);
Primitives set typedefine:
    tPrimSet: H₃ <prim I.D. type>;
        prim = h₃(prim I.D.);
```

**Table 1.** Comparison of collision detection methods.

| | Bounding volume hierarchy method | Common spatial tessellation method | OHC method |
|---|---|---|---|
| Broad phase detection at object-level | Pairwise | Non-pairwise | Non-pairwise |
| Broad phase detection at sub-object-level | Pairwise | Pairwise | Non-pairwise |
| Hierarchy complexity | Multi-levels | 1 level | 3 levels |
| Data storage and access | Efficient/Inefficient | Inefficient | Efficient |
| Topological Complexity | Dependent | Independent | Independent |
| Applicable to large number of moving objects | No | Yes | Yes |
| Applicable to large scale environment | Yes | No | Yes |

Where $H_1$, $H_2$ and $H_3$ represent the data sets for cells, objects, and primitives, respectively; $h_1$, $h_2$ and $h_3$ are the query functions returning instances of cells, objects and primitives from their sets; $H_1$ and $H_2$ are hash tables; $H_3$ is linked lists or vector.

The algorithm first fills the structure with cells occupied by at least one object. Tessellation and occupancy are determined by a coordinates hashing function that maps coordinates into cell indices. For applications that prefer a more concise structure that only contains the cells occupied by more than 2 objects, another optional hash table consisting of object-counters of the non-empty cells is checked before actually inserting a cell to the cascaded structure. Complexity of the filling process is $O(m)$, where $m$ is the total number of primitives.

The broad phase detection is finished after filling the structure with the data from all the objects and their primitives. The side length of the cubic cells is set to a few millimeters, which is the resolution of the broad phase detection.

The narrow phase detection is the primitive-to-primitive intersection test within each small cell that containing primitives of more than 2 objects.

For a given number of primitives, OHC achieved constant processing time in the broad phase test. However, the intersection test in the narrow phase is proportional to the output, which is the number of colliding primitive pairs.

To apply this collision detection method to different kinds of geometric objects such as triangles and voxels, a coordinates interpolation is necessary. The only exceptions are vertex primitives (particles). The interpolator samples the coordinates within the area or volume occupied by each primitive. We classify the occupancy test as node-based, polygonal-based or voxel-based, according to the primitives contained in the occupancy data structure. Note that applying node-based occupancy test for polygonal objects causes non-conservative collision detection, even if a distance test is added afterward, for polygons can intersect without having their vertices in very close ranges.

Let's consider a triangle primitive example, under a conservative condition that the maximum primitive side length is less than two times the cell size and, the coordinates at its three vertices plus one interpolation point at the geometric center are enough for locating all the cells occupied by the triangle. This simple interpolation guarantees no miss-detection.

When the distribution of primitive size shows a large variance, we apply adaptive interpolation - increase the degree of interpolation or subdivision, until the no-miss condition set upon the ratio between the size of primitives and of the cell is satisfied.

## 2.2. Soft tissue modeling

To achieve haptic rate deformation, we choose a first order numerical integrator to solve the ordinary differential equations in the mass spring modeling, and apply a stability penalty method to it. Higher order methods tend to be more accurate and stable while they advance slower in the integration.

Stability is an important concern in deformable modeling. The unstable behaviors have common characteristics: excess velocity, large acceleration, and oscillation, suggesting an excessively energized system.

The idea of adaptive stability control is to introduce a penalty function as a negative feedback to the deformation to avoid unstable behavior or provide restoration from the unstable phase. For a number of nodes $n \geq 1$, $N$ be the set of the nodes, and a certain node $i \in N$,

$$
C(\Omega_i) = \begin{cases} \dfrac{\Omega_i}{|\Omega_i|} |\Omega_t|, & \text{if } |\Omega_i| \geq |\Omega_t| \\ \Omega_i, & \text{if } |\Omega_i| < |\Omega_t| \end{cases}
\tag{2.1}
$$

Where $\Omega_i$ is an energy evaluation of node $i$, $|\Omega_t|$ is a threshold that can be optimized by experiments. This cut-off function saturates the energy of a set of nodes before it exceeds a given level. For $n = 1$, and energy estimation is based on velocity, equation 2.1 adjusts the integration time steps for individual nodes according to their current speed of movement.

Let $P$ be the collection of parameters used by the deformable modeling, such as time steps, stiffness, spring or damping coefficients, for $p_j \in P$, $p_j \in [p_j^{\min}, p_j^{\max}]$, and $\xi > 1$. Then, the adaptive penalty function is as follows:

$$
p_j = C(\Omega_1, \Omega_2, \ldots, \Omega_n) = \begin{cases} \max\left(\dfrac{p_j}{\xi}, p_j^{\min}\right), & \text{if } \sum_i^n |\Omega_i| \geq |\Omega^{\max}| \\ \min(p_j \cdot \xi, p_j^{\max}), & \text{if } \sum_i^n |\Omega_i| < |\Omega^{\min}| \end{cases}
\tag{2.2}
$$

This formula gradually and explicitly adjusts the selected simulation parameters by evaluating system energy and comparing it with a given range $[\Omega^{\min}, \Omega^{\max}]$. The effect of formula 2.2 is equal to applying a system-level brake that allows fast response at low energy status and prevents unstable behavior by slowing down the system reaction. Stability is substantially improved by applying these methods to our simulation. These methods increase the system tolerance to the numerical errors as well as larger time steps and stiffer spring constants.

There have been some applications of adding volume constraints to deformable models. Volume constraint is applied to a mass spring model in which elastic axes are reoriented [12]: volume of each element in a volumetric mesh is approximation by summation

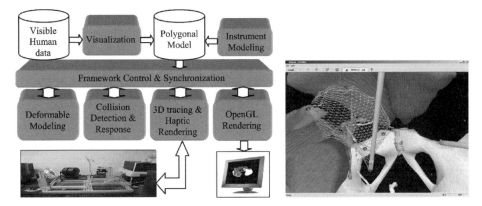

**Figure 2.** The block diagram of the prototype simulator.      **Figure 3.** The mesh stapling scene.

of the distance from vertices to the center of the element. The elastic force due to this volume change is then applied to the mass nodes on the vertices of the element.

In our simulation, volume preservation is advanced further into a new approach, which has a boundary constraint defined by mass spring structure plus a volume constraint - the elastic force generated due to an object's *total* volume change. Instead of piecewise estimation, volume is monitored as a state variable of the entire model and the constraint is applied equally to the mass nodes.

## 3. Framework implementation

The simulator is developed with VC++ on 2.8GHz dual-processor workstation. The system modules are shown in figure 2. The simulation program adopts up to 4 PHANToM$^{TM}$ devices for haptic rendering and instrument manipulation.

## 4. Results

This virtual environment consists of 18 objects, which are specified by laparoscopic surgeons. In the simulation shown in figure 3, the maximum number of surface triangles on the objects is tuned to 6k, after the visualization process. Deformation is being refreshed above 700Hz. The average frequency of instruments-to-tissues collision detection and collision response is 310Hz. As for the entire environment, the constant time of broad phase collision detection is 7ms/cycle. The total collision solution time, including primitive-to-primitive intersection test and collision response averaged 12ms/cycle.

## 5. Conclusion

The overall simulation achieved close to haptic feedback rates. The collision detection algorithm is capable of handling all collision detection problems encountered in this surgical simulation. The primitives input to this algorithm can be polygons, voxels or particles. The complexity of OHC collision detection algorithm is independent of the topological complexity of the objects, or the environment scale. OHC can be applied to the collision detection among highly deformable objects and a large number of moving objects. In broad phase detection, this algorithm extends the non-pairwise features beyond object-level, as well as increases the prune resolution of the broad phase detection from object-level to primitive-level.

## 6. Discussion

This algorithm makes no assumptions about its detection application and thus can be a generic solution to complicated situations. In addition, it can also be customized with additional performance increase for a given detection context. For example, among all the detection cases, if we assign faster timing or higher thread priority to instrument-to-tissue collision detection in a surgery simulation with haptic feedback requirement, OHC first fills its occupancy data structure with instruments objects. At this stage, only the cells occupied by instruments exist in the data structure. In the next step, OHC only adds tissue primitives into the existing cells - all the other primitives mapped into new cells are recognized away from the instruments and are excluded from further processing.

## Acknowledgements

This research is supported by Texas Higher Education Coordinating Board. Useful consultation with Robert Rege MD, and Mark Watson MD at UTSWMC is gratefully acknowledged.

## References

[1]  Digestive diseases in the United States: Epidemiology and Impact – NIH Publication No. 94-1447, NIDDK, 1994 (http://digestive.niddk.nih.gov/statistics/statistics.htm).
[2]  D. Jones, J. Wu and N. Soper, editors. Laparoscopic surgery: principles and procedures. Quality Medical Publishing, Inc., pages 3, 233-246, 1997.
[3]  http://www.nlm.nih.gov/research/visible/visible_human.html.
[4]  M. Lin and S. Gottschalk. Collision detection between geometric models: A survey. Proceeding of IMA Conference on Mathematics of Surfaces, pages 37-56, 1998.
[5]  P. Jiménez, F. Thomas, C. Torras. 3D collision detection: a survey. Computers and Graphics, 25(2), pages 269 - 285, 2001.
[6]  M. Lin and D. Manocha, editors. Interactive Geometric Computations Using Graphics Hardware: SIGGRAPH2002 Course Notes #31, 2002.
[7]  T. Uchiki, T. Ohashi and M. Tokoro. Collision detection in motion simulation, Computers and Graphics. 7 (3-4), pages 285-293, 1983.
[8]  M. Overmars. Point location in fat subdivisions. Information Processing Letter, 44, pages 261-265, 1992.
[9]  S. Frisken-Gibson. Using linked volumes to model object collision, deformation, cutting, carving and joining. IEEE Trans. Visualization and Computer Graphics, 5(4), pages 333-348, 1999.
[10] A. Gregory, M. Lin, S. Gottschalk, R. Taylor. Fast and accurate collision detection for haptic interaction using a three degree-of-freedom force-feedback device. Computational Geometry: Theory and Applications, 15(1-3), pages 69-89, 2000.
[11] S. Cotin, H. Delingette and N. Ayache. Real-time elastic deformations of soft tissues for surgery simulation. . IEEE Trans. Visualization and Computer Graphics, 5(1), pages 62-73, 1999.
[12] D. Bourguignon, M. Cani. Controlling anisotropy in masss-spring system. Proceedings of the 11th Eurographics Workshop, pages 113-123, 2000.

*Medicine Meets Virtual Reality 13*
*James D. Westwood et al. (Eds.)*
*IOS Press, 2005*

# Affordable Virtual Environments:
# Building a Virtual Beach for Clinical Use

Andrei SHERSTYUK, PhD, Christoph ASCHWANDEN and Stanley SAIKI, M.D.

*University of Hawaii*

**Abstract.** Virtual Reality has been used for clinical application for about 10 years and has proved to be an effective tool for treating various disorders. In this paper, we want to share our experience in building a 3D, motion tracked, immersive VR system for pain treatment and biofeedback research.

## 1. Introduction

Presently, Virtual Reality (VR) systems have a multitude of uses: architectural design, task training, vehicle design, education and certainly gaming and entertainment [1]. In most cases such VR application development requires expensive and unique hardware and software solutions that are developed for very specialized uses. This limits the general use of such systems to well-funded efforts of large institutions. There is a growing category of VR applications that can be effectively implemented on a relatively small budget. This new area is the use of VR in clinical applications. For a review of the current state of the art we refer readers to Hodges et al [2]. These applications address clinical approaches to a variety of anxiety disorders, post-traumatic stress disorder, substance abuse and chronic pain.

The purpose of this paper is to show that creating a clinical VR system is not as difficult as it may seem. Specifically, we want to share our experience in building a VR beach simulation to study the incorporation of virtual environments with biofeedback and psychotherapy in pain control.

## 2. Project specifications

The beach simulation is utilized to provide a relaxing, stress-free environment. The user can "walk" around and enjoy the scene that is populated with pleasant and engaging animated interactive objects. Overall, the scene is designed to convey the sense of peace and calmness. From the technical perspective, the following goals were defined: (a) creating 3D content; (b) stereo rendering at 25 fps; (c) tracking of user's head and hand for viewing and interaction; (d) navigation system; (e) 3D sound effects; (f) event scheduling incorporating user input.

## 3. VR Equipment

### 3.1. Computer system

To minimize cost a single PC configuration is used. Images are generated for left and right channels by a rendering engine and sent to HMD and VR console monitor. The sound server runs on the same PC and provides 3D positional playback of various sound effects, such as ocean waves crashing on the shore, bird cries, sounds of falling coconuts, etc. The entire beach simulator runs on a 2.4 GHz dual-processor computer at 25 frames per second in stereo mode. For the 3D engine, we used *Flatland* system, developed in the University of New Mexico under supervision of Thomas Caudell [3].

### 3.2. Motion tracking

For motion tracking, we used *Flock of Birds* by *Ascension, Inc*, which provides high accuracy tracking at 1.8 mm. The beach simulator communicates with the motion tracking system by reading translation and rotation data from two sensors: one for the head (camera in VR), and one for the hand, which allows an immersed person to use a virtual hand for interaction with objects on the scene.

### 3.3. Head Mount display

The choice of HMD is no doubt the most crucial for making the VR system as immersive and engaging as possible. From the user point of view, the most important factors are: stereo capability, field of view and image resolution. We have tried four stereo-capable HMDs: V8, Kaiser ProView, 5DT, nVisor SX from *NVIS Corporation* and have chosen the last one for its superior image quality (1280×1024 pixels) and wide field of view (60 deg diagonal).

## 4. Content

What does it take to make subjects believe that he or she is on a beach? For that, we need content – a set of objects and events that create the sense of "presence." Content may be created and delivered in a variety of ways. For instance, one can place a subject in the middle of a 3D cube and stream prerecorded video on all or some of its faces. That would create a realistic, but totally non-interactive environment. The opposite side of the scale is a completely synthetic CG environment, without video footage at all. In mixed systems, video sequences can be projected onto some objects of the CG environment. That technique works very well for indoor scenes, especially if the user can be restricted from looking at these video-textured objects from arbitrary angles. On the beach, the user is should free to walk and look in any direction. This was the main reason why we have chosen completely virtual settings. An additional advantage is the consistent level of representation of all objects. With uniform CG environments, there's no need to worry if a bird on a video background looks more realistic than a CG bird walking by the user on the foreground. All models and animations for this project were created by *Sprite Entertainment* [4]. Two snapshots from the beach scene illustrate their work.

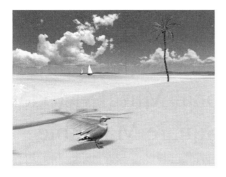 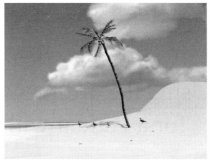

## 5.  Things to do on the virtual beach

On the virtual beach, one has no tasks to accomplish, no levels of game play to move up, and no specific time limits set. As on a real beach, people enter at will, spend some time and leave at will. The beach is there for them "living its own life." It is up to the user how far he or she wants to explore it. We programmed several events that happen in the scene to enhance a sense of presence. Here are some examples.

A large seagull lands near the beach chair, walks around it and takes off (see left figure). A crab crawls out of the ocean, approaches the chair and runs back into the water. Another seagull makes a wide circle in the sky. Coconuts drop from a palm tree with a *thump* sound. That happens twice during the session and each time when the user hits a palm tree while walking around. A flock of sea gulls lands on the distant shore (right figure). If the user tries to chase them, the birds take off with a loud noise. Dolphins jump up from the water at random times. Two butterflies fly around the beach, sitting occasionally on various objects. The user can catch a butterfly with the virtual hand - then the butterfly sits on the hand, flapping its wings slowly until released. For adventurous types, there are more attractions. Various seashells are lying on the shore, they can be picked up and examined. Fallen coconuts, palm tree leaves, straw hat and a couple of dry crabs are also interactive. One "not so dead" crab is hiding in the water that user can grab at his/her own risk. (The crab starts twitching when picked up). Overall, the scene provides enough activities to keep users interested for 20-30 minutes.

## 6.  Conclusions

Modeling and animation work was completed in 3 months by 3 CG artists. Programming was finished in 6 months, by 2 programmers. The whole project turned out to be a good example of how a low-budget production can yield effective and interesting results.

## References

[1]  F.P. Brooks, Jr., "What's Real About Virtual Reality?", IEEE Computer Graphics and Applications, vol. 19, no. 6, Nov./Dec. 1999, pp. 16-27.
[2]  L. F. Hodges, P. Anderson, G. C. Burdea, H. G. Hoffman, B. O. Rothbaum, "Treating Psychological and Physical Disorders with VR", IEEE Computer Graphics and Applications, vol. 21, no. 6, Nov./Dec. 2001, pp 25-33.
[3]  Flatland Project http://www.hpc.unm.edu/homunculus/.
[4]  Sprite Entertainment http://www.spritee.com/.

*Medicine Meets Virtual Reality 13*
*James D. Westwood et al. (Eds.)*
*IOS Press, 2005*

# Analysis of Masticatory Muscle Condition Using the 4-dimensional Muscle Model for a Patient with Square Mandible

Yuhko SHIGETA [a], Takumi OGAWA [a], Eriko ANDO [a], Shunji FUKUSHIMA [a],
Naoki SUZUKI [b], Yoshito OTAKE [b] and Asaki HATTORI [b]

[a] *The 2nd Department of Prosthetic Dentistry,*
*Tsurumi University School of Dental Medicine*
[b] *Institute for High Dimensional Medical Imaging,*
*Jikei University School of Medicine*

**Abstract.** The present study was conducted to ascertain characteristics of mandibular movements in patients with SQM, observe the kinetics of masticatory muscles using a four-dimensional (4D) muscle model, and kinetically investigate the etiology of Square Mandible (SQM). As results, 1, In the maximum opening position, location of the condyle was beyond the articular tubercle for volunteer, but within the mandibular fossa for SQM patient. 2, While the temporal muscle of volunteer was markedly expanded, that of SQM patient was not. 3, In both volunteer and SQM during left lateral excursion, the right mandibular condyle moved to a position slightly before the lowest point of the articular tubercle. The 4D muscle model showed that the cause of limited mouth opening in SQM patient was insufficient expansion of the temporal muscle, and not dysfunction of the opening muscles. Insufficient expansion of the temporal muscle stresses the masseter muscle and leads to hypertrophy of the masseter muscle and hyperplasia of the mandibular angle, resulting in the unique facial configuration.

## 1. Introduction

As the name suggests, Square Mandible (SQM) represents a facial configuration characterized by pronounced mandibular angles. Some individuals with SQM display painless limited mouth opening despite the absence of organic abnormality in the temporomandibular joint. Although protrusive and lateral movements are reportedly not limited, opening movements are restricted in patients with SQM [1]. While mandibular movements in SQM have been analyzed macroscopically and clinical findings have been obtained by palpation of the temporomandibular joint, no qualitative studies have yet been reported.

In patients with SQM, degree of mouth opening can be increased by coronoidotomy or coronoidectomy, suggesting that the cause is contracture of the temporal muscle. However, the most notable characteristic of SQM, the facial configuration, is caused by hyperplasia of the mandibular angle and hypertrophy of the masseter muscle. In other words, the temporal muscle is involved in the onset of SQM, while the masseter muscle

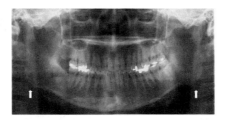

**Figure 1.** Radiographic images show square mandibles with hyperplasia of mandibular angle.

is involved in the clinical features of this condition. However, the relationship between the two muscles has not been clarified.

The present study was conducted to ascertain characteristics of mandibular movements in patients with SQM, observe the kinetics of masticatory muscles using a four-dimensional (4D) muscle model, and kinetically investigate the etiology of SQM.

## 2. Subjects and Methods

### 2.1. Subjects

Subjects were a healthy volunteer and a patient with square mandible. A volunteer was a 26-year old female who had no missing teeth and no morbid findings in clinical examination. A patient was a 37-year old female. Diagnostic imaging scarcely depicted any disc derangement, but a severely limited jaw opening was noted. As well, her facial appearance showed a characteristic square mandible facial configuration (Fig.1). She had not responded to drug and splint therapy.

### 2.2. Methods

The skull and mandible were reconstructed into a 3-dimensional (3D) bone model from the CT data and mandibular movements were recorded by a measurement device of MM-JI-E (Shofu Inc.). The bone model and the mandibular movements were combined using the 4D analyzing system [1].

The origin and halt of each masticatory muscle were positioned on the surface of the 3D bone model, and connected together with a string respectively.

In this system, the color of the string was designed to be passively changed in accordance with mandibular movements (Fig.2).

## 3. Results

### 3.1. Maximum opening position

In the maximum opening position, location of the condyle was beyond the articular tubercle for volunteer, but within the mandibular fossa for SQM patient. In other words, opening movements of SQM patient resemble hinge movements (Fig.3).

Also, while the temporal muscle of volunteer was markedly expanded, that of SQM patient was not. This could be explained by the difference in maximum interincisal dis-

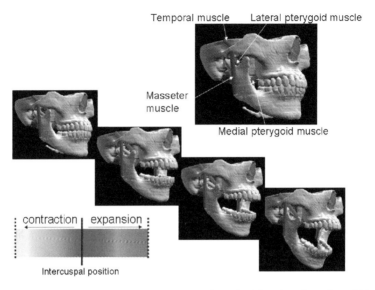

**Figure 2.** Color changes during expansion and contraction of muscles. The color of muscle model is red in the intercuspal position, and it changes from red to purple when expanded and to yellow when contracted.

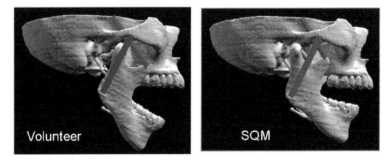

**Figure 3.** In the maximum opening position, the condyle of the SQM patient moves less than that of the volunteer.

tance, but also supports the notion that contracture of the temporal muscle is the cause of limited mouth opening in SQM patients [2]. As to the masseter muscle, maximum interincisal distance for SQM patients was shorter, but degree of expansion for SQM patient was slightly larger compared to healthy volunteer (Fig.4).

## 3.2. Left lateral excurtion

In both volunteer and SQM during left lateral excursion, the right mandibular condyle (mandibular condyle on the non-working side) moved to a position slightly before the lowest point of the articular tubercle, suggesting that the lateral pterygoid muscle was displaying basically normal function (Fig.5).

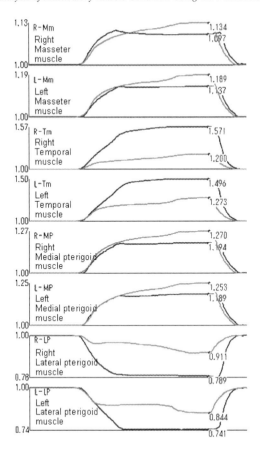

**Figure 4.** Activity of each muscle during opening and closing movement. In the maximum opening position, the SQM patient's temporal muscle is shorter than that of the volunteer. On the other hand, the masseter is expanded. (Green line : Volunteer, Red line : SQM).

## 4. Discussion and Conclusion

The present study analyzed mandibular movements of SQM patient with limited mouth opening, and investigated the kinetics of the masticatory muscles using a 4D muscle model. The results show that movement of the condyle was limited by some factor at opening, despite acceptable lateral excursion, and suggest that the mode of lateral movements in SQM patient may differ slightly from those in healthy individual.

Results of analysis using the 4D muscle model showed that the cause of limited mouth opening in SQM patient was insufficient expansion of the temporal muscle, and not dysfunction of the opening muscles. Insufficient expansion of the temporal muscle stresses the masseter muscle and leads to hypertrophy of the masseter muscle and hyperplasia of the mandibular angle, resulting in the unique facial configuration.

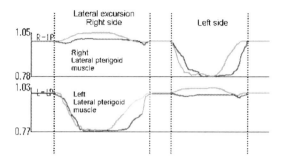

**Figure 5.** There was no difference in the condition of the lateral pterygoid muscle between the volunteer and SQM patient during lateral excursion to the right and left side (Green line : Volunteer, Red line : SQM).

## References

[1] Shigeta Y, Suzuki N, Otake Y et al. Four-Dimensional Analysis of Mandibular Movements with Optical Position Measuring and Real-time Imaging. Medicine Meets Virtual Reality 11 2003 : 315-317.
[2] Murakami K, Yokoe Y, Yasuda S et al. Prolonged Mandibular Hypomobility Patient with a "Square Mandible" Configuration with Coronoid Process and Angle Hyperplasia. J Craniomandib Pract 2000; 18 : 113-119.

*Medicine Meets Virtual Reality 13*
*James D. Westwood et al. (Eds.)*
*IOS Press, 2005*

# Automated Renderer for Visible Human and Volumetric Scan Segmentations

Jonathan C. SILVERSTEIN, Victor TSIRLINE, Fred DECH,
Philip KOUCHOUKOS and Peter JUREK

*Department of Surgery, The University of Chicago*
*e-mail: jcs@uchicago.edu*

**Abstract.** Creating a library of binary segmentation mask sequences for the abdominal anatomy hierarchy of SNOMED and developing a quick, flexible automatic method for generating iso-surface models from these named structure masks has been a primary goal in our research. This paper describes our development of a clear path for computing visualizations of arbitrary groups of organs from these masks (typically generated from Visible Human data). One use of these methods is teaching the anatomy of various organ systems in the human body using virtual reality environments.

## 1. Problem

The process of generating size-efficient, contiguous, high-quality surface structures from data masks has typically required multiple steps and iterations with human intervention at each transition. This is time-consuming and error-prone, but is necessary to achieve the National Library of Medicine's long-term goals in the Visible Human Project® [1].

We have developed an automatic, highly customizable technique for rapidly generating multiple combined polygonal iso-surfaces from pre-segmented binary mask slices of structures derived from the Visible Human Female cryosection. The generation of the polygonal models can be adjusted for nearly 50 different parameters.

## 2. Methods

Our standalone application, AutoSCAN, was written in C and C++ using open source libraries available for multiple platforms. It uses standard Visualization Toolkit (VTK) [2] classes, customized VTK procedures readily available on the Internet, and ImageMagick's [3] mogrify routine. It inputs slice data obtained directly from our library of Visible Human Female masks, CT or MRI scans, and generates 3D contour(s), decimates them, and writes them to standard file formats. Input slices may be coronal, saggital, or horizontal.

The data flow diagram (Table 1) illustrates the various modules that make up AutoSCAN. The full processing pipeline may be roughly divided into 3 steps: resizing, 3-D reconstruction, and optimization (including decimation). The images and data files

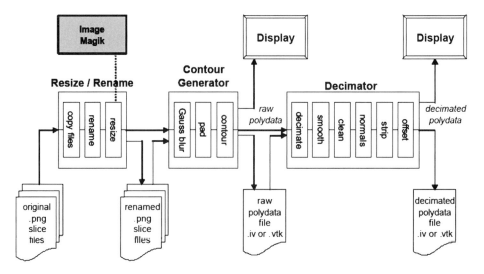

**Figure 1.** Data flow diagram for AutoSCAN application.

may be saved to disk at various steps so that re-parameterized re-runs can be performed without the need to go through what might be identical manipulations.

The Resize / Rename module in AutoSCAN enables resizing the input images if desired, before passing them to the VTK reconstruction methods. This is important because the high native pixel resolution of the Visible Human and new CT scaners can generate 3D datasets that exceed the power of desktop systems and typical contour resolution needs. The working image size is specified in the configuration file.

The Contour Generator performs a highly customizable Gaussian blur on the resized 3D pixel data and then pads the faces of the 3D array. The padding is done in order to ensure that the VTK contour filter generates a closed iso-surface. The application can later be rerun multiple times starting with this raw polydata and using different Decimator Module parameters. In the Decimator Module the polydata is first decimated and then smoothed and cleaned (outlying points are removed). Finally, vertex normals are generated to allow for Gouraud shading. Depending on one of the configuration parameters, the polydata is either merged into triangle strips or left unstripped to support the indexed face set section of an Open Inventor vertex list. Lastly a common reference coordinate system is generated from geometric offset parameters and the final data is saved as .iv or .vtk files.

## 3. Results

Full rendering of a single structure on a modern desktop computer takes on the order of minutes depending on the number of slices, the size of the slice images, and the complexity of the structure. Since AutoSCAN can save the raw polydata generated by the Contour Generator (the most computation intensive and time consuming portion of the entire application), this intermediate data can be quickly and easily reprocessed through the Decimator. In other words, the application can be restarted at the beginning of the Decimator module and produce the final data files in seconds. This greatly facilitates

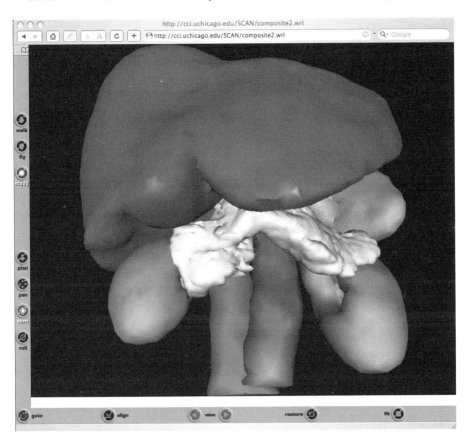

**Figure 2.** Example output of AutoSCAN application showing .wrl file rendered in browser with free cross-platform Cortona plugin (available at http://www.parallelgraphics.com/products/cortona).

minor decimation reconfigurations that may be needed in order to accommodate disparate organ topologies. Once initial contours have been generated, this feature enables the illustrator to use AutoSCAN as an interactive visualization tool, adjusting decimation parameters as needed to suit the specific visualization task.

Multiple overlapping structures can be created from multiple slice series in a single execution. The application is controlled entirely through a single configuration file with nearly fifty parameter input fields so a high degree of control over the various processes can be achieved. AutoSCAN has been successfully deployed on Linux, Windows and MAC OS-X. Figure 1 demonstrates the output using a free VRML client.

## 4. Conclusion/Discussion

Our results thus far have been very encouraging. Not only have we developed a single simple application that the medical illustrator can use interactively to view intermediate results of segmentation sessions, but the vast majority of the organ surface models that result are of excellent quality.

## Acknowledgement

This work was supported by NIH/National Library of Medicine grant R01-LM06756.

## References

[1]  www.nlm.nih.gov/research/visible/visible_human.htm.
[2]  Schroeder W, et al. The Visualization Toolkit: Object-Oriented Approach to 3D Graphics. Prentice Hall, 1995.
[3]  www.lsw.uni-heidelberg.de/manuals/ImageMagick.

Medicine Meets Virtual Reality 13
James D. Westwood et al. (Eds.)
IOS Press, 2005

# Distributed Collaborative Radiological Visualization using Access Grid

Jonathan C. SILVERSTEIN [a,c], Fred DECH [a], Justin BINNS [b], David JONES [b],
Michael E. PAPKA [b,c] and Rick STEVENS [b,c]

[a] *Department of Surgery, The University of Chicago*
*e-mail: jcs@uchicago.edu*
[b] *Mathematics and Computer Science Division, Argonne National Laboratory*
[c] *Computation Institute of The University of Chicago and Argonne National Laboratory*

**Abstract.** This paper describes early technical success toward enabling high quality distributed shared volumetric visualization of radiological data in concert with multipoint video collaboration using Grid infrastructures. Key principles are the use of commodity off-the-shelf hardware for client machines and open source software to permit deployment of over a large and diverse group of sites. Key software used includes the Access Grid Toolkit, the Visualization Toolkit, and Chromium.

## 1. Problem

Biomedical research, education, and the practice of medicine have become socially complex, team-oriented activities. The Advanced Biomedical Collaboration Testbed [1] is a NIH/National Library of Medicine funded project focused on improving efficiency and effectiveness across complex teams in complex environments using Grid technologies. One specific goal of the project is to leverage the Access Grid (AG) [2] and other remote visualization techniques [3] to enable distributed shared volumetric visualization of radiological data combined with multipoint video collaboration.

Our prior work toward this goal was developed on high-end graphics hardware, coupled with spatially immersive displays [4]. We demonstrated feasibility of implementing a variety of collaboration features using radiological data and virtual reality including: persistent server-client tele-collaboration; distributed application control with synchronization and audio sharing; model selection, transparency of elements; translate, rotate, scale; automatic DICOM import; segmentation; 3D region of interest selection; sampling precision; and an arbitrary clipping plane. However, the methods used previously proved to be too costly and esoteric to be practical for all but highly specialized sites. Largely because of these practical limitations, our goal of deploying high quality collaborative volumetric radiological investigation over a large and diverse group of institutions has yet to be realized. Here we present our early technical success toward achieving the vision using commodity off-the-shelf hardware for client sites (PCs, PC graphics and video capture cards, digital video cameras, and projectors) and open source software, which we believe, after further development, will be practical enough to be widely utilized.

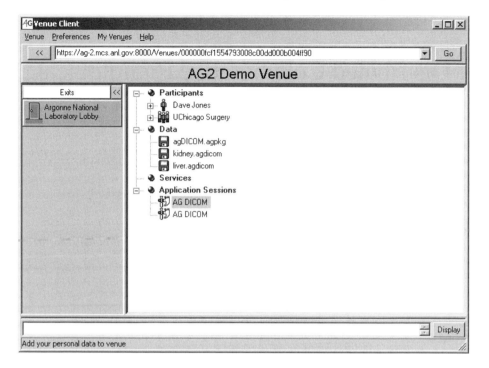

**Figure 1.** Screen capture of an Access Grid Venue Client in a venue running the AG DICOM application between Argonne National Laboratory and the University of Chicago.

## 2. Methods

The Access Grid is an ensemble of resources that supports group-to-group human inter-action across the Grid. It consists of large-format multimedia displays, presentation and interactive software environments, interfaces to grid middleware, and interfaces to re-mote visualization environments. More information about this internationally deployed infrastructure can be found at the Access Grid Project page [2]. The AG Toolkit and other tools used are open source.

Typical use of the AG today includes conducting high quality distributed meetings using multicast video and audio streams by joining Clients in peer-to-peer ad hoc net-works through the use of coordinating Venues. In addition to these "standard services", the Access Grid Toolkit provides the framework for much more sophisticated collabora-tive applications. Figure 1 is a screen capture of the Access Grid Venue Client version 2, which is the standard GUI used by each peer during an AG session. Here it is shown dur-ing a collaborative session between Dave Jones and the UChicago Surgery group node. The Venue Client permits ready access to other Participants, Data, Services, and Ap-plication Sessions that have joined the Venue regardless of what hardware platform on which the Venue Client is being run. In this case, one can see the DICOM data instances that individuals have uploaded to the venue as well as the currently running AG DICOM application sessions using the data (instances of the application described in this paper).

Our distributed collaborative radiological visualization application is constructed from four essential components:

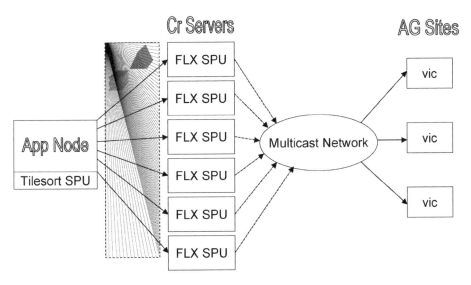

**Figure 2.** Example system flow for a 3 by 2 tiling (six streams generated) of a visualization from the server-side components to three client-side visualization display sites.

1. A Visualization Server
2. A server-side AG integration component
3. A client-side AG integration component & graphical user interface (GUI)
4. A specialized video client for client-side visualization display.

The Access Grid is used for GUI synchronization and application startup, which also initiates out-of-band (XML-RPC) communication for handling of high-frequency events and server state changes (i.e., mouse events). The Visualization Server utilizes XML-RPC interface for control, Chromium/FLX for high-resolution shared display, and VTK for volume rendering. Chromium is a system for interactive rendering on clusters of graphics workstations (http://chromium.sourceforge.net/). The server-side AG integration component provides necessary startup information in AG Shared Application data space and responds to load requests by retrieving data from the venue and passing it to the Visualization Server. The client-side AG integration component/visualization GUI provides: AG integration, retrieving startup data and allowing for 'one-click' startup from the venue client; a 'filter' for mouse/keyboard events from VIC client, to reduce event processing or provide explicit floor control; and the GUI interface for additional configuration options. Finally, the customized VIC client (a modified OpenMASH VIC tool) bonds multiple video streams to support high-resolution visualization while capturing mouse and keyboard events to allow client interaction. Figure 2 emphasizes the key architectural feature of multiple parallel video stream generation by the server-side components (Application Node and Chromium Servers), the sum of which represents the entire visualization, multicasting of the multiple streams, and reassembly as a single combined visualization in the customized vic clients. The out-of-band control (which flows in the opposite direction) is not shown.

The visualization server used to date consists of a Linux system running on a dual P4-Xeon (Intel) 1.8 GHz machine with 1 GB of RAM and an nVidia GeForce3-class video card. It utilizes the Visualization Toolkit's (VTK) [5] raycaster for volume rendering.

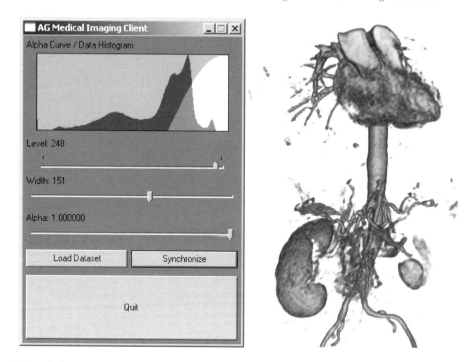

**Figure 3.** Screen capture of a GUI control window is shown on the left while screen capture from a shared visualization display is shown on the right. The data used on the right is a coronal section MR Angiogram enhanced with Gadolinium. In plane resolution is 1.3 mm pixels; slice resolution is 1.2 mm; and volumetric resolution is $256 \times 256 \times 56$.

The resulting graphics stream is broken up into several separate tiles that are rendered in parallel then encoded and broadcasted as standard H.261 [6]. A standard demonstration uses six H.261 streams creating a $3 \times 2$ tiling of streams, but it is possible to generate $n \times m$ streams.

The user interface is built upon the shared application API and communication methods that are defined as part the AG Toolkit v2.2. Standard VTK interactive commands and mouse events are transferred from the custom video client to the visualization server. These simple, frequent, low latency events are transmitted via XML-RPC (extensible markup language remote procedure calls) directly to the visualization server as part of the design to enable maximum interactivity between users. The visualization server then updates the resulting visualization image, which is broadcasted to the users. State changes made to the application via the user interface are coordinated with the AG venue server, which updates the user interface of all participants. The specialized video client, located as a shared application in the AG Virtual Venue, matches up the streams into one high-resolution $1056 \times 576$ image (constructed from a $3 \times 2$ tiling of $352 \times 288$ H.261 streams).

## 3. Results

The distributed shared application user interface consists of a segmentation window and level control sliders as well as a maximum opacity slider. See Figure 3. The features of the persistent server-client tele-collaborative application are: interactive control of the visualization by all participants in the session, multimodal communication, and the benefits of parallel rendering for larger datasets; and shared visualization with analysis tools including: image window mouse control of HPR and zoom, an ROI widget to limit rendering and allow roaming through subsections of data, and an arbitrary clipping plane; GUI control of segmentation window, level, and maximum opacity; complete synchronization of the GUI and the data window; and loading datasets.

## 4. Conclusion/Discussion

We've leveraged a content-rich, highly interactive shared visualization method and standard medical visualization tools, in combination, to enable collaborative manipulation of radiological data and multimodal communication simultaneously on commodity-off-the-shelf clients. The AG framework effectively integrates audio and video feedback between participating clients with the system. No highly specialized graphics hardware is required at any of the clients.

Our impression is that the Access Grid is increasingly affordable while collaborative visualization is increasingly important to biomedical research, education, and clinical care. Thus, because shared AG Applications make distributed collaborative biomedical visualization more feasible (among groups in the same institution and across geographically diverse institutions), academic medical centers may find AG technologies essential.

Future work on this application will include: expanding file input features, including support for standard and time-dependent DICOM studies, pre-segmented data, and other data types; deploying alternate renderers including parallel rendering, making this type of application update faster with higher resolution data; and deploying stereo rendering for nodes that support it.

## Acknowledgement

This work was supported in part by U.S. Department of Energy under Contract W-31-109-Eng-38 and by the NIH/National Library of Medicine, under Contract N01-LM-3-3508.

## References

[1]  ABC Testbed Project page (maintained by authors): http://cci.uchicago.edu/projects/abc.
[2]  The Access Grid Project page (maintained by authors): http://www.accessgrid.org.
[3]  Olson R., Papka ME. Remote Visualization Using Vic/Vtk, IEEE Visualization 2000 Hot Topics.
[4]  Dech F, Silverstein JC. Rigorous Exploration of Medical Data in Collaborative VR Applications. IEEE Computer Society Proc of 6th Ann Conf on Info Vis (2002).
[5]  Schroeder W, et al. The Visualization Toolkit: Object-Oriented Approach to 3D Graphics. Prentice Hall, 1995.
[6]  Karonis N, et.al. High Resolution remote rendering of large datasets in a collaborative environment. Future Generation Computer Systems (2003).

*Medicine Meets Virtual Reality 13*
*James D. Westwood et al. (Eds.)*
*IOS Press, 2005*

# Development of a Method for Surface and Subsurface Modeling Using Force and Position Sensors

Kevin SMALLEY and T. KESAVADAS [1]

*Virtual Reality Laboratory, Department of Mechanical and Aerospace Engineering,
State University of New York at Buffalo, Buffalo, New York 14260, U.S.A.
e-mail: ksmalley@buffalo.edu; kesh@buffalo.edu*

**Abstract.** Subsurface modeling of deformable objects, such as soft tissues and organs, involves the use of non-destructive methods of determining the properties of an object encased by a material. Some of the properties that can be determined from subsurface modeling include: shape, hardness, texture and possibly material. The ability to determine these properties is based on the accuracy of the method used and the properties of the surface encasing the object. As computers become more powerful and are able to produce even more realistic graphics, it will be possible to store and recreate precise duplicates of the original for later analysis. This paper will present a method of approximately modeling both the surface and an object below the surface of the skin by a method of palpation and then present this data in an interactive 3-D model.

## 1. Introduction

Being able to detect and localize hard or soft abnormal objects within tissue is a very essential procedure in medicine today, and is a reason why palpation is performed on patients (Peine et al. 1998). Palpation is a medical procedure where the fingers apply a gentle pressure to determine growths underneath the skin, changes in size of organs, and/or abnormal response. As of yet, the technology is nonexistent to combine the palpation process with the field of medical imaging.

By developing a method in which doctors can use a glove equipped with a force and position sensor connected to a regular desktop or laptop PC to generate a surface/subsurface model, a doctor can quickly analyze the situation and determine if further imaging tests are required. This will result in preventing unnecessary test from being performed and costly medical bills. In addition, since the sensors are positioned such that they sample the force applied during palpation with out adversely interfering with the procedure, the doctor can accurately determine how much pressure to apply.

This paper will present a method for approximately modeling both the surface and an object below the surface of the skin (subsurface) by a method of palpation, and then present this data in an interactive 3-D model.

---

[1] Author for communication.

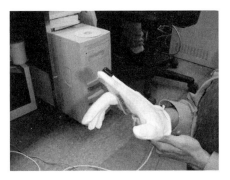

**Figure 1.** ModelGlove.

## 2. Previous Works

Review of past work indicates that some research has been done in the use of haptic devices in the area of subsurface modeling for medical applications and the reaction of the skin to palpation. One such research involves using haptic devices to train medical students. The training was done by modeling a virtual reality human torso and asking the students to find any tumors, which were either hard or soft (Dinsmore et al. 1997). Another method that has been researched calculates the response time of the skin, and underlying tissue, to palpation (Mayrose et al. 1998). This method presented by Mayrose takes into account the different mechanical properties of the skin and incorporates them into the calculations. The data collected from the experiment is stored in a database and used in conjunction with data obtained from the CT scan of each subject, prior to the palpation procedure, and is used to calculate the stiffness value of the tissue in the abdomen region.

While there has not been any attempt to model objects underneath a surface, there have been many studies into accurate reconstruction of surfaces. However, these surface approximations are usually generated from data obtained from laser scanners or from ordered data points obtained from coordinate measuring machine, hence is beyond the scope of this work. The method presented here samples data of soft organs and tissues as the user palpates using an instrumented glove called ModelGlove and then approximates surface/subsurface models based solely on this data is created.

## 3. Collecting Data Using Modelglove©

The ModelGlove (Kamerkar, 2004) (based on a Patent Pending glove by Mayrose, Chugh, and Kesavadas) consists of a force sensor attached to the bottom of the index finger and a position sensor attached to the top part of the same index finger (Fig. 1). This allows the force sensor to sample the force being applied by the user while still being able to record its location. The ModelGlove can easily sample data at 5 Hz, while remaining small and lightweight. In addition, the force sensors are very thin and flexible, and do not interfere with the palpation process performed by the user or the readings being sampled by the sensor. The user can also easily orient their hand in any direction to obtain readings without changing the data being recorded.

The use of the force sensor and position sensor in combination with each other is very important to recording accurate points. By using just the position sensor and tracing a surface, every point that is sample will be accepted and used in the model calculation.

However, by using the force sensor, we are essentially applying a filter to the data by only accepting coordinates that pass a force validation test. This validation test attempts to determine mathematically when a boundary interface has been reached, and only then is the position sampled and recorded for later calculation. By changing the values of the threshold force values, surface materials with varying stiffness values can be scanned (as opposed to only rigid objects many other techniques).

## 4. Methods for Creating the Model

Creation of both the surface and subsurface model involved similar steps. The only difference occurs in the way the data points are determined to be 'valid'. The five basic steps required to generate both models are: data collection and validation, sort data, arrange data into groups, calculate control points, and generate NURB surface.

### 4.1. Data Collection and Validation

The data was collected by running the gloved finger over the surface (and subsurface) several times. Depending on whether the surface or subsurface option is current, a specific data validation test is employed. For the surface option, if the force (surface threshold force value) sampled is greater than zero (meaning the user is in contact with a surface) it implies that the user is in contact with a surface, and the position will be sampled and stored.

Since the stiffness of a material is not always available, or is unknown such as the case with human skin and tissue, the use of Hooke's law would be impractical to use as a force validation test. Instead, when the subsurface option is selected, a force comparison test is used, and the current force is compared to the previous force collected to obtain a net change: $Force_{current} - Force_{previous}$.

For a net change above a preset value (the subsurface threshold force value), the program checks to see if the previous reading was a valid data point. If the previous point was not valid (a subsurface object was not encountered) the current point is ignored and sampling resumes. Should the previous point be a valid point, the current point will still be considered valid, and the current position will then be stored. Once the net change exceeds the set value, what was previously valid is now invalid (meaning the force change is too drastic).

There is a subsurface threshold force value to determine if a surface boundary is contacted, and a separate subsurface threshold force value to determine when the boundary is not in contact anymore.

In addition, there is a comparison check between the previous sampled position and the current position. If all three coordinates are approximately equivalent (a net change of 1/16" in any direction), it is assumed that the user has not moved and the point will be disregarded.

## 4.2. Sorting the Data

After all the data is collected, both the surface and subsurface data points must be sorted by increasing $x$ coordinate. This is performed using a Boolean sort function. Within the comparing function, value A is compared with value B, and the entire <vector> is sorted automatically by the comparison criteria. The STL sort method has been optimized to be very efficient, with a worse case run time of n(log n) when compared to other methods such as *qsort* which has a worst case time of n2.

## 4.3. Arranging the Data

Once the raw data has been sorted, it can now be grouped by it's $x$ coordinates into a 3-D <vector>, where the number of groups and the low and high values are preset by the program. The range for each group is calculated by subtracting the low value from the high value and dividing it by the number of groups - this value is now the range for each group. For the point to be included in that group, its $x$-coordinate must be greater than or equal to the low value and less than the high value for the range of each group, where $n$ is the current groups and $N$ is the total number of groups (Eq. 1).

$$\frac{(x_{high} - x_{low})}{N} \cdot (n - 1) \leq x_{coordinate} < \frac{(x_{high} - x_{low})}{N} \cdot n \tag{1}$$

## 4.4. Calculating the Control Points

With all the stored data now arranged in smaller groups of points, it is now possible to create control points for each group, upon which the surface and subsurface model will be based on. Control points are used to reduce the amount of computation required should a large collection of data points be encountered, and thus simplify the approximation of the models.

To create the general shape of the entire model, it can be thought of as creating a shape curve for each group by using a blending function. Then, by combining all of these shape curves, an approximate model can be created.

In order to generate this shape curve, we must first generate a collection of control points that are based upon the data points collected. Using the Bezier function (Equation 2), it is possible to generate a rectangular mesh of control points, where each curve (or group) has the same number of control points. In addition, the spacing of the control points along each of the approximated curves is obtained by changing the value of $u$ (where $0 \leq u \leq 1$). Since the number of control points for each group is pre-defined, the control points can be equally spaced across the curve.

$$P(u) = \sum_{i=0}^{n} \binom{n}{i} u^i (1 - u)^{n-i} P_i \tag{2}$$

Where: $\binom{n}{i} = \frac{n!}{i!(n-i)!}$
Where $P_i$ = position vector $n$ = number of data points $-1$.

In addition, it must be mentioned that by increasing the number of control point, the degree of the curve will also increase (where the degree is equal to number of control points plus 1), and oscillation can occur (Lee 1999).

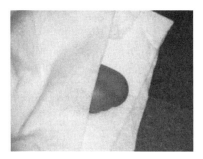

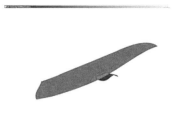

**Figure 2.** Spleen model under one layer of cotton batting.

**Figure 3.** Shaded image of spleen under one layer.

## 4.5. Generating the Surface

The surface is approximated using the NURB (Non-Uniform Rational B-spline) surface evaluator. A NURB surface is commonly used in graphics to create and describe smooth curves and surfaces that are based on polynomials. This evaluator is accessed through an OpenGL library and automatically generates a surface based on an array of control points, and the NURBS evaluator requires that each row have the same number of control points. While the NURB surface doesn't pass through the majority of the control points, the goal of this paper is to test the validity of approximating a surface and subsurface object.

## 5. Experiments and Results

In this section, a description of the experiments that were performed as well as the results obtained will be explained.

To test the modeling approach, a relatively hard object was placed within a softer object (Figure 2), and then both surface and subsurface was modeled through palpation (Figures 3). This test shows the ability of this method to model both surface and subsurface without knowing the stiffness value of either material. This experiment was performed by placing an object under one layer of cotton batting. Again, the models were generated by breaking the data into 16 groups and calculating 22 control points for each group. In another experiment lower part of the thigh was modeled (Fig. 4 and 5).

From the images shown, it is possible to model an object underneath a softer object without having prior knowledge to the stiffness value of the surface. Although the distance between the surface and subsurface cannot be exactly determined from the generated model, the general location and size of the object can be determined.

## 6. Conclusion and Future Work

Palpation is a very important technique for doctors to use to detect not only tumors or other growths, but muscles and organs within the body. While this paper presented a general method for visualizing a surface objects beneath a surface during palpation, it has the potential for being a very valuable medical tool.

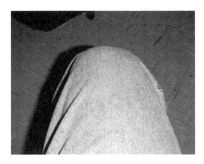

**Figure 4.** Lower part of the thigh.                    **Figure 5.** Modeled surface.

From the results presented, it has been shown that it is possible to generate an approximate NURB model of a surface and subsurface based only on force and position data, and the model can be saved for later viewing and comparison.

Finally, combining the method presented in this paper with the field of haptics can result in a method to not only help doctors analyze a situation, but help train future doctors. By adding the ability to feel what was modeled at a previous time, a doctor can make a better diagnosis of the problem or pass this information onto a specialist for later analysis.

### References

[1] Dinsmore M., et al, 1997. Virtual Reality Training Simulation for Palpation of Subsurface Turmors. *Rutgers University*.
[2] Kamerkar, Ameya, 2004. *An Interactive Touch based NURBS Modeler using a Force/Position Input Glove.* MS Thesis; University at Buffalo.
[3] Lee, Kunwoo. 1999. *Principles of CAD/CAM/CAE Systems*. Reading, MA.: Addison Wesley.
[4] Mayrose J., Chugh K., Kesavadas T., and Ellis D.G., 1998. A Non-Invasive System for Measuring Soft Tissue Response to Abdominal Palpation. *University at Buffalo*.
[5] Peine, William J., Robert D. Howe, 1998. Do Humans Sense Finger Deformation or Distributed Pressure to detect Lumps in Soft Tussue? *Proc. of the ASME Dynamic Systems and Control Division, ASME International Mechanical Engineering Congress and Exposition* 64:273-278.

*Medicine Meets Virtual Reality 13*
*James D. Westwood et al. (Eds.)*
*IOS Press, 2005*

# The Physiology and Pharmacology of Growing Old, as Shown in Body Simulation

N. Ty SMITH, M.D. [a] and Kenton R. STARKO [b]

[a] *Professor Emeritus, University of California, San Diego*
*e-mail: tsmith@ucsd.edu*
[b] *Director, Advanced Simulation Corporation*
*e-mail: advsim@whidbey.com*

**Abstract.** Geriatric medicine is becoming increasingly important, due to the aging of our population. Healthcare givers need methods that can teach efficiently and painlessly the complexities involved with aging. One important tool in this area comprises modeling and simulation. Accordingly, we present a detailed model and simulation of the aging process. To implement the aging process, we changed over 50 existing parameters that are part of a physiologic, pharmacologic multiple transport model of the human body. To evaluate the new patients, we imposed three stresses: anesthesia induction, hemorrhage and apnea. Five patients were used: a young healthy patient and four healthy, but elderly, patients, aged 65, 75, 85 and 95 years. We observed an age-related response to the stresses. The elderly patients fared worse with anesthetic induction and with hemorrhage, but better with apnea. Some independent data support our results.

## 1. Introduction

The increasing numbers of the elderly stress the expanding importance of geriatric medicine. In many geriatric medical areas, a good model and simulation can help deal with what can only become an increasing challenge. Because of the extensive and complex physiologic and pharmacologic considerations involved in the aging process, any model must contain considerable detail, as well as the potential for relatively easy expansion and modification. The considerations involved in the care of the elderly should be able to be implemented and studied in wide-ranging detail. In addition, the user should be able to practice on "patients," in a realistic way that allows not only a thorough understanding of the clinical picture of aging, but also a broad-based insight into the science behind the clinical picture.

## 2. Methods

BODY Simulation is a physiologic, pharmacologic multiple transport model of the human body. To enhance the understanding of the normal aging process we have added four

**Table 1.** Parameters that were changed to implement elderly patients.

| Cardiovascular | Respiratory | Miscellaneous |
|---|---|---|
| Blood pressure | Total lung capacity | Total body mass |
| Heart rate | Functional residual capacity | Individual tissue and organ masses |
| Stroke volume | Pulmonary compliance | Total blood volume |
| Cardiac output | Airway resistance | Hemoglobin concentration |
| Systemic vascular resistance | Tidal volume | Hepatic function (must be set by user) |
| Regional blood flows and resistances | Respiratory rate | Renal function (must be set by user) |
| Unstressed blood volumes of tissues and organs | Dead space | |
| Baroceptor reflexes (heart rate, mean arterial pressure, venous compliance and myocardial contractility) | $VO_2$ | |
| | AV $VO_2$ difference | |
| | $PaO_2$ | |

$VO_2$ = minute $O_2$ consumption; AV $O_2$ = arterial-venous $O_2$ difference; $PaO_2$ = arterial $O_2$ partial pressure.

new patients, age 65, 75, 85 and 95 years, to BODY's patient repertoire. In constructing these patients, we have taken into account the physiologic parameters listed in Table 1, as a function of age. The appropriate values for these parameters have been incorporated into the patient files for each age and are available to the user for examination and comparison with the corresponding parameters in a young adult. Over 50 parameters have been changed, directly or indirectly. No disease has been incorporated into the patients.

We examined 113 papers to glean information on parameters that can be changed in the BODY model. From the data, we calculated linear slopes for the parameters as a function of age, extrapolating to the higher ages, if necessary. We tried to use human data as much as possible, but rarely the gaps had to be filled with data from other animals.

We used three stresses to demonstrate the effects of "normal" aging. The stresses were: 1) the bolus injection of thiopental, to demonstrate kinetics and resulting overdosage in the elderly; 2) brisk hemorrhage, to demonstrate the marked response in the elderly to this stress, and 3) apnea. We implemented the three different stresses, on the five patients described above. Thus, there were 15 different runs, three each on five patients. We produced the same stress in each patient, for example, the same dose of thiopental injected over the same time period. With each stress, we plotted a different set of variables. Because of space limitations, we concentrate on hemorrhage. Hemorrhage was accomplished with a bleeding rate of 100 ml/minute for 10 minutes. No fluid was administered, nor was the patient connected to an oxygen source.

## 3. Results

Space constraints require our listing the results for only one stress. The results for hemorrhage are summarized in Table 2. A hemorrhage that will minimally affect a resting, recumbent young person can be fatal in the older patients. As age increases, the effects of thiopental become more pronounced. Thiopental doses that are normal for a young

**Table 2.** Lowest or highest values at end of hemorrhage.

| Var | SvO$_2$ | MAP | HR | CO | TBV | THb | PP O$_2$ BG | Myo O$_2$ | BG O$_2$ | Death |
|-----|---------|-----|----|----|-----|-----|-------------|-----------|----------|-------|
| YHM | 66 | 81 | 81 | 4.50 | 4.15 | 581 | 33 | 0 | 0 | No |
| 65 | 53 | 58 | 83 | 2.67 | 3.05 | 407 | 29 | 652 | 0 | No |
| 75 | 46 | 49 | 85 | 2.08 | 2.78 | 354 | 26 | 4,671 | 4,004 | No |
| 85 | 37 | 39 | 86 | 1.51 | 2.50 | 304 | 23 | 14,600 | 17,400 | Yes |
| 95 | 29 | 30 | 86 | 1.07 | 2.23 | 270 | 20 | 28,300 | 38,100 | Yes |

Var = variable; SpO$_2$ = arterial O$_2$ saturation; SvO$_2$ = venous O$_2$ saturation; MAP = mean arterial pressure; HR = heart rate; CO = cardiac output; TBV = total blood volume; THb = total hemoglobin; Myo O$_2$ = myocardial O$_2$ deficit; BG O$_2$ = Brain gray O$_2$ deficit.

person produce profound and prolonged anesthetic depth and cardiovascular depression in the elderly. The elderly patient, however, tolerates apnea better than the young patient.

## 4. Discussion

Aging affects nearly every tissue, organ, system and function of the body. With few exceptions, the manifestation is a deterioration of structure, function, or both. When elderly patients are compared with a young patient and with each other, one can detect the potential for increasing fragility in the initial, resting values. The best way, however, to examine the effects of aging is to subject patients of different ages to the identical stressful situation. One of the beauties of modeling/simulation is the ability to give precisely the same stress to each patient.

Remember that these are "healthy" elderly people, that is, they only manifest the effects of "normal" aging. The elderly are also more prone to many diseases that could widen the gap between young and old, including the response to stress.

The changes in these parameters affect not only the normal resting state of the patient, but should also impact the response to a drug or to a stress, such as hemorrhage. Simms [10] examined the response to hemorrhage in young through increasingly elderly rats. He observed that the mortality rate for elderly rats was 16 times greater than that for young rats, results that corroborate ours. Many factors conspire to make the elderly patient more susceptible to hemorrhage, including lower blood volume and decreased reactivity of baroceptors.

The future of the study of aging with modeling and simulation is exciting, given the increasing information on aging and the basic construction of BODY Simulation.

## References

[1]  Babb, T.G. and J.R. Rodarte, Mechanism of reduced maximal expiratory flow with aging. J Appl Physiol, 2000. **89**: p. 505-511.
[2]  Beere, P.A., et al., Aerobic Exercise Training Can Reverse Age-Related Peripheral Circulatory Changes in Healthy Older Men. Circulation, 1999. **100**: p. 1085-1094.
[3]  Bosy-Westphal, A., et al., The age-related decline in resting energy expenditure in humans is due to the loss of fat-free mass and to alterations in its metabolically active components. J Nutr, 2003. **133**: p. 2356-62.
[4]  Cleroux, J., et al., Decreased cardiopulmonary reflexes with aging in normotensive humans. Am. J. Physiol., 1989. **257**: p. H961-H968.

[5] Davy, K.P. and D.R. Seals, Total blood volume in healthy young and older men. J. Appl. Physiol., 1994. **76**(5): p. 2059-2062.
[6] DeLorey, D. and T. Babb, Progressive mechanical ventilatory constraints with aging. AM J RESPIR CRIT CARE MED, 1999. **160**: p. 169–177.
[7] Folkow, B. and A. Svanborg, Physiology of Cardiovascular Aging. Physiological Reviews, 1993. **73**(4).
[8] Olive, J.L., A.E. DeVan, and K.K. McCully, The effects of aging and activity on muscle blood flow. Dynamic Medicine 2002, 2002. **1**(2).
[9] Ritschel, W., Gerontokinetics. The pharmacokinetics of drugs in the elderly. 1988, Caldwell, NJ: Telfor Press, Inc. 114.
[10] Simms, H.S., The use of a measurable cause of death (hemorrhage) for the evaluation of aging. J Gen Physiol, 1942. **26**: p. 169-178.
[11] Slotwiner, D.J., et al., Relation of Age to Left Ventricular Function and Systemic Hemodynamics in Uncomplicated Mild Hypertension. Hypertension, 2001. **37**: p. 1404-1409.

*Medicine Meets Virtual Reality 13*
*James D. Westwood et al. (Eds.)*
*IOS Press, 2005*

# Physiologic and Chemical Simulation of Cyanide and Sarin Toxicity and Therapy

N. Ty SMITH, M.D.[a] and Kenton R. STARKO[b]

[a] *Professor Emeritus, University of California, San Diego*
*e-mail: tsmith@ucsd.edu*
[b] *Director, Advanced Simulation Corporation*
*e-mail: Kenton@advsim.com*

**Abstract.** The possibility of mass terrorism has become increasingly apparent. Accurate and relevant teaching tools are needed for healthcare givers and emergency personnel of all experience. We describe one of these tools, BODY Simulation, and its use in training caregivers to respond to chemical terrorism. We have implemented two chemical agents—cyanide and sarin, the latter a nerve agent—in a detailed whole-body model and simulation. In the simulation, each agent was administered to a healthy young adult, first without therapy, then with therapy, for a total of four runs. We recorded several variables, each appropriate to the agent used. The recorded variables included physiological variables in addition to the blood and brain concentrations of each agent and its antidotes. In addition, for cyanide, the compounds that resulted as the byproducts of therapy (methemoglobin, for example) were plotted. The results were consistent with those described in the literature, including agent concentrations and pathophysiologic changes.

## 1. Introduction

Simulation is particularly well suited for teaching how to treat the victims of chemical warfare. Neither animal models nor human models are acceptable for this purpose. We consider two possible chemical warfare agents: cyanide and sarin.

Cyanide (CN) works by blocking a site on cytochrome oxidase, so that the body cannot utilize $O_2$. The BODY model is well suited to handle this type of toxicity. It incorporates 14 compartments, of which eight are tissues or organs [1,2]. Each tissue compartment has its own $VO_2$ ($O_2$ consumption, or uptake), which is, of course, blocked by CN. Because CN's mechanism is the intracellular blocking of $O_2$ utilization, the arterial $O_2$ saturation will remain normal, until the patient is essentially terminal from hypoxia.

The human body uses four mechanisms to neutralize CN. The antidotes for CN use two of these mechanisms. The first mechanism used in therapy is the conversion of oxyhemoglobin ($HbO_2$) to methemoglobin (MetHb). MetHb has a strong affinity for CN, essentially "pulling" it out of the cells into the blood. Nitrites rapidly facilitate the formation of MetHb. Nitrite therapy is quick acting, but it can decrease blood pressure. More importantly, MetHb is toxic, since the patient has available proportionately less HbO2 to release $O_2$ to the tissues (MetHb binds $O_2$, but does not release it). The second protective mechanism involves the slower acting therapy with thiosulfate, which, by copiously supplying critical elemental sulfur, facilitates the conversion of cyanide into thiocyanate by the enzyme rhodanese. Rhodanese also converts cyanmethemoglobin (CNMetHb) into MetHb plus thiocyanate. The resulting thiocyanate is toxic, although considerably less so than cyanide.

Nerve agents, including sarin, work by forming a "permanent" bond with acetyl-cholinesterase. Acetylcholine accumulates, producing a cholinergic crisis, with combined muscarinic and nicotinic effects. The result is severe cardiovascular and respiratory dysfunction, with death occurring in a few minutes at high concentrations of the agent.

We describe a simulation system that can, for example, take the user through the primary pathophysiology of CN poisoning, as well as its treatment. The BODY models will simulate the blocking of $O_2$ consumption; the conversion by nitrite of $HbO_2$ to MetHb; the "transfer" of CN from tissue to blood, to bind with MetHb to form CNMetHb; the reduction in CN concentration in blood and tissue; the production of sulfur from thiosulfate; the production of thiocyanate from S- and CN, as well as from CNMetHb; and the blood and tissue concentrations of all these agents and chemicals, as well as their disposition. Blood and tissue concentrations of the toxic and antidote agents are displayed and plotted over time. One can also plot the Hb species that are involved: Hb, HbO2, MetHb and CNMetHb (the latter two are necessary, but toxic, byproducts of therapy), as well as the concentrations of nitrite, sulfate, sulfide, and thiocyanate, in the blood and tissues.

## 2. Methods

The BODY Simulation model is a whole-body physiologic, pharmacologic, multiple transport model. Originally developed as an anesthesia-related model, the principles and structure of the model result in versatility, as well as the ability to change and expand the model with relative ease. This has allowed us to implement the two terror chemical agents without the model's undergoing a major overhaul.

We did make certain modifications to the BODY Simulation model to be able to implement the terror agents. For cyanide, one change in the model was to create an agent (CN) that blocks the utilization of $O_2$. This block is dependent on the concentration of CN in the tissue. Of BODY Simulation's eight tissue or organ compartments, the most important are the heart and the brain-gray compartments. Over the short term, it is the concentration of CN in these two compartments, as modified by the slope and amplitude of the concentration-response curve, that produces the damaging effects. Two antidotes to CN were modeled: Na nitrite and Na thiosulfate. To enhance realism, we implemented two features. First, we broke the salts down into the negative ions, and then sulfate into elemental sulfur. For the second, we did make a significant change in BODY Simulation: the incorporation of five chemical equations. These equations were used to implement the sequences described in the last paragraph of the Introduction. For each of the equations, the user can adjust the rate constants, as well as the equilibrium constants, the latter in those equations that do not go completely to the right.

The following mass equations are used in BODY's modeling of the process of cyanide therapy. It should be emphasized that these equations are how the *process* is modeled.

1. $NO_2 + HbO_2 \leftrightarrow MetHb$
2. $S + SO3 \leftrightarrow SSO_3$

3. CN + MetHb → CNMetHb
4. S + CN ↔ SCN
5. CNMetHb + S → SCN + MetHb

Where S = sulfide ion; SO3 = sulfite ion; SSO3 = thiosulfate ion; and SCN = thiocyanate.

Since BODY Simulation does not specifically model carotid bodies, hypoxia-
induced changes in heart rate and ventilation were accommodated through changes in
the CN drug file (the drug-specific file in which the user can change any of the 46 agent
parameters).

For sarin, we modeled a neuromuscular blocking agent with profound cardiovascular
effects. For the antidote, we modeled an agent (pralidoxime chloride [2-PAM]) that an-
tagonizes sarin, using the concentration-additive concept of Loewe [3,4]. Atropine was
already available in the BODY Simulation.

Using these approaches for CN and sarin, we performed four simulation runs on the
same submodel of a healthy 75-kg adult male. The patient was resting and recumbent. We
used inspired concentrations from the literature. With each agent, we exposed the patient
to an inspired concentration, so that death would occur after ten minutes of continuous
steady-state exposure. We then did two more runs, using the same lethal concentration
but with therapy instituted at an appropriate time. For demonstration purposes, we have
chosen to continue exposure to the agent during therapy. No $O_2$ was administered, nor
was the patient ventilated.

All CN therapy was administered by an intravenous infusion via a syringe pump.
After brain and myocardial $O_2$ deficits became significant, (see below), we started an
infusion of Na nitrite, 30mg/ml in a 10 ml syringe at a rate of 400 mcg/min. After an
arbitrary three minutes, we started an intravenous infusion of Na thiosulfate, 250 mg/ml
in a 50 ml syringe, at a rate of 16.7 mg/kg/min. We shut off the Na nitrite as we began
the Na thiosulfate. This combination of therapy is said to be able to detoxify 30–40 times
the LCt50 (see below for explanation of LCt50) for cyanide).

The therapy that we used in these simulations is that used by the US military forces.
Some other countries use other agents and doses. All of our therapy was administered
intravenously, and this mode may vary by country or unit.

We began therapy for sarin with a bolus injection of 10 mg atropine (this was a severe
case of poisoning). We injected 15 mg/kg (2-PAM) about 30 seconds after the onset of
the apnea produced by the neuromuscular block.

## 3. Results

The results for untreated subjects are shown in Tables 1 and 2. The significant results for
CN include an increase in $SvO_2$ and pronounced myocardial and brain $O_2$ deficits. With
sarin, we observed marked decreases in arterial and venous $O_2$ saturation, mean arterial
pressure, heart rate, cardiac output, tidal volume and, again, pronounced myocardial and
brain $O_2$ deficits. Space limitations prevented our listing the results for treated subjects.

The muscarinic effects of sarin are treated by giving very large and frequent injec-
tions of atropine. The nicotinic effects can be treated with ventilation. One must still
try to reverse/break the bond between the agent and the acetylcholinesterase site. The
drug of choice in the US is 2-PAM. It is very important to administer 2-PAM as soon

**Table 1.** Results with untreated Cyanide Poisoning (Run 1).

| Var | Sp $O_2$ | $SvO_2$ | MAP | HR | RR | CNAo | CNBG | Myo $O_2$ | BG $O_2$ |
|---|---|---|---|---|---|---|---|---|---|
| Control | 97 | 71 | 86 | 72 | 12 | — | — | 0 | 0 |
| BG death | 97 | 82 | 82 | 73 | 7 | 0.00019 | 0.00016 | 58,700 | 106,000 |
| Myo death | 90 | 72 | 57 | 21 | 0 | 0.00018 | 0.00019 | 106,000 | 191,000 |

Var = variable; SpO2 = arterial O2 saturation (%); SvO2 = venous O2 saturation (%); MAP = mean arterial pressure (mm Hg); HR = heart rate; RR = respiratory rate; CNAo = aortic blood concentration of CN (vol%); CNBG = brain gray concentration of CN (vol%); Myo O 2 = myocardial O2 deficit; BG O2 = Brain gray O2 deficit.

**Table 2.** Results with untreated Sarin Poisoning (Run 3).

| Var | $SpO_2$ | $SvO_2$ | MAP | HR | CO | NMB | VT | Sarin Ao | Sarin BG | Myo $O_2$ | BG $O_2$ |
|---|---|---|---|---|---|---|---|---|---|---|---|
| Control | 97 | 71 | 86 | 72 | 5,440 | 0 | 586 | 0 | 0 | 0 | 0 |
| CV min | 97 | 62 | 48 | 29 | 3,400 | 0.002 | 470 | 0.0072 | 0.0067 | 3,015 | 8,888 |
| BG death | 22 | 18 | 63 | 44 | 4,300 | 0.95 | 0 | 0.0066 | 0.0072 | 4,9700 | 106,000 |
| Myo death | 14 | 18 | 21 | 7 | 610 | 0.97 | 0 | 0.0063 | 0.0067 | 106,000 | 203,000 |

Var = variable; SpO2 = arterial O2 saturation (%); SvO2 = venous O2 saturation (%); MAP = mean arterial pressure (mm Hg); HR = heart rate; CO = cardiac output; NMB = neuromuscular block level (arbitrary units); VT = tidal volume (ml); Sarin Ao = aortic blood concentration of sarin (vol%); Sarin BG = brain gray concentration of sarin (vol%); Myo O2 = myocardial O2 deficit (arbitrary units); BG O2 = Brain gray O2 deficit (arbitrary units); CV min = greatest cardiovascular depression.

as possible, because the process of "aging," which can take place in a matter of minutes or hours, depending on the nerve agent, will render the bond between agent and acetyl-cholinesterase permanent. The only recourse then is to wait out the regeneration of the enzyme, a matter of days to weeks of mechanical ventilation. Since aging for sarin does not occur until about five hours after exposure, it was not a consideration with the brief exposures and rapid therapy that we used with that agent.

## 4. Discussion

The following lists some of the qualitatively realistic observations that BODY Simulation allows one to make with cyanide poisoning and its therapy.

1. $SvO_2$ increases, while $SpO_2$ remains constant.
2. The body's stores of $NO_2$ and MetHb are rapidly depleted with overwhelming doses of CN .
3. MetHb does literally pull CN out of tissue.
4. The heart and brain accumulate $O_2$ deficits, even though the blood $O_2$ concentration is high; tissue $O_2$ concentrations actually increase.
5. Plots show the conversion of $HbO_2$ to MetHb and thence to CNMetHb, as well as the corresponding decrease in $HbO_2$.

Similarly, the realism with BODY Simulation during sarin toxicity and therapy is demonstrated by the following examples.

1. The signs of a cholinergic crisis are remarkably real and include bradycardia, hypotension and poor tissue perfusion, as well as a neuromuscular block.
2. The cardiovascular depression is so severe that myocardial and cerebral $O_2$ demand are not met.
3. Direct therapy of the muscarinic effects is difficult, requiring large doses of atropine.
4. In severe poisoning, what ultimately kills the victim is the neuromuscular block, with its resulting apnea.

This simulation demonstrates the pathophysiology and treatment of poisoning with the nerve agent sarin. The cholinergic crisis that occurs from the blocking of the acetylcholinesterase site is closely mimicked, as is the therapy with atropine and 2-PAM. It turns out that the signs of sarin poisoning are dramatic, yet easier to deal with, as compared with those of CN. This is because the signs and symptoms of nerve gas poisoning are much more predictable than those of CN toxicity. They also resemble some familiar therapeutic agents, such as neuromuscular blocking agents and their antagonists, such as neostigmine.

A quirk of CN renders it difficult to determine what its lethal concentration is for a given period of time in a simulation. Cyanide is one of the few chemical agents that do not follow Haber's law, which states that the Ct (the product of concentration and time) necessary to cause a given biological effect is constant over a range of concentrations and times. For this reason, the LCt50 (the vapor or aerosol exposure that is lethal to 50% of the exposed population) for a short exposure to a high concentration is different from that for a long exposure to a low concentration. Thus, one must find in the literature a range of values, each determined at a stated concentration and for a stated time. Fortunately, these data are available. The same problem – and solution – holds with sarin.

One of the many strong features of BODY Simulation is that each compartment has its own $VO_2$ ($O_2$ consumption). Each $VO_2$ decreases with anesthesia, and myocardial $VO_2$ changes directly with changes in heart rate or contractility. Compartmental $VO_2$ varies inversely with the compartmental concentration of CN, and is modified by the slope and amplitude of the concentration-effect curve in that compartment. This adds realism to the model.

Another important feature of BODY Simulation relates to two calculated variables that reflect the $O_2$ deficit in the heart and brain, respectively. We can continually calculate these variables that compare the $O_2$ supply with the $O_2$ demand, because BODY Simulation computes regional $VO_2$ values (as affected by CN), as well as the regional blood flow, the $O_2$ arterial partial pressure, the concentration of Hb, the arterial saturation, and the configuration of the Hb dissociation curve. When demand exceeds supply, the BODY model starts calculating the deficit. When the deficit exceeds 50,000, we say that there is reversible organ damage. When the deficit exceeds 106,000, we say that the damage is irreversible. The patient will either remain comatose, or die. This is a time-severity concept, as it is in real life – and death. These calculated variables are BODY Simulation's mechanism for determining death or severe physiological injury. This makes sense, because severe cerebral and myocardial hypoxia represents the final common pathway to death, as well as to injury in the organs involved.

These $O_2$-deficit plots make an excellent teaching tool. In BODY Simulation's Dynamic Plots, students can track the changes in the accumulated brain and myocardial deficits. Students can also determine when they have waited too long before starting therapy. The plots can also be part of a game of "chicken:" who can wait the longest before starting therapy. Students become much more aware of the time required to start therapy and for the therapy to take effect, as well as the factors involved in any kind of agent therapy.

## 5. Conclusion

We believe that true clinical skill comes best with an understanding of basic concepts and mechanisms. These concepts can be difficult with chemical injury, however, and realistic simulation eases the drudgery of learning. BODY Simulation is expected to help the process of learning and remembering.

## References

[1] Fukui, Y. and N.T. Smith, Interaction among Ventilation, the Circulation, and the Uptake and Distribution of Halothane. Use of a Hybrid Computer Model I. The Basic Model. Anesthesiology, 1981. **54**: p. 107-118.

[2] Fukui, Y. and N.T. Smith, Interaction Among Ventilation, the Circulation, and the Uptake and Distribution of Halothane. Use of a Hybrid Computer Model II. Spontaneous vs. Controlled Ventilation, and the Effects of $CO_2$. Anesthesiology, 1981. **54**: p. 119-124.

[3] Greco, W.R., G. Bravo, and J.C. Parsons, The search for synergy: A critical review from aresponse surface perspective. Pharmacol. Rev., 1995. **47**(2): p. 331-385.

[4] Loewe, S., The problem of synergism and antagonism of combined drugs. Arznemi. Forsch,1953. **3**: p. 285-290.

[5] Abraham R, Rudick V, Weinbroum A. Practical guidelines for acute care of victims ofbioterrorism: conventional injuries and concomitant nerve agent intoxication. Anesthesiology 2002;97(4):989-1004.

[6] Baskin S, Brewer T. Cyanide poisoning. Medical aspects of chemical and biological warfare,Chapter 10: US Army Medical Research Institute; 2000. p. 271-86, http://ccc.apgea.army.mil/reference_materials/textbook/HTML_Restricted/chapters/chapter_10.htm#cyanide.

[7] Sidell F. Nerve agents. Medical aspects of chemical and biological warfare, Chapter 5: US Army Medical Research Institute; 2000. p. 129-79, http://ccc.apgea.army.mil/reference_materials/textbook/HTML_Restricted/chapters/chapter_5.htm#nerveagents.

[8] van Heijst A. IOCS monograph on cyanide: IPCS; 1997. p. 1-49, htpp://www.inchem.org/documents.pims/chemical/pimg003.htm.

*Medicine Meets Virtual Reality 13*
*James D. Westwood et al. (Eds.)*
*IOS Press, 2005*

# Monitor Height Affects Surgeons' Stress Level and Performance on Minimally Invasive Surgery Tasks

Warren D. SMITH, Ph.D. [a],
Ramon BERGUER, M.D. [b] and Ninh T. NGUYEN, M.D. [c]

[a] *Biomedical Engineering, California State University, Sacramento,*
*6000 J Street, Sacramento, CA 95819-6019, USA*
[b] *Department of Surgery, University of California, Davis, School of Medicine*
*2221 Stockton Boulevard, Sacramento, CA 95817, USA*
[c] *Department of Surgery, University of California, Irvine, School of Medicine,*
*101 The City Drive South, Orange, CA 92868, USA*

**Abstract.** This study investigated the effect of monitor height on surgeons' workload and performance during simulated minimally invasive surgery (MIS).

Fourteen volunteer subjects (7 experienced, 7 inexperienced) performed a cutting task in a training box at a standard MIS station with the video monitor positioned in random order at, below ($-35$ degrees), and above ($+15$ degrees) the subject's eye level. Task time and error, difficulty and discomfort, head orientation, trapezius and neck muscle activity, and skin conductance were recorded.

The experienced subjects performed the task faster, with less error, and with less difficulty than did the inexperienced subjects.

For the experienced subjects, error decreased when the monitor was lowered. Difficulty and discomfort increased at the high monitor position. As the monitor was lowered, the head pitched forward, and paraspinal cervical muscle activity increased. Variability in sternocleidomastoid activity increased both at the low and high monitor positions.

The results show that monitor height affects both performance and workload. The monitor should be lowered to reduce error and task difficulty but not so low as to produce excessive neck flexion.

## 1. Introduction

Minimally invasive surgery (MIS) is associated with significant ergonomic problems for the surgeon, including increased pain and discomfort in the upper extremities and neck [1]. The development of complex MIS procedures such as laparoscopic gastric bypass and cardiac bypass is further challenging surgeons and members of the operating room team to work in visually and mechanically remote ways. Understanding the optimum layout of MIS equipment will help reduce unnecessary efforts by the surgeons and permit more rapid and safe operations.

The video monitor is one of the most important equipment items during MIS, since it provides the surgeon and the assistants with a view of the operating field. Lowering

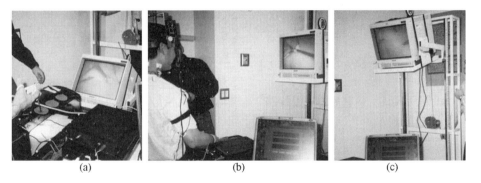

<table>
<tr><td>(a)</td><td>(b)</td><td>(c)</td></tr>
</table>

**Figure 1.** The experimental setup with the monitor at heights of (a) −35 degrees, (b) 0 degrees, and (c) +15 degrees. A subject is shown at the left in (b) standing at the trainer box. The 3DM orientation sensor is mounted on his head, and SCM skin surface electrodes are visible on his neck. Leads from EMG and skin conductance electrodes on the subject are plugged into the electronics boxes near the subject's right elbow. Outputs from the 3DM sensor and the electronics boxes feed into the laptop computer visible in the foreground that is running a custom-built LabVIEW virtual instrument.

the display below eye level may reduce eye strain and neck discomfort [2]. Yet, the operating room display often is mounted on a "tower" so that it can be seen above the other equipment and personnel. This study investigated the effect of monitor height on surgeons' workload and performance while they performed MIS tasks.

## 2. Methods

With IRB approval, 14 subjects performed a simulated MIS task in a training box at a standard MIS station. Seven of the subjects (6 male, 1 female, ages from 29 to 35 years) were experienced with MIS procedures (more than 50 laparoscopic cholecystectomies), and seven (5 male, 2 female, ages from 25 to 41) were inexperienced (fewer than 10 laparoscopic cholecystectomies). The task was to cut along a quarter-circle arc marked on a 2 cm × 2 cm square of 4-mm-thick foam rubber. Two trials were performed with the video monitor positioned in random order at each of three heights: level with the subject's eyes (0 degrees), −35 degrees below this height, and +15 degrees above this height. For each height, the monitor's horizontal position was adjusted to maintain a fixed distance from the subject's eyes, and it was tilted and to ensure that the screen remained perpendicular to the subject's line of sight.

For each trial, task time and cut error (area of deviation from the marked cut line) were recorded. For each monitor height, the subject was asked to rate the level of task difficulty and the level of discomfort on analog visual scales. Physiological variables were monitored from the subject by means of a custom-built LabVIEW-based (National Instruments, Austin, TX) virtual instrument (VI) on a laptop computer [3,4]. The subject's head orientation was monitored using a 3DM sensor (MicroStrain, Burlington, VT). Skin surface electromyogram (EMG) signals were recorded from the subject's right trapezius (Trap), sternocleidomastoid (SCM), and paraspinal cervical (Cerv) muscles. Skin conductance (SC), a measure of stress level, was monitored on the subject's right palm. Figure 1 shows the experimental station with the monitor at (a) −35 degrees, (b) 0 degrees, and (c) +15 degrees.

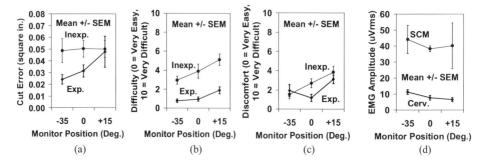

**Figure 2.** Effect for experienced (Exp.) and inexperienced (Inexp.) subjects of monitor position on (a) cut error, (b) self-assessed difficulty, and (c) self-assessed discomfort, and effect for experienced subjects on (d) EMG amplitude for SCM and Cerv neck muscle activity.

Comparisons of mean values for the experienced and inexperienced subject groups were performed using one-tail, grouped-data t-tests. Comparisons of mean values between monitor heights were performed using one-tail, paired-data t-tests. Comparisons of variance values were performed using one-tail F-tests. A level of significance of $P = 0.05$ was used.

## 3. Results

Figure 2 shows some of the experimental results (as plots of mean +/- standard error of the mean). Compared with the inexperienced subjects, the experienced subjects performed the task faster, with less error, and with less difficulty. The experienced subjects reported less discomfort than did the inexperienced subjects, but only for the monitor at 0 degrees, and they showed less variability in neck muscle (SCM and Cerv) activity, except at the high monitor position.

For the experienced subjects, error decreased when the monitor was lowered, but neither task time nor skin conductance changed with monitor height. Difficulty and discomfort increased at the high monitor position, and some subjects also reported increased discomfort at the low monitor position. As the monitor was lowered, the head pitched forward, and cervical muscle activity increased. Variability in SCM activity increased at both the low and high monitor positions.

## 4. Conclusions

Monitor height affects both performance and workload. The monitor should be lowered to reduce task error and difficulty and discomfort, but not be so low as to cause inordinate increases in neck muscle work and discomfort level.

## References

[1]  Berguer, R., Forkey, D., and Smith, W. Ergonomic problems associated with laparoscopic surgery, *Surgical Endoscopy*, Vol. 13, pp. 466-468, 1999.

[2] Menozzi, M., von Buol, A., Krueger, H., and Miege, C. Direction of gaze and comfort: discovering the relation for the ergonomic optimization of visual tasks. *Ophthalmic Physiol. Opt.*, Vol. 14, pp. 393-399, 1994.

[3] Smith, W., Chung, Y., and Berguer, R. A virtual instrument ergonomics workstation for measuring the mental workload of performing video-endoscopic surgery. *Studies in Health Technology and Informatics*, Vol. 70, pp. 309-315, 2000.

[4] Berguer, R., Chen, C., and Smith, W. A virtual instrument ergonomics workstation to measure surgeons' physical stress. *Studies in Health Technology and Informatics*, Vol. 62, pp. 49-54, 1999.

502

*Medicine Meets Virtual Reality 13*
*James D. Westwood et al. (Eds.)*
*IOS Press, 2005*

# A New Platform for Laparoscopic Training and Education

Vidar SØRHUS, PhD [a,b], Eivind M. ERIKSEN, MSc [a],
Nils GRØNNINGSÆTER, BA [a], Yvon HALBWACHS, MSc [a],
Per Ø. HVIDSTEN, MSc [a], Johannes KAASA, MSc [a], Kyrre STRØM, PhD [a],
Geir WESTGAARD, PhD [a] and Jan S. RØTNES, MD PhD [a,c]

[a] *SimSurgery AS*
*url: www.simsurgery.com*
[b] *Ullevål University Hospital, Oslo, Norway*
[c] *Interventional Centre, Rikshospitalet, Oslo, Norway*

**Abstract.** A new platform for laparoscopic training and education is presented. Fundamental requirements about a flexible haptic interface, specter of training areas, skill assessment, educational content, and level of realism are presented and discussed. The new system, including a new and flexible haptic interface and a broad specter of training modules combined with the use of multimedia content, is described.

## 1. Introduction

More than a decade ago, VR training was presented as the future in minimal invasive surgical training and education [1]. Later, VR training has been proven to be a useful tool for training basic laparoscopic skills [2]. Even though several VR training products are available, VR training is not widely used in laparoscopic training and education.

There are probably many reasons why this is the case. The focus on cost makes it important to demonstrate cost effectiveness when investing in a VR system. Cost of surgical education and cost reductions related to systematic use of simulators are difficult to estimate and need to be compared to surgical outcome [3]. To establish a systematic educational program, in order to make use of simulators in surgical education an integrated part of the program, may be a difficult and complex task. The educational programs are already filled up, and to add new elements or replace existing elements and to set up the necessary resources may require strategic decisions in the management of the educational programs. Another reason is that available systems do not provide sufficient realism, training content, or other specific features.

In this paper, we describe requirements that need to be fulfilled in order to provide a sufficient educational value to defend the cost of investment and establishment of VR-based training as part of a surgical educational program. To meet the needs and requirements from the users, we propose a new platform for laparoscopic training and education. Section 2 describes the set of requirements, and section 3 describes the solutions that are used to meet these requirements.

## 2. System Requirements

In this section, we describe a set of requirements that the new platform is based on.

### 2.1. Flexible Surgical Interface

The surgical interface (haptic system with or without force feedback) is an important component in the simulator-based laparoscopic trainer. The anatomical organs, interactions between instruments and anatomies, and changes in the tissue are purely simulated and virtual, whereas the surgeon's interaction with the laparoscopic instruments needs to be represented with a physical interface. Such surgical interface systems need to resemble the laparoscopic situation as realistic as possible. This include both instrument maneuver, force and tactile feedback, realistic response in the visual display (measured positions and orientations), and realistic setup of the instruments (patient and port setup).

One limitation with the current interface systems that are used in laparoscopic surgery simulation is the limited flexibility regarding port placement. Because the instrument orientation and position are measured in the pivot point (gimbal), the flexibility of the surgical interface is limited to the physical positioning of the pivot point.

### 2.2. All Basic Skill Areas

To become a real competitor to different kinds of (home made and commercial) box trainers, a VR trainer must contain the full range of basic skill areas. According to SAGES [4], these include: 1) Camera navigation, 2) Dexterity – instrument manipulation, 3) Dissection, 4) Suturing and knot tying, 5) Hemostasis, and 6) Organ exposure. If not all of these areas are covered by a training system, additional components are needed. This makes the conversion to a simulator-based educational program more complicated and costly.

Individually, the different skill areas may be more realistically practiced with other means than a simulator-based system. But once the complete (basic skill) set of training is provided in one system, the value as a component in a systematic educational program becomes significant. Training on hemostasis and organ exposure is in fact more feasible in a VR trainer than in a physical trainer.

### 2.3. Abstract and Procedure Realistic Training Tasks

The first and most validated VR training system, the MIST [5], contained abstract training only. Later, other VR trainers have been developed with more or less realistic environments. It is not obvious that procedure realistic environments increase the efficiency of laparoscopic training, especially for the most basic skill training. With abstract environment it is easier to focus on specific skills that are relevant in all kinds of laparoscopic surgery. Two examples are the basic concepts of camera navigation and the fulcrum effect. On the other hand, a procedure realistic environment may be more exciting, allow more emotional stress, and for more advanced skills, add educational elements. An example on the latter is the traction of the gallbladder during clipsing of the cystic duct in the cholecystectomy procedure.

## 2.4. Skill Assessment

The fundamental idea behind the introduction of VR-based training in the education of laparoscopic surgeons is to replace the 100 years old Halstedian principle "see one, do one, teach one" [6] with a systematic approach inspired by the use of flight simulators in the education of pilots. The education and evaluation of the trainee are to some extent transferred from the senior surgeon to the simulator system. Therefore, it is very important that education by VR trainer must be evaluated using validated metrics and measures that reflect the user's competence level [7].

## 2.5. Port Placement and Anatomy Exploration

Because the visual and haptic realism are limited due to available technologies, the main emphasis has been on the basic skills. As eligible technologies are being developed, it is likely that port placement, anatomy exploration, and anatomical variations will be more and more important in the future training systems.

## 2.6. Learning Platform

One of the opportunities with digital simulators is that it is easily combined with all kinds of additional educational material, like e-learning packages, case studies, multimedia material, procedure descriptions, device documentation, etc. As a consequence of the introduction of systematic education of laparoscopic surgery outside the OR with training based on VR trainers, it is reasonable that the users will require educational systems that provide complete educational material on electronic form.

## 3. Results and Discussion

Based on the system requirements described in the previous section, we have developed a new platform for laparoscopic training and education. The new platform includes both a new surgical interface system and a new software system for VR training. Below, we will describe the different components of the new platform and how the different requirements are met.

This system includes a new and flexible surgical interface SimPack™(patent pending) with an emulated patient element with free port placement and generic instrument devices with electromagnetic tracking sensors. The surgical interface system has no force feedback. Today, a flexible haptic interface with force feedback does not seem to be possible within reasonable cost. Therefore, we concluded that it is more to gain on flexibility than on force feedback. Because the instrument position and orientation is measured by tracking sensors on the instrument devices instead of locating the measuring devices in a gimbal, it is possible to resemble a body surface with any number of potential port placements (Figure 1).

The new platform includes modular software for easy update of new training modules. The system has individual applications for administration, training in roaming mode, and training in session mode. In the session mode, it is possible to require that the user exceed a certain performance level, before he/she can continue to the next set of training exercises.

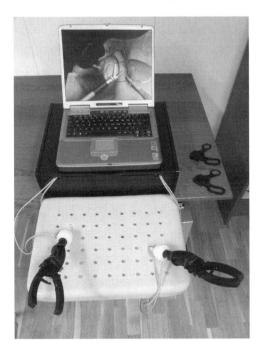

**Figure 1.** SimPack™, a new and flexible surgical interface.

The current training modules include camera navigation, instrument manipulation, suturing and knot tying, dissection, and hemostasis, utilizing a simulator engine based on SimSurgery's Sim3DM® technology [8] (Figure 2).

We suggest that the most basic skills can be learned in an abstract environment, whereas more advanced skills can, and in some cases should, be learned in procedure realistic environments. Because our focus has been on optimal learning, we have on purpose omitted use of "semi-realistic" environments (e.g. use anatomical textures on abstract shapes) in any exercise. Therefore, the current training modules contain exercises in either a purely abstract environments or in procedure realistic environments (Figure 3).

Skill assessment is accomplished by recording a broad range of errors and measures [7]. This is of course one of the strengths of digital trainers compared to physical trainers. For example, in a digital trainer it is possible to distinguish between a square and a granny knot, which is difficult in a physical trainer.

Some of the measures are already validated in similar exercises in existing trainers. New measures (in new exercises) need additional studies to test if they are valid metrics in skill assessment.

Since training on port placement and anatomy exploration are included as training modules in the system, the digital platform will demonstrate its scalability compared to physical platforms. Training modules on port placement and procedure specific anatomy exploration require a flexible haptic interface, as described above (Figure 4). A more comprehensive multimedia material for describing the different anatomies and procedures will also be needed. Therefore, the new platform contain extensive tutorials for

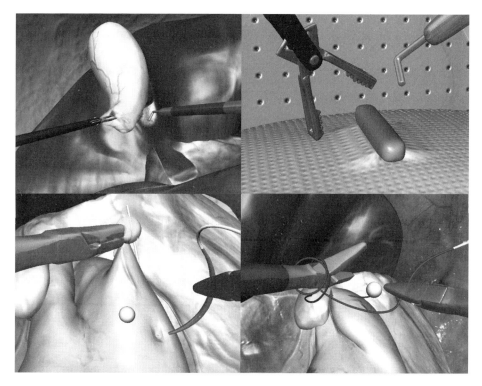

**Figure 2.** Exercise screenshots. Upper left: Dissect gallbladder. Upper right: Retract and dissect. Lower left: Lift and stitch. Lower right: Guided surgeons knot.

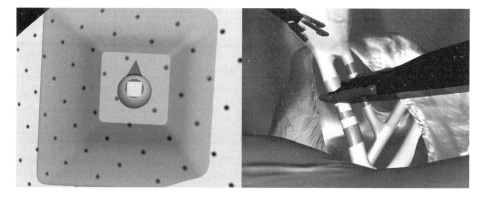

**Figure 3.** Exercises in abstract and realistic environments. Camera exercises in abstract environment (left) and apply clips exercise in realistic environment (right).

each exercise including descriptions of the purpose of the exercise, how to perform it, the metrics that are used, and the surgical context where it applies. In addition, preinstalled and locally added multimedia content about procedures, techniques, devices, etc. makes this a comprehensive learning platform for laparoscopic surgery.

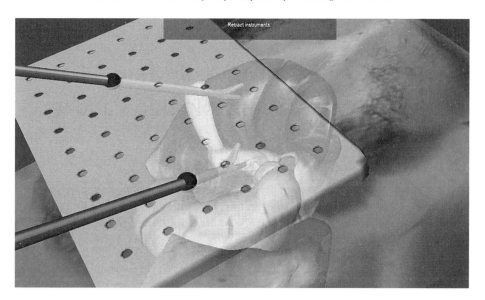

**Figure 4.** Example on how a flexible surgical interface can be used to enhance the realism in laparoscopic trainer. Example is from the initial part of the "Dissect Gallbladder" exercise.

## 4. Conclusion

We have presented a new platform for laparoscopic training and education, including new solutions on both hardware and software. A flexible surgical interface yields new possibilities in learning laparoscopic port placement and anatomy exploration. Together with a modular software system including simulator-based skill training and multimedia content, the result is a comprehensive learning platform for laparoscopic surgical education.

## References

[1] Satava RM. Virtual reality surgical simulator: The first steps. *Surg Endosc* 1993; 7:203–5.
[2] Seymour NE, Gallagher AG, Roman SA, O'Brien MK, Bansal VK, Andersen DK, and Satava RM. Virtual reality training improves operating room performance: Results of a randomized, double-blinded study. *Ann Surg* 2002; Vol 236, 4:458–64.
[3] Babineau TJ, Becker J, Gibbons G, Sentovich S, Hess D, Robertson S, and Stone M. The "Cost" of Operative Training for Surgical Residents. *Arch Surg* 2004; 139:366-70
[4] SAGES curriculum outline. http://www.sages.org/sg_pub28.html.
[5] www.mentice.com.
[6] Haluck RS and Krummel TM. Computers and virtual reality for surgical education in the 21st century. *Arch Surg* 2000; 135:786-92.
[7] Satava RM, Cuschieri A, and Hamdorf J. Metrics for objective assessment - Preliminary summary of the Surgical Skills Workshop. *Surg Endosc* 2003; 17:220-6.
[8] www.simsurgery.com.

*Medicine Meets Virtual Reality 13*
*James D. Westwood et al. (Eds.)*
*IOS Press, 2005*

# Virtual Reality Testing of Multi-Modal Integration in Schizophrenic Patients

Anna SORKIN [a], Avi PELED [b] and Daphna WEINSHALL [a]

[a] *Interdisciplinary Center for Neural Computation,*
*Hebrew University of Jerusalem, Israel*
[b] *Institute for Psychiatric Studies, Sha'ar Menashe Mental Health Center,*
*& Faculty of Medicine, Technion, Israel*

**Abstract.** Our goal is to develop a new family of automatic tools for the diagnosis of schizophrenia, using Virtual Reality Technology (VRT). VRT is specifically suitable for this purpose, because it allows for multi-modal stimulation in a complex setup, and the simultaneous measurement of multiple parameters.

In this work we studied sensory integration within working memory, in a navigation task through a VR maze. Along the way subjects pass through multiple rooms that include three doors each, only one of which can be used to legally exit the room. Specifically, each door is characterized by three features (color, shape and sound), and only one combination of features – as determined by a transient opening rule – is legal. The opening rule changes over time. Subjects must learn the rule and use it for successful navigation throughout the maze. 39 schizophrenic patients and 21 healthy controls participated in this study.

Upon completion, each subject was assigned a performance profile, including various error scores, response time, navigation ability and strategy. We developed a classification procedure based on the subjects' performance profile, which correctly predicted 85% of the schizophrenic patients (and all the controls). We observed that a number of parameters showed significant correlation with standard diagnosis scores (PANSS), suggesting the potential use of our measurements for future diagnosis of schizophrenia. On the other hand, our patients did not show unusual repetition of response despite stimulus cessation (called perseveration in classical studies of schizophrenia), which is usually considered a robust marker of the disease. Interestingly, this deficit only appeared in our study when subjects did not receive proper explanation of the task.

## Introduction

Schizophrenia is a very debilitating disease, involving multiple and diverse symptoms, none of which is unique to schizophrenia. There is no biological marker to diagnose schizophrenia, and today the diagnosis is achieved primarily by psychiatric evaluation, which relies on symptoms, medical history, interview and observation. This procedure is difficult and somewhat unreliable, since each patient manifests a different sub-set of symptoms, whose evaluation in turn may differ even across expert observers.

In this paper we describe a new tool for the diagnosis of schizophrenia, which is essentially a computer game based on Virtual Reality Technology (VRT), including real time interactions and multi-modal stimulations. We believe that VRT is specifically suitable for studying schizophrenia for a number of reasons: (i) Schizophrenia involves primarily high-level brain functions [1,2], and therefore some of its symptoms may be only manifested in a natural complex setup, with a strong sense of presence. (ii) Moreover, by incorporating visual and auditory modalities and visual-motor skills within one task, multiple parameters can be measured during one behavior, rather than in a separate manner, revealing true correlations among functions. (iii) Finally, by replacing the traditional "boring" testing procedure with a "fun" game in a virtual environment, we may be able to overcome the notorious low motivation and lack of concentration exhibited by schizophrenic patients.

By way of background, schizophrenia is a devastating mental disorder with no known cure. The symptoms are usually classified as positive or negative. Positive symptoms include hallucinations (mostly auditory, though visual, tactile or olfactory rarely occur) and delusions (false unshakable beliefs). Hallucinations and delusions are so strong that they dominate the perception, actions and behavior of the patient. Negative symptoms consist of disorganized thinking & speech, social withdrawal, absence of emotion & expression, and reduced energy, motivation & activity. Typically, negative symptoms are more subtle and harder to define; they may be misinterpreted as personality traits, or may be confused with a reaction to certain life situations.

In the current study we sought to measure aspects of sensory integration within working memory (WM), known to be deficient among schizophrenic patients [3]. These patients also exhibit decreased ability to adjust to change (known as perseveration, or the repetition of response despite stimulus cessation) [4]. We therefore designed a virtual maze, with rooms that include a number of different doors, identified by a few features. The task is to navigate in the maze by opening only the "correct" door in each room, as defined by a fixed combination of features – the opening rule; remembering the rule puts load on the working memory of the subject. Moreover, the rule changes abruptly, which challenges the subject's ability to adapt to change.

Our main result in this study is the establishment of a routine that can distinguish patients from controls based on their performance profile, including multiple measurements collected during the VRT task. We measured errors scores, aspects of response time, and a variety of parameters reflecting the subject's navigation ability and decision strategy. We then developed a classification procedure, which modeled the distribution of the normal population, and then computed the probability to observe a given profile given this distribution. Finally, we fixed a single threshold to classify a profile as healthy or not. This procedure predicted correctly 85% of the participating patients (in a leave-one-out paradigm), and all the control subjects.

Our second main finding concerns perseveration – in our tests, patients adapt their response well (like controls) to change of stimuli when they are given proper explanation and training about the experiment. Perseveration as measured in classical studies of schizophrenia appears only when no initial explanation about the task is given, and thus seems related more to task understanding than to adaptability to change.

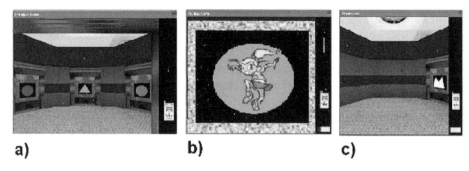

**Figure 1.** The virtual maze. *a*) "Challenge" room with 3 doors. *b*) Feedback when the correct door is opened. *c*) "Delay" room.

## Experiment 1: Working Memory

### Design

The main experiment involves a computer game, requiring navigation in a virtual maze with "challenge" and "delay" rooms. Each "challenge" room has three doors, only one of which can be legally used to exit the room, while each "delay" room has a single door. The goal of the game is to reach the end of the maze as fast as possible, which only happens after all the rooms have been legally exited (by opening the correct door).

Each door in a "challenge" room is associated with up to three distinct features - shape (triangle, square or circle), color (red, green or blue) and sound (3 different sounds), see Figure 1a. The sound is played when the subject examines the door. At each point in time, there is a certain "opening rule" which determines which door should be used to exit a "challenge" room. For example, the rule may say that only red doors can be opened, in which case any red door, regardless of its shape or sound, can be used. There will always be only one such door in each "challenge" room. The subject has to figure out the correct rule and open only the appropriate door (with the correct combination) in each "challenge" room.

We created four experimental conditions by manipulating two factors: the number of features which define the opening rule (1 or 2), and the presence or absence of a distractor feature on the doors (a door feature that is not used in the opening rule), see Table 1. The rule changes over time as indicated by a visual cue. When the correct door is chosen, the subject receives a reward (cigarette or chocolate icon) and gets encouragement (a dancing figure clapping hands), see Figure 1b.

In between challenge rooms, the subject passes through a few "delay" rooms with only one door. A door in a "delay" room is also associated with a colored shape and sound, different from those used on doors in challenge rooms (see Figure 1c). "Delay" rooms are included in order to increase the load on the subject's working memory.

### Methods

*Procedure:* 39 schizophrenic patients and 21 healthy controls matched by age and education level participated in the study. All subjects volunteered and received payment. The patients were evaluated using the standard PANSS (Positive and Negative Symptoms

**Table 1.** Four rule types used in the experiment.

| Number of features | No distractor | Distractor present |
|---|---|---|
| 1 | Sound | Sound + Color as distractor |
| 2 | Sound & Shape | Sound & Shape+ Color as distractor |

Scale). The experiment included a training phase, followed by the actual game. Training consisted of 3 stages: First, subjects learned how to open doors legally without movement. Second, they learned how to navigate in the maze at the desired speed. Finally, they practiced on a game-like session, with emphasis on achieving best performance (rather than speed). Subjects were encouraged to verbalize their strategy, were reminded of the ultimate goal, and received rich positive feedback from the experimenter.

*Equipment:* The sense of reality was obtained with 3D glasses, head tracker and joystick. Subjects used the joystick to navigate and open doors. The navigation button enabled movement in four directions: forward, backward, left and right. A change in the direction of movement could also be made by turning the head.

*Data Analysis:* We collected a vector of 26 parameters for each subject based on some continuous physical measurements. These included errors scores and Response Time (RT), the position and direction of gaze of each subject at any time, and the subject's rate of improvement with time. The 26 parameters define a subject's performance profile and can be divided to three groups: WM & Integration, Navigation & Strategy, and Learning.

- The *WM & Integration group* includes various errors scores, perseveration and distractor effect. In calculating error scores we distinguished between: (i) errors made during learning the rule (after the rule has changed); (ii) errors made while using the rule; (iii) the number of consecutive errors. Among all the erroneous choices, perseveration errors include all the repeated selections of a previous incorrect choice, or any erroneous choice which is consistent with a previous "opening rule" that has already changed. Perseveration was measured as the ratio between the number of perseveration errors and the total number of errors. Finally, the distractor effect was measured as the difference in error rate between two conditions: distractor is present less distractor is absent (the rows in Table 1).

- The *Navigation & Strategy group* includes three components: response time, navigation profile and strategy parameters. The navigation profile of a subject includes a combined measure of navigation speed with the number of collisions with walls and movements' histogram (e.g., forward, backward, rotation). The subject's decision strategy is measured by the number of doors inspected in each room, and the time spent looking at each door. To assess the selection strategy of a subject, we compared the histogram of locations of selected doors with the histogram of locations of correct doors.

- The *Learning group* measures the rate of subject's improvement with time on WM & Integration parameters, RT and navigation speed.

All the data was normalized so that, within the control group, each parameter is distributed with zero mean and standard deviation 1. A subject is noted to differ from the control group on a given parameter if his absolute value exceeds 2 in the normalized distribution.

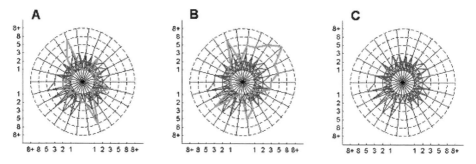

**Figure 2.** This plot shows subjects' performance profiles in polar coordinates. Each parameter corresponds to a certain angle $j$, and the radius $r$ reflects the subject's measurement value in the normalized coordinates system for that measurement. Thus a subject's profile corresponds to a close curve through 26 $(r, j)$ pairs. **A, B)** The personal profile of two patients, respectively, is shown in red. **C)** The performance profiles of all 21 control subjects, shown in blue, concentrate by definition in the area $r \leq 2$.

## Results

The patients group showed a very large variance in all the measured parameters. Each patient differed from the control group in a unique subset of parameters. To illustrate, two examples of individual performance plots are shown in Figure 2. There, patient A performed within the control range on all but two parameters, while patient B deviated in a wide range of parameters (concentrated in the upper right corner), most of which belong to the WM & Integration group of parameters.

The biggest difference between patients and controls (involving more than half of the patients) was manifested in increased errors rate when using the rule, increased consecutive errors, and large head rotation. The increased errors rate when using the rule in the patients group was maintained through both the training and experimental sessions. Some patients, however, showed large improvement during the training stage.

Generally, the patients' group demonstrated decreased ability to ignore irrelevant information. Accordingly, in the distractor conditions (right column of Table 1), they had higher errors rate. In addition, a noticeable number of patients showed one (or more) of the following deficits: increased errors rate during rule learning, elevated RT, and poor selection strategy. Overall, the patients were significantly slower than the controls; it was expressed in RT, speed and time spent looking on doors. However, they also showed a much bigger improvement than controls in RT and navigation speed. Finally, there was no marked difference between the groups in decision strategy or movement profile.

One of our most surprising finding is the similarity between patients and controls in the perseveration measure. Recall that in the relevant literature, perseveration is one of the strongest indicators of the disease. However, our approach to scoring perseveration differs from the classical procedure in two ways: First, we measure perseveration by a ratio, the number of perseverative errors divided by the total number of errors. This is because when the number of total errors is elevated, the number of perseverative errors should be expected to increase as well, irrespective of the source of error. Indeed, the numbers of total and perseverative errors showed very high correlation (0.87). Second, in our experiment subjects received a detailed explanation about the task, as well as extensive training. This difference might explain the discrepancy between our results and the relevant literature; to test this hypothesis, we designed an additional experiment, as reported below (experiment 2).

We also tested the correlation between our measurements and the subjects' PANSS scores, revealing a number of significant correlations ($p<0.01$): (i) Error rates when using the rule were significantly correlated with 5 positive and 4 negative symptoms. (ii) Consecutive error rates were correlated with 6 negative symptoms. (iii) Distractor effect for the sound rule was correlated with 6 positive symptoms, while distractor effect for the sound & shape rule was correlated only with one positive symptom – conceptual disorganization. (iv) Elevated RT was correlated with 6 negative symptoms. (v) Poor selection strategy was correlated with 6 positive symptoms.

## Experiment 2: Perseveration

This experiment was designed to investigate the reason for the absence of perseveration in experiment 1, a surprising result in light of the relevant literature, and specifically the relation between task understanding and perseveration. The experiment was conducted in the same virtual maze used in Experiment 1, with one-feature rule – color, and without a distractor. Subjects were told that the goal of the game is to find the correct door by which to exit each room. Two experimental conditions were compared: (i) subjects were not told what defines a legal door; and (ii) subjects were told that the correct door is defined by color, and that the correct color may change. In this experiment we measured high perseveration errors only in one condition: patients that did not receive explanation about the task. This finding implies that perseveration as measured in the classical literature may indicate a deficiency in problem solving, rather than the patients' inability to adjust to changes (as is usually believed).

## Summary and Discussion

We use VRT to design a complex environment for the diagnosis of schizophrenia. The technology made it possible to collect multiple measurements during a complex behavior, including multi-modal interaction and high load on working memory. In addition, the technology allowed us to conduct the experiment as a game and engage the patients in the task, which improved the subjects' concentration and motivation.

The most important finding of this study is that schizophrenic patients can be reliably separated from controls based on their performance profile in our VRT maze. To do this, we estimate the distribution of performance profiles using the control population only. For simplicity, we make the false assumptions of parameter independence, and that each parameter has normal distribution. We then compute the probability to receive a certain performance profile, and fix a threshold to discriminate between the controls and the patients in a leave-one-out paradigm. Specifically, we fix a probability value which separates best the control and patient populations, using 38 out of the 39 subjects, and check the prediction regarding the remaining patient. This procedure successfully predicts 33 out of 39 patients (85%). A closer look at the performance profile of the misclassified patients reveals that they fall in the normal range on almost all the parameters studied. A possible explanation may be that not all schizophrenic patients exhibit a working memory deficiency, as measured by our current experiment. Thus the final diagnostic routine should evaluate a wider spectrum of cognitive functions.

Two additional findings are worth noting: (i) Some of the measured parameters showed significant correlation with standard measures of schizophrenia (based on personal interviews), leading us to hope that similar tests may be able to replace subjective interviews in future diagnosis of the disease. (ii) The notion of perseveration should be further clarified. Our results indicate that standard measures or perseveration indicate a deficiency in problem solving, rather than a patient's inability to adjust to change. However, we have observed an interesting dissociation between patients' ability to learn a new rule, and their ability to recover from a mistake (which somewhat paradoxically appears harder for the patients' population than the mere learning of a new rule). This may be a better indication of preservation as originally intended, i.e., one's decreased ability to adjust to change.

## References

[1]  Friston KJ, Frith CD. Schizophrenia: a disconnection syndrome? Clin Neurosci 3(2):89-97, 1995.
[2]  Peled A. Multiple constraint organization in the brain: a theory for schizophrenia.
     Brain Res Bull Jul 1;49(4):245-50, 1999.
[3]  Silver H, Feldman P, Bilker W, Gur RC. Working memory deficit as a core neuropsychological dysfunction in schizophrenia. Am J Psychiatry, 160(10):1809-16, Oct 2003.
[4]  Crider A. Perseveration in schizophrenia. Schizophr Bull. 23(1):63-74, 1997.

*Medicine Meets Virtual Reality 13*
*James D. Westwood et al. (Eds.)*
*IOS Press, 2005*

# Emotional and Performance Attributes of a VR Game: A Study of Children

Sharon STANSFIELD [a], Carole DENNIS [b] and Evan SUMA [a]

[a] *Computer Sciences, Ithaca College, Ithaca, NY 14850*
[b] *Occupational Therapy Departments, Ithaca College, Ithaca, NY 14850*

**Abstract.** In this paper we present the results of a study to determine the effect and efficacy of a Virtual Reality game designed to elicit movements of the upper extremity. The study is part of an on-going research effort to explore the use of Virtual Reality as a means of improving the effectiveness of therapy for children with motor impairments. The current study addresses the following questions: 1. Does a VR game requiring repetitive motion sufficiently engage a child? 2. Are there detrimental physiological or sensory side-effects when a child uses an HMD-based VR? 3. Are the movements produced by a child while playing a VR game comparable to movements produced when carrying out a similar task in the real-world?

Based on study results, the enjoyment level for the game was high. ANOVA performed on the results for physical well-being pre- and post-VR showed no overall ill-effects as perceived by the children. Playing the game did not effect proprioception based on pre- and post-VR test scores. Motion data show similar, but not identical, overall movement profiles for similar tasks performed in the real and virtual world. Motor learning occurs in both environments, as measured by time to complete a game cycle.

## 1. Introduction

The idea of using Virtual Reality (VR) to assist in the rehabilitation of persons with disabilities was first introduced more than a decade ago. Since that time, several researchers have explored the use of VR for a diverse set of rehabilitation activities, including training in the use of motorized wheelchairs [1]; rehabilitation of balance disorders [2]; training spatial skills for mobility-impaired children [3]; and rehabilitation of cognitive and motor impairments caused by stroke [4]. Since most children play computer or video games, the use of VR as a rehabilitation tool for children with disabilities seems particularly promising. A VR therapy game could engage a child in play while delivering the needed therapy in a more palatable manner. Indeed, Reid [5] has shown that allowing children with severe handicaps to "participate" in virtual play activities from which they would normally be excluded in the real-world increases their sense of self esteem and self image. There is also evidence that spatial skills acquired by exploring a virtual world transfer to the real-world [6] and that motor tasks practiced in a virtual environment improve the performance of the same real-world tasks [7].

We are exploring the use of Virtual Reality to improve the effectiveness of therapy for children with motor impairments (for example, CP.) Our presumption (like those before us) is that VR can provide engaging "games" that will motivate the child to repetitively produce the desired therapeutic movements. Previous work in this area has been lacking in two ways: First, there has been no systematic study of the physiological and/or sensory effects of using VR on children (especially when a head-mounted display is used.) Second, the size of the population studied in most cases has been relatively small, making it difficult to generalize the results. As a first step in our work, we are addressing the first question: Does using VR have negative effects on children, and, equally important, do children enjoy playing VR games.

## 2.  Study Design and Method

### 2.1.  Experimental Setup

The virtual reality equipment used for the study consisted of a head-mounted display (HMD) and two position trackers: one tracker was mounted on the HMD and was used to update the virtual scene as the child moved his/her head. The other tracker was mounted on the child's hand and was used to update the position of the virtual hand and to permit the child to interact with the virtual game. The VR game consisted of a fantasy castle with 5 blocks displayed in front of the child. The child was instructed to "touch" each block with their virtual hand after it began to rotate. The rotating block then changed into an animated object (such as a rocket that blasted off accompanied by sound effects.) A cycle consisted of touching all five randomly positioned blocks sequentially and each child played 6 cycles. Data from the tracker worn on the hand was recorded during each reach (to the rotating block and back to the lap.)

### 2.2.  Method

Twenty four children between the ages of five and twelve participated. Sixteen were male and eight were female. All children were prescreened for normal vision and motor skills. Children used their non-dominant hand for all tasks. Each experiment was comprised of the following phases: The child first filled out a survey to record their level of motivation and current sense of well-being (i.e. were they dizzy, nauseous, etc.) The child then took a pre-VR proprioception test in order to quantify his/her proprioceptive motor skills. Each child was randomly assigned to one of two groups. Depending on his/her group, the child either played the VR game and then performed a real-world pointing test or the reverse. During the pointing test the child was instructed to point at each of five blocks mounted in front of him/her, with the sequence changed for each cycle. A cycle consisted of pointing at all blocks and there were six cycles. During each cycle, the motion of the child's hand was recorded and each data point was time-stamped to provide timing data. For both groups, the proprioception test was then re-administered. Finally, the child filled out a post-VR survey to record his/her enjoyment of the game and any changes in how they felt physically.

## 3.  Results and Discussion

Emotional attributes: All children indicated high motivation to play the game in the pre-experiment questionnaire and indicated they thought it would be fun (average response to

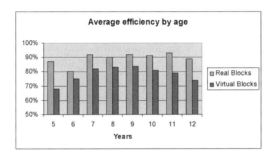

**Figure 1.** Chart showing efficiency of movements.

this question was 4.30/5.0.) Post experiment responses indicate that the children thought the game was fun (average response was 4.35/5.0) and that they would like to play the game again (average response 4.48/5.0). ANOVA performed on the results for well-being pre- and post-VR showed no overall ill-effects (i.e., increased nausea, dizziness, trouble walking or seeing) as perceived by the children.

Performance attributes: ANOVA was performed on the results of the pre-VR and post-VR proprioception test data. Separate analyses were performed for each group (those who took the proprioception test immediately after playing the VR game and those who took the test after also performing the real-world pointing test.) No significant effect on proprioception was found for either group.

We also compared the average time to complete a cycle for cycles two (real world timing: 15.05 sec, VR game: 39.4 sec) and five (real world: 13.77 sec, VR game: 37.3 sec.) Performance in both cases improved (real world: 1.27 sec, VR game: 2.09 sec.) This indicates that learning occurred in both situations.

Figure 1 charts the average efficiency of movement by age. (We assign an efficiency score as the ratio of distance to travel in a straight line from the lap to the block over actual distance traveled during the reach.) Movement within the VR game appears to be less efficient than in the real-world task. There may be several reasons for this: We observed that children moved their arms and hands more during the VR game. For example, some of the children followed the rotations of the block with their finger, while others raised their hands and moved them as they visually acquired the block to be touched. Other children found that they could cause the virtual block to transform by swiping their hand through it either from above or from the side – a motion they did not perform in the real world. In our next set of planned experiments, we will attempt to control for these variations. We will also compare movements for real, static blocks, virtual, static blocks, and virtual spinning blocks to attempt to extract whether the difference in motions was due to the nature of virtual reality itself or whether the differences in the two tasks (simply pointing at static blocks vs. attempting to make something interesting happen) was the primary cause of the additional movements.

## References

[1]  Inman, D., Loge, K., and Leavens, J. "VR Education and Rehabilitation." *Communications of the ACM.* 40(8):53-58. 1997.
[2]  McComas, J and Sveistrup, H. "Virtual reality applications for prevention, disability awareness, and physical therapy rehabilitation in neurology: Our recent work." *Neurology Report.* 26:55-64. 2002.

[3]  Stanton, D., Foreman, N. and Wilson, P. "Uses of Virtual Reality in Clinical Training: Developing the Spatial Skills of Children with Mobility Impairments." *Virtual Environments in Clinical Psychology and Neuroscience.* Riva, G., Wiederhold, B. and Molinari, E. (Eds.) Ios Press. Amsterdam. 1998.

[4]  Wann, J., Rushton, S., Smyth, M., and Jones, D. "Virtual environments for the rehabilitation of disorders of attention and movement," *Virtual Reality in Neuro-Psycho-Physiology,* Riva, G. (ed), Ios Press: Amsterdam. 1998.

[5]  Reid, D. "Virtual Reality and the Person-Environment Experience." *CyberPsychology and Behavior.* 5(6):559-564. 2002.

[6]  Wilson, P. Foreman, N., and Tlauka, M. "Transfer of spatial information from a virtual to a real environment in physically disabled children." *Disability and Rehabilitation.* 18(12):633-637. 1996.

[7]  Rose, F., Attree, A. and Brooks, B. "Virtual Environments in Neuropsychological Assessment and Rehabilitation." *Virtual Reality in Neuro-Psycho-Physiology,* Riva, G. (ed), Ios Press: Amsterdam. 1998.

*Medicine Meets Virtual Reality 13*
*James D. Westwood et al. (Eds.)*
*IOS Press, 2005*

# Virtual Reality Training Improves Students' Knowledge Structures of Medical Concepts

Susan M. STEVENS [a], Timothy E. GOLDSMITH [a], Kenneth L. SUMMERS [b],
Andrei SHERSTYUK [c], Kathleen KIHMM [c], James R. HOLTEN [b],
Christopher DAVIS [b], Daniel SPEITEL [c], Christina MARIS [d], Randall STEWART [d],
David WILKS [d], Linda SALAND [d], Diane WAX [d], PANAIOTIS [e], Stanley SAIKI [f],
Dale ALVERSON [d] and Thomas P. CAUDELL [d]

[a] *Department of Psychology, University of New Mexico*
[b] *Center for High Performance Computing, University of New Mexico*
[c] *University of Hawaii Telemedicine and Simulation*
[d] *Health Sciences Center, University of New Mexico*
[e] *Department of Music, University of New Mexico*
[f] *School of Medicine, University of Hawaii*
[g] *Department of Electrical and Computer Engineering, University of New Mexico*

**Abstract.** Virtual environments can provide training that is difficult to achieve under normal circumstances. Medical students can work on high-risk cases in a realistic, time-critical environment, where students practice skills in a cognitively demanding and emotionally compelling situation. Research from cognitive science has shown that as students acquire domain expertise, their semantic organization of core domain concepts become more similar to those of an expert's. In the current study, we hypothesized that students' knowledge structures would become more expert-like as a result of their diagnosing and treating a patient experiencing a hematoma within a virtual environment. Forty-eight medical students diagnosed and treated a hematoma case within a fully immersed virtual environment. Student's semantic organization of 25 case-related concepts was assessed prior to and after training. Students' knowledge structures became more integrated and similar to an expert knowledge structure of the concepts as a result of the learning experience. The methods used here for eliciting, representing, and evaluating knowledge structures offer a sensitive and objective means for evaluating student learning in virtual environments and medical simulations.

## 1. Introduction

Virtual reality (VR) immerses people into incredible worlds that offer unique and potentially fruitful educational experiences. Medical students can learn standard or complex procedures without worrying about harming people or animals in the process. Project TOUCH (Telehealth Outreach for Unified Community Health) is one example of work aimed at developing and testing VR technologies to enhance medical training. The TOUCH project is a multi-year collaboration between The University of Hawaii and The University of New Mexico.

Earlier TOUCH studies used a problem-based learning (PBL) [1–3,10,11] case that was designed to demonstrate an evolving epidural hematoma in a patient following a car crash. The interactive patient simulation allowed students to dynamically determine the outcome of the case scenario. A rule based artificial intelligence (AI) engine allowed realistic signs and symptoms of the hematoma patient to unfold over time and responded to the actions of the participants. Students were fully immersed within the virtual environment and also observed by others from outside the virtual world. Immersed students wore a head-mounted display with trackers, allowing them a sense of presence and interaction within the virtual environment. Team members within the virtual environment were able to see each other as full human figures (avatars) and could interact as if they were physically present, even when separated by significant distances. Students could examine and treat the virtual patient, independently controlling their viewpoint and motion within the virtual world.

## 1.1. Validation of Student Learning

The focus of the current study investigated the extent of student learning within VR training. Although several previous studies have used VR to train medical students [e.g., 13, 14], only a few studies have demonstrated the effectiveness of VR training in a medical setting by performing controlled studies [7–9,12,15,17]. Some of these studies have found significant improvements in performance in student learning for those using VR compared to those using traditional methods of learning [15]. The current study was designed to evaluate the effects of VR training on an objective outcome measure of student learning.

Research in cognitive science has shown that domain-specific learning is well characterized by the way students have the central concepts of the domain organized in memory [4]. More expert individuals have well-structured and coherent conceptual organizations, whereas novices show memory structures that are less coherent and defined by surface-level rather than semantic dimensions of the domain. Further, studies have shown that training effectiveness can be measured by examining how similar students' knowledge structures are to an expert's [6]. Within the medical field, previous studies have suggested that medical expertise may also be characterized by the nature and organization of conceptual knowledge [18].

In the current study we investigated whether medical students' knowledge structures would improve as a result of their diagnosing and treating a patient in a virtual environment. We used the same hematoma case described above, but now students diagnosed and treated the patient individually while immersed in the virtual environment. We compared students' knowledge structures of a set of core concepts from the hematoma case to an expert knowledge structure both prior to and after VR training. We hypothesized that students' knowledge structures would become more similar to an expert's knowledge structure as a result of virtual training on the hematoma case.

## 2. Participants

Participants were forty-eight medical students (28 males, 20 females) from the University of New Mexico and the University of Hawaii. All of the participants were volunteers and were compensated $100 for their participation. Students ranged from their first to their fourth year in medical school, with a mean of 2.96 years.

## 3. Materials

### 3.1. Flatland

Flatland served as the software infrastructure [5]. It is an open source visualization/VR application development environment, created at the University of New Mexico. Flatland allows software authors to construct, and users to interact with, arbitrarily complex graphical and aural representations of data and systems. It is written in C/C++ and uses the standard OpenGL graphics language to produce all graphics.

### 3.2. Artificial Intelligence (AI)

The AI component was a forward chaining IF-THEN rule based system that specified the behavior of objects in the VR world. The rules governing the physiology of the avatar were obtained from subject matter experts. The rules were coded in a C computer language format as logical antecedents and consequences. The AI loops over the rulebase, applying each rule's antecedents to the current state of the system, including time, and testing for logical matches. Matching rules are "fired," modifying the next state of the system. Time is a special state of the system that is not directly modified by the AI, but whose rate is controlled by an adjustable clock. Since the rate of inference within the AI is controlled by this clock, the user (or student) is able to speed up, slow down, or stop the action controlled by the AI. This allows a user to learn from his/her mistakes by repeating a scenario.

## 4. Procedure

### 4.1. Virtual Reality

Participants were tested individually in a lab room. After reading and signing a statement of informed consent, students were oriented to the VR equipment with the help of an assistant. After the orientation, the students were directed to a web site where they filled out a demographic questionnaire and then watched an instructional video on the use of the VR equipment. The web site also contained links to interactive, labeled diagrams of the VR equipment and links to head-injury reference materials such as brain section diagrams, schematics, short video animations and textual information. When the students were finished watching the video, they were shown additional reference materials and allowed to practice using the VR equipment until they felt comfortable locomoting and manipulating objects. The students were then directed back to the web site for step-by-step instructions for the experiment.

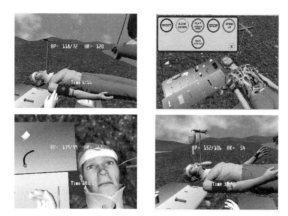

**Figure 1.** A depiction of what the students saw in the virtual environment (VE).

The experiment was designed to simulate a problem-based learning session that involved an automobile crash; participants were instructed to act as if they were the initial responders at the crash scene. The participants first completed a pre-experiment knowledge assessment exercise (described below). Next, they read a web-based, textual orientation to the clinical scenario and, based on this, were asked to complete a list of known and anticipated problems. Third, they were given 30 minutes to enter the virtual environment (see Figure 1) and to perform a physical exam on the virtual patient. On completion of this, they exited the virtual environment and documented their physical exam findings on the web site. After documenting their physical exam, they read a summary of the expected physical exam findings and were asked to document their assessment and plan. Next, they read a case conclusion, explaining the virtual patient's injuries, follow-up or confirmatory studies and the expected actions to be taken once the patient arrived at an ER. Finally, the participants completed the knowledge assessment exercise a second time.

## 4.2. Assessment of Knowledge Structures

Five subject matter experts identified 25 central concepts associated with the hematoma case. The experts then performed a semantic association task where they were asked to identify a small subset of the 25 concepts that were most related to a target concept. Each of the 25 concepts served in turn as the target concept. The resulting association ratings were averaged and submitted to Pathfinder [16], which generated an expert knowledge network. The 25 concepts were represented as nodes in the network and the links between nodes reflected the semantic relatedness of the concepts (see Figure 2). This expert knowledge network served as a referent against which students' knowledge networks were assessed.

The participants rated the semantic relatedness of 72 concept pairs using a 5-point Likert scale, with "1" indicating less related and "5" indicating more related. This subset of pairs was derived from the expert knowledge network; 36 pairs of related concepts came from the 36 linked concepts in the expert network and 36 unrelated pairs were used as foils.

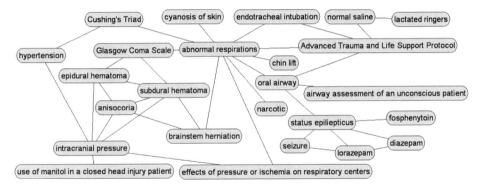

**Figure 2.** Expert knowledge network of the 25 core hematoma concepts.

## 5. Results

Each student's raw relatedness ratings were correlated with the experts' averaged relatedness ratings. The correlation was $r = 0.77$ for pre-training and $r = 0.76$ for post training, both highly statistically significant ($p < 0.01$). The high correlations implied that students had considerable knowledge about the hematoma concepts prior to training. This conclusion is also confirmed by comparing the mean rating of the related pairs (4.25) with the mean rating of the unrelated pairs (1.96) on the set of relatedness ratings before training.

Pathfinder was used to derive pre- and post-training knowledge networks for each student from his/her relatedness ratings. The student's knowledge networks were then compared to the expert knowledge network using a method that produced a similarity index ($s$) that varied from 0 to 1. The mean similarity scores were $s = 0.72$ before training and $s = 0.74$ after training. A matched t-test on these differences resulted in $t = -1.51$, $p = .139$. The pre/post difference likely failed to reach standard significance because of a ceiling effect; the students were already performing at a high level before training. To assess this, we used $s = .80$ as a cutoff value and selected the subset of students ($N = 36$) who had similarity to expert scores below this level on the pretest knowledge structures (i.e., students who were less knowledgeable about the concepts). A matched t-test for these 36 students on the difference between the similarity to expert scores before and after training resulted in $t = -2.577$, $p = .014$.

## 6. Discussion

Although previous studies have used VR to train medical students, there is a dearth of studies examining objective measures of student learning. Based on work from cognitive science, we suggest that changes in students' organization of core domain concepts as a function of VR training may be an important index of learning. Further, students who actively generate hypotheses, practice procedures, and offer justifications for their actions acquire deeper knowledge than students who simply read about cases [10]. These are the kinds of VR learning environments that we aim to create under Project TOUCH.

In the present study, a single virtual training exercise with an avatar suffering from a hematoma resulted in students reorganizing their semantic structure of a set of core of hematoma concepts. By focusing on those students who were lower in their knowledge of the concepts before training, we found that students' knowledge structures became significantly more similar to an expert's knowledge structure after training. Clearly more research using controlled studies is needed to tease apart what particular aspects of the training produced the changes in knowledge. But in general we suggest that the method used here for eliciting, representing and evaluating knowledge structures offers a sensitive, objective and valid means for evaluating student learning in virtual environments.

## Acknowledgments

The project described was supported partially by grant 2 D1B TM 00003-02 from the Office for the Advancement of Telehealth, Health Resources and Services Administration, Department of Health and Human Services. Its contents are solely the responsibility of the authors and do not necessarily represent the official views of the Health Resources and Services Administration.

## References

[1]   Alverson, D. C., Saiki, S. M., Jacobs, J., Saland, L., Keep, M. F., Norenberg, J., Baker, R., Nakatsu, C., Kalishman, S., Lindberg, M., Wax, D., Mowafi, M., Summers, K. L., Holten, J. R., Greenfield, J. A., Aalseth, E., Nickles, D., Sherstyuk, A., Haines, K. & Caudell, T. P. (2004). Distributed interactive virtual environments for collaborative experiential learning and training independent of distance over Internet2. In *Medicine Meets Virtual Reality 12, Studies in Health Technology and informatics, 98, 7-12,* J. Westwood et al. (Eds.). Amsterdam: IOS Press.
[2]   Anderson, A. (1991). Conversion to problem-based learning in 15 months. In D. Boud & G. Feletti, (Eds.) *The challenge of problem based learning* (pp. 72-79). New York: St. Martin's Press.
[3]   Bereiter, C. & Scardamalia, M. (2000). Commentary on Part I: Process and product in problem-based learning (PBL) research. In: D. H. Evensen and C. E. Hmelo (Eds.) *Problem-based learning: A research perspective on learning interactions* (pp. 185-195). Mahwah, NJ: L. Erlbaum Associates.
[4]   Bransford, J. D., Brown, A. L. & Cocking, R. R. (Eds.) (1999). *How people learn: Brain, mind, experience and school.* Washington, D.C.: National Academy Press.
[5]   Caudell, T. P., Summers, K. L., Holten, J. IV., Takeshi, H., Mowafi, M., Jacobs, J., Lozanoff, B. K., Lozanoff, S., Wilks, D., Keep, M. F., Saiki, S. & Alverson, D. (2003). A virtual patient simulator for distributive collaborative medical education. *Anat Rec (Part B: New Anat), 270B,* 16-22.
[6]   Goldsmith, T. E. & Kraiger, K. (1996). Applications of structural knowledge assessment to training evaluation. In J. K. Ford & K. Kraiger, (Eds.) *Improving training effectiveness in organizations* (pp. 73-96). Hillsdale, NJ: Erlbaum.
[7]   Grundman, J. A., Wigton, R. S. & Nickol, D. (2000). Controlled trail of a web based virtual reality program in teaching physical diagnosis skills to medical students. *Journal of General Internal Medicine, 15 (suppl.1),* 33.
[8]   Hoffman, H. G., Patterson, D. R. & Carrougher, G. J. (2000). Use of virtual reality for adjunctive treatment of adult burn pain during physical therapy: A controlled study. *The Clinical Journal of Pain, 16,* 244-250.
[9]   Holcomb, J. B., Dumire, R. D., Crommett, J. W., Stamateris, C. E., Fagert, M. A., Cleveland, J. A., Dorlac, G. R., Dorlac, W. C., Bonar, J. P., Hira, K., Aoki, N. & Mattox, K. L. (2002). Evaluation of trauma team performance using an advanced human patient simulator for resuscitation training. *The Journal of Trauma, 52 (6),* 1078-1086.
[10]  Jacobs, J., Caudell, T. P., Wilks, D., Keep, M. F., Mitchell, S., Buchanan, H., Saland, L., Rosenheimer, J., Lozanoff, B. K., Lozanoff, S., Saiki, S. & Alverson, D. (2003). Integration of advanced technologies to enhance problem-based learning over distance: Project TOUCH. *Anatomical Record (Part B: New Anat.), 270B,* 16-22.

[11] Kaufman, A., Mennin, S., Waterman, R., Duban, S., Hansbarger, C., Silverblatt, H., Obenshain, S., Kantrowitz, M., Becker, T., Samet, J. & Wiese, W. (1989). The New Mexico experiment: Educational innovation and institutional change. *Acad Med, 64*, 285-294.

[12] Lee, S. K., Pardo, M., Gaba, D., Sowb, Y., Dicker, R., Straus, E. M., Khaw, L., Morabito, D., Krummel, T. M. & Knudson, M. M. (2002). Trauma assessment training with a patient simulator: A prospective, randomized study. *The Journal of Trauma-Injury, Infection and Critical Care, 55(4)*, 651-657.

[13] Reznek, M., Harter, P. & Krummel, T. (2002). Virtual reality and simulation: Training the future emergency physician. *Academic Emergency Medicine, 9(1)*, 78-87.

[14] Riva, G. (2003). Applications of virtual environments in medicine. *Methods of Information in Medicine, 42(5)*, 524-534.

[15] Riva, G. (2002). Virtual reality for health care: The status of research. *CyberPsychology & Behavior, 5(3)*, 219-225.

[16] Schvaneveldt, R. W. (Ed.) (1990). *Pathfinder associative networks: Studies in knowledge organization.* Westport, CT: Ablex.

[17] Torkington, J., Smith, G. T., Rees, B.I. & Darzi, A. (2001). Skill transfer from virtual reality to a real laparoscopic task. *Surgical Endoscopy, 15*, 1076-1079.

[18] van de Wiel, M. W. J., Boshuizen, H. P. A., Schmidt, H. G. & Schaper, N. C. (1999). The explanation of clinical concepts by expert physicians, clerks and advanced students. *Teaching and Learning in Medicine, 11(3),* 153-163.

*Medicine Meets Virtual Reality 13*
*James D. Westwood et al. (Eds.)*
*IOS Press, 2005*

# Emphatic, Interactive Volume Rendering to Support Variance in User Expertise

Don STREDNEY [a], David S. EBERT [b], Nikolai SVAKHINE [b], Jason BRYAN [a],
Dennis SESSANNA [b] and Gregory J. WIET [c]

[a] *OSC – Ohio Supercomputer Center, Columbus, Ohio*
[b] *Purdue University, West Lafayette, Indiana*
[c] *Department of Otolaryngology, The Ohio State University and Children's
Hospital, Columbus, Ohio*

**Abstract.** Various levels of representation, from abstract to schematic to realistic, have been exploited for millennia to facilitate the transfer of information from one individual to another. Learning complex information, such as that found in biomedicine, proves specifically problematic to many, and requires incremental, stepwise depictions of the information to clarify structural, functional, and procedural relationships.

Emerging volume-rendering technique, such as non-photorealistic representation, coupled with advances in computational speeds, especially new graphical processing units, provide unique capabilities to explore the use of various levels of representation in interactive sessions.

We have developed a system that produces images that simulate pictorial representations for both scientific and biomedical visualization. The system combines traditional and novel volume illustration techniques. We present examples from our efforts to distill representational techniques for both creative exploration and emphatic presentation for clarity. More specifically, we present our efforts to adapt these techniques for interactive simulation sessions being developed in a concurrent project for resident training in temporal bone dissection simulation. The goal of this effort is to evaluate the use of emphatic rendering to guide the user in an interactive session and to facilitate the learning of complex biomedical information, including structural, functional, and procedural information.

## 1. Introduction

The importance of variation in the presentation of information has been widely established. A constructivist perspective on learning purports that students need to establish meaning, either implicitly or explicitly, to understand and integrate new information [1–3]. Spiro and Feltovich have demonstrated that re-presentations of the same information under different organizational schemes and representations may reduce and prevent reductive biases and oversimplification which often occur in learning complex material [8,16]. Although the gradual increase in variability of task complexity and representation initially decrease a learner's performance in training, it has been demonstrated to ultimately increase learning and transfer [9,13].

Because all constructive modeling of knowledge varies from individual to individual, understanding how students impose meaning and structure is essential to curriculum

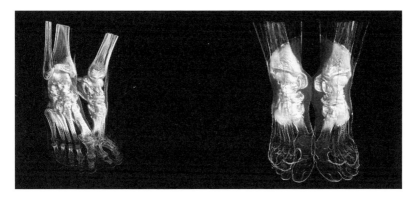

**Figure 1.** Two representative examples of emphatic volume rendering of the tarsal joints. Note illustrative technique to de-emphasize the external anatomy of the feet.

development that truly facilitates learning. This is one of the basic tenets of constructivism. One cannot simply consider the domain knowledge as something apart from the student. For instance, implicit learning is often occurring. Implicit learning is where a student is imposing his or her own structural classification of learned information, often with previously learned structure. A critical assessment of the level of constructive proficiency of the student would facilitate when to use an appropriate representation. However, personal assessment is difficult and it is often inefficient to tailor a curriculum to one specific student's model and unique phenotypical approach to learning. Ideally, the student should mediate the level of representation to facilitate their construction of the information. By allowing the student to influence the level of representation, we gain new insight into how there are formulating the structure and meaning of new information.

Recent results in volume rendering techniques, including incredible levels of realism and non-photorealistic rendering provide methodologies to present visualizations that can be self-titrated to the individuals levels of conceptual proficiency. Coupled with real-time performance for complex operations, current technologies present opportunities to exploit the constructivist view and allow the student to influence their own learning through control of the representation. Coupled with non-deterministic simulations that present new information in an experiential way, these emerging systems have the capacity to facilitate natural inquiry at one's own pace, with the student in control.

## 2. Background and Significance

Researchers at OSC have been actively involved in the development of surgical training simulations [6,10,11,14,17,18,25–27] as well as interactive volume visualization that support multimodal and multiscale analysis, manipulation and dissemination [5,19,20, 22]. Recently, OSC has collaborated with researchers at Purdue University to investigate the use of novel volume rendering techniques to cue and focus user attention to facilitate the dissemination of information graphically [24].

Through this collaboration, we have developed a volume illustration system that incorporates both realistic and illustrative rendering, a domain-specific, illustration specific framework, with a high-level, more natural user interface that can accommodate variance in student learning. It is important to point out that all of the various levels of

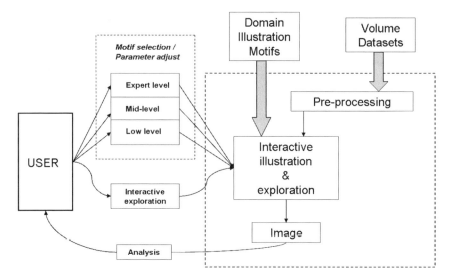

**Figure 2.** Overview of the components of, and user interaction with, the system.

representations can be derived from the same volume data set. Our objective is to provide an intuitive interface for users with various backgrounds to be able to rapidly and easily generate required imagery. The resulting images and animation allow for variance in user learning for education, training, and simulation environments.

## 3. Methods

Novel volume rendering techniques are the extension of texture-based volume rendering [5] using graphics hardware for accelerated rendering [7]. Also, two-dimensional transfer functions [12] are used for better implicit feature selection, if explicit data segmentation is not provided. The illustrative effect is achieved by selective enhancement application: we use a set of transfer functions that map volume values to the magnitude of a particular effect and, thus, makes it possible to distinguish the materials not just by opacity and color, but also by rendering technique.

The interface incorporates three levels of interaction: a low level, a mid-level, and a high level. The low user-level is for software developers, experienced illustrators, and system builders. The mid-level interface is for illustrators and experienced end-users that want to make adjustments once they understand the controls. The high-level interface is designed for the end user, and in our current application focus, it would be for medical students, surgical residents, physicians and surgeons.

More recently, we have been exploring the integration of these visualizations into an interactive tutorial previously developed for temporal bone dissection simulation for use in resident training [4,21,25–27]. This current effort seeks to exploit the illustrative techniques of the above system, however, in a way that titrates the representational qualities to the level of expertise of the user in real-time (see Figures 3–6). We have started with the integration of emphatic volume rendering for use in learning structural and functional relationships. Based upon our success, we will then employ these techniques to our procedural training sessions.

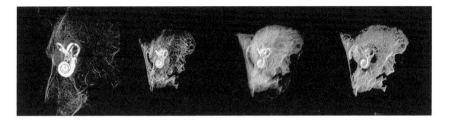

**Figures 3–6.** Left to right: Simple, intermediate, and complex representations of the otic capsule.

To learn structural and functional relationships, the temporal bone dissection simulation environment allows the user to enter an intelligent tutorial to learn and test their proficiency regarding the shape and configuration of requisite structures relevant to various techniques used in temporal bone surgery. These structures have been previously segmented. In addition, the dissection simulation tracks metrics that include number of visits to the tutorial, time to task, structures requested to view and previous dissections performed by experts. These metrics will be used to statistically classify level of expertise, which will then determine the level of representation to be presented.

Currently, we establish three levels of representation:

- Simple/schematic,
- Intermediate/combined (schematic and complex representations are used simultaneously in the same representation), and
- Complex/realistic.

Several pre-defined pixel and vertex shaders that emphasize or de-emphasize illumination and realism are being developed. Again, all levels of representation will be derived from a single volume data set. User's will be able to return to a more simplified presentation should that be required.

In the tutorial a morphometric tool is provided to interactively control a sectioning plan to explore the structures and their relationships. When this tool is selected, we can control a "sphere of influence" where various levels of representation can be implemented (See Figure 1). This tool allows a more detailed representation in the area being investigated, while surrounding areas are subjugated.

## 4. Results

The Figures 3–6 show the various levels of representation currently available. In Figure 3, a more schematic/simplistic representation of the cochlea and semicircular canals are portrayed. The surrounding bone is de-emphasized in complexity to focus the user on just the relationships of the two structures. In Figure 4 and 5, a more complex representation of the same area is employed, Figure 5 using more of a maximum intensity projection of the surrounding bone. Finally, Figure 5 shows a more realistic representation.

## 5. Conclusion

We have presented our current efforts to exploit volume rendering techniques for use in presenting various representations of structures in interactive learning environments.

These efforts present the groundwork for learning environments that dynamically accommodate variance in learning expertise while using a common data set. Further efforts include controlled studies with medical students and residents to validate the efficacy of this design to facilitate learning.

## Acknowledgements

We would like to thank Dr. Kimerly Powell at the Cleveland Clinic Foundation for the microCT images of the otic capsule used in Figures 3–6. Portions of this research, Validation/Dissemination of Virtual Temporal Bone Dissection, is supported by a grant from the National Institute on Deafness and Other Communication Disorders, of the National Institutes of Health, 1 R01 DC06458-01A1.

## References

[1]   Bruner J, (1966) Toward a Theory of Instruction, Cambridge, MA: Harvard University Press.
[2]   Bruner J, (1973) Going Beyond the Information Given, New York: Norton.
[3]   Bruner J, (1996) The Culture of Education, Cambridge, MA: Harvard University Press.
[4]   Bryan J, Stredney D, Sessanna D, Wiet GJ, (2001) "Virtual Temporal Bone Dissection: A Case Study", Proc. of IEEE Visualization, San Diego, CA, 2001:497-500.
[5]   Cabral B, Cam N and J Foran, (1994) "Accelerated volume rendering and tomopgraphic reconstruction using texture mapping hardware. ACM Symposium on Volume Visualization.
[6]   Edmond CV, Heskamp D, Sluis D, Stredney D, Wiet GJ, Yagel R, Weghorst S, P Oppenheimer, Miller J, M Levin and L Rosenberg, (1997) "ENT Endoscopic Surgical Training Simulator", Proc. MMVR5, Morgan et al, (Eds.), IOS Press, Amsterdam, 518-528.
[7]   Engel K and T Ertl. (2002) Interactive high-quality volume rendering with flexible consumer graphics hardware. STAR-State of The Art Report. Eurographics.
[8]   Feltovich PJ, Spiro RJ and RL Coulson (1989) The Nature of Conceptual Understanding in Biomedicine: The Deep Structure of Complex Ideas and the Development of Misconceptions. In D. Evans and V. Patel (Eds.), The Cognitive Sciences in Medicine (pp. 113-172). Cambridge, MA: MIT Press (Bradford Books).
[9]   Fried LJ and KJ Holyoak, (1984) Induction of category distributions: a framework for classification learning, Journal of Experimental Psychology: Learning, Memory and Cognition 10:234-257.
[10]  Hiemenz L, McDonald JS, Stredney D and D Sessanna, (1996) "A Physiologically Valid Simulator for Training Residents to Perform an Epidural Block," Proc.15th Southern Biomedical Engineering Conference, March 29-30.
[11]  Hiemenz L, Stredney D and P Schmalbrock, (1998) "Development of a Force Feedback Model for an Epidural Needle Insertion Simulaton," Proc. MMVR 6, Westwood et al, (Eds), IOS Press, Amsterdam:272-277.
[12]  Kniss J, Kindlmann G and C. Hansen. (2001) "Interactive volume rendering using multi-dimensional transfer functions and direct manipulation widgets". In Proceedings Visualization: 255.262, October.
[13]  Peterson MJ RM Meagher Jr. RM, Chait H and S Gillie, (1973) The abstraction and generalization of dot patterns,Cognitive Psychology 4:378-398.
[14]  Rosenberg LB and D Stredney, A Haptic Interface for Virtual Simulation of Endoscopic Surgery Proc. MMVR4, Weghorst et al. (Eds), IOS Press, Amsterdam; 1996:371-387.
[15]  Saltz JH, Catalyurek UV, Kurc TM, Gray M, Hastings S, Langella S, Narayanan S, Martino R, Bryant S,, Peszynka M, Wheeler M, Sussman A, Beynon M, Hansen C, Stredney D, Sessanna D, (2003) "Driving Scientific Applications by Data in Distributed Environments," International Conference on Computational Science:255-364.
[16]  Spiro RJ, Feltovich PJ, Coulson RI and DK Anderson, (1989) Multiple analogies for complex concepts: antidotes for analogy-induced misconception in advanced knowledge acquisition, In S Vosniadou & A Ortony (Eds.) Similarity and analogical reasoning, Cambridge: Cambridge University Press.

[17] Stredney D, Sessanna D, McDonald JS, Hiemenz L and L Rosenberg, (1996) "A Virtual Simulation Environment for Learning Epidural Anesthesia" Proc. MMVR4,Weghorst et al. (Eds), IOS Press, Amsterdam;164-175.

[18] Stredney D, Wiet GJ, Yagel R, Sessanna D, Kurzion Y, Fontana M, Shareef N, Levin M, Martin K and A Okamura, (1998) "A Comparative Analysis of Integrating Visual Representations with Haptic Displays", Proc. MMVR6, Westwood et al, (Eds.) IOS Press, Amsterdam:20-26.

[19] Stredney D, Crawfis R, Wiet GJ, Sessanna D, Shareef N and J Bryan, (1999) "Interactive Volume Visualization for Synchronous and Asynchronous Remote Collaboration," Proc. MMVR7, Westwood et al, (Eds.) IOS Press, Amsterdam:344-350.

[20] Stredney D, Agrawal A, Barber D, Crawfis R, Feng WC, Hou J, Panda DK, Sadayappan P, Powell K , Schmalbrock P, Sessanna D, Wiet GJ, Shareef N and J Bryan, (2000) "Interactive Medical data on Demand: A High-Performance Imaged Based Approach Across Heterogeneous Environments", Proc. MMVR8, Westwood et al, (Eds.) IOS Press, Amsterdam:327-333.

[21] Stredney D, Wiet GJ, Bryan J, Sessanna D, Murakami J, Schmalbrock P, Powell K, and DB Welling, (2002) "Temporal Bone Dissection Simulation – An Update", Proc. MMVR10, JD Westwood et al, (Eds.) IOS Press, Amsterdam:507-513.

[22] Stredney D, Bryan J, Sessanna D andn T Kerwin, (2003) Facilitating real-Time Volume Interaction,Proc. MMVR2003, Westwood (Eds.) IOS Press, Amsterdam:329-335.

[23] Svakhine N and D. Ebert. (2003) Interactive volume illustration and feature halos. Pacific Graphics '03 Proceedings, 15(3):67-76.

[24] Svakhine N, Ebert DS and D Stredney, (2004) "Illustration Motifs for Effective Medical Volume Illustration", in Submission, CG&A.

[25] Wiet GJ, Bryan J, Dodson E, Sessanna D, Stredney D, Schmalbrock P and B Welling, (2000) "Virtual Temporal Bone Dissection," Proc. MMVR8,Westwood et. al., (Eds). IOS Press Amsterdam: 378-384.

[26] Wiet, G.J., Stredney D, Sessanna and J Bryan. (2001) "Volume-based Temporal Bone Dissection Simulator," AAO-HNSF/ARO Research Forum, Annual Meeting of the American Academy of Otolaryngology-Head and Neck Surgery Foundation, Denver, Colorado, September 9-12

[27] Wiet GJ, Stredney D, Sessanna D, Bryan J, Welling DB and P Schmalbrock, "(2002) Virtual Temporal Bone Dissection: An interactive surgical simulator, Otolaryngology-H&NS, Vol. 127, No.1:79-83.

532

*Medicine Meets Virtual Reality 13*
*James D. Westwood et al. (Eds.)*
*IOS Press, 2005*

# First Clinical Tests with the Augmented Reality System INPRES

Gunther SUDRA [a], Rüdiger MARMULLA [b], Tobias SALB [a], Sassan GHANAI [b],
Georg EGGERS [b], Bjoern GIESLER [a], Stefan HASSFELD [b],
Joachim MUEHLING [b] and Ruediger DILLMANN [a]

[a] *Department for Computer Science - IRF*
*Universität Karlsruhe (TH), 76128 Karlsruhe, Germany*
[b] *Department of Cranio-Maxillofacial Surgery*
*University of Heidelberg, 69120 Heidelberg, Germany*

**Abstract.** In this paper we present the results of the first patient experiment in craniofacial surgery of the INPRES system - an augmented reality system on the basis of a tracked see-through head-mounted display.

## 1. Introduction

In the last decade research and development in computer aided surgery has been focused on preoperative problems and navigation tools. As a result of this, preoperative planning and simulation is supported quite well by computer based tools. By now some of these systems are already available for clinical use, for example in craniofacial surgery and neurosurgery [1–4].

Tools for intraoperative navigation are also available [5], most of them commercial. However these systems have one disadvantage: the surgeon has to turn his head from the computer monitor to the patient and vice versa [6]. To close this gap we present our augmented reality system INPRES. The expression "augmented reality" is associated with systems that can merge computer-generated virtual data with real-world information into a single coherent perception. There exist different approaches in several fields, using projectors, microscopes, half-silvered mirrors and see-through-devices [7–11]. Only few of them are reported to be used in clinical tests [12].

The main functionality of our system is to support the surgeon with relevant information directly in the operation field. For INPRES we use a head mounted display for the superimposition of the patient and virtual data. With these technique we can offer the surgeon important anatomical information from radiological image processing, preoperative planning or simulation software by presenting them as virtual data.

In this paper we will present our results of the first clinical tests with the augmented reality system INPRES. Section 2 states the experimental environment and explains the methods used for INPRES. Emphasis will lie on the registration and calibration process. The following section shows the results of our first clinical test. We will finish the paper with a conclusion including an overview on future work.

## 2. Methods

Clinical evaluation is done to acquire feedback on relevant issues from clinical end users of the system on the one hand and from engineers and computer scientists involved in the development on the other hand. Using INPRES under "real" conditions will point out the strengths of the system and demonstrate the weaknesses. In this article we will concentrate on the technical aspects.

### 2.1. Setup

For the overlay of real world scenes and virtual data we are using a commercial Sony Glasstron LDI-100E device. Calibration is done using a rigid body and an active pointer. The position of the glasses, the patient, the pointer and the calibration object is tracked via an optical NDI Polaris navigation system. All trackers are using passive retroflective target markers. In case of the patient the markers are mounted on a bite splint or adapted to a bone screw adapter. For detection of occlusion we use an optional mini stereo camera system which is mounted on top of the glasses. Data processing is performed with a Linux Pentium 4 - 3 GHz system.

### 2.2. Data Processing

The first step that has to be done is the acquisition of tomographic data, e.g. the data of a computer tomograph (CT). For intra-operative registration of the tracker coordinate system (TKS) and patient coordinate system (PKS) the patient has to wear a bite splint with artificial landmarks. The positions of these landmarks have to be segmented. By now this is done with an interactive segmentation tool. In addition the region of interest which should be visualized has to be segmented, too. The segmented regions are meshed using the marching cubes algorithm. Result of this processing is a 3D data structure. The number of points of the resulting data set should not be too large – otherwise the visualization framerate of INPRES could be negatively affected. Further processing of the data, like a reduction of the point cloud, could be done with a compatible software package, e.g. KasOP [13] or MEDIFRAME [14].

### 2.3. Registration

Registration is necessary to calculate the fixed translation from TKS to PKS. Therefore the patient and an active Pointer have to be tracked. Tracking of the patient is done via a passive marker consisting of three spheres which reflect the infrared-light from the NDI Polaris navigation system. The active pointer is equipped with infrared diodes and can also be detected by the navigation system. The bite-splint has to be encountered with the active pointer and a button has to be pressed to get each marker position. This can be done by the surgeon or a surgical nurse. Computation is done using a least-square point matching algorithm on the real-world and virtual marker-positions. Afterwards the quality of the registration can be specified by the root mean square error.

## 2.4. Calibration

Calibration of the display device is necessary for proper optical appearance of the pre-sented virtual data [15,16]. During calibration, parameters like position and orientation of the device in relation to the eyes, field of view, etc. are determined. These parameters are unique for each person and INPRES session. As calibration device we use an acrylic rigid glass body with passive markers. A two-dimensional cross is plotted on the body and a symbolic z-axis is added. During the calibration process, the surgeon has to overlay a computer generated virtual cross with the real world cross presented on the rigid body. For correct overlay regarding position and orientation the surgeon has to move himself appropriately. This procedure has to be undertaken five times for each eye with different positions of the virtual crosses. Position and orientation of the calibration object and the display device are acquired for each overlay and used for computation of the optimal calibration.

## 2.5. Visualization

Sending slightly different overlay information to the two displays in the see-through device induces a correct three-dimensional visualization of the virtual scene. For surgical use we can display for example anatomical images, pathological structures or results of preoperative planning and simulation like symmetry considerations and distraction planning for facial reconstruction [17].

## 3. Results

In an earlier evaluation phase the INPRES system has been tested intensively in labo-ratory environment [18–21]. This evaluation included aspects of accuracy, behaviour in respect to time and usability in the operation room. Some results are listed in table 1 [22].

Due to this results a positive vote to our request submitted to the ethics commission in Heidelberg was received in December 2003.

In May 2004 clinical studies in cranio-maxillofacial surgery have been initiated at the Department of Oral and Maxillofacial Surgery/University of Heidelberg. The first clinical case was a cyst removal from the lower jaw. Two surgeons evaluated the INPRES system for about 15 minutes during this clinical trial. Two engineers observed the tech-nical process of INPRES and assisted the registration and calibration process. Registra-tion had to be repeated once for good results. Both surgeons calibrated successfully with first trial. No problems occurred during the operation. Visibility of the virtual cyst was excellent and overlay correct. Maximum deviation was approximated about 1-2 mm.

**Table 1.** Results of accuracy tests performed with INPRES in a laboratory environment.

| Feature tested | Average deviation | Max. deviation | Min. deviation | Standard deviation |
|---|---|---|---|---|
| INPRES (overall system) | 1.46 mm | 4.07 mm | 0.42 mm | 0.88 mm |

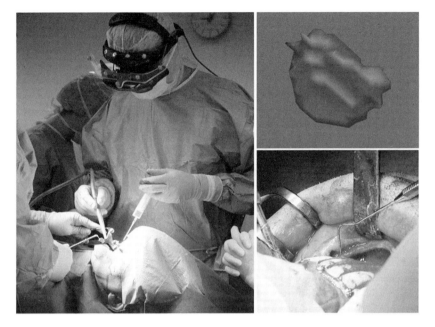

**Figure 1.** left: surgeon using the INPRES system, top right: segmented cyst, bottom right: patient after removal of the cyst.

## 4. Conclusion

The result of this first clinical testing showed that the precision and manageability of the system meets clinical demands in selected operations. Displaying virtual objects directly in the surgical site will have an impact on the work of surgeons. With regard to ergonomics the system offered a crucial advantage compared to previous navigation systems: firstly, the surgeon does not have to alternately watch the surgical site and the monitor, and secondly, no navigation instruments with large infrared tracking markers are used anymore. The fact that the complete usual instruments – to go from the scalpel, the drill, the oscillating saw to the raspatory – could be applied and be easily guided along the projected lines, had been considered to be a significant improvement by the operating team.

## 5. Further Work

From the technical point of view there are two main topics we are working on. First topic is the realization of a state of the art human-machine-interface. At the moment the surgeon interacts with the system through an operator who receives the commands and informs the surgeon about the status of the system. In order to decrease reaction time we plan to integrate speech recognition and speech output. Additional we will enable interaction with a sterile miniature keypad, which could be handled by the operator. The system status will be visualized directly in the display device. A limitation to selected information seems to be adequate.

Second topic is the improvement of the calibration process using new hardware devices. The construction of a tool called calibration bank is planned. It consists mainly of a maneuverable calibration object and a head clamp. Using this new device we hope to reduce the effect of tremor during calibration process and improve therefore total accuracy of the system.

## 6. Discussion

The INPRES system provides the surgeon with visual information from preoperative planning data in a reasonable way. Further improvements of accuracy can be obtained by modifying the calibration process. A better manageability will be achieved using a state of the art man-machine-interface and a new see-through display instead of the six year old Sony Glasstron.

## References

[1]  Jendrysiak, U., Gregg, S. and Weinert, J.: Virtual Access Planning for Neurosurgery with NeurOPS, Proceedings of Conference: Computer Assisted Radiology (CAR), Tokyo, Japan, June 1997.
[2]  Stein, W.: Computertomogrammbasierte 3D-Planung für die dentale Implantologie. Ph. D. Thesis, Universität Karlsruhe (TH), Germany, 1999.
[3]  Brock, O. and Kathib, O.: Real-Time Replanning in High-Dimensional Configuration Spaces Using Sets of Homotopic Paths. Proceedings of Conference: IEEE International Conference on Robotics and Automation (ICRA), San Francisco, CA, April 2000.
[4]  Schorr, O., Raczkowsky J., Woern H.: Simulation for Preoperative Planning and Intraoperative Application of Titanium Implants, Proceedings of the International Symposium on Surgery Simulation and Soft Tissue Modeling (IS4TM), France, 2003.
[5]  Grimson, E., Leventon, M., Ettinger, G. et al: Clinical Experience with a high Precision Image-Guided Neurosurgery System. Proceedings of Conference: Medical Image Computing and Computer-Assisted Intervention (MICCAI), Boston, MA, 1998.
[6]  Goebbels G., Troche K. , Braun M. et al: Development of an Augmented Reality System for intraoperative navigation in maxillo-facial surgery. Proceedings AR/VR-Statustagung Leipzig, 2004.
[7]  Hoppe, H., Däuber, S., Raczkowsky, J. et al: Intraoperative Visualization of Surgical Planning Data using Video Projectors. Proceedings of Conference: Proceedings of Conference: Medicine Meets Virtual Reality (MMVR), Newport Beach, CA, 2001.
[8]  Edwards, P., King, A., Hawkes, D. et al: Stereo Augmented Reality in the Surgical Microscope. Proceedings of Conference: Medicine Meets Virtual Reality (MMVR), Newport Beach, CA, 1999.
[9]  Birkfellner, W., Figl, M., Huber et al.: Calibration of a Head-Mounted Operating Microscope for Augmented Reality Visualization in CAS. Proceedings of Conference: Computer Assisted Radiology and Surgery (CARS), Berlin, Germany, June 2001.
[10]  Rosenthal, M., State, A., Lee, J.et al: Augmented Reality Guidance for Needle Biopsies: A Randomized, Controlled Trial in Phantoms. Proceedings of Conference: Medical Image Computing and Computer-Assisted Intervention (MICCAI), Utrecht, The Netherlands, 2001.
[11]  Liao, H., Nakajima, S., Iwahara, M.et al: Intra-operative Real-Time 3-D Information Display System Based on Integral Videography. Proceedings of Conference: Medical Image Computing and Computer-Assisted Intervention (MICCAI), Utrecht, The Netherlands, 2001.
[12]  Hoppe H., Marmulla R., Raczkowsky J. et al: Spatial Augmented Reality for Head Surgery: First Clinical Results, Proceedings of the International Symposium on Computer Aided Surgery around the Head, 2003.
[13]  Haag C., Brief J., Schorr O. et al: Clinical evaluation of the operation planning system KasOp using the "phantom" - new aspects of pre- and intraoperative computer-assisted surgery, Computer Assisted Radiology and Surgery (CARS), London, 2003.

[14] S.Seifert, O. Burgert, R. Dillmann: MEDIFRAME - An Extendable Software Framework for Medical Applications, Surgetica Grenoble France 2002.

[15] Ghanai S., Eggers G., Marmulla R. et al: Calibration of a stereo see-through head-mounted display, Workshop Medical Robotics, Navigation and Visualization, Remagen, 2004.

[16] Genc Y. et al. Practical solutions for calibration of optical see-through devices. Tagungsband: IEEE and ACM International Symposium on Mixed and Augmented Reality (ISMAR), Seiten 169-175, Darmstadt, 2002. IEEE CS Press.

[17] Burgert O., Seifert S., Salb T. et al: A System for Preoperative Planning of Soft Tissue and Bone Implantats, Computer Assisted Radiology and Surgery (CARS), London, 2003.

[18] Salb, T., Brief, J., Burgert, O. et al: An Augmented Reality System for Intraoperative Presentation of Planning and Simulation Results. Proceedings of 2nd Workshop: European Advanced Robotic Systems Development - Medical Robotics, Pisa, Italy, September 1999.

[19] Salb, T., Brief, J., Burgert, O. et al: Intraoperative Presentation of Surgical Planning and Simulation Results using a Stereoscopic See-Through Head-Mounted Display. Proceedings of Conference: Stereoscopic Displays and Applications, Part of Electronic Imaging / Photonics West (SPIE), San Jose, CA, January 2000.

[20] Salb, T., Burgert, O., Gockel, T. et al: Comparison of Tracking Techniques for Intraoperative Presentation of Medical Data using a See-Through Head-Mounted Display. Proceedings of Conference: Medicine Meets Virtual Reality (MMVR), Newport Beach, CA, January 2001.

[21] Brief, J., Hassfeld, S., Salb T. et al: Clinical Evaluation of a See-Through Display for Intraoperative Presentation of Planning Data. Proceedings of Conference: Israeli Symposium on Computer-Integrated Surgery, Medical Robotics and Medical Imaging (ISRACAS), Haifa, May 2000.

[22] Salb T., Brief J., Burgert O. et al: Evaluation of INPRES – Intraoperative Presentation of Surgical Planning and Simulation Results Proceedings of Conference: Medicine Meets Virtual Reality (MMVR), Newport Beach, CA, January 2003.

*Medicine Meets Virtual Reality 13*
*James D. Westwood et al. (Eds.)*
*IOS Press, 2005*

# Construction of a High-Tech Operating Room for Image-Guided Surgery using VR

Naoki SUZUKI [a], Asaki HATTORI [a], Shigeyuki SUZUKI [a], Yoshito OTAKE [a],
Mitsuhiro HAYASHIBE [a], Susumu KOBAYASHI [b], Takehiko NEZU [c],
Haruo SAKAI [d] and Yuji UMEZAWA [e]

[a] *Institute for High Dimensional Medical Imaging, The Jikei Univ. Sch. of Med.,
4-11-1 Izumihoncho, Komae-shi 201-8601, Tokyo, Japan*
[b] *Dept. of Surg., The Jikei Univ. Sch. of Med.*
[c] *Dept. of Anesthesiology, The Jikei Univ. Sch. of Med.*
[d] *Dept. of Neurosurgery, The Jikei Univ. Sch. of Med.*
[e] *Dept of Otorhinolaryngology, The Jikei Univ. Sch. of Med.*

**Abstract.** This project aimed to construct an operating room to implement high dimensional (3D, 4D) medical imaging and medical virtual reality techniques that would enable clinical tests for new surgical procedures. We designed and constructed such an operating room at Dai-san Hospital, the Jikei Univ. School of Medicine, Tokyo, Japan. The room was equipped with various facilities for image-guided, robot and tele- surgery. In this report, we describe an outline of our "high-tech operating room" and future plans.

## 1. Preface

We aimed to construct an operating room equipped with all devices utilizing high dimensional (3D, 4D) medical imaging techniques that enable the study of new surgical procedures; ones that indicate the directions of future surgical operations. This ideal operating room has been designed as a place to examine through clinical testing the various image-guided surgery systems and robotic surgery devices that have been developed to date. The room was built in the new operations building of Dai-San Hospital, Jikei University. Moreover, this operating room installed equipment with the intention of utilizing new robotic surgery techniques such as tele-surgery. This report describes the outline of this "high-tech operating room for image-guided surgery" and reviews future plans.

## 2. Methods

This operating room was designed and constructed to provide new functions such as 3D and 4D image applying real-time imaging and medical use VR technology that would be able to ascertain the structures of affected regions. In this operating room, a C-arm typed CT (Siemens-Asahi Medical Technologies Ltd.) for acquiring the 3D structures in the operating view and a non-metal operating table with movable type rail (MAQUET GmbH & Co. KG) that does not interrupt CT measurements were installed. As well, enable the fusion of various data streams, an optical 3D position sensor (Optotrak: Northern Digital Inc.), arm-type monitors for an operator's view, a computer for processing images, a large-size transparent monitor were hung from the ceiling of the operating room. Four liquid crystal display (LCD) arm-type monitors to provide an operator's view, designed and manufactured in consideration of surgical clarity, were installed around the operating table. The monitors were installed using a multi-joint arm, so that an operator would be able to freely choose from various information on images in the immediate proximity of the operating view. Moreover, it was equipped with a sterilization lever, and the LCD monitor could move wherever the operator needed it during the operation. The large-size transparent monitor aims to share information among staff in the operating room. This system can provide various images during the operation using the 40 inch-transparent hologram screen and the LCD projector, both hanging from the ceiling. The large-sized transparent screen was used to avoid there being any large dead angle in the operating room. Moreover, to prevent exhaust dust from the LCD projector's fan polluting the air-conditioning in the operating room, it was built into an exclusively designed transparent-globular form acrylic case, and exhausted to outside the operating room with a duct connected to the case. All image outputs to these displays are performed from the computer console in the operating room. We also decided to install a duct to exhaust the dust generated by fans in the equipment installed in the console, such as the Graphic Workstation, the PC, and the controller for 3D position sensors, would not be discharged in the operating room. Furthermore, we assumed that surgery, such as an endoscopic, that needs the operator to look at a monitor will increase; so we decided to use diffused green lighting that can have its brightness adjusted, instead of the usual operation room lighting, to aid the operators concentration. A complete view of this operating room is shown in Figure 1, and the computer console located in the operating room is shown in Figure 2. It is possible to output the images from each computer to optional display units by the matrix switcher in the console. Figure 3 shows the ceiling-mounted transparent hologram screen and projector.

Further, our research institute and this model operating room are connected by an optical fiber link, which makes it possible to utilize in the operating room a visual super-computer (ONYX3400: Silicon Graphics Inc.) installed in the research institute.

We have developed two different image display systems for surgical navigation using these equipments. One is a video see-through type display, and the other is an optical see-through type display. These systems enable surgeons to observe a patient's inner structure during surgery. The systems are composed of the ceiling-hanged LCD monitor and the optical 3D position sensor. Both the monitor and the objective inner structure are registered by an optical sensor. The video see-through type data fusion display also has a small size video camera on the back of the monitor. The monitor displays in 3D a patient's inner structure, which is superimposed onto a captured surgical field image. The optical see-through type data fusion display has a semi-transparent mirror in front of the monitor. The image displayed on the monitor is projected onto the mirror. As well, the surgeon's head position is measured by a 3D position sensor and the data fusion image is synchronized to the view of the surgeon. The surgeon is able to observe the surgical field and the inner structure of the patient through the mirror from various viewpoints.

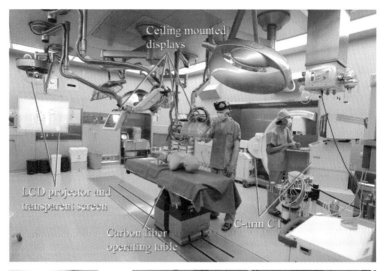

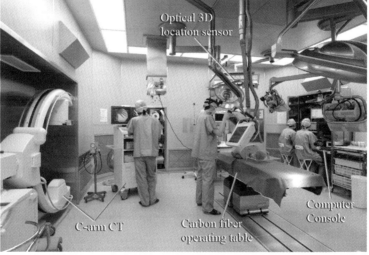

**Figure 1.** Overviews of the high-tech operating room from different points of view.

## 3. Results and Discussion

Figure 4 shows the appearance of the video see-through type display that uses a liver phantom (a) and an elbow model (b). The inner structural models are superimposed onto the captured surgical view. The appearance of the optical see-through type display is shown at Figure 5. The surgeon's head position is measured by a 3D position sensor (a). The surgeon is able to observe the patient's inner structure from various viewpoints.

In completing this operating room, we provided a new site for clinical studies that would not only clinically evaluate the data fusion and robotic systems involved in endoscopy, which have been developed to date, but one that would also construct a correspondence with the robotic surgery system or with tele-surgery, both areas we believe will increase in popularity. We intend to undertake research and better develop each system, and so more fully demonstrate the features of this operating room.

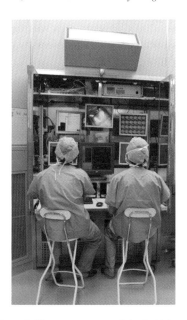
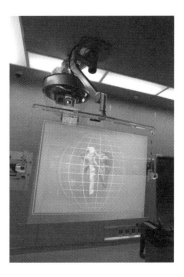

**Figure 2.** The computer console in the high-tech operating room.

**Figure 3.** The transparent hologram screen and the sealing formula LCD projector.

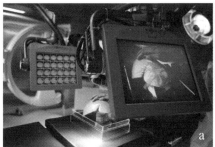
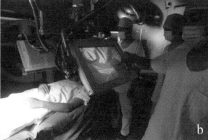

**Figure 4.** An appearance of the video see-through type display using a liver phantom model (a) and an elbow model (b). The reconstructed organ models are superimposed onto the captured surgical view.

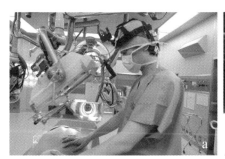
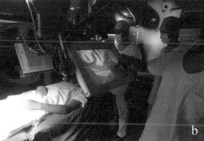

**Figure 5.** An appearance of the optical see-through type display using a head model. The 3D position sensor is attached to the surgeon's head (a) and tracks the position of the surgeon's head. The surgeon is able to see the actual surgical view and the reconstructed inner structures simultaneously.

This operating room was completed on 17 July 2003. This research was supported of the Maintenance Enterprise of the High-Tech Research Center, the Ministry of Education, Culture, Sports, Science and Technology, Japan.

## References

[1] Suzuki N, Hattori A, Suzuki S, Otake Y, Hayashibe M, Kobayashi S, Sakai H, Umezawa Y. Design and construction of a high-tech navigation operating room for various image-guided surgeries. J JSCAS 2003; 5(3): 257-8.
[2] Otake Y, Suzuki N, Hattori A, Suzuki S, Hayashibe M, Kobayashi S. Development of image display devices for the data fusion system at open surgery. J JSCAS 2003; 5(3): 349-50.

*Medicine Meets Virtual Reality 13*
*James D. Westwood et al. (Eds.)*
*IOS Press, 2005*

# Tele-Surgical Simulation System for Training in the Use of da Vinci™ Surgery

Shigeyuki SUZUKI [a], Naoki SUZUKI [a], Mitsuhiro HAYASHIBE [a], Asaki HATTORI [a],
Kozo KONISHI [b], Yoshihiro KAKEJI [b] and Makoto HASHIZUME [b]

[a] *Institute for High Dimensional Medical Imaging, The Jikei University School of
Medicine 4-11-1 Izumihoncho, Komae-shi, Tokyo, 201-8601, Japan*
[b] *Center for Integration of Advanced Medicine and Innovative Technology, Kyushu
University Hospital, Fukuoka, Japan*

**Abstract.** Laparoscopic surgery including robotic surgery allows the surgeon to be
able to conduct minimally invasive surgery. A surgeon is required to master difficult skills for this surgery to compensate for the narrow field of view, limitation
of work space, and the lack of depth sensation. To counteract these drawbacks, we
have been developing a training simulation system that can allow surgeons to practice and master surgical procedures. In addition, our system aims to distribute a
simulation program, to provide a means of collaboration between remote hospitals,
and to be able to provide a means for guidance from an expert surgeon. In this paper, we would like to show the surgery simulation for da Vinci™ surgery, in particular a cholecystectomy. The integral parts of this system are a soft tissue model
which is created by the sphere-filled method enabling real-time deformations based
on a patient's data, force feedback devices known as a PHANToM™ and the Internet connection. By using this system a surgeon can perform surgical maneuvers
such as pushing, grasping, and detachment in real-time manipulation. Moreover,
using the broadband communication, we can perform the tele-surgical simulation
for training.

## 1. Introduction

Recently robotic surgery systems such as the da Vinci™ and the ZEUS™ (Intuitive
Surgical Inc.) have been applied in clinical situations. The surgeons can conduct operations with minimally invasive surgery (MIS) and with accurate manipulation. However,
because of the narrow field of view, it is necessary for surgeons to master the handling
of the instruments and to simulate and practice surgical procedures as well as the general laparoscopic surgery. Moreover the difficulty level of the surgical techniques is increased by the difference in the handling of the tools between robotic surgery and general laparoscopic surgery. Hence, the simulation system of MIS for surgical training can
allow surgeons to enhance their skills in the surgery. In this study, we aimed to develop a
surgical training simulation that can provide a method of training and mastering surgical
procedures with the da Vinci™ system. The target operation of our system as the first
stage is a cholecystectomy. In addition, we aimed to develop a tele-surgery simulator and
construct a training simulation center that enables a surgeon to distribute the simulation

program, to provide a means of collaboration between remote hospitals, and to be able to allow an opportunity for guidance from an expert surgeon.

## 2. Related Work

The soft tissue model that has the ability of the real-time and quantitative deformation is needed to develop the surgery simulation. For construction of soft tissue modeling for surgery simulation, traditionally, physically-based models such as Finite Element Method (FEM) are used [1–3]. Although FEM can represent an accurate deformation of the model according to the organ's physical phenomenon, the conventional FEM has difficulty performing in a real-time, interactive simulation except for the specified deformable region, and with automatic modeling. In telling contrast to FEM for modeling, there is also the ChainMail algorithm [4] for constructing a deformable organ model. Although this algorithm is very simple and can perform real-time simulations without using a high performance workstation, there are difficulties when it comes to ensuring the user of quantitative deformation such as volume conservation. In addition, some of MIS simulation including robotic surgery are now commercial applications [5,6]. Their application can allow the doctor to practice the basic skills and the surgical procedures for laparoscopic surgery, and they are of great interest. However they cannot install the patient data whenever necessary. So that means it is difficult for them to provide a simulation scene that will satisfy the surgeon's requirements.

We also have contributed to the development of surgery simulation [7–9]. For open surgery and tele-surgery simulation, we think that real-time and interactive simulation is the most important thing. Hence, our system has been focusing on real-time simulation.

## 3. Method

Our tele-training simulation system is a client-server one, in order to allow multiple remote accesses and get full control over the interaction between the users at the server. The server side has a super computer with the multiple CPU, Onyx3400 (Silicon Graphics Inc.), which computes all the simulation processes. The user side needs only to prepare the force feedback devices, an ordinary personal computer is suitable to control them, and the appropriate software to compile or download the client program. The connection between the server and the user is through an optical fiber line via the Internet. At first, the user executes remote login procedure using secure shell (SSH) protocol. After the authentication of the user, the communication with the server program is initiated. Fig. 1 shows the global network system for tele-virtual surgery. The user can access the specific program on the server from this network.

To apply the surgery simulation program in wide area, the user side has to equip the force feedback device that can obtain easily without requiring a special manufacturing. Therefore, the daVinci$^{TM}$ operation console in our system consists of PHANToM$^{TM}$ Desktop (SensAble Technologies Inc.), which has gained widespread use. To emulate the da Vinci$^{TM}$ forceps manipulation in this system, the tip motion of the daVinci forceps is calibrated from the handling of the PHANToM$^{TM}$. In addition, one of the functions of this system is to indicate a warning to the user through a beep if the user's manipulation is mistaken and records the user's score on the server.

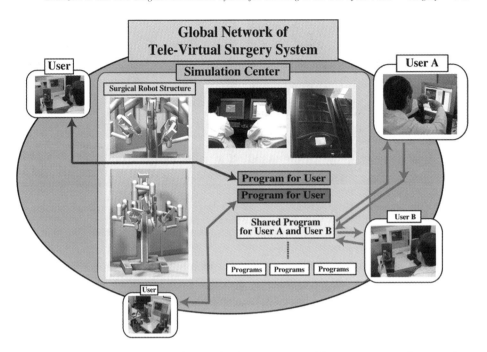

**Figure 1.** The global network system for tele-virtual surgery system. The user can access the appropriate program on the server from the Internet.

In our research, we constructed a soft tissue model known as a sphere-filled model for real-time simulation. This model was developed through current research [9]. This model consists of a group of small rigid spheres of the same radius, with triangle polygons at the surface. As well, this model can be constructed automatically and quickly because we fill the inside of the organ's contour with element spheres, if the organ's region can be determined. That is, our system has no problem providing the user patient's organ model.

The deformation shows the interaction of the internal spheres. If a collision is detected between a sphere (**$Sn$**) and its neighboring sphere, **$Sn$** is changed as follows:

$$\delta Sn = \text{length} * \textbf{\textit{vector}}/\text{distance} \tag{1}$$

where **$Sn$** is the positional vector of the spheres, **$\delta Sn$** is the displacement vector, ***vector*** is the vector from the neighboring sphere to **$Sn$**, length is the overlap between **$Sn$** and the neighboring sphere, and distance is the length between **$Sn$** and the neighboring sphere. Then, if a collision is detected between **$Sn$** and an external force is generated, the effect of gravity is generated for the sphere's movement (**$\delta Sn +$** = ***gravity***, where ***gravity*** is the constant vector). This model automatically calculates the connection between a sphere and a polygon at the organ's surface in the model construction step. Hence, by following the internal spheres' movements, the surface can show the deformation.

In this study, a gallbladder is reconstructed with 2 mm radius spheres while a liver is reconstructed with 6 mm spheres, in order to represent the deformation responding to the organ's shape and size. Fig. 2 shows the reconstructed soft tissue model.

Detachment procedures for a gallbladder are as follows;

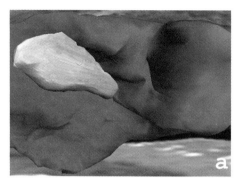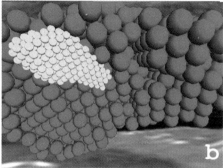

**Figure 2.** The reconstructed liver and gallbladder model. a shows the texture mapped organ model using the surface rendering method. b shows the internal spheres of each organ.

1) The spheres of the gallbladder model, which belong to the contact region between the liver and the gallbladder, are calculated.
2) The collision between the calculated spheres and the electrical scalpel are detected as the left forceps grasp the gallbladder.
3) The detected spheres move the vector from the sphere's center to the left forceps's grasp point on the organ surface.
4) The gallbladder is removed from the liver by repeating procedures 1) to 3).

Regarding the da Vinci$^{TM}$ modeling, the whole structures of the da Vinci$^{TM}$ and forceps, such as long tip forceps, cadiere forceps, round tip scissors and cautery with a spatula, are measured. Then these are reconstructed as the three dimensional CAD data.

## 4. Result

Fig. 3 shows the deformation of the gallbladder model as a time-sequence image for removal of the gallbladder. In this figure, the left forceps is manipulated for the grasping procedures while the right is used for the dissection. Then, the force feedback parameter was computed and transmitted to PAHTNoM$^{TM}$ device on the basis of the sphere-filled model's algorithm [9]. The visual feedback was about 30 Hz and the haptic feedback was about 1,000 Hz for a local area network environment. If the forceps are in contact with the liver surface or a collision between forceps is detected, this system indicates a warning. In addition, the gallbladder model can show the deformation within 1.0 percent volume error at most when the model experiences deformations by pushing.

Thus, this system allows surgeons to perform and practice surgical procedures such as grasping and detachment, for training in the use of da Vinci$^{TM}$ surgery, in particular cholecystectomy. Moreover, by using our simulation system, surgeons can perform a manipulation similar to the da Vinci$^{TM}$ forceps' operation. In addition to these, by using a broadband line via the Internet, we have performed tele-surgical simulation for training between Fukuoka and Tokyo, a distance of about 1,000 kilometers.

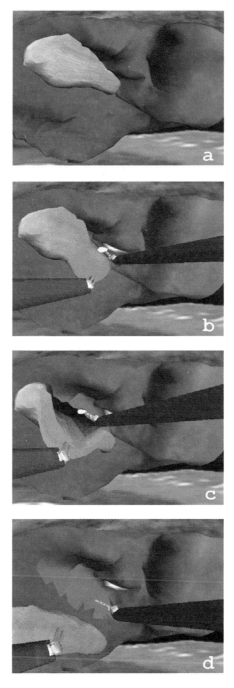

**Figure 3.** The deformation of the gallbladder model for cholecystectomy. The left forceps manipulation is grasping while the right is dissection.

## 5. Discussion

Our tele-surgical simulation system consists of the soft tissue model created by the sphere-filled method, commercial force feedback devices, and the Internet line. By using our system, surgeons can perform and practice surgical procedures, and we have realized tele-virtual surgery over a long distance. In this system, the indication as a warning message is useful for the surgeon not only to get a sense of the depth, but also understand and validate the user's surgical techniques objectively. In addition, with respect to the soft tissue model, the size selected was the best choice for real-time and quantitative deformation in the gallbladder model, although the number of internal spheres depends on the computing capability.

The target of our current research is training simulation for robotic surgery and work is underway to achieve our purpose, but it will be possible to apply to the general laparoscopic surgery. In the near future, we will be able to improve the performance of other surgical maneuvers including general laparoscopic surgery. We will complete the server system for tele-training simulation and have plans to construct a training center for the distribution of training programs on a global scale.

## References

[1]  S. Cotin, H. Delingette, and N. Ayache, "Real-time elastic deformations of soft tissues for surgery simulation," IEEE Transactions on Visualization and Computer Graphics, vol. 5, no. 1, pp. 62-73, 1999.
[2]  C. Mendoza and C. Laugier, "Tissue Cutting Using Finite Elements and Force Feedback," Lecture Notes in Computer Science 2673, Surgery Simulation and Soft Tissue Modeling, pp. 175-182. 2003.
[3]  J. Berkley, G. Turkiyyah, D. Berg, M. Ganter, and S. Weghorst, "Real-Time Finite Element Modeling for Surgery Simulation: An Application to Virtual Suturing," IEEE Transactions on Visualization and Computer Graphics, vol. 10, no. 3, pp. 314-325, 2004.
[4]  S.F. Firsken-Gibson, "Using Linked Volumes to Model Object Collisions, Deformation, Cutting, Carving, and Joining," IEEE Transactions on Visualization and Computer Graphics, vol. 5, no. 4, pp. 333-348, 1999.
[5]  The LapSim System, http://www.surgical-scinece.com
[6]  The SimSurgery$^{TM}$ Educational Platform (SEP) for robotic surgery, http://www.simsurgery.no
[7]  N. Suzuki, A. Hattori, T. Ezumi, A. Uchiyama, T. Kumano, A. Ikemoto, Y. Adachi, and A. Takatsu, "Simulator for virtual surgery using deformable organ models and force feed-back system," Medicine Meets Virtual Reality, pp. 227-233, 1998.
[8]  N. Suzuki, A. Hattori, S. Suzuki, MP. Baur, A. Hirner, S. Kobayashi, Y. Yamazaki, and Y. Adachi, "Real-time surgical simulation with haptic sensation as collaborated works between Japan and Germany," Lecture Notes in Computer Science 2208, Proc. Medical Image Computing and Computer-Assisted Intervention-MICCAI2001, pp. 1015-1021, 2001.
[9]  S. Suzuki, N. Suzuki, A. Hattori, A. Uchiyama, and S. Kobayashi, "Sphere-Filled Organ Model for Virtual Surgery System," IEEE Transactions on Medical Imaging, vol. 23, no. 6, pp. 714-722, 2004.

*Medicine Meets Virtual Reality 13*
*James D. Westwood et al. (Eds.)*
*IOS Press, 2005*

# Homeland Security and Virtual Reality: Building a Strategic Adaptive Response System (STARS)

Christopher SWIFT, Joseph M. ROSEN, Gordon BOEZER, Jaron LANIER,
Joseph V. HENDERSON, Alan LIU, Ronald C. MERRELL, Sinh NGUYEN,
Alex DEMAS, Elliot B. GRIGG, Matthew F. McKNIGHT,
Janelle CHANG and C. Everett KOOP

*Dartmouth-Hitchcock Medical Center, One Medical Center Drive*
*Lebanon, NH 03756, United States of America*

**Abstract.** The advent of the Global War on Terrorism (GWOT) underscored the need to improve the U.S. disaster response paradigm. Existing systems involve numerous agencies spread across disparate functional and geographic jurisdictions. The current architecture remains vulnerable to sophisticated terrorist strikes. To address these vulnerabilities, we must continuously adapt and improve our Homeland Security architecture. Virtual Reality (VR) technologies will help model those changes and integrate technologies. This paper provides a broad overview of the strategic threats, together with a detailed examination of how specific VR technologies could be used to ensure successful disaster responses.

## 1. Introduction

### 1.1. Asymmetric Threats

The United States emerged from the Cold War as a preponderant power with no near-term competitor [1]. As the threat of nuclear conflict faded, however, new subnational and transnational threats challenged the emerging international order [2]. Failed states and terrorist syndicates undermined Westphalian archetypes. As Al Qaeda rose to new prominence, the global threat axis shifted from "superpower contests to a much older struggle: that between North and South, between the powerful and the weak" [3]. Homeland security eclipsed national security.

From David and Goliath to the Greeks at Marathon, the discourse of weak against strong is as old as the recorded history of armed conflict. Yet two dynamics amplify the contemporary threat. The first is the compression of time and space by global communications and transportation networks [1]. The second is the progressive proliferation of Chemical, Biological, Nuclear, Radiological and Explosive (CBRNE) weapons technologies [4]. Together, these trends create a dynamic geopolitical environment in which otherwise marginal insurgents can punch above their weight while minimizing the prospect of strategic blowback.

It is, however, an exaggeration to suggest that transnational terrorism poses an un-qualified existential threat to the United States. Short of a global thermonuclear war or unforeseen environmental cataclysms, the continued survival of the nation is not easily challenged. What is at risk is the *will* of the nation—our capacity to sustain popular con-sent for national policy in the face of political intimidation. As Prussian strategist Karl von Clausewitz observed, war is "a struggle of moral and physical forces by means of the latter" [5].

The threat posed by a Strategic Economic Attack (SEA) underscores the importance of those moral forces. Simultaneous bioterrorist strikes in multiple metropolitan areas, for example, would require swift isolation and treatment. Prolonged quarantines could impair regional deliveries of critical goods and services. Combined with a concurrent cyber offensive on U.S. banks and securities markets, the nation might witness massive losses in economic productivity, personal wealth and public confidence.

Against that backdrop, the strategic value of an effective, coordinated disaster re-sponse should not be understated. Victory in the Global War on Terrorism (GWOT) will require not just the ability to thwart terrorist attacks, but also the capacity to reduce the scope and political significance of such events if they do occur. Failure to learn this les-son now will only invite costly reforms in the future. Failure to act will threaten the will of the nation.

This paper explores the role of Virtual Reality (VR) technologies in meeting Home-land Security challenges. It does so in five stages. First, it will examine the past history and future implications of Biological Warfare (BW). Second it will identify existing vul-nerabilities in the U.S. disaster response architecture. Third, it will discuss the charac-teristics of a Strategic Adaptive Response System (STARS) for homeland defense [6]. Fourth, it will explore VR applications in STARS and the benefits accruing from the same. Finally, it will conclude by briefly assessing the integration of current technologies and the impetus for future change.

## 1.2. Biological Warfare

The germ theory of disease marked a revolution in the capacity to identify and contain the spread of deadly pathogens. Yet the rise of epidemiology and prophylactic vaccination also witnessed the systematic application of scientific knowledge in the production and weaponization of biological agents. With the exception of Germany, all of the major belligerents in World War Two maintained robust BW programs [7]. British anthrax tests precipitated the prolonged evacuation of remote Scottish islands. Japanese experiments on Chinese civilians still underscore contemporary friction between Beijing and Tokyo.

Military strategists note numerous limitations on the use of BW in conventional warfare. Among them are "the potential unpredictability of the effects of a BW attack, and the required incubation period between a target's exposure to BW agents and the onset of disease. . ." [7] In Trinitarian conflicts, uncertainty enhances deterrence. BW is therefore a terminal option—the poor man's nuclear bomb [7].

These dynamics are radically different in asymmetric war. Uncertainty matters less when insurgents operate within the target society, or when the attack has no swiftly dis-cernable return address. What is more, many of the characteristics that render BW un-suitable in conventional military operations make them especially desirable for terrorist attacks [8]. Silence conspires against early detection. Infection enhances public hysteria.

The 2000 TOPOFF exercises in Denver, Colorado, and subsequent simulations by ANSWER and Dartmouth College illuminated the threat BW could pose to U.S. security [8]. There are, however, notable differences between BW agents. Some are deadly but not terribly infectious. Others are highly infectious but seldom lethal. Pathogens that fall into these categories are tactical in scope: they harm those infected. As with the anthrax attack on the U.S. Congress, public apprehension would likely reinforce rather than challenge the will of the nation.

A strategic BW weapon, by comparison, would be lethal, drug-resistant and highly infectious. Anthropomorphic infections would also be difficult to distinguish from naturally occurring phenomena. Early symptoms from a staged release of SARS, for example, would resemble those of common seasonal ailments. Transmitted through the global transportation network, SARS's long incubation period might swiftly outpace the public health infrastructure and precipitate the need for economically deleterious quarantines [9]. Even limited outbreaks would carry serious consequences, as evident from the experience of Hong Kong and Toronto.

## 2. Disaster Management

### 2.1. Existing Vulnerabilities

The threat of terrorist attacks with CBRNE weapons underscored the Bush Doctrine [4]. Though highly controversial, this renewed focus on strategic pre-emption correctly acknowledged the difficulty of deterring non-state actors and focused instead on interdicting Al Qaeda operations. By privileging offensive operations outside the continental United States (OCONUS), the Bush Administration hoped to prevent further attacks on CONUS itself.

There is much to be said for taking the fight to one's adversary. The challenge, however, is to do so while simultaneously enhancing our capacity for self-defense. Despite widespread official concern regarding CBRNE attacks, there is considerable dissonance between the current structure of the U.S. disaster response system and the threat posed by transnational terrorism. Notwithstanding significant increases in Homeland Security funding, the scope and structure of our emergency response system remains little different from that first developed during the Regan administration.

The U.S. government established the National Disaster Management System (NDMS) in 1983 with the object of coordinating a federal response in the event of a major natural or transportation disaster [10]. Drawing resources from the Department of Defense, Health and Veteran Affairs, planners designed a system capable of evacuating and treating as many as 100,000 casualties in remote locations. The resulting architecture proved suitable for numerous applications, be they from an earthquake or support for OCONUS military operations.

In an age of asymmetric warfare, however, NDMS doctrine contains two notable deficiencies. First, unlike conventional disasters, an effective disaster response may require isolation and containment, rather than evacuation and treatment. This is particularly true for events involving Chemical, Biological or Radiological agents, whose spread threatens civilians and first responders alike. Absent adaptive doctrines and adequate planning, responding to certain terrorist events could ultimately exacerbate rather than ameliorate the crisis.

Second, NDMS is an echelon-based system. Local personnel are the first to respond. State and federal support arrives only after decision-makers declare an emergency. Hence by 'the time a crisis is detected, the scale of it is appreciated, and federal resources are put into play, it may be too late' [10]. Though appropriate for natural disasters, this incremental operational tempo could prove devastating in a swiftly escalating bioterrorist event.

## 2.2. Strategic Adaptive Response System

We believe the United States should transform the current disaster response paradigm through informational superiority and network-based organization [11]. To do so, it must establish a Strategic Adaptive Response System (STARS) that facilitates the coordination of resources, personnel and expertise within and across numerous jurisdictions. The object is not to centralize or federalize the emergency Command and Control ($C^2$) system, but to knit the current patchwork quilt of agencies, capabilities and personnel into a dynamic and highly flexible net-centric architecture.

STARS would possess three key characteristics. First, it would employ an "integrated grid of sensors, communications networks and shared resources... [to] provide local first responders with the information richness and reach necessary to mount an instantaneous, fully integrated disaster management operation" [9]. Though each individual asset would maintain its own unique characteristics, the broader architecture would build upon "an overriding philosophy of designing for effected integrated functionality" [11].

Second, STARS would establish a distributed, multi-nodal $C^2$ network flexible enough to respond to multi-modal, multi-site events, yet robust enough to resist attacks on the U.S. critical information infrastructure [12]. For this reason, major communications nodes should be mobile or deployed to geographically isolated locations. Aircraft and naval vessels with global satellite uplinks are an obvious choice, particularly in instances where infectious disease, computer viruses, or other threats overwhelm the primary communications and transportation networks.

Finally, STARS would employ the core elements of Cybercare to treat isolated casualties from remote locations [10]. Videoconferencing and other telemedicine technologies would allow infectious disease experts to diagnose BW victims from institutions across United States [11]. Teleoperation applications would allow surgeons to provide treatment in crisis where casualty tempos outpace the scope and scale of local medical personnel [13]. Mobile robots would allow the collection of medical informatics from "hot zones" while minimizing potential exposure among emergency personnel.

To be sure, technology cannot replace human observation, analysis and judgment. It can, however, facilitate the rapid dissemination of critical information—thus reducing the fog and friction that often hamper crisis operations [11]. What is more, new software and hardware could amplify the effectiveness of existing personnel. EMTs using personal data assistants (PDAs) equipped with global positioning system (GPS) technology, for example, can identify victims and perform triage while simultaneously uploading information to incident commanders [14]. Combined with Radio Frequency Identification Devices (RFIDs), these and other point of care technologies could substantially enhance existing triage systems.

## 3. Virtual Reality

### 3.1. Training, Education and Simulation

Although the importance of such systems is recognized within the U.S. Government, state and local officials remain ill prepared for a CBRNE attack. Research by the Federation of American Scientists found that "physicians. Nurses, emergency medical workers, police and fire officials feel unprepared for a WMD emergency—particularly at the level of cities and counties" [15]. To address these apparent shortcomings, we must first rethink out approach to disaster response, as well as the manner in which we train first responders.

Training, education and simulation technologies will play a central role in implementing and sustaining STARS. Computer-based Training (CBT) and interactive video-conferencing and simulations will reduce the time necessary for hands-on training while improving the knowledge base first responders bring to field exercises and actual emergencies. Using standardized, interactive curricula, small cadres of trainers could supplement CBRNE response training a local fire and police departments whenever necessary.

VR will be a critical element in educational applications. The Virtual Terrorism Response Academy (VTRA), for example, creates a reusable virtual learning environment to prepare emergency responders to deal with high risk, low frequency events. Currently under development at Dartmouth Medical School, the academy trains through apprenticeship, allowing first responders to pursue a broad spectrum of relevant skill under the guidance of instructors who are both master practitioners and master trainers. The mentors are real experts videotaped according to courseware designs. Their tutorials are available to first responders at any time or location via the Internet or CD-ROM [16].

### 3.2. Wide-Area Virtual Environments

Simulations present another important VR application. Just as war games are invaluable in evaluating military operations, simulated disasters will allow the diverse, diffuse elements of STARS to identify and correct failings in the response architecture. Joint exercises would occur across a Wide-Area Virtual Environment (WAVE) in which participants would interact with each other and shared data sources [17]. Combined with remote sensing, Unmanned Aerial Vehicles (UAVs) and Unmanned Ground Vehicles (UGVs), crisis coordinators could interact directly with the incident cite. Moreover, secure satellite communications would allow them to do so from various isolated locations, be it a hospital, a regional emergency center or even a naval vessel deployed on the other side of the world.

Drills employing WAVE systems would also improve "jointness" among the various elements of the homeland security architecture. In simulation, first responders and incident commanders could assume each other's roles. Fire fighters, police officers and EMTs might use simulations for local and regional cross training. Decision makers could gain first-hand experience of the diverse resources, skills, and tasks necessary to ensure an effective disaster response. Properly configured, WAVE might enhance coordination not just in the tactical and operational spheres, but also in the domains of public policy and national strategy.

## 4. Conclusions

As the threat of transnational terrorism grows, so does the need for STARS. Building this system poses numerous challenges, however. The ideal network must be net-centric, distributed and robust. The ideal first responders must be well rounded, prepared for any eventuality and capable of working jointly. A centralized, federally controlled emergency management system will not produce these characteristics. Instead, the optimal solution is to establish a dynamic milieu in the varied and often highly diffuse elements of the U.S. disaster response infrastructure can communicate, coordinate and operate with one another.

This objective is not achievable absent the implementation of cutting-edge technologies. Against that backdrop, VR represents a sea change in our ability to accumulate, organize and employ numerous data-streams. The ability to interact with incident site in real time from numerous remote locations will provide first responders and those responsible for their oversight with powerful tools. Combined with the broad dissemination of low-cost, high-yield training curricula, simulation could provide an invaluable means of defense against an audacious adversary.

The purpose of STARS is to prevent tactical strikes from assuming strategic proportions. While it may not be possible to prevent terrorist attacks, it is possible to ameliorate deleterious economic, social and political outcomes. The latter objective remains crucial, both for the protection of our homeland and for the preservation of U.S. leadership in the international community.

## References

[1] Z. Brzezinski, *The Choice: Global Domination or Global Leadership*. New York, NY: Basic Books, 2004.

[2] S. J. Tangredi, "Globalization and Sea Power: Overview and Context," in *Globalization and Maritime Power*, S. J. Tangredi, Ed. Washington, DC: National Defense University, 2002, pp. 1-39.

[3] T. Barkawi, "On the pedagogy of 'small wars'," *International Affairs*, vol. 80, pp. 19-38, 2004.

[4] G. W. Bush, "National Security Strategy of the United States," The White House, Washington, DC September 17 2002.

[5] K. V. Clausewitz, *On War*. Princeton, NJ: Princeton University Press, 1976.

[6] Concept developed by Christopher Swift and Joseph M. Rosen, Dartmouth College.

[7] S. B. Martin, "The Role of Biological Weapons in International Politics," *Journal of Strategic Studies*, vol. 25, pp. 63-98, 2002.

[8] J. M. Rosen, C. E. Koop, and E. B. Grigg, "Cybercare: A System for Confronting Bioterrorism," *The Bridge*, vol. 32, pp. 34-50, 2002.

[9] J. M. Rosen, G. Boezer, C. Swift, M. F. McKnight, E. B. Grigg, and C. E. Koop, "Red Threats, White Space and Blue Response: Building a Strategic Adaptive Response System (STARS)," Dartmouth College, Hanover, NH September 2004.

[10] J. M. Rosen, E. Grigg, S. McGrath, S. Lillibridge, and C. E. Koop, "Cybercare NDMS: An Improved Strategy for Biodefense Using Information Technologies," in *Integration of Health Telematics into Medical Practice*, M. Nerlich and U. Schaechinger, Eds. Amsterdam: IOS Press, 2003, pp. 95-114.

[11] J. M. Rosen, E. B. Grigg, M. F. McKnight, C. E. Koop, S. Lillibridge, B. L. Kindberg, L. Hettinger, and R. Hutchinson, "Transforming Medicine for Biodefense and Healthcare Delivery: Developing a Dual-Use Doctrine that Utilizes Information Superiority and Network-Based Organization," *IEEE Engineering in Medicine and Biology*, vol. 23, pp. 89-101, 2004.

[12] Concept developed by Jaron Lanier. http://www.advanced.org/jaron/.

[13] T. Lange, D. J. Indelicato, and J. M. Rosen, "Virtual Reality in Surgical Training," *Surgical Techniques and Outcomes*, vol. 9, pp. 61-79, 2000.

[14] Concept developed by Ronald C. Merrill, Virginia Commonwealth University.

[15] H. Kelly, V. Blackwood, M. Roper, G. Higgins, G. Klein, J. Tyler, D. Fletcher, H. Jenkins, A. Chisolm, and K. Squire, "Training Technology against Terror: Using Advanced Technology to Prepare America's Emergency Medical Personnel and First Responders for a Weapons of Mass Destruction Attack," Federation of American Scientists, Washington, DC September 9 2002.

[16] Program developed by Joseph V. Henderson, Interactive Media Laboratory, Dartmouth Medical School.

[17] Concept developed by Alan Liu, Surgical Simulation Laboratory, U.S. Uniformed Services University.

*Medicine Meets Virtual Reality 13*
*James D. Westwood et al. (Eds.)*
*IOS Press, 2005*

# Haptic Interaction and Visualization of Elastic Deformation[1]

F. TAVAKKOLI ATTAR, R.V. PATEL and M. MOALLEM

*Canadian Surgical Technologies and Advanced Robotics (CSTAR)*
*and Department of Electrical and Computer Engineering*
*University of Western Ontario, London, Ontario, Canada N6A 5B9*
*e-mail: ftavakko@uwo.ca; rajni@eng.uwo.ca; mmoallem@engga.uwo.ca*

**Abstract.** In this paper, we represent a new method to model real-time local and global deformations on a variety of three-dimensional sculptured surfaces governed by physical principles. The deformable objects are highly elastic with linear behavior in the range of typical haptic forces. A deformation model is developed for incompressible material based on a mapping technique and the superposition principle. The law of energy conservation is used to calculate real-time force reflection. Using the divergence theorem, force reflection is calculated for volumetric deformations.

## 1. Introduction

In developing interactive deformable models for accurate haptic applications such as surgical simulation, the speed, reliability, and realism are very important. Methods for physically-based modelling of deformable objects have been studied widely in recent years. Witkin and Baraff [4] summarize the methods and principles of physically-based modelling. In general, there are two different approaches for modelling deformable objects, the mass-spring model and the finite-element model. Gibson [1] gives a comprehensive survey on this subject. The mass-spring model requires relatively little computation time. This model has had good success in creating visually satisfactory animation. Waters [5], Lee *et al.* [6], and Platt and Badler [7] use mass-spring models for computer animation. Despite the success in some animation applications, mass-spring models are not physically accurate. This makes them unsuitable for simulations that require accuracy. Furthermore, substituting material constants such as the *elasticity modulus (E)* and *Poisson's ratio (ν)* with a set of spring constants creates undesired approximations. In addition, certain constraints, such as incompressibility, are not expressed in the model. More accurate physical models are finite-element models (FEMs) that treat deformable objects as a continuum. FEMs can model complex soft tissue deformations more accurately, and equations of equilibrium can be developed based on mechanical properties of soft tissue. However, the use of FEM in computer graphics has been limited because

---

[1]This research was supported by the Ontario Research and Development Challenge Fund under grant 00-May-0709 and an infrastructure grant from the Canada Foundation for Innovation awarded to the London Health Science Centre (Canadian Surgical Technologies and Advanced Robotics).

of computational requirements. In practice, it is difficult to apply FEM in real-time systems. Various methods have been introduced by researchers to speed up FEM, including, condensation [8], preprocessing [3], adaptive FEM [9], and hybrid methods [10]. In general, these methods improve the speed of simulation, but with the cost of significant preprocessing and reduction of accuracy.

The key objective of this research is to achieve a trade off between accuracy and computational speed for real-time simulation. The developed methods essentially depend on force-deformation relationships. Classical mechanical engineering solutions for force-deformation are based on the concept of activity of the system, which means that the deformation is calculated based on the force exerted by the user. Solving the obtained equations of equilibrium between force and deformation is computationally very expensive [1]. Conversely, the developed methods in this research are based on the key fact of passivity in haptic systems. It is generally assumed that a human operator interacting with a haptic interface behaves passively in the sense that he or she does not introduce energy in the system [2]. The position of the tip of the haptic device is the only information transmitted by the device. Consequently, the deformation must be driven based on the displacement of the haptic contact point and not the force [3]. This consideration leads to the possibility of developing new methods, customized for haptic systems and computationally efficient for real-time applications.

In our work, the materials are assumed to be perfectly elastic with small elasticity modulus. We concern ourselves with materials that have the ability to recover their original size and shape when the forces producing the deformation are removed. Perfect elastic behaviour can be observed in many artificial materials, such as rubber, and many biomaterials, such as Abductin, Resilin, and Elastin [11].

## 2. Method

The governing algorithm in this research is developed based on the passivity of haptic systems and works continuously in a loop. The penetration of the haptic tip into a deformable object is calculated by a collision detection method based on a ray tracing technique. By having the amount of penetration into the deformable object, a distribution of deformation for incompressible materials is estimated using the superposition principle and a mapping technique. In the next step, the amount of energy required to result in the volumetric deformation in the object is estimated based on the law of energy conservation and the divergence theorem to finally calculate the force reflection.

In order to represent the shape of the external surface of the objects, we use a parametric surface representation. Any of the known parametric surface representation techniques such as Bezier, B-Spline or NURBS can be used to produce points on the surface.

## 3. Experiments

Implementation of the system was accomplished using the GHOST SDK$^{TM}$ libraries [12] on a PHANToM$^{TM}$ haptic device, and experiments on a variety of geometries with different material properties were conducted. The effect of different model variables such as elasticity modulus, poisson's ratio, magnitude of the penetration vector, shape of geom-

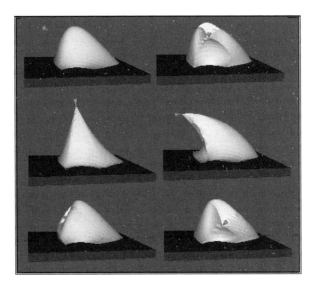

**Figure 1.** A sequence of images from a real-time simulation. The model is a B-spline surface with 530 vertices.

etry, and the location of contact point on force reflection has been investigated in or-der to evaluate the system performance. Experiments show that for materials with small elasticity modulus such as Elastin, the amount of force reflection is small and increases linearly by increasing the amount of penetration. Fig. 1 is one example of the result of our implementations. All experiments were performed on a Windows 2000 Pentium 4 computer with a single processor running at 1.6 GHz.

## 4. Conclusion

This paper has presented novel approaches for collision detection, distribution of defor-mation, and force reflection estimation in haptic environments. The concept of passivity makes these methods very efficient for haptic interaction. The methods are applicable for a variety of objects with 3D sculptured surfaces in the range of the typical haptic forces found in applications such as surgical simulations.

## References

[1] S. F. F. Gibson and B. Mirtich, "A survey of deformable modeling in computer graphics," Tech. Report no. TR-97-19, *MERL-Mitsubishi Electric Research Laboratory*, November, 1997.
[2] M. L. McLaughlin, J. P. Hespanha and G. S. Sukhatme, *Touch in Virtual Environments*, Haptics and the Design of Interactive Systems, IMSC Press Multimedia Series, 2002.
[3] S. Cotin, H. Delingette and N. Ayache, "Real-time elastic deformations of soft tissue for surgery simula-tion," *IEEE Transactions on Visualization and Computer Graphics*, vol. 5, no. 1, pp. 62-73, 1999.
[4] A. Witkin and D. Baraff, "An introduction to physically based modelling," course notes, Carnegie Mellon University, Pittsburgh, 1994.
[5] K. Waters, "A physical model of facial tissue and muscle articulation derived from computer tomogra-phy," In *Proceedings of Visualization in Biomedical Computing*, vol. 1808, pp. 574-583. SPIE, 1992.
[6] Y. Lee, D. Terzopoulos and K. Waters, "Realistic modelling for facial animation," *Proceedings of SIG-GRAPH 95*, pp. 55-62. ACM SIGGRAPH, 1995.

[7] S. Platt and N. Badler, "Animating facial expressions," *Computer Graphics*, vol. 15, no.3, pp. 245-252, 1981.

[8] M. Bro-Nielsen, "Finite elements modeling in surgery simulation," *Proceedings of IEEE*, vol. 86, issue 3, pp. 490-503, March 1998.

[9] X. Wu, M. S. Downes, T. Goktekin, and F. Tendick, "Adaptive nonlinear finite elements for deformable body simulation using dynamic progressive meshes," *Proceedings of Eurographics*, vol. 20, no. 3, pp. 349-358, 2001.

[10] S. Cotin, H. Delingette and N. Ayache, "A hybrid elastic model allowing real-time cutting, deformations and force feedback for surgery training and simulation," *Visual Computer Journal*, vol. 16, no.8, pp. 437-452, 2000.

[11] Y.C. Fung, *Biomechanics, Mechanical Properties of Living Tissues*, 2nd ed., Springer-Verlag, New York, 1993.

[12] GHOST® SDK, Programmer's Guide, version 4.0, SensAble Technologies, Inc.® , MA, rev. 2002.

560
Medicine Meets Virtual Reality 13
James D. Westwood et al. (Eds.)
IOS Press, 2005

# Segmenting Deformable Surface Models Using Haptic Feedback

Praveen THIAGARAJAN [a], Pei CHEN [a], Karl STEINER [a],
Guang GAO [b] and Kenneth BARNER [b]

[a] *Delaware Biotechnology Institute, University of Delaware 15,
Innovation Way, Newark, DE 19711*
[b] *Department of Electrical and Computer Engineering, University of Delaware
140 Evans Hall, Newark, DE 19716*

**Abstract.** Clinically relevant segmentation often incorporates physician insight in
the segmentation process (eg. overestimation of tumors). This is a primary reason
in the continued use of per-slice based segmentation approaches. Segmenting structures directly by interacting with a volume space provides the advantages of being
time efficient and accurate in contrast to per-slice based methods. In this approach
volume navigation and parameter specification become critical towards the accuracy of the results obtained. In this paper we present some preliminary results in our
research towards segmentation using a haptic device for navigation and parameter
specification in an immersive environment. To incorporate the physician's requirements we model the results as a deformable surface model and the user interacts
with the surface to obtain the final segmentation.

## 1. Introduction

Segmentation is the first step in parsing desired regions in the data from an imaging
modality. This processing step identifies the contents and shapes of the different objects
present in the image dataset. Radiation treatment planning and evaluation, intraoperative
surgical guidance and surgical rehearsal and training, all depend on this step of segmentation. The per-slice based nature of the current segmentation methods provide a cumbersome interface to the problem of semi-automatic segmentation. This results in the
segmentation process being inefficient in terms of time and accuracy.

Segmentation approaches like region growing [1] and level sets [2] are capable of
segmenting in three dimensions directly and thereby overcome the shortcomings of per-
slice based methods. But, navigation in a three dimensional environment and parameter
definition become critical to the successful application of these approaches. Our research
is in the direction of using a haptic input device (PHANToM) in an immersive environment to perform segmentation and define some of these parameters. Further, we also explore the modification of results from a segmentation process by deforming the resulting
surface model with the aid of haptic feedback. This allows the incorporation of heuristics
of a physician for a specific case.

Several groups have investigated the use of haptic feedback for segmentation purposes [3,4] and have found haptic feedback to be useful. Our segmentation approach is

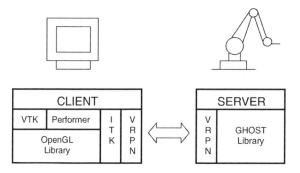

**Figure 1.** System Architecture.

novel in its attempt to use haptic feedback as a guide to specify the parameters for the segmentation process and in deforming the segmentation results.

## 2. Interactive Segmentation

### 2.1. System Overview

Our system design consists of two modules a client and server (Figure 1). This design allows the haptic interface to be portable between different systems. The server handles the force calculations and provides the tracking information. The server and client use the VRPN (Virtual Reality Peripheral Network) layer to communicate with each other over the network (TCP/IP). The client is the interface to the user. It is built using ITK, VTK and OpenGL to allow quick prototyping of different segmentation approaches. The display is stereo capable and allows rendering of the volume to represent the data space. The network communication bandwidth between the server and the client does not introduce any noticeable lag in the system.

### 2.2. Haptic Interaction and Deformation

We use force feedback to allow the user to feel the boundaries in the data space and place seeds in the data space. The gradient provides a suitable boundary model for our application. For a given volume, we calculate the force feedback from the haptic device based on the gradient information in the image ($\mathbf{F}=\nabla\mathbf{I}$). We use a mass spring loaded force model and non-linearly map ($\mathbf{N}$) the gradient magnitude to the force feedback ($\mathbf{F}=\mathbf{N}(\nabla\mathbf{I})$). The non-linear mapping serves for enhancing high gradient components, while suppressing the lower ones. This is a user defined component and can be changed during the segmentation process. Since images are typically noisy, we perform smoothing of the data ($\mathbf{F}=\mathbf{N}(\mathbf{S}(\nabla\mathbf{I}))$) to obtain consistent force feedback results during navigation. We use seeded segmentation approaches in the form of level sets and region growing. The seeds are placed by tracking the haptic probe. As the user sweeps the volume within an object of interest in the volume, guided by the haptic feedback, we track a series of probe locations. This information is used to set the parameters such that these regions are included in the final result. Depending upon the nature of the required seg-

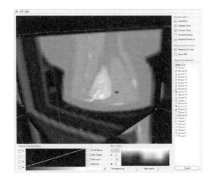
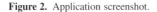

**Figure 2.** Application screenshot.

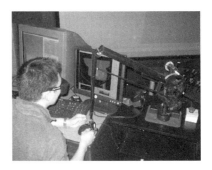

**Figure 3.** Haptic feedback setup.

mentation, the segmentation process can be chosen between a region growing (colon) or level-set (kidneys) approach.

Once we obtain an initial segmentation result we model the surface as a free form deformable model [5]. We then use the haptic device to produce deformations on this surface model to fine tune the final result. The same haptic feedback model as in the segmentation process is used here to guide the deformations. Image data is currently not used as part of the deformation model. Figure 2 shows the application screenshot and Figure 3 shows the hardware setup.

## 3. Conclusions and Future Work

In our current implementation, we have found that the use of force feedback while roaming the volume enables the user to set seed locations quickly. Tracking the probe location, while the user roams the data and using this information to determine some of the segmentation parameters, has shown to reduce the time taken towards setting and exploring the parameter space. We have found that the region growing based approaches work well for segmenting tubular structures and level sets work well for organs and tumors spanning higher intensity values in the image.

The results towards surface deformations are preliminary and we need further enhancements to incorporate a more advanced sculpting process [6]. We are also considering an alternative in the form of using the information in the binary image directly as a volume rendered component. This approach has the advantage of producing local deformations, compared to the global changes in the deformable surface model.

### Acknowledgements

This work has been supported under NIH-NCRR Grant 2P20016472-04. We would like to thank our collaborators at Christiana Care Health System for providing data and useful discussions.

# References

[1]  R. Huang and K. Ma, RGVis: Region Growing Based Visualization Techniques for Volume Visualization, Proceedings of Pacific Graphics 2003 Conference.

[2]  A. Lefohn, J. Cates, R. Whitaker: Interactive, GPU-Based Level Sets for 3D Segmentation. MICCAI 2003.

[3]  M. Harders and G. Szekely. New Metaphors for Interactive 3D Volume Segmentation. Conference proceedings of EuroHaptics 2001.

[4]  S. Senger. Haptic Feedback to Facilitate Interactive Segmentation of Volumetric Data Sets. Medicine Meets Virtual Reality, Newport Beach, CA, Jan. 2002.

[5]  S. Hu, H. Zhang, C. Tai and J.Gua. Direct Manipulation of FFD: efficient explicit solutions and decomposable multiple point constraints. The Visual Computer, Springer, August 2001.

[6]  M. Heiland et al.. Realistic haptic interaction for computer simulation of dental surgery. In Heinz U. Lemke et al. (eds.): Proc. CARS 2004, International Congress Series 1268, Elsevier, Amsterdam, 2004.

564

*Medicine Meets Virtual Reality 13*
*James D. Westwood et al. (Eds.)*
*IOS Press, 2005*

# Parametric Model of the Scala Tympani for Haptic-Rendered Cochlear Implantation

Catherine TODD and Fazel NAGHDY

*School of Electrical, Computer and Telecommunications Engineering,*
*Faculty of Informatics, University of Wollongong,*
*Northfields Avenue, Wollongong, NSW 2500, Australia*

**Abstract.** A parametric model of the human scala tympani has been designed for use in a haptic-rendered computer simulation of cochlear implant surgery. It will be the first surgical simulator of this kind. A geometric model of the Scala Tympani has been derived from measured data for this purpose. The model is compared with two existing descriptions of the cochlear spiral. A first approximation of the basilar membrane is also produced. The structures are imported into a force-rendering software application for system development.

## 1. Motivation

Cochlear implantation is a delicate surgical procedure aimed at restoring hearing to the profoundly deaf. Electrical stimulation of the auditory nerve provides the recipient with the sensation of sound. To enable this facility, an electrode array embedded in a silastic carrier is inserted into the cochlear structure, located within the inner ear. Primary passage for insertion is the lower chamber of the cochlear spiral; the Scala Tympani (ST), with the Scala Vestibuli (SV) as a secondary option.

In the current work, a parametric model of the ST and Basilar Membrane (BM) are derived from previously measured data [1–3,5]. This paper describes the method and results associated with three-dimensional model development. It is the first stage in the development of a surgical simulator for visual and haptic-rendering of the cochlear implant insertion process. The end result will provide considerable benefits to both novice and skilled surgeons. Insertion of the implant into the virtual, patient-specific model may be carried out in a risk-free environment. The system will offer quantitative evaluation of insertion forces and torques, real-time electrode array location, insertion depth and trauma analysis, which has previously been subjective. Information of this type may lead to improvements in electrode array design, as well as pre- and post- operative planning.

The cochlear structure is notably small, anatomically complex and differs in tilt and length between individuals. This makes it hard to model precisely, and on an individual basis. It also makes the process of parameter selection and extraction a difficult one.

## 2. Method

In this work, a virtual model of the human ST is produced using the Finite Element Modelling (FEM) software package ANSYS (Leap Australia). Previously published ST measurements [1–3,5] were analysed for three-dimensional surface reconstruction of this chamber. A combination of these were used to derive a final model; including ST cross-sectional height, width information, Organ of Corti (OC) length, radial displacement about the modiolar axis, change in ST height from base to apex and intra-cochlear tilt.

Mean height and width measurements of the ST [1] are extrapolated to the average length of the OC, 35.58 mm [2]. Results in [1] and [2] are combined to give cross-sectional measurements as a function of angular displacement about the modiolar axis. Height and width information is mapped to percentage lengths at each quarter turn, as well as 1.5 mm along the cochlear path, to the length of the OC (or 2.63 cochlear turn).

The cochlear spiral begins at an angular displacement of 13.47° [3], the location of the Round Window (RW) and common insertion site. At each defined cross-section, a value for radius (from modiolus to OC) is added by combining actual radii in [3] with percentage lengths in [2], to each quarter turn. Each side of the cross-section is approximated by a parabola, although the BM surface is kept flat and perpendicular to all height measurements. OC location is considered to be along the inner edge of the BM, where BM measurements were taken from [6]. Intra-cochlear tilt and a constant 10° height inclination after the first turn are also included.

To parameterise the model, width and height measurements for each cross-section were calculated from percentages of the initial cross-section. Values for radii defined at each quarter turn were calculated as percentages of OC length. Consequently, in order to replicate the ST and BM models for each individual, ST cross-section width, height and cochlear (OC) length must be measured (from CT scans). The three parameters are entered into a spreadsheet to automatically generate ST cross-section co-ordinates along its length. Co-ordinates are then imported into ANSYS, splines are drawn between the points and areas are defined between intersecting splines, to give a surface description of the ST.

## 3. Results

A three-dimensional surface representation of the ST and BM, modelled separately, are produced in this work (refer Fig. 1a). Representations of the Contour Array (Cochlear Ltd) and straightening stylet are also produced. The final design for each structure produced using ANSYS is saved in VRML format, modified and imported into the Reachin API (ReachinDirect, Inc) for force modelling and visual representation during the simulation. Accuracy of the final ST model produced in this work is discussed in the next section.

## 4. Discussion

Cross-section areas and spline lengths representing the inner and outer ST walls and the BM were compared with measured results [1,2], revealing similarities between the data.

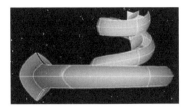

**Figure 1a.** Parameterised model of ST.

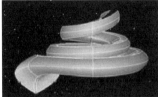
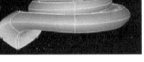

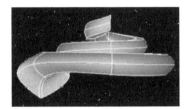

**Figure 1b.** Helico-spiral model.          **Figure 1c.** Archimedian spiral model.

The design was also compared to two mathematical models produced previously [4,5]. Three-dimensional spirals in [4] and [5] approximate the central path of the cochlear. Parametric data for ST cross-sections produced in this work were added to each spiral and the outcome is shown in Figures 1b and 1c respectively.

Cross-sections from this work plotted along the helico-spiral path in [4] gave a favourable three-dimensional representation of the ST and BM, which was similar to the model produced in this work. However, when the same cross-sections were interpolated along the Archimedean spiral in [5], the model produced inaccuracies at the helicotrema. The spiral in [5] actually traces an electrode array trajectory which differs from the central path of the cochlear. This may explain such inconsistencies between results.

## 5. Future Work

Current and future work is aimed at facilitating insertion of the Contour Array into the ST, including partial and full removal of the straightening stylet. Insertion and restoration forces associated with this process, as well as visual changes in topology, are also being modelled. The user will be provided with force-feedback information at both the graphical and haptic interfaces. Varying degrees of magnification will also be offered, as in the real procedure. There is also scope to model the membranous Cochlear Partition as a whole and the SV as an alternative chamber for insertion.

## 6. Conclusions

In this work, an anatomically accurate, reproducible model of the ST and BM is produced. A unique process is applied for determining width and height of ST cross-sections at each quarter turn, based on measured data. In order to reproduce the model, initial ST cross-section width and height, and cochlear (OC) length must be measured from CT. These parameters are entered into a spreadsheet to give all ST coordinates along its length, which are plotted in ANSYS. A three-dimensional surface reconstruction of the ST and BM is thus derived. The geometric model is used in haptic simulation of cochlear implant surgery. Outcomes of this work include fast and accurate derivation of a patient-specific model of the human cochlear, for use in pre-operative planning and simulator development.

## References

[1] S-H Hatsushika, RK Shepherd, YC Tong, GM Clark, S Funasaka, 'Dimensions of the Scala Tympani in the Human and Cat with Reference to Cochlear Implants', The Annals of Otology, Rhinology & Laryngology, 99:871-876, 1990.
[2] A Kawano, HL Seldon, GM Clark, 'Computer-Aided Three-Dimensional Reconstruction in Human Cochlear Maps: Measurement of the Lengths of Organ of Corti, Outer Wall, Inner Wall, And Rosenthal's Canal', Ann Otol Rhinol Laryngol, 105:701-709, 1996.
[3] LT Cohen, J Xu, SA Xu, GM Clark, 'Improved and Simplified Methods for Specifying Positions of the Electrode Bands of a Cochlear Implant Array', The American Journal of Otology, 17:859-865, 1996.
[4] SK Yoo, G Wang, JT Rubinstein, MW Vannier, 'Three-Dimensional Geometric Modeling of the Cochlea Using Helico-Spiral Approximation', IEEE Transactions on Biomed. Eng., 47(10):1392-1402, 2000.
[5] DR Ketten, MW Skinner, G Wang, MW Vanner, et al., 'In Vivo Measures of Cochlear Length and Insertion Depth of Nucleus Cochlear Implant Electrode Arrays', The Annals of Otology, Rhinology & Laryngology, 107(11):1-16, 1998.
[6] E Givelberg, M Rajan, J Bunn, 'Detailed Simulation of the Cochlea: Recent Progress Using Large Shared Memory Parallel Computers', Center for Advanced Computing Research (CACR) Technical Report, CACR-190, July 2001.

*Medicine Meets Virtual Reality 13*
*James D. Westwood et al. (Eds.)*
*IOS Press, 2005*

# Three Dimensional Electromechanical Model of Porcine Heart with Penetrating Wound Injury

Taras USYK and Roy KERCKHOFFS

*Department of Bioengineering, The Whitaker Institute for Biomedical Engineering,*
*University of California, San Diego, La Jolla, CA 92093-0412, USA*
*e-mail: taras@bioeng.ucsd.edu*

**Abstract.** The aim of this study is development a prototype computational model of the pig heart that can be used to predict physiological responses to a penetrating wound injury. The pig has been chosen for this model studies because it shares many anatomical similarities with humans.

Three-dimensional cubic Hermite finite element meshes based on detailed measurements of porcine anatomy combined into an integrated anatomic model. The pig ventricular model includes detailed left and right ventricular geometry and myofiber and laminar sheet orientations throughout the mesh [1].

The cardiac mesh was refined and monodomain equations for action potential propagation solved using well-established collocation-Galerkin finite element methods [2]. The membrane kinetic equations for the action potential model was based on detailed cellular models of transmembrane ionic fluxes and intracellular calcium fluxes in canine ventricular myocytes and human atrial myocytes. We modified the anisotropic myocardial conductivity tensor on the endocardial surface of the ventricles by making use of a surface model fitted to measured of Purkinje fiber network anatomy.

The mechanical model compute regional three-dimensional stress and strain distributions using anisotropic constitutive laws referred to local material coordinate axes defined by local myofiber and laminar sheet orientations. Passive myocardial mechanics modeled using exponential orthotropic strain energy functions. Active systolic myocardial stresses computed from a multi-scale model that uses crossbridge theory to predict calcium-activated sarcomere length- and velocity-dependent tension filament tension.

Since the electrical and mechanical models use a common finite element mesh as the parent parametric framework and both models are solved within our custom finite element package, it is straightforward to couple these models, as we have recently done for a model of coupled ventricular electromechanics [3].

We apply the coupled electromechanical model to predict alterations in regional diastolic and systolic wall mechanics associated with rhythm disturbances and possible arrhythmias with decreased blood volume, tamponade, myocardial injury, and regional ischemia caused by a penetrating wound.

## 1. Introduction

The heart is a complex three-dimensional structure in which the biophysics of myocyte excitation and the mechanics of crossbridge interaction are coordinated to produce ventricular pumping. Much is known about the cellular basis of the cardiac action potential and the uniaxial mechanics of cardiac muscle contraction, but relating these properties to the regional pattern of activation and mechanics in the intact ventricles remains a difficult problem. While some variables, such as regional strains and epicardial activation patterns have been measured in the intact heart [4], practical experimental methods for mapping three-dimensional distributions of other important variables such as stress, strain energy, or transmembrane potential are still not available.

The pig has been chosen for these model studies for the same reason that many investigators have used the pig as an experimental model system; namely that it is a well characterized experimental model for cardiovascular physiology and pathophysiology, and it shares many anatomical similarities with humans.

Cardiac function of the heart with penetrating wound injury causes regional alterations in stress strain and material properties, rhythm disturbances and possible arrhythmias with decreased blood volume.

A recent computational model of normal electromechanics [3] and the effects of ventricular pacing [5,6] showed good agreement with experimental measurements in anesthetized dogs. The goal of present study was to develop and validate a numerical electromechanical model of the pig heart and investigate how penetrating wound injury effect on global cardiac function and regional stress strain distribution during cardiac cycle. Such model will be useful tool in diagnostic and treatment soldiers with penetrating wound injury.

## 2. Methods

Three-dimensional model of porcine left and right ventricular anatomy with a detailed Purkinje fiber network, myofiber and sheet architecture was based on measurements [1]. The resulting 90 – element tricubic Hermite mesh was refined to obtain 720 – element mesh, which had 3042 degrees of freedom and was used as the computational domain for simulating passive inflation, electrical impulse propagation and active contraction of the left and right ventricles. The injured region was chosen at left ventricular free wall. The shape of this region was assumed cylindrical.

In the present analysis, the resting myocardium was modeled as a nonlinear, orthotropic and nearly incompressible material [7]. The passive properties of myocardium were taken from previous study [7] on the dog heart. Stiffness of injured region was increased by 20%, since we assume that passive property of the injury were stiffer, similar to severe ischemic region. We model penetrating wound injury similar to ischemic model described earlier by Mazhari et al [8]. Pressure boundary conditions were specified on the left and right ventricular endocardial surfaces, with left ventricular end diastolic pressure 11.0 mmHg, which was consistent with experimental observation.

Nonlinear membrane ionic kinetics was modeled using the two-variable modified FitzHugh-Nagumo [9,10] equations, and impulse propagation was modeled using a monodomain formulation [9,10]. The contribution of the Purkinje fiber network to ventricular conduction was modeled by adding an extra diagonal diffusion tensor, representing conductivity along the Purkinje fibers [3] on the lumenal surfaces of the endocardial elements. Electrical activation time was defined as the instant when transmembrane potential reached 40 mV and it was used to initiate regional systolic tension development following a constant delay of 8.4 ms [11]. This latter time (electrical activation time plus 8.4 msec) we refer to as "contractile activation time". In order to model electrical propagation, we applied an initial stimulus at the left and right bundle brunch of Purkinje fiber network, located on the left and right ventricular side of the septum, similar to our earlier model of normal activation [3]. Diffusion coefficients were chosen same as in previous model [3], but we apply zero diffusion in injured region of the heart.

The model of active contraction includes length-, time- and calcium-dependent active contractile stresses with transverse active stress components [7]. To model active contraction in injured region myofiber calcium sensitivity was reduced with a step transition across the injured boundary [8,12].

A Windkessel model for arterial impedance was coupled to ventricular pressure and volume to compute the hemodynamic boundary conditions. Ventricular cavity volume constraints were imposed during the isovolumic phases [3]. The formulation and solution of the electromechanical model have been described in detail previously for the case of normal activation [3] and ventricular pacing [5,6].

## 3. Results

The calculation of the model of passive and active mechanics required 650 Mb of main memory and ran for approximately one hour and 8 hours respectively on a single processor of a Silicon Graphics Origin 2100. The model of electrical propagation required 1.76Gb of main memory and ran for approximately 12 hours on this platform.

The convergence of the reaction-diffusion problem for electrical impulse propagation is determined in part by the kinetics of the ionic model, which determines the sharpness of the wavefront upstroke. Hence, ionic models with faster kinetics than the FitzHugh-Nagumo model used by us do require additional spatial mesh refinement. Adopting a more detailed membrane kinetics, with a realistic upstroke rate, require approximately 96000 elements mesh, which increase calculation time approximately by 3000 times. To make such model practical it is necessary to parallelize the model code, which will require modifications to the algorithm such as imposing boundary conditions explicitly and using parallel solver.

The time for 90% activation of the left ventricle was 55 ms for normal activation after external simulation of the His bundle. Excitation spreads rapidly from the His bundle to the right and left bundle branches and significantly slower through the rest of the myocardial tissue. Wavefront progress around the cavity is much more rapid then the spread toward the epicardium. Those results agree with experimental activation data from long-axis sections of the human heart [13]. Figure 1 shows initial activation time during normal activation (*a*) and activation of the model with penetrating wound injury (*b*). In the model with penetrating wound injury activation time at septal and right ventricular wall are similar to normal activation. At left ventricular free wall excitation spreads around the injured region with no activation at the center of it.

Figure 2 shows that during mitral valve closure there were smaller fiber strains due to stiffer material properties of the injured region. During active contraction there were significantly larger fiber strains at the wounded region (See Figure 2). Computed strains show that the tissue shortened rapidly at the early activated regions and shortening was preceded by prestretching of the tissue. This prestretching was a result of passive stretch-

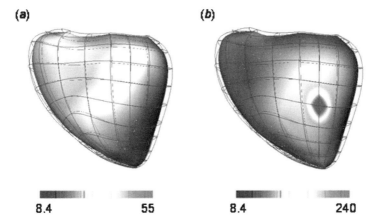

**Figure 1.** Initial activation time (ms) during normal activation (*a*); activation of the model with penetrating wound injury (*b*).

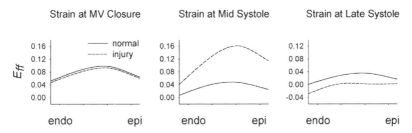

**Figure 2.** Fiber strains at left ventricular free wall at the location of injury during mitral valve (MV) closure, mid systole and late systole with reference state at the beginning of diastole.

ing of the late-activated regions in response to the contraction of the tissue activated earlier. At the injured region we found no contraction and passive stretching was significant due to contraction of surrounded tissue. Figure 3 represent circumferential, longitudinal and radial strain components during mitral valve closure, mid systole and late systole. At mid systole circumferential and longitudinal strain components were significantly larger for model with penetrating wound injury than for normal model, because of absent active forces at the wounded area.

## 4. Future work

A penetrating wound injury will most likely result in e.g. blood loss, tamponade, increasing heartbeat frequency, and a change in contractility. To account for these effects the finite element model will be integrated with a complex circulatory model, developed at the University of Washington [14], which contains the following sub-models: 1) varying elastance models for the atria (for a realistic preload) [15]; 2) pericardial load (for cardiac tamponade) [16]; 3) systemic and pulmonary circulations (for a realistic afterload) [17]; 4) baroreceptors (for the feedback on beating frequency/contractility) [16]; 5) ventilatory exchange (for pleural pressure acting on pericardium) [17] and 6)

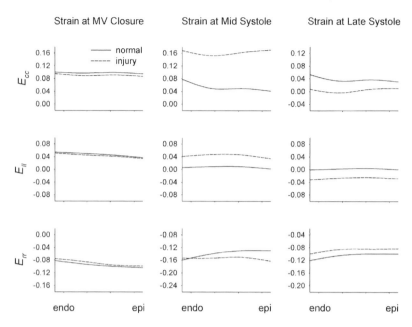

**Figure 3.** Circumferential, longitudinal and radial strains at left ventricular free wall at the location of injury during mitral valve (MV) closure, mid systole and late systole at the beginning of diastole.

blood/tissue gas exchange and blood $O_2$/$CO_2$/pH handling (for feedback on beating frequency/contractility).

The coupling between the finite element model and the circulatory model will take place through the right and left ventricular cavity pressures. Generally, throughout the whole cardiac cycle, cavity pressures will be estimated for each new timestep and prescribed both in the finite element model and circulatory model. When the difference in cavity volumes from the finite element model ($V_{FE}$) and the circulatory model ($V_{circ}$) is small enough, the next timestep will be entered. Otherwise, a new pressure will be estimated using $dp/dV$ relations from both models. This iteration cycle will be repeated until $V_{FE}-V_{circ}$ is small enough.

## 5. Conclusion

This study represent computational electromechanical model of the porcine left and right ventricles during normal conditions and with penetrating wound injury. Depending on the area and location of the injury such a model can define impact from penetrating wound on the cardiac function and can give prediction to physician how severe this impact is.

## Acknowledgements

This work was supported by a grant from the DARPA, executed by the U.S. Army Medical Research and Materiel Command/TATRC Cooperative Agreement, Contract # W81XWH-04-2-0012.

# References

[1] Stevens C, Hunter PJ. Sarcomere length changes in a model of the pig heart. Prog Biophys Molec Biol 82:229-241, 2003.

[2] Rogers JM, Courtemanche M, McCulloch AD. Finite element methods for modeling impulse propagation in the heart. In: Panfilov AV, Holden AV, editors. Computational Biology of the Heart. Sussex: John Wiley and Sons, Ltd.; 1996.

[3] Usyk TP, LeGrice IJ, McCulloch AD. Computational model of three-dimensional cardiac electromechanics. Comput Visual Sci. 4(4):249-257, 2002.

[4] Moore CC, Lugo-Olivieri CH, McVeigh ER, Zerchouni EA. Three-dimensional systolic strain patterns in the normal human left ventricle: characterization with tagged MR imaging. Radiology. 214: 453-466, 2000.

[5] Usyk TP, McCulloch AD. Electromechanical model of cardiac resynchronization in the dilated failing heart with left bundle branch block. Journal of electrocardiology. 36: 57-61, 2003.

[6] Usyk TP, McCulloch AD. Relationship between regional shortening and asynchronous electrical activation in a three-dimensional model of ventricular electromechanics. Journal of Cardiovascular Electrophysiology. 14:196-202, 2003.

[7] Usyk TP, Mazhari R. and McCulloch AD Effect of laminar orthotropic myofiber architecture on regional stress and strain in the canine left ventricle. J. Elasticity. 61: 143-164, 2000.

[8] Mazhari R., McCulloch AD. Integrative models for understanding the strucural basis of regional mechanical dysfunction in ischemic myocardium. Annals of Biomedical Engineering. 28: 979-990, 2000.

[9] Rogers JM, McCulloch AD. A Collocation-Galerkin finite element model of cardiac action potential propagation. Transactions on Biomedical Engineering. 41: 743-757, 1994.

[10] Rogers JM, McCulloch AD. Nonuniform muscle fiber orientation causes spiral wave drift in a finite element model of cardiac action potential propagation. Journal of Cardiovascular Electrophysiology. 5: 496-509, 1994.

[11] Wyman BT, Hunter WC, Prinzen FW, McVeigh ER. Mapping propagation of mechanical activation in the paced heart with MRI tagging. Am J Physiol. 276(3) (Heart Circ. Physiol): 881-891, 1999.

[12] Allen DG, Orchard CH. Myocardial contractile function during ischemia and hypoxia. Circ. Res. 60: 153-168, 1987.

[13] Durrer, D, van Dam RT, Freud GE, Janse MJ, Meijler FL, Arzbaecher RC: Total excitation of the isolated human heart. Circulation;41(6):899-912, 1970.

[14] Neal M, Bassingthwaighte J., Usyk T, McCulloch A, Kerchoffs R. A highly integrated physiology (HIP) cardiovascular/respiratory model used to simulate cardiac injury. MMVR13: The Magical Next Becomes the Medical Now. January 26-29, 2005 The Westin Long Beach Hotel Long Beach, California (in press).

[15] Rideout VC. Mathematical computer modeling of physiological systems. Englewood Cliffs, NJ: Prentice Hall, 1991, 261 pp.

[16] Sun Y, Beshara M, Lucariello RJ, Chiaramida SA. A comprehensive model for rightleft heart interaction under the influence of pericardium and baroreflex. Am J Physiol Heart Circ Physiol. 272: H1499H1515, 1997.

[17] Lu K, Clark JW, Ghorbel FH, Ware DL, Bidani A. A human cardiopulmonary system model applied to the analysis of the Valsalva maneuver. Am J Physiol Heart Circ Physiol. 281: H2661H2679, 2001.

*Medicine Meets Virtual Reality 13*
*James D. Westwood et al. (Eds.)*
*IOS Press, 2005*

# Beyond VR:
# Creating the Augmented Physician

Kirby G. VOSBURGH

*CIMIT/Massachusetts General Hospital/Harvard Medical School*
*65 Landsdowne St., Cambridge, MA 02465 USA*
*e-mail: kirby@bwh.harvard.edu*

**Abstract.** The ongoing shift of high tech capability from the specialist to the primary physician and the merging of medical and surgical therapies will demand more sophisticated measurement and control, but more positively, it will be possible to differentiate each individual situation and tailor treatment to provide an optimum result for each person, for each condition, in each environment, if these could all be measured, understood, and effected. The effective augmentation of the caregiver's physical, sensory, and cognitive capabilities will require more transparent, nuanced, and adaptive interfaces to information and to its therapeutic application. While the enhancement and classification of digitized findings is a beginning, the key may be better tracking and presentation of the chronological course, particularly the prior events which set the physiologic or morphologic data in context. Systems engineering approaches will define paths toward optimized, autonomous treatment, where the most rapid progress may be made through functional partitioning using scale-independent models, and the delineation of intermediate stages between today's macroscopic presentation of disease and molecular-scale treatment. These stages will comprise the steps toward useful patient avatars; our task is to fill in, with successively more powerful models, the convergence of large scale and small scale information, as it is used to support diagnostic and therapeutic decisions.

## 1. The Challenge to Medical (Information) Technology

For the next decade, the physician will face increasing complexity. Both information and treatment options will be presented across a daunting range of physical scales, from nano to macro. Vast volumes of information will be available, often without useful indexing or condensation. Even worse, practical therapeutic endpoints will remain obscure due to the combination of long disease time spans and the inadequacy of current cellular and animal models to predict progress toward beneficial human outcomes. The ongoing shift of high tech capability from the specialist to the primary physician and the merging of medical and surgical therapies will demand more sophisticated measurement and control, but more positively, it will be possible to differentiate each individual situation and tailor treatment to provide an optimum result for each person, for each condition, in each environment, if these could all be measured, understood, and effected. Finally, these challenges arise in the context of societal pressures for reduced cost and greater equality of access, and improved quality.

## 2. A Strategy for Progress

How will we, as technologists, help the caregivers? Although nothing in medicine is ever simple, or simply connected, let us concentrate on two major areas of opportunity: diagnosis and therapy. The major developments in anatomic radiology (CT, MRI, digital angiography...) have been diagnostic. These techniques have become a prominent feature in the healthcare landscape because they enable the more efficient routing of patients though care choices. This benefit manifests as the selection of the optimal care path, and particularly the avoidance of useless interventions, such as the reduction in negative laparotomies for suspected appendicitis [1]. The key in the care pathway is the prognosis for cure, with the associated factors of choices and well understood weights for risks and costs.

It's not just a matter of improved anatomic segmentation and showing function through false colour. Rather, the augmentation of the caregiver's physical, sensory, and cognitive capabilities will require more transparent, nuanced, and adaptive interfaces to information and to its therapeutic application. While the enhancement and classification of digitized findings is a beginning, the key may be better tracking and presentation of the chronological course, particularly the prior events which set the physiologic or morphologic data in context.

While the overall understanding of disease and its biologic pathways is the ultimate aim of medical research, this knowledge is now so incomplete that most treatment paradigms go only "halfway" as Lewis Thomas bluntly said [2]. Now, a dozen years later, we have an even more complex situation. Thomas's confident statement that "it now seems likely that a single centrally placed genetic anomaly will be found as the cause of all human cancers." doesn't resonate as firmly in a world of mass proteomic serum screening. While Thomas may yet be proven right regarding the etiology of cancer, the implication that all patients might be managed in the same way seems a distant goal.

Rather, it appears likely that empirical systems-engineering approaches will define paths toward optimized (and eventually autonomous) treatment, where the most rapid progress may be made through functional partitioning using scaleable models, and the delineation of intermediate structural or physiomic stages and states between today's macroscopic presentation of disease and molecular-scale treatment. These stages will comprise the steps toward useful patient avatars. Our task is to fill in, with successively more powerful models, the convergence of large scale and small scale observations and interventions, as they interact with the body's manifold cross coupled structures and systems.

## 3. The path to useful models and avatars

From the standpoint of the caregiver, a model is a useful way to parameterize, record and present information. A particular benefit is that is can (potentially) incorporate information of a variety of characters and scale. For example, a useful model for hemorrhagic shock might include gross observations of circulation (arterial blood pressure, cardiac output, etc.) but also blood chemistry factors such as oxygen saturation or cytokine levels. It is the human physician's ability to work across theses scales and disparate observations that is so difficult to mirror in the digital world. Models provide the structure to enable digital processing to emulate human observation, memory, and cognitive ability.

As the basic biologic processes are understood and described, the resultant knowledge structure will provide the armature for the contextual integration and display new information as state changes of the model. As if the development of an integrated model were not sufficiently challenging, the models have to accommodate realistic "real-world" conditions. Thus, for example, an improved model of the functions of the spleen might incorporate not only its normal biochemical function, but its response to external trauma. From where we are starting today, this will take time.

In the interim, the increasingly sophisticated models being developed by the physiome projects [3,4] will be valuable in practical use. In addition to their utility in archiving and mining data, one likely possibility is the positioning of these models as "strong priors" for improving the quality of the measured data [5]. For relatively stable processes, such as associated with chronic disease, the useful statistical power of measurements can be augmented through the assumption that they represent a small change in a stable prior model. This approach has been followed in the longitudinal analysis of radiologic findings for patients with neurological diseases, such as multiple sclerosis [6].

A key factor in implementing such systems is to reduce measurement bias due to variations in metrology. The biases inherent in the use of the model (which, almost by definition, does not represent the diseased state) must be accommodated in the prognostic estimates, generally by characterizing the goodness of the statistical fit.

## 4. Supporting the Therapeutic Intervention

The caregiver is generally in the position of attempting to understand and respond to a change in the patient's underlying health. While there is great power in being able to assume that most human beings of a given age and gender with normal history are similar, the potential for differentiating care for each individual is one of the most exciting and powerful recent trends. This goes beyond simple comparative findings ("the tumor appears to have grown by 20%") to utilize new tools with greater analysis power. Thus the concept is based on improved sensors with much enhanced digital processing capabilities. Consider these examples:

*Enhanced Image Guided Therapy.* The direct use of radiologic techniques to guide therapy [7] has recently been improved through the use of registered "augmented reality" capability. Examples of this include intraprocedural registrations of multiply acquired MR Images; particularly showing functional MRI images such as diffusion tract imagery in relationship to the anatomic components [8]. This has reached new levels in the direct fusion of modalities, as in PET/CT, which the anatomic and functional images are acquired simultaneously.

*Biological Signals.* This type of progress does not always require large scale imaging systems, if molecular contrast can be used. For example, Frangioni and co-workers [9] have shown the utility of such contrast systems with optical detection which easily delineates vascular and lymph structures, as much as a centimeter below the skin surface, with the potential for displaying them in real time to better set margins of surgical resection.

It has been said that the sign of a first rate mind is to be able to function despite holding two diametrically opposite positions. Modern medicine abounds in such opportunities, and most notably in considering the impact of bio-genetic information on clinical medicine. On one side there are the results of data mining through such techniques as protein panel serum measurements, while on the other there is painstaking analysis such as the description of the cascade of angiogenesis. Despite the limits to our understanding of either the empirical or scientific information, clinical benefits are manifest. As examples, consider the effective titration of pharmacologic therapies for ovarian cancer through observation of proteomic markers [10], or the correlation of specific genetic markers with the effectiveness of treatment of breast cancer treatment using tamoxifen [11]. In these cases, as in an increasing number of others, Evidence Based Medicine approaches will give validated support to change clinical practice.

*Patient-Specific Sensing.* In the past decade, progress has been made in management of patients utilizing new sensors and increasingly capable analysis of physiologic signals. As in the case of biological signals, both empirical and fundamental studies have been pursued. A prominent example of data archiving and analysis has been the PhysioNet system [12], an open-source annotated archive of gold standard-level signals from intensive care units. The power of higher bandwidth and more sophisticated analysis is exemplified in a recent study [13] of prognostic recognition of epileptic seizures using patient specific algorithms. It appears that, even for patients with refractory disease, a large percentage may be enabled to lead more normal lives through this individualized early detection and therapeutic nerve stimulus to abort the seizure.

## 5. Technical Challenges and Opportunities

Among the many technical issues, two stand out:

*Context and Trends.* Augmenting reality, perhaps through composite or fused displays, is a means for communication. The context of information is often vital to using it correctly. How can semi-automated systems decide which contextual information is relevant in a real-time diagnostic or treatment situation? How should it be shown? Is there a better way to show trends than a simple chart? Is it possible to make models powerful enough that they can absorb and represent complex processes and potential therapeutic responses, and thus stimulate and support more timely and beneficial decisions?

*Upward integration.* How do we design and implement systems that work for a particular condition, but can be generalized to cover many conditions? If we are not successful, the field will be limited by the costs of constantly re-developing sensors, algorithms, software systems, displays, and so on... The field is not sufficiently mature that standards seem appropriate, but it may be possible to structure open source development environments where many of the components can be re-used, as is now done for radiologic image processing software [14].

## 6. Summary: Thoughts on Helping the Physician

Why are there relatively few augmented reality systems in clinical use today, after much more than a decade of effort? Are physicians techno-phobic?... No. Rather, they adopt anything that works, amazingly quickly. As technologists, our challenge is to identify and implement those possible systems that satisfy this craving for patient benefit.

We should seek to provide technical enhancements to the performance of the expert user, that is, to constructively change their behavior by providing better, more timely, and more useful data. The concept of usability is paramount. Recent studies of the use of physiologic data in "first responder" management of trauma emphasize this point, by asking: when has this patient's status deteriorated to the point that a life saving intervention is necessary [15]?

Augmented reality is in its infancy in helping physicians reach higher levels of performance, but there is little question that its capabilities will be needed to help all caregivers manage the burgeoning information and more complex therapeutic choices in medicine for the next decade.

## References

[1] Rao, PM, JT Rhea, RA Novilline, AA Mostafavi, CJ Macabe, Effect of computed tomography of the appendix on treatment of patients and use of hospital resources, *NEJM 1998;338(3).141-6.*

[2] Thomas, Lewis, NIH is "Century's Finest Invention" *The Scientist 1992;6(20):0.*

[3] Bassingthwaighte, JB Strategies for the physiome project *AmBiomed Eng 2000;28(8):1043-58.* See also http://www.virtualsoldier.net/.

[4] Hunter, PJ Borg, TK Integration from proteins to organs: the Physiome Project *Nature Reviews/Molecular Cell Biology 2003;4:237-243.*

[5] See, for example, Leventon, Michael "Statistical Models for Medical Image Analysis" *MIT Ph.D Thesis, 2000.*

[6] Meier DS. Guttmann CR. Time-series analysis of MRI intensity patterns in multiple sclerosis *Neuroimage 2003; 20(2):1193-209.*

[7] Vosburgh KG. Jolesz FA. The concept of image-guided therapy. *Academic Radiology 2003; 10(2):176-9.*

[8] Ruiz-Alzola J. Westin CF. Warfield SK. Alberola C. Maier S. Kikinis R. Nonrigid registration of 3D tensor medical data. *Medical Image Analysis.2002;6(2):143-61.*

[9] Kim S. Lim YT. Soltesz EG. De Grand AM. Lee J. Nakayama A. Parker JA. Mihaljevic T. Laurence RG. Dor DM. Cohn LH. Bawendi MG. Frangioni JV. Near-infrared fluorescent type II quantum dots for sentinel lymph node mapping. *Nature Biotechnology.2004;22(1):93-7,* and references cited therein.

[10] Penson RT. Oliva E. Skates SJ. Glyptis T. Fuller AF Jr. Goodman A. Seiden MV. Expression of multidrug resistance-1 protein inversely correlates with paclitaxel response and survival in ovarian cancer patients: a study in serial samples. Gynecologic Oncology. 2004;93(1):98-106.

[11] Nowell,S, C. Sweeney, M Winters, A Stone, NP Lang, LF Hutchins, FF Kadlubar, CB Ambrosone. Association Between Sulfotransferase 1A1 Genotype and Survival of Breast Cancer Patients Receiving Tamoxifen Therapy *J Natl Cancer Inst 2002; 94: 1635-1640.*

[12] http://www.physionet.org/.

[13] Shoeb A. Edwards H. Connolly J. Bourgeois B. Treves ST. J. Patient-specific seizure onset detection. *Epilepsy & Behavior. 5(4):483-98, 2004 Aug.*

[14] The Insight Segmentation and Registration Toolkit, National Library of Medicine, see http://www.itk.org/.

[15] Holcomb, JB unpublished lecture at Advanced Technology Applied to Combat Casualty Care (AT-ACCC 2004); see also Holcomb, JB, Methods for improved hemorrhage control. *Critical Care 2004;8(Suppl2):S57-60.*

*Medicine Meets Virtual Reality 13*
*James D. Westwood et al. (Eds.)*
*IOS Press, 2005*

# Stiffness and Texture Perception
# for Teledermatology

Kenneth J. WALDRON [a], Christopher ENEDAH [a] and Hayes GLADSTONE [b]

[a] *Department of Mechanical Engineering, Stanford University*
[b] *Dermatologic Surgery, Stanford University Medical Center*
*e-mail: {kwaldron, cenedah, hayes.gladstone}@stanford.edu*

**Abstract.** The goal of the teledermatology project currently being carried out at Stanford University is to deliver tactile images of the human skin to a dermatologist at a remote location, in real time. In order to make a diagnosis, dermatologists typically need to obtain data regarding the skin texture and the mechanical properties of any lesions on a patient's skin. For example, pre-cancerous or weather-damaged skin typically feels rougher than normal skin and the profile and stiffness of the underlying tissue may shed light on the nature of a skin disease.

## 1. Introduction

Skin cancers are a very common disorder, particularly in areas where the population is predominantly light skinned. At some point in their lives, approximately one in five Americans will be diagnosed with some form of skin cancer. This increases to one in four in Australia and New Zealand, with incidence of the deadly melanoma type being about one in thirty [8].

Teledermatology is important in serving sparsely distributed rural populations. Specialist dermatologists are located in central hospitals, often far from the patients needing diagnostic services. It is very expensive to transport the patient to the specialist's location in these circumstances. Diagnosis of a skin lesion requires both inspection, using high definition video, and palpation. It is the palpation part of this information we are seeking to address in this study.

The overall system configuration we propose to use is shown in Figure 1. The master and slave robot are envisaged as being commercially available, six-axis devices, such as those available from SensAble Technologies. The haptic probe mounted on the slave device, and the haptic display mounted on the master device will be designed for this specific application and are the subjects of this paper. Two types of haptic information must be transmitted to the specialist for this purpose. Skin texture requires the sensing, transmission and display of high spatial frequency, low spatial amplitude data. Skin profile, as needed to evaluate lumps in or under the skin, requires transmission and display of relatively low frequency, high amplitude data. Sensing of mechanical properties such as stiffness is also important.

In the profile detection domain, the raw haptic feedback from a slave to a master haptic robot will provide, in principle, profile information. However, given the bandwidth

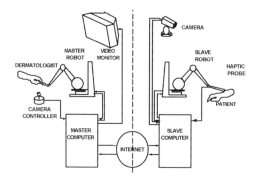

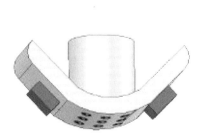

**Figure 1.** Schematic configuration of teledermatology system. The left side of the figure is located at a central medical facility. The right hand side is a local medical provider's office.

**Figure 2.** CAD generated drawing of probe with accelerometers and piezoelectric sensor attached

limits of currently available devices, of the order of 100 Hz [7], it is likely that little more than gross geometric form will be discerned by this means. Since mechanical properties are important in diagnosis of skin lesions, a sensor designed to detect this information is being developed. Khaled *et al.* [5] have used ultrasound to detect and measure the physical properties of forms within the skin. The use of ultrasound does provide a way of detecting tissue transitions and measuring mechanical properties. Although it conveys nothing about texture, for the moment, we are pursuing use of a mechanical probe because of its relative simplicity and capacity for integration with a texture sensor, but the ultrasound option is certainly interesting.

Previous experiments have looked at texture perception using accelerometers. In reference [1], Howe and Cutkosky experimented with various scanning velocities and normal forces and were able to gather textural data in the form of vertical acceleration only.

## 2. Device Description

The texture and stiffness perception probe, shown in Figure 2, comprises a piezoelectric sensor and a pair of accelerometers mounted in quadrature. The piezoelectric sensor was made by attaching electrodes etched on a flexible membrane to either side of Polyvinylidene Fluoride (PVDF) film. 3M's 9703 tape, which is electrically conductive in the 'z-axis', was used to maintain an electrical connection between the electrodes and the PVDF film. The PVDF film and conductive adhesive used were 28 microns and 50 microns thick respectively. Figure 2 shows a schematic of the piezoelectric array of electrodes. Application of force to the sensor results in the formation of an electric charge across the affected electrodes, the piezoelectric effect. The pattern of electrodes allows isolation of the impacted electrode pair. A 3 × 3 array was formed of the electrodes, which are 1mm in diameter and spaced 2.5 mm apart. The piezoelectric sensor is shown adhered to the bottom of the probe in Figure 2.

The accelerometers are dual-axis, 1.5 g devices sensitive to both static and dynamic accelerations and are mounted so that the axes of interest are in quadrature. In this configuration, taking the summation or difference of the sensed accelerations yields normal and tangential components, which respectively, are measures of feature amplitudes and the frequency with which features occur on the skin surface. To improve sensitivity of the probe, its mass was kept to a minimum and a spring was used to decouple it from the manipulator arm. The bottom of the probe, the sensing surface, was covered with 3M's Greptile tape (not shown in diagram). The tape's surface is one of small-scale, criss-crossed, parallel ridges. Its textured, non-adhesive surface magnifies local vibrations as the probe is dragged across a target surface [1]. This surface choice is not ideal for the piezoelectric sensor but a compromise is reached by improving its sensitivity through careful design of its signal conditioning circuit.

## 3. Method

A mathematical model of the probe is needed to properly relate sensor data to the skin properties being sensed. The probe is modeled as a particle mounted to a moving frame *via* a long, soft spring. The model is depicted in Figure 3, below. The probe frame is moved over the skin surface with constant velocity, $v_P$ and transmits force to the probe body in the horizontal direction by means of the spring, $k_P$ which is assumed to be very stiff for the purpose of the present analysis. The probe body is pressed against the skin with constant force $F_P$, achieved in practice, by means of a long, soft spring. Let the unloaded skin profile relative to a reference line be $y(x)$ where $x$ is the distance traveled by the probe, and let the local stiffness of the skin in the vertical direction be $k_S$ with the corresponding local damping be $b_S$. If Y is the height of the probe above the reference then, in the vertical direction, $k_S(y - Y) + b_S(\dot{y} - \dot{Y}) - F_P = m_P \ddot{Y}$ or $m_P \ddot{Y} + b_S \dot{Y} + k_S Y = F_P + b_S v \dot{y} + k_S y$. Reasonable values for the skin properties may be estimated by conducting simple experiments. We can then estimate behavior when passing over a bump of given height etc.

Bumps and texture in the skin cause variations in the contact force between the probe and skin that are detected by the piezoelectric sensors, and accelerations of the probe body that are detected by the accelerometers. These forces and accelerations are, of course, dependent on the mechanical properties of the skin and the underlying tissues.

Pushing the probe a known distance into human tissue and measuring the resulting reaction force as the tissue pushes back, it is possible to gain a measure of the tissue's stiffness. Dermatologists use a number of methods to perceive tissue stiffness. One method is to squeeze the tissue between the index finger and thumb. Simply pressing on the tissue also gives the required feedback. Acquiring low frequency stress data presents a significant challenge as PVDF possesses both pyroelectric and piezoelectric properties. The proposed stiffness acquisition method requires stress information of roughly 1 Hz or less, pyroelectric effects due to warm bodies fall within a similar frequency range. The capacitance of each pair of electrode is proportional to the area of overlap between them and inversely proportional to the sum of PVDF and adhesive thicknesses. The electrode pairs each have a very small area of overlap resulting in small capacitance values of 0.66 pF and relatively high voltage generation under stress. The piezoelectric film, essentially a capacitor in series with a voltage source, exhibits high output impedance and requires a high-impedance amplifier to convert its output to a low impedance signal suitable for use with measuring devices. A differential charge amplifier circuit (see Fig-

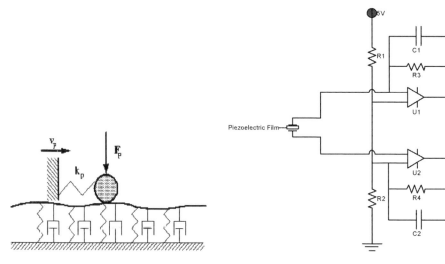

**Figure 3.** Model of skin compliance and damping. The probe is modeled as a particle held against the skin by the constant force, $F_P$.

**Figure 4.** Differential charge amplifier circuit.

ure 4 for a schematic) was used to transform the piezoelectric film's output charge to a low impedance voltage signal.

The charge amplifier's output is dependent only on the feedback capacitance and the piezoelectric charge and is given by $V_{out} = Q/C_1$, where Q is charge generated by applied force. The charge amplifier circuit prevents errors due to cable capacitance while the differential design reduces line noise through common mode rejection. The time constant of the circuit is given by the product of $C_1$ and $R_3$. Small time constant values improve performance at high frequency, which favors texture perception. Conversely, a large time constant is needed for stiffness measurement. The cutoff frequency was chosen to prevent the piezoelectric film from responding to thermal effects.

## 4. Results

Texture perception experiments for the pair of accelerometers and the piezoelectric film were conducted by scanning the surface of interest with the probe mounted on a robotic manipulator programmed for a straight, level trajectory. The scan speed was approximately 4 cm/s. Scanning was performed by bringing the probe into contact with the test materials which were laid flat on a hard smooth surface. Scans were carried out of sandpapers of various grit levels. Grit is a measure of the number of abrasive particles that appear in a square inch of sandpaper and of the size of these particles. Sandpaper grit has been used in roughness discrimination tests, for instance in [x]. The 3 levels of grit used were 180, 320 and 600 with 180 being the coarsest and 600 being the finest.

The FFT of the time domain data was taken for each signal. The frequency contents of these signals are plotted as power spectra below. Howe and Cutkosky [1] make note of a 'critical speed' needed for adequate signal output for texture perception of a given material. Although this possibility was not investigated, changing the stroking speed did not strongly affect signal amplitude.

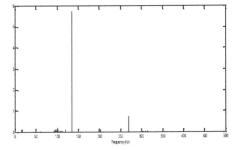

**Figure 5a.** Reference spectral data presents vibratory information due only to manipulator's motion. Indicates resonant frequency of 135 Hz.

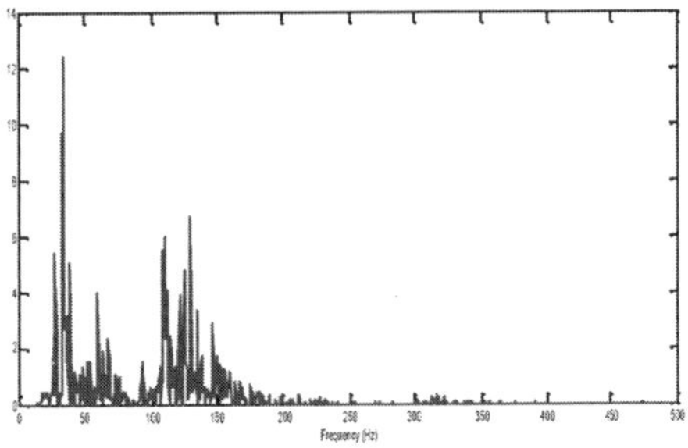

**Figure 5b.** Frequency content of vibratory data from a scan of 180 grit sandpaper.

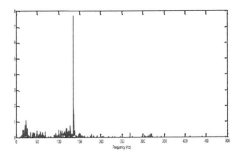

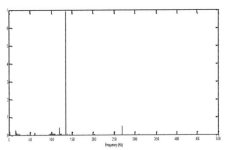

**Figure 5c.** Frequency content of vibratory data from a scan of 320 grit sandpaper.

**Figure 5d.** Frequency content of vibratory data from a scan of 600 grit sandpaper.

Figures 5a through 5d are power spectral plots of the vibratory information of the various sandpaper grits. They indicate the difference in levels of coarseness of the sandpapers. Reference data taken of the robotic arm's motion is shown in Figure 5a indicating a resonant frequency of roughly 135 Hz for the vibration sensing element of the device. Plots of power spectral data for normal vibration are shown below for different sandpaper grades. The 180 grit paper produced significantly more excitation than 320 grit sandpaper. The plots indicate significant differences in excitation levels for the 3 grades of sandpaper used in the test.

Figures 6a through 6c are power spectral plots of stress information gathered from the piezoelectric sensor as the probe scanned the sandpaper surfaces. The plots show differences of a few orders of magnitude in the signal amplitudes for the 3 types of sandpaper used in the experiment.

Buttazzo *et al.* [2] describe a method for measuring stiffness with a force sensor. Using this method, the probe is advanced into the skin and the position D1 at force threshold F1 is recorded. The probe is advanced further until a 2nd force threshold F2 is reached at position D2. The stiffness S is given by S = (F2 – F1)/(D2 – D1). Force threshold, F1 is the amount of force needed to indicate surface contact. A second method for measuring stiffness is to advance the probe into the skin a fixed distance say 1mm, measuring the force at each point. A measure for stiffness is obtained from the slope of the Force vs. Distance curve with a steep slope indicating stiff tissue. A larger time

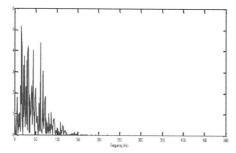

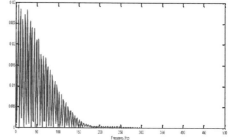

**Figure 6a.** Frequency content of stress data from a scan of 180 grit sandpaper.

**Figure 6b.** Frequency content of stress data from a scan of 320 grit sandpaper.

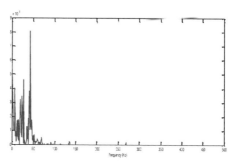

**Figure 6c.** Frequency content of stress data from a scan of 600 grit sandpaper.

constant is required for stiffness perception purposes. This is achieved by modifying the RC components of the charge amplifier circuit described earlier in the paper.

## 5. Conclusion

The above results show that relatively high frequency signals from the piezoelectric sensor and the accelerometers can be used to discern relative roughness of skin surfaces. Results also indicate that a quantitative measure on the stiffness of a given human tissue can be obtained by using the method outlined above. Because the electrode array does a good job of pinpointing source of force, additional spatial information on bump profiles or distance between bumps can be obtained from the piezoelectric sensor. An added benefit of using two approaches for texture perception is that one set of data may be used to validate the other.

As discussed by Gordon and Cooper in their 1975 paper [11], texture perception can be further complicated when undulations, gradual surface changes, occur on the surface. This is because receptors present in the skin will respond not only to surface roughness but also to undulations. A similar problem is faced by a robotic texture perception system which needs to maintain light contact with a constant force magnitude and proper probe orientation in order to accurately perceive surface roughness. Because stress data is required for both contact and roughness information, this may appear to be a problem. However, because textural information comes in the form of low amplitude, high frequency stress data while contact information is usually present in low frequency data. Monitoring this low frequency information and ensuring that contact force lies in the desired range during scanning is one way to maintain contact pressure. Information on the geometry of the skin could also be gathered this way. To maintain probe orientation, static acceleration from the second axis of the accelerometer could be monitored to ensure the probe remains normal to the surface.

## References

[1] Howe, R.D. and Cutkosky, M.R. "Sensing Skin Acceleration for Slip and Texture Perception". In *Proceedings of IEEE Conference on Robotics and Automation*, Scottsdale, Arizona, May 14-16, 1989, pp. 145-150.

[2] Buttazzo, G., Bicchi, A. and Dario, P. "Robot Tactile Perception". In *Sensor-based robots: Algorithms and Architectures*, pp 25-39.

[3] Fraden, J. "Piezoelectric Effect". In *Handbook of Modern Sensors*.

[4] Hayward, V., "Display of Haptic Shape at Different Scales". In *Proceedings of Eurohaptics* 2004, Munich, pp. 20-27.

[5] Khaled, W., Reichling, S., Bruhns, O.T., Boese, H., Baumann, M., Monkman, G., Egersdoerfer, S., Klein, D., Tunayar, A., Freimuth, H., Lorenz, A., Pessavento, A., Ermert, H., "Palpation Imaging Using a Haptic System for Virtual Reality Applications in Medicine". In *Proceedings of Medicine Meets Virtual Reality 12*, Newport Beach, 2004, pp. 147-153.

[6] Okamura, A.M. and Cutkosky, M.R. "Haptic Exploration of Fine Surface Features". In *Proceedings of the IEEE International Conference on Robotics and Automation*, 1999.

[7] K. Tollon, K.J. Waldron, W.L. Heinrichs, "Performance Characteristics of the Immersion Bimanual Surgical Simulation Interface". Presented at *Medicine Meets Virtual Reality* 12, Newport Beach, January 2004.

[8] Burton, R.C., "Malignant Melanoma in the Year 2000". In *CA-A Cancer Journal for Clinicians*, Vol. 50, No. 4, 2000, pp. 209-213.

[9] Krishna, G.M. and Rajanna, K., "Tactile Sensor Based on Piezoelectric Resonance". In *IEEE Sensors Journal*, Vol. 4, No. 5, 2004, pp. 691-697.

[10] Howe, R.D. and Cutkosky, M.R. "Dynamic Tactile Sensing: Perception of Fine Surface Features with Stress Rate Sensing". In *IEEE Transactions on Robotics and Automation*, April 1993.

[11] Gordon, I. and Cooper, C. "Improving One's Touch". In *Nature*, 1975

586

*Medicine Meets Virtual Reality 13*
*James D. Westwood et al. (Eds.)*
*IOS Press, 2005*

# Linking Human Anatomy to Knowledgebases: A Visual Front End for Electronic Medical Records[1,2]

Stewart DICKSON [a], Line POUCHARD [a], Richard WARD [a], Gary ATKINS [b],
Martin COLE [c], Bill LORENSEN [d] and Alexander ADE [e]

[a] *Oak Ridge National Laboratory*
[b] *Fisk University*
[c] *University of Utah*
[d] *GE Global Research*
[e] *University of Michigan*

**Abstract.** A new concept of a visual electronic medical record is presented based
on developments ongoing in the Defense Advanced Research Projects Agency Virtual Soldier Project. This new concept is based on the holographic medical electronic representation (Holomer) and on data formats being developed to support
this. The Holomer is being developed in two different visualization environments,
one of which is suitable for prototyping the visual electronic medical record. The
advantages of a visual approach as a front end for electronic medical records are
discussed and specific implementations are presented.

## 1. Introduction

The President's Information Technology Advisory Committee June 2004 report calls for
federal leadership to create needed technological innovations "to enable development
of 21st century electronic medical records" [1]. In July, Department of Health and Human Services Secretary Tommy Thompson and National Coordinator for Health Information Technology David Brailer announced a framework for strategic action for delivering "consumer-centric and information-rich" health care [2]. Concepts important to
this vision for 21st century medical care include: medical information moves with consumers, care is delivered electronically as well as in person, medical care is provided
with fewer medical errors and with less variation utilizing the electronic medical record.
The report expresses the hope that "sophisticated decision-support tools that help identify treatments....best suited to a given patient would be available to help reduce unnec-

---

[1]This work was supported by a grant from the DARPA, executed by the U.S. Army Medical Research and
Materiel Command/TATRC Cooperative Agreement, Contract # W81XWH-04-2-0012.

[2]The submitted manuscript has been authored by the U.S. Department of Energy, Office of Science of the
Oak Ridge National Laboratory, managed for the U.S. DOE by UT-Battelle, LLC, under contract No. DE-AC05-00OR22725. Accordingly, the U.S. Government retains a non-exclusive, royalty-free license to publish
or reproduce the published form of this contribution, or allow others to do so, for U.S. Government purpose.

essary treatments and to ensure prevention procedures, both of which will result in better outcomes [2]." One component of that vision for future medical care is decision support tools to help the physician in diagnosis. Another component needed is a visual user interface that collects varied types of information, for example text, charts, imagery such as CT and MRI, and three-dimensional (3D) reconstructions. We refer to this component as the Visual Electronic Medical Record (VEMR).

The Defense Advanced Research Projects Agency (DARPA) Virtual Soldier Project (VSP) is working on these issues in the context of providing medical care on the battlefield. The DARPA VSP is investigating methods to predict outcomes from wounding that will revolutionize medical care for the soldier. This research is expected to have a significant impact on civilian medical care. The goal of the VSP is prediction of outcomes of penetrating wounds, which will be based on comparison of results from complex mathematical models with experimental data. In the not too distant future, this will allow prediction of consequences of a wound using a soldier's post wound imaging along with pre-wound clinical data including baseline x-ray CT.

To provide a visual environment for encapsulating the results of this prediction, the VSP is developing a holographic medical representation (or Holomer) to be used to connect a 3D model of the soldier's body, based on x-ray CT, with anatomical and physiological information for purposes of improving medical diagnosis and treatment both on and off the battlefield. This visual-based prediction and medical record for the soldier can become, in the not too distant future, a first prototype for the VEMR, where a patient's vital signs, imagery, and other information is keyed to the locations in the anatomy of the medical complication. We discuss here the development of the VSP Holomer and its modifications for use in the civilian medical community as a VEMR.

## 2. Method

To address the problem of linking visual representation of the anatomy to a knowledgebase of information and prediction tools, the VSP is developing the Holomer. The Holomer will connect a 3D model of the soldier's body, based on X-ray CT, with anatomical and physiological information for purposes of improving medical diagnosis and treatment both on and off the battlefield. The Holomer coupled with predictive modeling software will facilitate a new level of integration in medical procedures and create a prototype for a truly interactive VEMR.

To demonstrate the Holomer concept, a 3D model was created from segmented and annotated National Library of Medicine Visible Human male photographic data [3]. The 3D model is displayed in SCIRun [4] using existing volume visualization techniques (Fig. 1), and is linked to knowledgebases using a specially developed module, referred to as the HotBox. The HotBox interacts with the geometric model via a 3D widget (the probe or blue sphere seen in Fig. 1) which is user controlled such that it can be moved to any location in the model. This provides the user with a means to input the location of interest. Given the location from the user controlled 3D widget, the HotBox implements the linkage to the 3D anatomy and the many levels of information provided in the knowledgebases.

Presently the information returned by the Hotbox is the tissue at the location of the probe and the adjacent tissues (see Fig. 2). In the future, this information could also

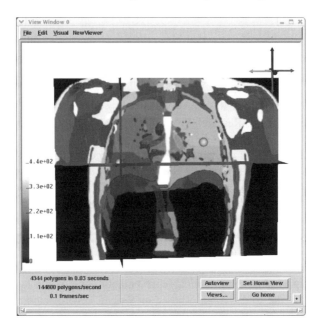

**Figure 1.** Thorax anatomy displayed in the SCIRun visualization environment. The blue sphere is the 3D widget (probe).

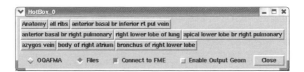

**Figure 2.** The Hotbox interface returns the tissue located at the 3D widget (probe), i.e. right lower lobe of the lung, and all adjacent tissues.

include a list of a patient's allergic reactions to drugs or allergens, or records of visits to the physician, or vital signs recorded during a hospital stay.

Different forms of information content from text-based to 3D imagery can be linked in the Holomer, thus providing a unique visual-based electronic medical record which the medic or physician can utilize for purposes of diagnosis and treatment. The specific focus of this unique visual approach to medical informatics in the VSP is penetrating wounds to the heart.

To develop the SCiRun-based Holomer, we have prototyped this concept using a visual front end developed using Visualization ToolKit (VTK) software [5]. The Visible Human (male) photographic data were used to create surface models and associated label maps for the thorax. For a soldier who has received a projectile wound, the wound is described using an Extensible Markup Language (XML) file standard based on a wound ontology developed by the VSP. Information in the wound ontology is used to show the regions of stunned and ablated tissue as the projectile enters the body and either lodges in an organ or exits the body. Information on the properties of the wounded tissue and various physiological and tissue material properties can be entered by the physician and

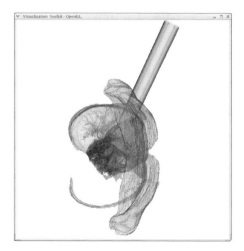

**Figure 3.** VTK-based visualization environment for prototype development. The wound has the projectile stopping in the left ventricle.

stored in this XML file to control the display of the region of wounded tissue. Figure 3 demonstrates a wound to the left ventricle of the heart, where the wound track is shown as a series of concentric cylinders representing tissue which has been ablated or simply stunned by the projectile.

In the future the wound description could be obtained from comparison of post trauma ultra sound (US) with baseline US or X-ray CT imagery for this soldier. The combination of the comparison of the wounded region and the baseline would then be automatically encoded into the wound ontology instance or wound XML file that controls the visual interface. Existing XML standards for medical records (such as HL7) would also be used for integrating standard medical records data. We will demonstrate how this can be done in connection with the wound ontology XML developed under the VSP.

When applied to a patient in a hospital setting, the interface could capture and display the patient's vital signs, making it possible for the physician to keep a detailed record of the patient's physiological responses during surgery or during recovery. The visualization of the physiological data (see Fig. 4) is accomplished using standard ICU monitor software, which we demonstrate here with simple Tcl/Tk plotting program which interfaces with the original VTK Holomer.

The advantage of this simple demonstration based on VTK is that it can be used to develop more sophisticated interfaces such as the SCIRun visualization interface being developed for the VSP and for prototyping a civilian VMER which is based on electronic medical record standards, yet incorporating new standards for the visual representation of information, such as the wound ontology XML and the physiological (vital signs) data format.

## 3. Results

A prototype of the HotBox has been developed within SCIRun. The HotBox, which comes from animation software [6], is a menu activated by placing the cursor at a par-

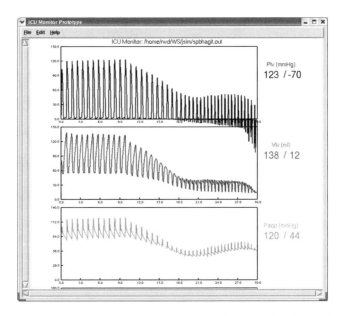

**Figure 4.** The prototype ICU Monitor screen displaying physiological results, in this case, for a model of the physiology in the thorax with injury to the left ventricle at 10 s. In clinical medical implementation, this display would show patient vital signs.

ticular point in the 3D space (anatomy). The menu provides the user with a multitude of options based on retrieving the anatomical structure at the spatial point from the "Master Anatomy" list created from segmenting and labeling the Visible Human data. For example, a menu item can be selected to invoke a connection, by Web services, to the Foundational Model of Anatomy [7] to provide the anatomical structures adjacent to the structure at the cursor location.

Physiological information from measured vital signs will also be available via the Web service from the HotBox menu. In addition, we have also developed an alternative approach for connecting to knowledgebases that is independent of SCIRun and can be run on PC platforms. In this approach the 3D images are created using VTK [5].

We have found that the VSP VTK-based Holomer concept has been useful in developing the more sophisticated visual Holomer based on SCIRun. It can also serve as a useful prototype development environment for a civilian version of the VEMR integrating significant new concepts such as the wound ontology XML and the physiological (vital signs) monitor with standard patient medical record. Further, the Holomer coupled with predictive modeling software will facilitate a new level of integration in medical procedures and create a prototype for a truly interactive VEMR.

## 4. Conclusions

We described the prototype concept of the HotBox, which can be integrated into the SCIRun Holomer to provide a link between 3D anatomy and knowledgebases of anatomical information, physiological response (vital signs) data and other standard medical records. We further describe a development environment based on VTK which has been used to prototype the SCIRun-based Holomer. The VTK-base visual interface is platform independent and has served well as a prototype for a new type of visual electronic medical record, one based on a 3D representation of the individual soldier or patient, providing unique visual access to the patient or soldier's condition, be it a wound or a disease.

The prototype Holomer being developed within the VSP is a unique demonstration of the concept of a "Visual Electronic Medical Record". Visual electronic medical records will improve the ease and use of medical records data by the physician, providing an interactive interface to records based on 3D anatomical reconstruction of the patient. Using the Holomer, a physician or medic will have access, at the touch of a button, to all available information about a patient or wounded soldier, greatly facilitating accurate and efficient diagnosis of medical conditions.

## References

[1] President's Information Technology Advisory Committee (PITAC) Report, "Revolutionizing Health Care through Information Technology", June 2004,
(http://www.itrd.gov/pitac/reports/20040721_hit_report.pdf).

[2] Tommy G. Thompson and David J, Brailer, "The Decade of Health Information Technology: Delivering Consumer-centric and Information-rich Health Care: Framework for Strategic Action, July 2004, (http://www.hhs.gov/onchit/framework/).

[3] See: National Library of Medicine Web site: http://www.nlm.nih.gov/research/visible/.

[4] SCIRun: A Scientific Computing Problem Solving Environment, Scientific Computing and Imaging Institute (SCI), 2002 (http://software.sci.utah.edu/scirun.html).

[5] See: http://www.kitware.com/vtk.html.

[6] Pouchard, LC, Dickson, SP (2004) "Ontology based three-dimensional Modeling for Human Anatomy" ORNL Technical Report ORNL/TM-2004/139.

[7] Rosse, C. and Mejino, JLV. (2003) "Ontology for Bioinformatics: The Foundational Model o of Anatomy". *Journal of Biomedical Informatics 36*:478-500.

592

*Medicine Meets Virtual Reality 13*
*James D. Westwood et al. (Eds.)*
*IOS Press, 2005*

# Simulating the Continuous Curvilinear Capsulorhexis Procedure During Cataract Surgery on the EYESI™ System

Roger WEBSTER, Ph.D. [a], Joseph SASSANI, M.D. [b], Rod SHENK [a],
Matt HARRIS [a], Jesse GERBER [a], Aaron BENSON [a], John BLUMENSTOCK [a],
Chad BILLMAN [a] and Randy HALUCK, M.D. [c]

[a] *Department of Computer Science, Caputo Hall, Millersville University,*
*Millersville, PA. USA 17551*
[b] *Department of Ophthalmology, Penn State University College of Medicine,*
*Milton S. Hershey Medical Center, Hershey, PA USA 17033*
[c] *Department of Surgery, Penn State University College of Medicine,*
*Milton S. Hershey Medical Center, Hershey, PA USA 17033*

**Abstract.** This paper describes a technique for simulating the capsulorhexis procedure during cataract surgery on the EYESI™ system. The continuous curvilinear
capsulorhexis technique can be a difficult procedure for beginning ophthalmology
surgeons. In the initial phase of tearing the tissue, the tear vector is tangential to
the circumference of the tear circle. However, without the proper re-grasping of the
flap of torn tissue close to the tear point, the tear vector angle quickly runs down-
hill possibly causing severe damage to the tissue. Novice surgeons tend to try to
complete the capsulorhexis without the time consuming re-grasping of the tissue
flap. Other factors such as anterior bowing of the lens diaphragm, patient age, and
shallow anterior chambers add to the problematic nature of the procedure. The tissue area is modeled as a curvilinear mesh of nodes and springs. Deformation is
accomplished via a physically based particle model utilizing a heuristic algorithm
to constrain the deformation calculations to the locality of the tear area to speed
up computations. The training software alerts the user of any potential tear problems before they occur thus instructing the novice surgeon. The EYESI™ hardware
system (from VRMagic GmbH) provides the user with stereoscopic images thus
providing 3D viewing. Our capsulorhexis simulator software models a number of
tear problems and anomalies to provide a useful training environment without the
dangers of using live patients.

## 1. Introduction

Eye surgery necessitates sub-millimeter precision and demanding hand-eye coordination
in a very small workspace, thus making it difficult to simulate. Some researchers have
developed eye surgical simulators [1,2] but none have attempted to model the capsulorhexis procedure during cataract surgery. Our capsulorhexis simulator uses complex
3D graphical models, a high fidelity eye simulator hardware platform, and a mathemati-

cal model of various tissue tear problems to provide a training environment without danger to patients. The continuous curvilinear capsulorhexis technique, developed by Gimbel and Neuhann, has become the standard method of anterior capsulectomy for phacoemulsification [3]. The capsulorhexis procedure begins by making a small incision with a cystotome in the center of the lens and generating a radial flap of tissue to grasp. The surgeon grasps the folded over flap of tissue and begins to tear in a circular motion such that the tear force vector is tangential to the circumference of the tear circle [4]. Angled forceps are used to grasp and pull the tissue circumferentially. All too often, beginning surgeons attempt to complete the capsulorhexis procedure without the proper re-grasping of the flap of torn tissue close to the tear point. This error in technique can cause the tear to run peripherally. If the surgeon attempts to redirect it by traction directed in a radial fashion toward the center of the lens, the tear only propagates further peripherally. It may even extend to the posterior capsule resulting in the complication of vitreous loss and/or the dropping of lens material into the posterior segment of the eye, necessitating more extensive corrective surgery. Anterior bowing of the lens diaphragm as well as a shallow anterior chamber can accentuate this peripherally directed tear phenomenon [5,6].

## 2. Methods and Tools

There are basically three major paradigms for modeling soft tissue in surgical simulation: Finite Element Models (FEMs), mass-springs models, and hybrid approaches [7,8]. Although many researchers have used mass-spring models successfully to model cloth animations, VR facial expressions, and abdominal organs, there appears to be a movement afoot to use more hybrid models and algorithms to avoid issues of numerical instability and prohibitive computational complexity. We use a modified hybrid mass-springs system to take advantage of the computational speed and simplicity. The tissue area is modeled as a curvilinear mesh of nodes and springs. Deformation is accomplished via our physically based particle model utilizing the mass-springs-damper connectivity with our modified implicit predictor to speed up calculations during each time step. The dynamics equation for each mass point is: $m_i x_i = -\gamma_i x_i + \sum g_{ij} + f_i$ Where: $m_i$ is the mass at point $x_i \in R^3$, $-\gamma_i x_i$ is the damping force to prevent instabilities, $g_{ij}$ is the linear Hookian force exerted on mass i by the spring between $i$ and $j$, $f_i$ is the sum of the external forces acting on mass $i$ (gravity, pushing, pulling, and tearing the tissue). Combining the vectors of all mass points produces: $Mx + Dx + Kx = f$, where $M$ is the mass matrix, $D$ is the damping matrix, $K$ is the stiffness matrix, and $f$ is the aggregate force vector. As the system progresses through time dt, the first order differential equations are: $v = M^{-1}(-Dv - Kx + f)$, $x = v$, where $v$ is the velocity vector. To get around the computational expense of solving a linear system at each time step, we incorporate an approximate solver, that pre computes the solution to a linear system [9]. In addition, we incorporate a heuristic algorithm to constrain the deformation calculations to the locality of the tear area to speed up the computations. As the mesh is pulled, a heuristic routine determines the direction of the tear based on the force vectors acting on the mesh. The parameters of this routine can be adjusted to model various capsule characteristics.

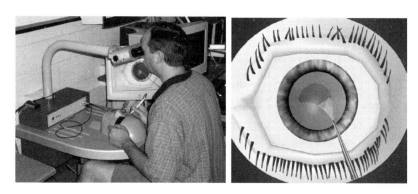

**Figure 1.** (left) The EYESI™ hardware system (right) Virtual instrument tearing the tissue.

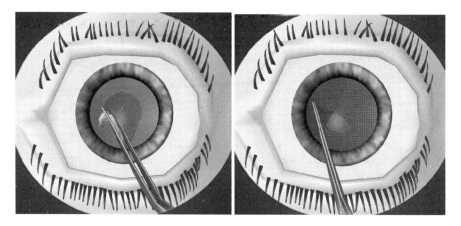

**Figure 2.** (left) The tissue after the tear has progressed too far radially (right) Modified hybrid mass-springs model used for tearing the membrane.

## 3. Results

Our training simulator software runs on the EYESI™ hardware system from VRMagic GmbH (see Figure 1). The training software has a data collection module that collects various metrics such as: time spent on the capsulorhexis procedure, tissue tear metrics, re-grasping time, and severe tear errors. Another software module records the motions of the user, which are used to replay the technique, thus showing the resident or mentor what the user did during the training session. Our training system provides a useful tool for beginning ophthalmology surgeons to experiment and test their skills before interaction with live patients.

## Acknowledgments

This project is funded, in part, by the National Science Foundation under grant number EIA-0116616, the Neimeyer-Hodgson Grants Program, the Havemeier-Gibson Endowment for Computer Science, MU Faculty Grants program, and by the Penn State University College of Medicine Department of Ophthalmology.

# References

[1] Michael Sinclair, J. Peifer, R. Haleblain, M. Luxenberg, K. Green, D. Hull, *"Computer-simulated Eye Surgery - A Novel Teaching Method for Residents and Practitioners"*, Ophthalmology, Vol. 102, Number 3, March 1995, pps. 517-521.

[2] Clemens Wagner, M. Schill, R. Manner, *"Collision Detection and Tissue Modeling in a VR-Simulator for Eye Surgery"*, Eighth Eurographics Workshop on Virtual Environments (2002), Barcelona, Spain, May 30-31, 2002, pps. 27-36.

[3] Norman Jaffe, M. Jaffe, G. Jaffe, Cataract Surgery and its Complications, Sixth Edition, Mosby Press, St. Louis, Baltimore, 1977, pps. 50-97.

[4] Ehud Assia, D. Apple, J. Tsai, E. Lim, *"The Elastic Properties of the Lens Capsule in Capsulorhexis"*, American Journal of Ophthalmology, Vol. 111, No. 5, May, 1991, pps. 628-632.

[5] James Morgan, R. Ellingham, R. Young, G. Trmal, *"The Mechanical Properties of the Human Lens Capsule Following Capsulorhexis or Radio Frequency Diathermy Capsulotomy"*, Archives of Ophthalmology, Vol. 114, September 1996, pps. 1110-1115.

[6] H.J. Burd, S.J. Judge, J.A. Cross, Numerical Modeling of the Accommodating Lens, *Vision Research*, Vol. 42, 2002, pps. 2235-2251.

[7] Sarah Frisken and B. Mirtich, A Survey of Deformable Modeling in Computer Graphics, *MERL Technical Report TR-97-19*, November 1997, http://www.merl.com/reports/TR-97-19/.

[8] Roger Webster, R. Haluck, B. Mohler, R. Ravenscroft, E. Crouthamel, T. Frack, S. Terlecki, J. Sheaffer, Elastically Deformable 3D Organs for Haptic Surgical Simulators, *Proceedings of the Medicine Meets Virtual Reality Conference*, MMVR 2002, Newport Beach, California, January 23-26, 2002, IOS Press, pps. 570-572.

[9] Mathieu Desbrun, G. Debunne, A. Barr, M, Cani, Interative Multi-Resolution Animation of Deformable Models, *Proceedings of the Annual ACM SIGGRAPH Conference*, ACM Press, Los Angeles, California, August 1999, pps. 82-89.

596

*Medicine Meets Virtual Reality 13*
*James D. Westwood et al. (Eds.)*
*IOS Press, 2005*

# Using an Approximation to the Euclidean Skeleton for Efficient Collision Detection and Tissue Deformations in Surgical Simulators

Roger WEBSTER, Ph.D. [a], Matt HARRIS [a], Rod SHENK [a], John BLUMENSTOCK [a],
Jesse GERBER [a], Chad BILLMAN [a], Aaron BENSON [a] and Randy HALUCK, M.D. [b]

[a] *Department of Computer Science, Caputo Hall, Millersville University,*
*Millersville, PA. USA 17551*
[b] *Department of Surgery, Penn State College of Medicine, Milton Hershey*
*Medical Center, Hershey, PA USA 17033*

**Abstract.** This paper describes a technique for efficient collision detection and deformation of abdominal organs in surgical simulation using an approximation of the Euclidean skeleton. Many researchers have developed surgical simulators, but one of the most difficult underlying problems is that of organ-instrument collision detection followed by the deformation of the tissue caused by the instrument. Much of the difficulty is due to the vast number of polygons in high resolution complex organ models. A high resolution gall bladder model for instance can number in the tens of thousands of polygons. Our methodology utilizes the reduction power of the skeleton to reduce computations. First, we recursively compute approximations to the Euclidean skeleton to generate a set of skeletal points for the organ. Then we pre-compute for each vertex in each polygon the associated skeleton point (minimal distance discs). A spring is then connected from each vertex to its associated skeleton point to be used in the deformation algorithm. The data structure for the organ thus stores for each skeletal point its maximum and minimum distances and the list of associated vertices. A heuristic algorithm using the skeleton structure of the instrument and the skeleton of the organ is used to determine instrument collisions with the organ.

## 1. Introduction

This paper describes an efficient method for performing real-time collision detection and object deformation in surgical simulations. Our method utilizes the reduction power of the skeleton to reduce computations for collision detection and deformation. The skeleton is used to speed up the detection of collisions, and to handle deformations. The skeleton is created by recursively computing approximations to the Euclidean skeleton to generate a set of skeletal points for the organ. The refined approximation skeleton is then fit to a Bezier curve to smooth out the data points and ensure an equally spaced distribution of points. A data structure is built containing information about each skeleton point, the

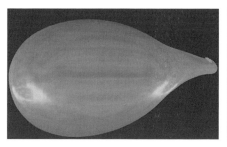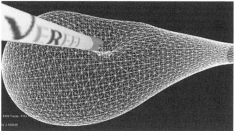

**Figure 1.** (left) Gallbladder model (right) Wireframe showing real-time tool-tissue deformation.

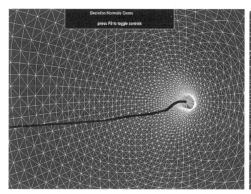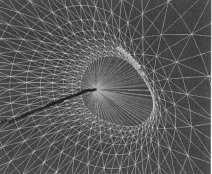

**Figure 2.** (left) Skeleton points (right) Wireframe showing skeleton points with connector springs attached to all vertices associated with the skeleton point.

associated vertices, and a hierarchy of springs for use in the deformation algorithm. Collision detection utilizes the adjacency information included in the skeleton data structure to prune away vertices and faces from consideration.

## 2. Methods and Tools

The software runs on a conventional Windows XP™ workstation with a 2.0 GHz Pentium™ processor (or higher) and an OpenGL™ graphics accelerator such as the Nvidia Geforce™ board. The application software makes calls to our proprietary object oriented software toolkit called MUOpenGL, which is an easy to use API (Application Programmers Interface) that calls OpenGL™ graphics routines. The toolkit provides additional functionality on top of OpenGL™ and has various objects and methods to rapid prototype simulation systems. The skeleton is created by gathering approximated distance information for a finite set of interior points in the model. For each interior point, the Euclidean distance to the closest point of each face of the model is calculated, grouping together exterior points that are equidistant within some epsilon of error. A heuristic algorithm is used to determine the interior points whose group of closest exterior points is distributed on opposite sides of the model. These interior points form the first approximate skeleton.

The algorithm is then recursively rerun on the approximate skeleton points at progressively higher resolutions to improve the accuracy of the skeletal points. Finally, the approximated skeleton is fit to a cubic Bezier spline to smooth out the data points and ensure an evenly distributed set of skeleton points. Each vertex in the model is then attached to a skeleton point by a Hookian spring. For every skeleton point, the distance of its farthest associated vertex is saved. Collision detection is done by first calculating the distance from the colliding object to each skeleton point. If the distance is greater than the maximum distance for that skeleton point, then all of the vertices associated with that skeleton point are pruned away from consideration. If the distance is less than the maximum distance, then triangle intersection tests are performed against the tool and faces that contain vertices attached to the skeleton point. When collisions occur, vertices are translated along the vector towards their skeleton point, with neighbors being progressively deformed based upon vertex displacement.

To smooth the skeletal points we use a Bezier cubic spline function of the form:

$$f_i(t) = \sum_{k=0}^{B} C_{i-k} B_k(t)$$

with basis polynomials

$$b_0(t) = 1/6(-t^3 + 3t^2 - 3t + 1) \quad b_1(t) = 1/6(3t^3 - 6t^2 + 4)$$
$$b_2(t) = 1/6(-3t^3 + 3t^2 + 3t + 1) \quad b_3(t) = 1/6(t^3)$$

## Acknowledgments

This project is funded, in part, by the National Science Foundation under grant number EIA-0116616, the Noonan Grants Program, the Willard O. and Dr. Catherine Gibson Havemeier Endowment in Computer Science, MU Faculty Grants program, and by the Penn State University College of Medicine.

## References

[1] H. Blum, "Biological Shape and Visual Science", Journal of Theoretical Biology, 38 (1973) 205-287.
[2] Richard Robb, "An Axial Skeleton Based Surface Deformation Algorithm for Patient Specific Anatomic Modeling", Proceedings of the Medicine Meets Virtual Reality Conference, MMVR 2000, Newport Beach, California, January 20-24, 2000, IOS Press, pps. 53-58.
[3] G. Borgefors, I. Nystrom, and G. S. D. Baja, "Computing Skeletons in Three Dimensions", Pattern Recognition, 32:1225-1236, 1999.
[4] H. Li and A.M. Vossepoel, "Generation of the Euclidean Skeleton by a Bisector Decision Rule on a two-Shortest-Vector Distance Map", in: H.J.A.M. Heijmans, J.B.T.M. Roerdink (eds.), Mathematical Morphology and its Applications to Image and Signal Processing, Computational Imaging and Vision Series, vol. 12, Kluwer, Dordrecht, 1998, 151-158.
[5] T.C. Lee and R. L. Kashyap, "Building Skeleton Models via 3-D Medial Surface/axis Thinning Algorithm" CVGIP: Graphical Models and Image Processing, 56(6): 462-478, November 1994.
[6] Roger Webster, R. Haluck, B. Mohler, R. Ravenscroft, E. Crouthamel, T. Frack, S. Terlecki, J. Sheaffer, "Elastically Deformable 3D Organs for Haptic Surgical Simulators", Proceedings of the Medicine Meets Virtual Reality Conference, MMVR 2002, Newport Beach, California, January 23-26, 2002, IOS Press, pps. 570-572.

Medicine Meets Virtual Reality 13
James D. Westwood et al. (Eds.)
IOS Press, 2005

# Virtual Surgical Planning and CAD/CAM in the Treatment of Cranial Defects

John WINDER [a], Ian McRITCHIE [a], Wesley McKNIGHT [b] and Steve COOKE [c]

[a] *Health and Rehabilitation Sciences Research Institute, University of Ulster*
[b] *Electrical and Mechanical Engineering, University of Ulster, Newtownabbey*
[c] *Department of Neurosurgery, Royal Victoria Hospital, Belfast*

**Abstract.** The purpose of this work was to enhance the clinical outcome in the neurosurgical treatment of cranial defects and fibrous dysplasia. Cranial defects require repair using a variety of materials to protect the brain and provide a good cosmetic outcome for the patient. Virtual neurosurgery and CAD/CAM techniques have been employed to increase the implant 3-dimensional accuracy. The source data was 3D Computed Tomography scans. The CT scans were visualised using surface shading and rotation with volume rotation and re-sizing being used to review the complete data set. The volume data was manipulated using 3D image editing and surface modelling. Physical models of the patients' skulls were created using computed numerical milling which provided a physically accurate template for the production of a cranial implant. This has led to improved fitting for titanium plates requiring less theatre time and in the case of fibrous dysplasia a change in the operative technique from a two stage operation to one stage.

## 1. Introduction

The purpose of this work is to describe and illustrate the application of virtual neurosurgery and computer assisted design/manufacturing techniques to the treatment of fibrous dysplasia. Virtual neurosurgery is defined as the simulation, planning and practice of a neurosurgical procedure on computer. We developed this methodology to enable surgeons to experiment and review surgical techniques in cases that required special attention. In all cases, surgery was on the skull and therefore the imaging modality used for planning was CT.

### 1.1. Repair of Cranial Defects

The repair of cranial defects requires two clinical outcomes; protection of the brain and good cosmetic appearance. Accurate fitting of the implant contributes to these outcomes. The materials used for repair include methyl methacrylate resin, hydroxyapatite bone cement [1] and titanium [2]. Each of these materials requires manual handling during the operation to model the implant. The contour and fit of the implant is adjusted intraoperatively which is time consuming and may introduce inaccuracy. The challenge was to exploit existing 3D image processing and CAD/CAM technologies using commercially available software for accurate surgical planning and manufacture of cranial implants.

The aim of this approach is to improve the physical accuracy of the implant and reduce manual input within the design process.

## 1.2. Surgical Treatment of Fibrous Dysplasia

Fibrous dysplasia is a benign bone disease that usually occurs in childhood when growth is rapid. The disease causes excess bone growth especially in regions of the skull and face and sometimes the long bones and is found equally between males and females. Generally, it is not dangerous in itself, but may lead to complications where the bone growth impinges on other structures such as brain tissue and nerves. The bone growth may be extensive causing an unsightly appearance and may require correction. In these cases surgical intervention is used to either reduce the size of the bone growth or to remove the diseased tissue completely.

Fibrous dysplasia may be managed by conservative curettage or debridement of the affected area [3]. This procedure is used to reduce the volume of the diseased tissue. The disease may also be managed successfully by radical resection of the diseased bone. Depending on the location of the diseased area, follow-up reconstruction using an autologous bone graft of healthy tissue from another part of the patient's body may be performed. The reconstruction aspect of the surgery may take place at a second operation.

## 2. Methods

Patients underwent a custom 3D CT scan and their data were transferred to a 3D imaging workstation for surgical planning. The CT imaging was performed on a Philips AV-E1 single slice helical scanner with a slice acquisition thickness of 3.0 mm, reconstructed at 1.0 mm intervals. The scan range depended on the location of the disease but generally ranged from the supra-orbital ridge to the top of the cranium. Virtual neurosurgery was used in six cases of fibrous dysplasia in adults and children ranging in age from 5 to forty-five years.

## 2.1. Virtual Neurosurgery

Bone tissue was segmented from soft tissue by simple image pixel thresholding. A surface shaded representation of the skull was presented on the computer screen to the neurosurgeon. The range of functionality required to interact with the data was as follows:

- Data surface shading;
- Data volume rotation and re-sizing;
- Manual drawing of lines on the skull surface;
- Cutting and removing bone by image editing;
- Storing of test operations for review.

This computer-based surgical planning assisted the surgeon in determining the fixation points and shape of the implant. The software functionality required to interact with the data was as follows: data surface shading; data volume rotation and re-sizing; volume distance and area measurements; cutting and removing bone by image editing; storing of test operations for review. Figure 1 (a-c) shows the procedural steps for virtual surgical planning and manufacture of implants. The CT data was rendered and surface modelled

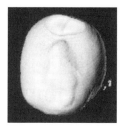 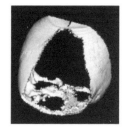 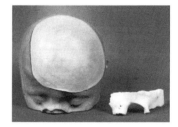

**Figure 1.** (a-c) showing a) surface shaded CT scan, b) the results of the virtual operation performed by the surgeon and c) the CNC milled model and acrylic implants created for defect repair.

to produce a data set suitable for either medical rapid prototyping or computer-controlled milling [4]. The milled model was used as a template for the construction of custom cranial implants from either titanium or acrylic resin.

## 3. Results

50 patients have had a titanium or acrylic resin cranioplasty implanted over a period of 8 years at the Department of Neurosurgery, Royal Victoria Hospital, Belfast, Northern Ireland. Defect size ranged from 3 cm to 12 cm at its greatest dimension. Physical accuracy of the models was +/- 2.0 mm. However, the anatomical accuracy is defined by the CT scan parameters. Neurosurgeons have anecdotally noted improved accuracy of fit and reduced theatre time with the potential for significant impact on patient care and health economics. For instance, the conventional surgical treatment of fibrous dysplasia generally requires two operations, firstly, to remove the diseased bone and, secondly, to repair the defect. In six cases, the virtual surgical planning allowed the surgeon to resect the diseased area and fit the implant in a single operation as the implant was prepared before the operation.

## 4. Conclusion

We have presented a successful computer based methodology for accurate surgical planning and cranial implant design. We have used 3D imaging and CAD/CAM technology which has improved the physical accuracy of the implant and patient cosmetic outcome.

## References

[1] Arriaga MA, Chen DA, 2002. Hydroxyapatite cement cranioplasty in translabyrinthine acoustic neuroma surgery. Otolaryngol Head Neck Surg., 126(5), 512-517.
[2] Winder RJ, Cooke RS, Gray J, Fannin T, Fegan T, 1999. Medical rapid prototyping and 3D CT in the manufacture of custom made cranial titanium plates. Journal of Medical Engineering and Technology, 23(1), 26-28.
[3] Zenn MR, Zuniga J, 2001. Treatment of fibrous dysplasia of the mandible with radical excision and immediate reconstruction: case report. J Craniofac Surg., 12(3), 259-63.
[4] Joffe J, Nicoll, Richards, Linney, A, Harris M, 1999. Validation of computer assisted manufacture of titanium plates for cranioplasty. Int J Oral Maxillofac Surg., 28, 309-13.

*Medicine Meets Virtual Reality 13*
*James D. Westwood et al. (Eds.)*
*IOS Press, 2005*

# New Approaches to Computer-based Interventional Neuroradiology Training

Xunlei WU, Vincent PEGORARO, Vincent LUBOZ, Paul F. NEUMANN,
Ryan BARDSLEY, Steven DAWSON and Stephane COTIN

*The Simulation Group, CIMIT, MGH, Harvard Medical School*

**Abstract.** For over 20 years, interventional methods have substantially improved the outcomes of patients with cardiovascular disease. However, these procedures require an intricate combination of visual and tactile feedback and extensive training periods. In this paper, a prototype of endovascular therapy training system is presented. A set of core simulation components applicable to most vascular procedures has been designed and integrated into a real-time high-fidelity interventional neuroradiology training system for the prompt treatment of ischemic stroke. We believe it will improve the quality of training and the speed of learning without putting patients at risk.

## 1. Introduction

### 1.1. Background

Stroke is the third leading cause of death in the US. Each year, more than $750,000$ strokes result in over $150,000$ deaths [1]. The main therapy for ischemic stroke is catheterization, allowing direct lytic therapy to dissolve the clot and restore the flow. Following femoral arterial puncture, a guidewire-catheter combination is advanced under fluoroscopic guidance through the iliac arteries, into the aortic arch, and inside the common carotid artery. This allows entry into the internal carotid artery and the cerebral circulations in the brain. This guidance is provided by intravascular angiogram, obtained during contrast agent (CA) propagation, which defines the abnormal areas, guides the instrument movement, and verifies the treatment. Because the treatment is delivered only under image-based guidance, the dedicated skill of instrument navigation and the thorough understanding of vascular anatomy are critical to avoid irreversible complications. Unfortunately, the best training environments have been actual patients who have had a stroke. Additionally, the shortage of trained interventional neuroradiologists means that many ischemic stroke patients do not have access to care.

In 2004, a decision by the FDA regarding appropriate levels of training for physicians who perform high-risk procedures in the cerebral circulation mandated that physicians train to proficiency before treating humans.A For the first time, a major part of this mandated training includes simulation. Future trends in procedural education are therefore likely to increase the role of high-fidelity simulation for medical training.

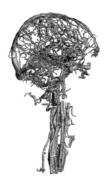 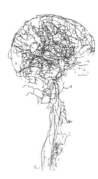

**Figure 1.** *Left*: Segmented vasculature. *Right*: Geometric skeleton generated from the vascular isosurface.

## 1.2. Previous Work

A few VR systems focusing on interventional radiology (IR) have been developed or commercialized [10,7,9,3]. The core architecture has remained the same. In this paper, we propose new approaches for rendering, physics-based modeling, and anatomical representations that will lead to a real-time high fidelity simulation system for more effective IR skill training.

## 2. Methodology

### 2.1. Semi-automatic Segmentation

At first we need to segment the cerebrovascular system from a CTA scan. The segmentation task is particularly challenging due to the small vessel diameter and the close proximity of vessels to the skull. We used a combination of anisotropic filtering and morphological operators, e.g. dilation and erosion provided in *Amilab*[1] to eliminate bony structures, skin, and sinuses. The result of the segmentation on a CTA dataset of $0.586 \times 0.586 \times 0.5 \ mm^3$ can be seen on the left side of Figure 1. A few discontinuities in the network due to artifacts will be resolved to generate a complete 3D vascular model.

After obtaining the isosurface of the vascular network, the medial axis is computed. Geometric skeletons are defined as the locus of the centers of maximal spheres within a shape, and provide a mean of describing the topology of the model. This information is required by the one-dimensional flow model in Section 2.4 and contrast agent propagation algorithm in Section 2.5. We also used *Amilab* to generate the centerlines and, with the help of a physician, to label each vessel as shown in the right half of Figure 1.

### 2.2. Incremental Finite Element Model for Catheter/Guidewire

In this simulator, we have developed physics-based flexible instrument models representing a variety of intravascular devices, suitable for vessels from 3 to 20 *mm* diameter. Current methods represent flexible instruments as a set of connected rigid elements [5], or by

---

[1] http://serdis.dis.ulpgc.es/amilab.

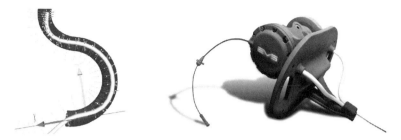

**Figure 2.** *Left*: Model the catheter/guidewire deformation by 3D beam elements with collision response. *Right*: The optical tracking device for catheter/guidewire can be concealed inside a patient mannequin.

linear elastic FEM [9]. A common drawback of current methods is the inability to capture the essential characteristics of wire-like structures, including high tensile strength and low resistance to bending. To improve the accuracy of previously proposed models, we have developed new mathematical representations based on three-dimensional beam theory, where the large number of parameters for each element will allow the representation of a library of commonly employed catheters or guidewires. Key characteristics to model mechanical properties include: cross-sectional area, effective shear area, Young's modulus, Poisson's ratio, and cross-section/polar moment of inertia. By using an incremental approach to update the stiffness matrix at every time step, highly non-linear behavior of catheter/guidewire can be realisticly simulated. Furthermore by controlling the number of elements, we are able to ensure real-time deformation while maintaining reasonable accuracy.

### 2.3. Sequential Quadratic Programming for Collision Response

Navigating through the vasculature of this system requires an instrument tracking device and a collision response (CR) method between the vasculature and instrument models. In our previous work [3], as well as that of others [8,4], once contact has been determined, forces or boundary conditions are applied to the deformable catheter/guidewire model. Since the catheter has many contacts against the vessels, an Octree based collision detection (CD) algorithm has been implemented. Because sliding occurs at the point of contact, Lagrange multiplier techniques or penalty forces will not constrain the flexible body correctly and may induce oscillations. Our approach relies on sequential quadratic programming (SQP), combining FEM and CR together. A set of inequality constraints, based on the distance between catheter nodes and neighboring vessel triangles, are added to the set of FEM equations. Our catheter model and CR are shown in the left half of Figure 2.

### 2.4. One-dimensional Vascular Flow Computation

Clinically turbulent flow is a diagnostic aid for IR procedures, but rarely observed under stroke therapy where the small diameter of vessels combined with limited flow rates reduces the occurrence of turbulence. In addition, the average resolution of a fluoroscopic image is on the order of $0.3mm$, making it difficult to observe turbulence or transaxial flow pattern. Hence, one-dimensional fluid flow model along the vessel axes should provide enough information for a training system. To compute such vascular flow, we

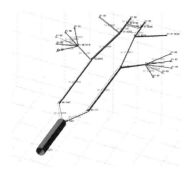 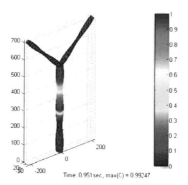

**Figure 3.** *Left*: Real-time 1D vascular flow simulation using vascular graph. *Right*: Contrast agent propagation computed in a simplified bifurcation according to an advection diffusion model.

have implemented a simplified one-dimensional FEM representation proposed in [3].The blood flow in each element is modeled as an incompressible viscous fluid flowing through a cylindrical pipe, and can be calculated from the Naiver-Stokes equation. The resulting equation, called Poiseuille Law [6], is solved by linear FEM. This computation runs very efficiently and provides real-time simulation of vascular flow. The left half of Figure 3 shows the flow computation results with vessel median axes with radii ranging from 2 to 6*mm*.

### 2.5. 3D Particle-based Real-time Angiography Simulation

Contrast agent (CA) is often used during medical imaging to highlight specific parts of the body under X-ray, CT, and MRI. Upon injection, CA is carried by blood cells and circulates through the vasculature until it is eliminated in the kidneys and liver. We computed the transportation of CA by an advection equation in terms of the CA concentration $C(x, t)$ distribution parameterized by the curvilinear coordinate $x$ and time $t$,

$$\frac{\partial C(x,t)}{\partial t} + u(x,t)\frac{\partial C(x,t)}{\partial x} = r(t) \tag{1}$$

where $r(t)$ is the injection rate of contrast agent and $u(x, t)$ is the averaged laminar flow velocity along the axial direction of each vessel. Mixture transition of multiple fluids and the transversal velocity profile are not considered. We numerically solved (1) by forward-in-time and center-in-space finite difference schemes whose accuracy is linear in temporal domain and quadratic in space.

To visualize an angiogram, we used a set of equally spaced 3D particles to represent the vessel's internal volume as in Section 2.1. The intensity values of particles are then mapped to $C(x, t)$ at each sampling point along the vascular graph. The final rendering stage combines one updated particle system for CA propagation and one volumetric texture map for the surrounding anatomy as described in Section 2.6. This approach uses mainly GPU power and runs at an interactive frame rate.

### 2.6. Real-time Simulation of Fluoroscopic Rendering

We have developed a new volume rendering approach for the simulation of fluoroscopic images directly using CT. With OpenGL as a rendering library, a ray casting method using specific blending is implemented to approximate the X-ray attenuation process. The volume rendering algorithm creates a set of parallel slices onto which the corresponding part of the volume intersects. The slices are rendered as a 2D texture-mapped polygon by approximating the beam attenuation described by the discretized Beer's Law,

$$I = I_0 e^{-\sum_j \mu_j d_j} \qquad (2)$$

with $I_0$ the input intensity, $\mu_j$ the linear attenuation coefficient sampled at slice $j$, and $d_j$ the slice thickness along the ray. This method greatly reduces computation times by using OpenGL and specific texture map operations.

### 2.7. Catheter/Guidewire Motion Tracking Device

We have developed an optic catheter/guidewire tracking device that passively recreates haptic sensation, since most feedback in IR is visual. The tracking device is embedded inside a full-size patient mannequin, therefore naturally recreates the OR environment as shown in the right of Figure 2. This improves the level of realism during training. The virtual vasculature is accessed through a standard sheath on the left or right femoral artery. Once a real catheter is inserted into the sheath, the system starts tracking the instrument's 2 DOF's motion. Passive haptic feedback – friction – is provided by a set of anatomically correct Teflon tubing phantoms.

Currently, only one instrument – catheter or guidewire – can be tracked at a time. A major difficulty, when tracking two or more nested devices, is that access to the inner device is mechanically impossible without modifying the instrument [7]. This challenge will be thoroughly investigated in the future as well as the validation of tracking accuracy.

## 3. Results

We have developed new approaches for fluoroscopic rendering, physics-based instrument modeling, and high reslution anatomical representations and integrated them into a real-time interventional neuroradiology simulator for skill training. Our simulator is implemented on a P4 3.0 GHz PC equipped with 1 GB main memory and NVIDIA GeForce FX5900 Ultra graphic card. It is capable of rendering 256 slices of a $512^3$ volume with more than one million 3D particles at 29 FPS depending on user interaction. This frame rate includes fluoroscopic rendering, collision detection and response, catheter/guidewire deformation, and CA advection. The left half of Figure 4 shows the full simulation system and the right half illustrates the simulated contrast agent propagation through a volumetric cerebro-vasculature model.

## 4. Conclusions and Future Work

In summary, a set of endovascular simulation components have been developed and integrated into a training system for the treatment of stroke. This system allows multiple levels of skill acquisition using interventional instruments. This prototype emphasizes high fidelity visual feedback and physically accurate CR and CA propagation. Due to its cost-effective design and system compactness, such a system would lead to cross-specialty

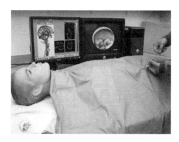
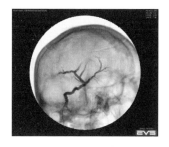

**Figure 4.** *Left*: The high-fidelity interventional neuroradiology skill training simulator. *Right*: 3D fluoroscopic rendering of CA propagating through a cerebrovascular model within a CT head model.

interventional training. Also, this platform increases accessibility to medical institutions and hospitals.

In the future, we will extend the catheter model to interventional balloon and stent by mass-spring network or as a set of radial elements [2]. Upon completion, our prototype will undergo face validity from our hospital collaborators and then comprehensive validation study. We will also incorporate an educational curriculum providing various scenarios. These improvements should reveal full potentials of this simulator including procedural planning.

## Acknowledgments

This work was supported by Telemedicine and Advanced Technology Research Center (TATRC) through grant number DAMD-17-02-2-0006. We thank Dr. Karl Krissian from SPL and Dr. James Rabinov in MGH for providing us valuable feedback on anatomical segmentation.

## References

[1] American Heart Association. Heart and stroke facts statistics: Statistical supplement. American Heart Association, Dallas, Texas, 1999.

[2] R. Balaniuk and K. Salisbury. Soft-tissue simulation using the radial elements methods. In *Proc. International Symposium on Surgery Simulation and Soft Tissue Modeling*, pages 48–58, 2003.

[3] S. Dawson, S. Cotin, D. Meglan, D.W. Shaffer, and M.A. Ferrell. Designing a computer-based simulator for interventional cardiology training. *Catheterization and Cardio. Intervention*, 51(4):522–527, 2000.

[4] A. Deguet, A. Joukhadar, and C. Laugier. A collision model for deformable bodies. In *International Conference on Itelligent Robots and Systems*. IEEE, 1998.

[5] R. Featherstone. The calculation of robot dynamics using articulated-body inertias. *International Journal of Robotics Research*, 2(1):13–30, 1983.

[6] A. Guyton and J. Hall. *Textbook of Medical Physiology*. Saunders Elsevier, 10th edition, 2000.

[7] U. Hoefer, T. Langen, J. Nziki, F. Zeitler, J. Hesser, U. Mueller, W. Voelker, and R. Maenner. Cathi - catheter instruction system. In *Computer Assisted Radiology and Surgery (CARS), 16th International Congress and Exhibition*, pages 101 – 06, Paris, France, 2002.

[8] P. Meseure, J. Davanne, L. Hilde, L. France, F. Triquet, and C. Chaillou. A physically-based virtual environment dedicated to surgical simulation. In *Surgery Simulation and Soft Tissue Modeling (IS4TM)*, pages 38–47, June 12-13 2003. Juan-les-pins, France.

[9] W.L. Nowinski and C.K. Chui. Simulation of interventional neuroradiology procedures. In *Int. Workshop on Medical Imaging and Augmented Reality (MIAR)*, pages 87–94. IEEE Computer Society, 2001.

[10] N. Subramanian and T. Kesavadas. A prototype virtual reality system for preoperative planning of neuro-endovascular interventions. In *Proceedings of Medicine Meets Virtual Reality 12th*, pages 376–80, 2004.

*Medicine Meets Virtual Reality 13*
*James D. Westwood et al. (Eds.)*
*IOS Press, 2005*

# CAD Generated Mold for Preoperative Implant Fabrication in Cranioplasty

J. WULF [a], L.C. BUSCH [a], T. GOLZ [a], U. KNOPP [b], A. GIESE [b],
H. SSENYONJO [b], S. GOTTSCHALK [c] and K. KRAMER [d]

[a] *Department of Anatomy, University of Luebeck,*
*23538 Luebeck, Germany*
[b] *Department of Neurosurgery, University of Luebeck,*
*23538 Luebeck, Germany*
[c] *Department of Neuroradiology, University of Luebeck,*
*23538 Luebeck, Germany*
[d] *Department of Computer-Aided Engeneering, University of Applied Sciences,*
*23562 Luebeck, Germany*
*e-mail: joergwulf@yahoo.de*

**Abstract.** Intraoperative fabrication of acrylic cranial implants may be difficult and will increase operation time. In addition forming implants directly on the defect, intracranial tissues are exposed to heat of polymerization and residual monomer, that occurs, when autopolymerizing methyl methacrylate is used intraoperatively. Furthermore the cosmetical result may be unacceptable. Preoperatively formed acrylic implants may reduce these disadvantages compared to conventional techniques in cranioplasty. We will present methods for preoperative fabrication of cranial implants for a cadaver specimen. Implants were fabricated using a Rapid prototyping (RP) models of the skull built by Fused Deposition Modeling (FDM). In addition a mold of the defect was generated by CAD techniques, that can serve as a template for implant design.

## 1. Introduction

Trauma, calvarian tumors, infected craniectomy bone flaps and defects following decompressive surgery are the main reasons for large cranial defects. The indication for reconstruction of these defects are cosmetic reasons and/or protection against mechanical impact. The intraoperative free-hand modeling of skull implants turns out, in particular with very large defects, as cosmetically and technically difficult. In addition the operation time is often prolonged, which is medically [1–3] and economically unfavorable. Laboratory pre-manufactured implants reduce such disadvantages [4].We report a technique of Rapid Prototyping (RP) for custom reconstruction of large cranial defects using Fused Deposition Modeling (FDM) which is based on routine radiographic diagnostics.

A thermoplastic material extruded as a wire is used by a 3D-plotter to reconstruct the bony skull defect based on CT data. Using CAD technique an anatomical model and a negative mold of the defect is reconstructed, which can be created based on CT data

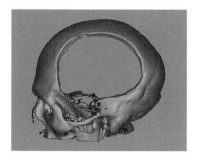

**Figure 1.** Virtual model showing the defect.

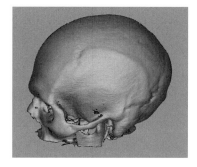

**Figure 2.** Mirror image of healthy side.

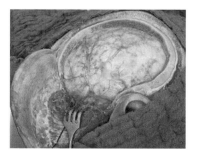

**Figure 3.** Intraoperative view on bony defect.

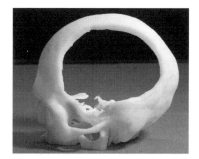

**Figure 4.** FDM model of defect side.

or be recreated by an approximation of a mirrored image of the unaffected contralateral side (Figure 1 and Figure 2).

## 2. Methods

Anatomical models can serve as templates for laboratory fabricated implants. Furthermore the negative mold of the defect can be used to form directly methyl methacrylate (Palacos®) reconstructions. This technique has been used to reconstruct large defects based on 1mm spiral CT images and data sets.

   In a cadaver specimen a surgical craniectomy (Figure 3) was performed and a negative mold of the defect that was built using Fused Deposition Modeling. The mold was based on the preoperative imaging data taking into account the modified mirror image of the contralateral side using "free hand" CAD assisted design (Figure 5).The CAD data of the mold cold be transferred to .STL-file format by means of which it is possible to generate rapid prototyping models, e.g. using FDM techniques. Furthermore a positive FDM-model was built (Figure 4). Different acrylic implants were built using a negative mold. In addition laboratory fabricated implants were built by means of a wax pattern formed on the FDM model in order to form a properly contoured shape. The wax pattern than was invested in gypsum and wax was removed. The resulting mold then was used for acrylic implant fabrication. The different implants were radiographically imaged and the reconstructions were compared to the preoperative images by an overlay technique.

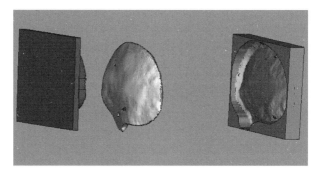

**Figure 5.** CAD generated virtual implant with upper and lower part of mold.

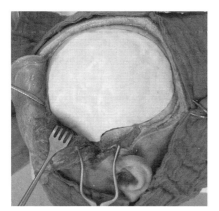

**Figure 6.** Intraoperative fit of implant on defect.        **Figure 7.** CT image of implant on defect.

## 3. Results

Our results demonstrate that FDM generated anatomical models and negative molds of the defects provide a rapid and highly accurate method of custom implants of skull defect reconstructions (Figure 6 and Figure 7) which is based on routine CT data and commercially available hardware and CAD software components. It is a cost-effective alternative to industrially produced implants. The implant fabrication can be performed preoperatively by the operating surgeon.

## References

[1] Taub PJ, Rudkin GH, Clearihue WJ 3rd, Miller TA. Prefabricated alloplastic implants for cranial defects. Plast Reconstr Surg 2003;111:1233-40.
[2] Cooper PR, Schechter B, Jacobs GB, Rubin RC, Wille RL. A pre-formed methyl methacrylate cranioplasty. Surg Neurl 1977;8:219-21.
[3] Dumbrigue, HB, Arcuri MR, LaVelle WE, Ceynar KJ. Fabrication procedure for cranial prosthesis. J. Prosthet Dent 1998; 79:229-31.
[4] Gronet PM, Waskewicz GA, Richardson C. Preformed acrylic cranial Implants using fused d modeling: A clinical report. J Prosth Dent; 90:429-33.

*Medicine Meets Virtual Reality 13*
*James D. Westwood et al. (Eds.)*
*IOS Press, 2005*

# Effect of Binocular Stereopsis on Surgical Manipulation Performance and Fatigue When Using a Stereoscopic Endoscope

Yasushi YAMAUCHI [a] and Kazuhiko SHINOHARA [b]

[a] *National Institute of Advanced Industrial Science and Technology (AIST),*
*Tsukuba Central 6, 1-1-1 Higashi, Tsukuba 305-8566, Japan*
[b] *School of Bionics, Tokyo University of Technology,*
*1404 Katakura, Hachioji, Tokyo 192-0982, Japan*

**Abstract.** We compared performance in three kinds of endoscopic tasks – a peg-board, incision, and suturing – under the monoscopic (2D) and stereoscopic (3D) visual conditions conducted for 1 hour in total. We also evaluated the degree of fatigue from the aspects of subjective and objective consciousness using the critical flicker frequency (CFF) test together with a questionnaire of fatigue. A total of eight subjects showed higher performance when using the 3D display than the 2D display in all three tasks and, simultaneously, improvement in performance as a result of learning effect. No difference of fatigue was found depending on the display conditions both in the CFF test and questionnaire.

## 1. Objective

For medical stereoscopic imaging, the usefulness of the presentation of depth information and the issues of picture quality and fatigue have been discussed. Opinion of stereoscopic endoscopes has been divided among medical professionals, partly because of differences in the types of endoscope used and the evaluation methods employed. For example, the report on an endoscopic trainer by Taffinder et al. [1] revealed a remarkable improvement in the accuracy of forceps manipulation. Clinical findings on cholecystectomy by Hanna et al. [2], however, revealed no difference in performance between novel stereoscopic endoscopy and conventional monocular endoscopy. Further, no studies have deeply investigated fatigue experienced during observation of stereoscopic endoscope images.

We have previously attempted to evaluate performance of a pegboard task by using a laparoscope that allows switchover between monoscopic (2D) display and stereoscopic (3D) display [3]. The purpose of this study is to evaluate the effect of binocular stereopsis in laparoscopic surgical tasks: a pegboard, incision, and suturing. Also, the subjective and objective fatigue was assessed.

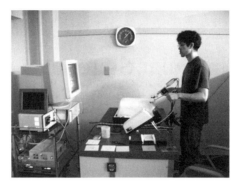

**Figure 1.** Stereoscopic endoscope and training box.

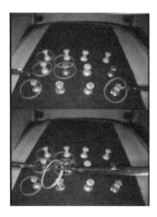 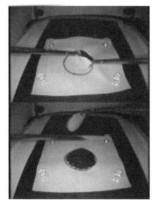 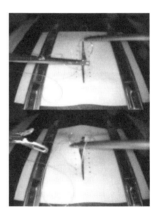

**Figure 2.** Experimental tasks in the training box.

## 2. Methods

The stereoscopic endoscope that we used was an SK-1057-3D-A laparoscope (Shinko Optical Co. Ltd, Tokyo, Japan). A liquid-crystal shutter (120 Hz) placed in front of the CRT switched the left and right images. The observer was required to wear polarized glasses. The system also provided 2D images by presenting the left (or right) images to both eyes. Thus, the optical condition of the 2D image, including its quality, color and FOV was identical to that of the 3D image, except stereopsis.

Tasks were performed in a laparoscope manipulation training box (MATT trainer, Limbs & Things). The endoscope was fixed and the distance from the subject to the monitor was about 1.1 m (Fig. 1).

Subjects were asked to perform three kinds of tasks in the training box: A (pegboard, 8 min.), B (cutting, 6 min.), and C (suturing, 10 min.) (Fig. 2) [4]. Each task was carried out twice in the order of ABCABC, requiring about one hour in total. The subjects were eight healthy individuals with no previous experience in surgical manipulations of an endoscope. Before experiments, they were allowed to practice only once for each task. The order of the 2D/3D was set at random by the subject. An interval of two weeks or more was placed between both 2D/3D experiments.

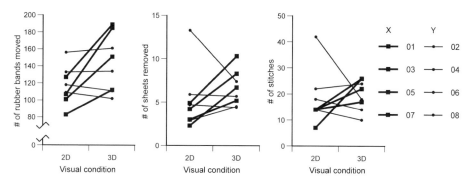

**Figure 3.** Results of task performance for eight subjects. Thick lines: group X (3D before 2D). Thin lines: group Y (2D before 3D).

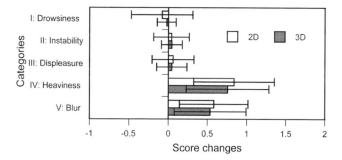

**Figure 4.** Score changes in "Subjective Symptom Test of Fatigue (SSTF)" before and after the tasks. Marked subjective fatigue was observed in category IV and V. However, no significant difference was found between the 2D display and the 3D display in any question ($p > 0.05$).

The subjective symptoms of fatigue were indexed using "Subjective Symptom Test of Fatigue (SSTF)" [5], consists of 25 questions about fatigue, rated on a scale of 1–5. The questions in SSTF can be categorized into five categories: "I: Drowsiness", "II: Instability", "III: Displeasure", "IV: Heaviness", and "V: Blur." Meanwhile, as an objective assessment of eye fatigue, we employed critical flicker frequency (CFF) test. Entry of SSTF and CFF were conducted before and after the each experiment.

## 3. Results

The group that performed tasks with the 2D before the 3D (group X) performed markedly better with the 3D than 2D (paired t-test, $p < 0.01$), regardless of the kind of task. In contrast, the group that performed tasks with the 3D before the 2D (group Y) showed no marked difference in performance ($p > 0.05$) (Fig. 3). In SSTF, the degree of fatigue after the experiments was markedly elevated for "IV: Heaviness" (fatigue of the muscular systems), and "V: Blur" (fatigue of the visual system) (Fig. 4). The rate of change in CFF value after the experiments with that before was $1.01 \pm 0.02$ and $1.02 \pm 0.02$ with the 2D and the 3D, respectively. However, no difference of fatigue was found depending on the display mode, in both SSTF and CFF test ($p > 0.05$).

## 4. Discussion

The difference in the results between group X and group Y, which was due to the order of display conditions, suggests that improvement in the manipulation performance as a result of using the 3D display and improvement in performance as a result of learning took place simultaneously. That is, in group Y, the effect of observing the 3D display probably compensated for the learning effect. Large individual variations in performance were also found.

The results of this study suggests that, as for the current stereoscopic endoscope, continuous use of about one hour presents almost no problem of fatigue attributed to binocular stereopsis. It should be noted, however, that in the experiments of this study, the endoscope was fixed. There is a possibility of having "motion sickness" if someone else manipulates an endoscope as in an actual operation.

## References

[1] Taffinder N, Smith SG, Huber J, Russell RC, Darzi A: The Effect of a Second-generation 3D Endoscope on the Laparoscopic Precision of Novices and Experienced Surgeons. Surgical Endoscopy 13:1087-1092, 1999.

[2] Hanna GB, Shimi SM, Cuschieri A: Randomized Study of Influence of Two-dimensional versus Three-dimensional Imaging on Performance of Laparoscopic Cholecystectomy. Lancet 351:248-251, 1998.

[3] Yamauchi Y, Shinohara K: Study on Evaluation Indexes of Surgical Manipulations with a Stereoscopic Endoscope. Lecture Notes in Computer Science 3217:1083-1084, 2004.

[4] Derossis AM, Fried GM, Abrahamowicz M, Sigman HH, Barkun JS, Meakins JL: Development of a Model for Training and Evaluation of Laparoscopic Skills. The American Journal of Surgery 175:482-487, 1998.

[5] The Industrial Fatigue Research Committee of Japan Society for Occupational Health: Subjective Symptom Test of Fatigue– New Version. Digest of Science of Labour 57:295-314, 2002.

*Medicine Meets Virtual Reality 13*
*James D. Westwood et al. (Eds.)*
*IOS Press, 2005*

# A Dynamic Friction Model for Haptic Simulation of Needle Insertion

Yinghui ZHANG and Roger PHILLIPS

*Department of Computer Science, The University of Hull,*
*Kingston upon Hull, HU6 7RX, UK*

**Abstract.** This paper describes a new friction model, termed the *brush model*, suitable for haptic simulations of needle insertion in virtual environments. A novel two-layer surface contact model is presented that provides real-time rendering of friction forces at haptic refresh rates. A significant modification to the brush model is also presented, leading to a new friction model, termed the *fixed bristle brush model*. Simulation results show that the two models can accurately reflect the experimentally observed friction characteristics. This paper presents a simulation of friction during needle insertion; results agree with the experimental observations.

## 1. Introduction

Needle insertion is one of the less invasive medical procedures. Kataoka et al. [1] classified the forces acting on the needle during insertion into three types: the tip force, the friction force acting on the wall of the needle shaft, and the clamping force acting on the side wall of needle shaft in the normal direction. Simulating these forces is essential for training surgeons with needle insertion in haptic-based virtual environments. However, friction force simulation has remained somewhat primitive. Friction models used in various simulations of needle insertion typically use some forms of static friction model [2]; these models do not satisfactorily simulate the dynamic behavioural effects of friction caused by the reversal and variations of insertion velocity. The disadvantages with static friction models, such as the Coulomb model, the Karnopp model and their modified versions, are that they characteristically do not capture many of the friction phenomena observed experimentally, and consequently the tactile responses of simulators using them tend to lack reality. Furthermore, using either the velocity threshold or friction threshold for switching between the sticking and sliding friction modes may result in implementation problems and incorrect simulation results.

The goal of our work is to develop a dynamic friction model which produces realistic virtual experiences for training surgeons. The advantages of the new model are:

1) displacement dependent;
2) smooth transition between static and dynamic friction;
3) zero velocity detection not required;
4) captures most of the friction phenomenon;
5) takes account of normal load;
6) efficient enough for real-time haptic rendering of friction.

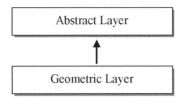

**Figure 1.** The two-layer architecture of the surface contact model.

## 2. Method

From a microscopic viewpoint, no surfaces are truly smooth in real world, all surfaces are rough. The friction force between surfaces is contributed by the contact forces developed at asperity junctions. Our new friction model [3], termed the brush model, is based on the interaction of asperities. It features a novel two-layer surface contact model. The next subsection presents a description of the surface contact model. The mathematical derivation of our model for the simulation of friction is described in Section 2.2. The modification of the brush model, as well as the fixed bristle brush model, is presented in Section 2.3.

### 2.1. Surface Contact Model

In the surface contact model, a novel two-layer architecture is developed, see Fig. 1. In the geometric layer, which is the underlying layer of the contact model, the interaction between asperities is simplified by supposing one surface is stationary and smooth with the other surface being covered with flexible bristles which make contact with the smooth surface. A brush-like behaviour of flexible bristles is employed to define how the contact surfaces interact. Based on this, a mathematical equation is derived in the abstract layer which is the upper layer of the contact model, describing the relationship of the normal load and the number of bristles in contact.

The two-layer architecture of the surface contact model presents advantages in terms of the computational efficiency, namely,

1) explicit collision detection between bristles and the opposite surface is not required;
2) the location of bristles is not required;
3) the model is not constrained by surface geometry; the contact surfaces can be flat or curved surfaces.

This feature distinguishes our friction model from other asperity-based friction models such as the bristle model [4].

Fig. 2 illustrates the geometric layer in which surface $A$ is covered with flexible bristles that are able to slide against the stationary surface $B$. The length of bristles is governed by a probability distribution $\varphi(h)$, where $h$ is the height of a bristle. These bristles are distributed randomly over the surface are of $A$ in contact with surface $B$. According to the Coulomb's law, the friction force developed between contacting surfaces is determined only by the true contact area. Therefore, the distribution of bristles does not have any significant effects on the resulting friction forces; and the model does not need to know the actual locations of bristles on surface $A$. When the relative motion starts, bris-

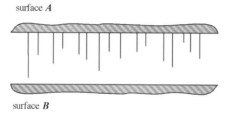

surface *A*

surface *B*

**Figure 2.** The geometric layer of the surface contact model describing the interaction of contacting surfaces.

tles in contact will bend to generate the tangential resistance. This tangential resistance is simulated by the Dahl's spring model. When the deflection of a bristle exceeds the maximum deflection displacement, the bristle snaps, and is then replaced by another bristle at the same position. The snap distance is randomly varied for the set of bristles. Physically this variation in snap distance is analogous to the variations between asperities on the actual surface. In the contact model, the snap distance is supposed to be governed by the uniform probability distribution; and all bristles have uniform tangential stiffness.

The frictional force of the contacting surfaces is calculated by summing together the effects of all the bristles of surface *A* that actually make contact with surface *B*.

To model the influence of changing normal load, the interacting bristles deform in the normal direction to carry the normal pressure. In the surface contact model, the contact area of each bristle is supposed to remain constant; and all bristles have uniform normal stiffness. As the normal pressure increase, more bristles will come in contact with the opposite surface; similarly, the number of contacting bristles will decrease when the normal pressure decreases. The number of bristles in contact, therefore, varies with the changes of the normal force; and hence the overall friction force varies.

Let $\varsigma$ denote the number of bristles in contact, and $N$ denote the normal load. We suppose the height of bristles is governed by the exponential distribution [5], e.g. $\varphi(h) = \sigma^{-1}e^{-h/\sigma}$, where $\sigma$ is the standard deviation and mean of the distribution. For most metal surfaces in manufacturing, $\sigma$ takes the value of $10^{-6}$ m [6]. A mathematical method has been developed to describe the relationship between the number of bristles in contact and the normal load, namely,

$$\varsigma = \frac{N}{\sigma_\perp \sigma}$$

where $\sigma_\perp$ is the uniform normal stiffness of bristles. We have proved that this relationship holds both for the contact between two flat surfaces and the contact between curved surfaces.

## 2.2. Friction Calculation

Let $z_\lambda$ denote the deflection of bristle $\lambda$. The motion of bristle $\lambda$ is modelled as

$$\frac{dz_\lambda}{dt} = \frac{dx}{dt}, \quad |z_\lambda| < \delta_\lambda$$

where $x$ is the relative displacement of the contacting surface, and $\delta_\lambda$ is the maximum deflection displacement of bristle $\lambda$. When the deflection $|z_\lambda|$ exceeds $\delta_\lambda$, bristle $\lambda$ snaps and $z_\lambda$ will be reset to zero. Let $\sigma_0$ denote the uniform tangential stiffness of bristles, the local friction at each asperity junction, by using the Dahl's model, is then given by

$$f_{local} = \sigma_0 z_\lambda + \sigma_1 \frac{dz_\lambda}{dt}$$

where $\sigma_1$ is the damper coefficient. The addition of a damper term is to prevent the oscillation which occurs in the sticking phase when velocity is at a small level around zero. In the brush model, the damper coefficient is chosen as an exponential form in velocity,

$$\sigma_1(v_\lambda) = \sigma_1 e^{-v_\lambda/v_s}$$

which is characterized by the parameter $\sigma_1$ and $v_s$. $v_s$ is also known as the Stribeck velocity which may take a value of $10^{-3}\,\mathrm{ms}^{-1}$ for most simulations. For the contact without the presence of lubrication, the dry friction force of the solid-to-solid contact surfaces is calculated by summing up the local frictions generated at asperity junctions,

$$F = \sum_{1 \leq \lambda \leq \varsigma} \left( \sigma_0 z_\lambda + \sigma_1 e^{-v_\lambda/v_s} \frac{dz_\lambda}{dt} \right)$$

To take account of the viscous friction for the lubricated surfaces, an additional term which is proportional to velocity needs to added to give,

$$F = \sum_{1 \leq \lambda \leq \varsigma} \left( \sigma_0 z_\lambda + \sigma_1 e^{-v_\lambda/v_s} \frac{dz_\lambda}{dt} \right) + \sigma_2 \frac{dx}{dt}$$

where $\sigma_2$ is the viscous coefficient.

The brush model is characterized by the parameters $\sigma_0$, $\sigma_1$ and $\sigma_2$. A mathematical method to determine the parameter $\sigma_0$, and $\sigma_1$ has been developed. This method is derived based on the physical properties of surfaces which are available in literature for a wide range of materials.

In summary, the brush model is given by

$$F = \sum_{1 \leq \lambda \leq \varsigma} \left( \sigma_0 z_\lambda + \sigma_1 e^{-v_\lambda/v_s} \frac{dz_\lambda}{dt} \right) + \sigma_2 \frac{dx}{dt}$$

$$\frac{dz_\lambda}{dt} = \frac{dx}{dt}, \quad |z_\lambda| < \delta_\lambda,$$

$$\varsigma = \frac{N}{\sigma_\perp \sigma},$$

$$\sigma_1 = (\mu_s - \mu_d)\sigma_\perp \sigma \, e v_s^{-1}$$

$$\sigma_0 = 4\mu_d \sigma_\perp \sigma \delta^{-1}, \quad \delta = \max\{\delta_\lambda\}$$

where $\mu_s$, $\mu_d$ are the static and dynamic friction coefficients respectively.

## 2.3. Modification

By correspondingly varying the number of bristles in contact, the brush model takes account of the influence of changing normal load. However, this causes the computational costs of the brush model to fluctuate, which is an undesirable feature particularly for simulations in haptic-based virtual environments. A modification has been made to the brush model, leading to a new friction model, termed the *fixed bristle brush model*.

It is known that when surfaces come into contact, asperities compress to carry out the normal load. It is reasonable to assume that the compression of asperities gives rise to the increase of hardness of asperities. To overcome the shortcoming of the brush model, we suppose that the number of bristles in contact remains constant so that the computational costs would not wave but instead both the normal stiffness and the tangential stiffness vary with the normal load. The relationship between the normal and tangential stiffness and the normal load has been developed. The fixed bristle brush model is, therefore, given by,

$$F = \sum_{1 \leq \lambda \leq \varsigma_0} \left( \sigma_0 z_\lambda + \sigma_1 e^{-v_\lambda / v_s} \frac{dz_\lambda}{dt} \right) + \sigma_2 \frac{dx}{dt}$$

$$\frac{dz_\lambda}{dt} = \frac{dx}{dt}, \quad |z_\lambda| < \delta_\lambda,$$

$$\sigma_1 = \frac{e(\mu_s - \mu_d)}{\varsigma_0 v_s} N,$$

$$\sigma_0 = \frac{4\mu_d}{\varsigma_0 \delta} N, \quad \delta = \max\{\delta_\lambda\}$$

where $\varsigma_0$ is the fixed number of bristles in contact. It is worth noting that the fixed bristle brush model has two more parameters less than the brush model.

## 3. Results

Various simulations have been performed to investigate the dynamic behaviours of our friction models. The simulation results show that our friction models capture accurately most friction phenomena observed experimentally. A full exposition of the behaviour and features of our model is provided elsewhere [7].

To assess fidelity generated by the models in a haptic-based virtual environment, simulations are also performed with the comparison with the Karnopp model. The results show that our models provide a more realistic feel to users than the Karnopp model.

The simulation of friction forces after puncture during the needle insertion is also performed by using the fixed bristle brush model. The physical dimension of the needle is chosen as that in [8]. The simulation result clearly shows the tendency that the friction force grows with the needle penetration after puncture, due to the effects of the increasing normal pressure on the side wall of the needle shaft and the viscous friction, see Fig. 3. This agrees with the experimental results [8].

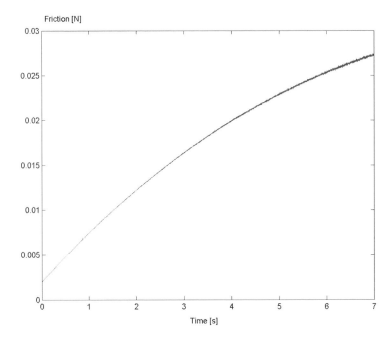

**Figure 3.** Friction force increases with the needle penetration after puncture.

## 4. Conclusion

Two friction models for accurate simulation of static and dynamic friction have been described. Simulation results show that the models capture the dynamic behaviours of friction. The models also take account of normal load which is essential for the simulation of needle insertion.

   We are developing virtual environments applications that use our friction models, for example, virtual environment trainers for various interventional radiological procedures.

   Our friction models has a relatively low demand on computation, thus they provide good fidelity in simulation of friction, it appears to be suitable for a wide range of virtual environment applications that demand high quality tactile responses.

## References

[1] Kataoka, H., Washio, T., Chinzei, K., Mizuhara, K., Simone, C., Okamura, A., Measurement of the tip and friction force acting on a needle during penetration. MICCA 2002, pp.216-23.
[2] Alterovitz, R., Pouliot, J., Taschereau, R., Hsu, I., Goldberg, K., Simulating needle insertion and radioactive seed implantation for prostate brachytherapy. MMVR 2003, pp.19-25.
[3] Zhang, Y., Phillips, R., Efficient and accurate simulation of friction using a multi-asperity surface contact model. EuroHaptic 2004.
[4] Haessig, D. A., Friedland, B., On the modelling and simulation of friction. J. of Dynamic Systems, Measurement and Control. Vol. 113, No. 3, (1991) pp. 354-62.
[5] Greenwood, J. A., Williamson, J. B. P., Contact of nominally flat surface. Proc. Roy. Soc. London, Ser. A 295 (1966), pp. 300-319.
[6] Bjorklund, S., A random model for micro-slip between nominally flat surfaces. J. Tribology, Vol. 119, (1997) No. 4.

[7] Zhang Y. and Phillips R., A Multi-asperity Surface Contact Model for the Simulation of Friction in Virtual Environments, University of Hull, pre-publication draft, (2004), 16 pp.

[8] Washio, T., Chinzei, K., Needle force sensor, robust and sensitive detection of the instant of needle puncture. MICCAI 2004, pp. 113-120.

*Medicine Meets Virtual Reality 13*
*James D. Westwood et al. (Eds.)*
*IOS Press, 2005*

# Enhanced Pre-computed Finite Element Models for Surgical Simulation

Hualiang ZHONG, Mark P. WACHOWIAK and Terry M. PETERS
*Robarts Research Institute, London, Canada*
*{hzhong,mwach,tpeters}@imaging.robarts.ca*

**Abstract.** Soft tissue modeling is an important component in effective surgical simulation systems. A pre-computed finite element method based on elastic models is well suited to modeling soft tissue deformation. This paper address two principal issues: the flexibility of the pre-computed FE method and the approximation approach to non-linear elastic models. We describe a dynamic mechanism of the reconfiguration of the contacted nodes and the fixed boundary, without re-computing the inverse of the global stiffness matrix. The flexibility of the pre-computed models is described for both linear and non-linear elastic models.

## 1. Introduction

Medical simulation systems based on CT or MRI images are becoming increasingly attractive for planning and guidance of minimally invasive surgical procedures. By using such a system, surgeons are able to rehearse various approaches to carefully plan procedures. This kind of simulation system requires visual and physical realism as well as computational efficiency. Among the several key features in the development of a surgical simulator, realistic simulation of soft tissue deformation under external forces is of crucial importance. The finite-element method (FEM) is a standard technique for solving many problems in continuum mechanics, and can accurately simulate deformation and haptic intervention. However, solving the large-scale system of equations required by FEM is time consuming and not efficient for real time simulation, especially for complex organs where a finer mesh is required to capture the deformation of its surface details. Because real-time performance is one of the most important features in a surgery training and planning system, much of the progress in real-time FEM has been motivated by work in surgical simulation [2,3,12].

Based on the linear elasticity of soft tissue, Cotin et al [4] introduced a preprocessing step in which the FE solver calculates the displacements of each free node for a sequence of input data sets, and then generates tensor matrices to connect the displacements of free nodes with those of contacted surface nodes. This method can provide simultaneous visual and force feedback as well as higher accuracy (the same as that of the linear elastic FEM model). One of its drawbacks is that it works well only in a pre-defined area. For example, a surgeon interacting with such a system needs complete flexibility in the manner with which he interacts with simulated organs. He should not be restricted to a single area. In this case, the method suffers because the global equations must be solved in real time. In addition, linear elastic models are not rotationally invariant and are limited to small perturbations. To alleviate these problems, some non-linear models have been proposed. For example, Picinbono [12] employed the St. Venant-Kirchhoff model, where the elastic energy $W$ is denoted by $W = \lambda (tr\, E)^2/2 + \mu (tr\, E^2)$ and the Green-St. Venant strain tensor $E$ is denoted by $E = (\nabla U + \nabla U^t + \nabla U^t \nabla U)/2$, where $U$ is a displacement vector, and $\lambda$ and $\mu$ are the Lamé coefficients. In this case the linear tensor matrix approach in [4] is no longer valid. While our work described here is related to [3,4], we clarify the concept of tensor matrices and extend it to polynomials for non-linear elastic models. To overcome the restriction of pre-defined area imposed on the pre-computed model [4,5], we describe a direct method to calculate and update the tensor matrices for linear elastic models, and propose an affine mapping for non-linear models.

## 2. Methods

A deformable model is a mathematical description of the geometry of an object and its deforming mechanism. Like many other continuous problems, soft tissue deformation is usually addressed by discretization. For example, the finite element method divides the problem domain into discrete elements, each containing several nodes. The unknown displacements of these nodes are subject to the elastic model, imposed force, and boundary constraints, and usually are calculated by solving a set of linear/non-linear algebraic equations. The displacements of the internal points in the element are obtained by interpolating the nodes' displacements. Since the force and boundary constraints are imposed on each element through its shape functions, the element type and its geometric representation are crucial for precise results, as well as for minimizing computation time.

In our experiments, we segment a volume of a brain phantom from a MRI data set through a morphological approach, and smooth its surface with a spherical kernel Gaussian filter. Based on the segmented image, we generate a geometric representation of the surface by employing the marching cubes algorithm [8]. After smoothing and decimating, we obtain a mesh consisting of 40,466 triangles and 20,211 points. Since the shapes of these triangles are not suited to FEM computation, the ICEM® package was used for regularization. From the surface triangles, ICEM generated a solid 3D tetrahedral representation of the brain phantom. The final mesh included 3,921 nodes and 11,741 tetrahedrons. To prevent translation, we assume that the bottom part of the phantom has been fixed and that the external force has been applied at its apex.

The pre-computed model takes advantage of available FEM software packages for a variety of elastic models, but its real time behavior should be independent of the software employed at the pre-computation stage. In a virtual environment, a user's interaction is reflected through the movement of contacted points between the surgical tool and the organ surface. Our system accepts the movements of such points as prescribed displacements for its boundary constraints, and its outputs include both displacement and haptic feedback.

### 2.1. Mechanism of the Pre-computed FE Model for Linear Elastic Models

In FEM, the linear elastic model can generate the following matrix equation for each element $e_i$: $K^{e_i} D^{e_i} = F^{e_i}$, where $K^{e_i}$ is the stiffness matrix ($12 \times 12$ for tetrahedron), and $D^{ei}$ and $F^{ei}$ are the vectors of the displacements and forces of the element's nodes. After assembling these individual forces at each node, the global equation can be written as

$$K (d_1 d_2 \ldots d_{3n})^T = (F_1 F_2 \ldots F_{3n})^T \tag{1}$$

where $F_i$ are external forces, and $K$ is the assembled global stiffness matrix.

Similar to the condensation technique used in [3] which separates all the nodes into the internal and surface components to reduce the size of $K$ for efficiency, here we consider flexibility, and divide all the nodes into to three sets: the contacted nodes, the free nodes, and the fixed boundary nodes, denoted by $P_K = (p_1 p_2 \ldots p_k)$, $P_R = (p_{k+1} \ldots p_m)$, and $P_B = (p_{m+1} \ldots p_n)$, respectively. Then the above global equations are reduced to

$$\tilde{D} = \tilde{K}^{-1} \tilde{F}, \tag{2}$$

where $\tilde{K}$ is a $3m \times 3m$ matrix obtained from $K$ by removing the rows and columns corresponding to the set of the fixed nodes. $\tilde{D}$ and $\tilde{F}$ correspond to all other nodes except the fixed ones. Without loss of generality, we write $\tilde{K}^{-1}$ as

$$\tilde{K}^{-1} = \begin{pmatrix} A_{3k \times 3k} & B_{3k \times 3(m-k)} \\ C_{3(m-k) \times 3k} & D_{3(m-k) \times 3(m-k)} \end{pmatrix} \tag{3}$$

where $A_{3k \times 3k}$ corresponds to the contacted nodes $P_K$. To simplify this expression, we ignore gravity so that the external forces at the free nodes $P_R$ are zero. The above equations yield:

$$(F_1 F_2 \ldots F_{3k})^T = A^{-1}_{3k \times 3k}(d_1 d_2 \ldots d_{3k})^T \tag{4}$$

Combining (2) and (4), we obtain:

$$\begin{pmatrix} d_1 \\ \ldots \\ d_{3m} \end{pmatrix} = \tilde{K}^{-1}_{3m \times 3k} A^{-1}_{3k \times 3k} \begin{pmatrix} d_1 \\ \ldots \\ d_{3k} \end{pmatrix} = \begin{pmatrix} I_{3k \times 3k} \\ C_{3(m-k) \times 3k} A^{-1}_{3k \times 3k} \end{pmatrix} \begin{pmatrix} d_1 \\ \ldots \\ d_{3k} \end{pmatrix} \tag{5}$$

where $\tilde{K}^{-1}_{3m \times 3k}$ represents the $3k$ columns corresponding to the set $P_K$. In contrast to the aforementioned procedure [4] where the FEM solver needs to run $3k$ times to generate a tensor matrix for each node, the above method generates each tensor matrix directly from the inverse of the global stiffness matrix $\tilde{K}_{3m \times 3m}$. When the set of the contacted nodes $K$ is replaced by another set $K_1$, we only need to renumber A, B, C, D in $\tilde{K}^{-1}_{3m \times 3m}$ and then to recalculate $A^{-1}$.

In addition to allowing the contacted nodes to be displaced in real time (30 frames/sec), the above approach also allows users to dynamically add the boundary conditions during the simulation. We may first fix $l$ ($l \geq 3$) nodes to generate the global inverse $\tilde{K}^{-1}_{3(n-l) \times 3(n-l)}$. During the simulation, additional free nodes $p_j \in P_R$ are fixed by the user, and we extend $A_{3k \times 3k}$ to $A_{3(k+1) \times 3(k+1)}$ to include three extra rows and columns for $p_j$. Equation (4) is then replaced by:

$$(F_1, \ldots, F_{3k}, F_j, F_{j+1}, F_{j+2})^T = A^{-1}_{3(k+1) \times 3(k+1)}(d_1, \ldots, d_{3k}, d_j, d_{j+1}, d_{j+2})^T$$

$$= A^{-1}_{3(k+1) \times 3k}(d_1, \ldots, d_{3k})^T \tag{6}$$

Therefore the analytic linear relationship between displacements of the contacted nodes and free nodes can be specified as:

$$(d_1 d_2 \ldots d_{3m})^T = \tilde{K}^{-1}_{3m \times 3(k+1)} A^{-1}_{3(k+1) \times 3k} (d_1 d_2 \ldots d_{3k})^T \tag{7}$$

### 2.2. Polynomial Interpolation to the Non-linear FE Model

From the last section, we know that the tensor matrix method is valid because the relationship between the force and displacement on each element is linear and this linearity propagates in FE methods. Suppose $S = \{s_1, s_2, \ldots, s_k\}$ is a set of the contacted nodes, and the displacement of a free node $p$ is denoted by $d_p$. Compared to the linear elastic model where $d_p$ is expressed exactly in linear terms of $\delta s_i$, hyper-elastic material models can only generate implicit functions $G_p(d_{\{q, q \in Q_p\}}, \delta s_1, \ldots, \delta s_k) = 0$, where $Q_p$ is the set of $p$'s neighbor nodes. Thus, at the pre-processing stage, an analytic solution for $d_p$ usually cannot be obtained. Instead, we seek an approximation of the $d_p$. Taking a polynomial basis $\{1, x, y, z, xy, yz, zx, x^2, y^2, z^2\}_S$, denoted by $\{1, X_{\{j, s_i\}}\}_{j=1, \ldots, 9; s_i \in S}$, we expand the function $d_p$:

$$d_p \cong a_0 + \sum a_{j,p}^{(s_i)} X_{j,s} \tag{8}$$

To calculate the coefficients $a_{j,p}^{(s_i)}$ for a better approximation, we assume the maximal displacement of the contacted points before the surface ruptures is $R(x_r, y_r, z_r)$. We partition the interval $[0, R]$ into $N$ ($N \geq 9k+1$) subintervals, and sample at each $\frac{iR}{N}$. We set these values as prescribed boundary displacements into the FE model, then use the FE solver to calculate the displacements $(\delta x_p, \delta y_p, \delta z_p)$ of each free node $p$. After generating $N$ sets of displacements for the free node $p$, we can solve the following equations for the coefficients $a_{i,p}$:

$$(\delta x_p^1 \delta x_p^2 \ldots \delta x_p^N)^T = (S_1 S_2 \ldots S_{3k})(a_{0,p} a_{1,p} \ldots a_{9k,p})^T \tag{9}$$

where $S_\nu$ is defined by $S_\nu = (1, X_{j,s_i}^\nu)_{j=1, \ldots, 9; s \in S}$ and $X_{j,s_i}^\nu$ is the value of $X_{j,s_i}$ at $\nu R/N$. Here we may simply invert $S$ to obtain $a_{i,p}$ if $N = 9k + 1$. Alternatively, (9) may be solved using the least squares method. Similar to the linear case in [4], both the generation of the sampled data sets and the solution of the coefficients for each $p$ occur at the preprocessing stage, while the real time simulation only involves multiplying the coefficient vector with the displacements of contacted nodes.

### 2.3. St. Venant's Principle and Affine Mapping

For a non-linear elastic model, the linear relation (5) is no longer valid. To meet the surgeon's requirement for interacting with the model in arbitrary regions, we employ St. Venant's Principle in elastic theory to obtain an approximate result. St. Venant's Principle [6] states that statically equivalent systems of forces produce the same stresses and strains within a body except in the immediate region where the loads are applied. It suggests that the stress change in local vicinity is virtually independent of other part of the body. Suppose $T = \{t_1, t_2, \ldots, t_k\}$ is another set of the contacted nodes close to the set $S$ discussed previously. We separate the vicinity $V$ containing both $S$ and $T$. Suppose also that $b_1$ and $b_2$ are two nodes on the boundary $\partial V$ of $V$, and $s = (x_s, y_s, z_s)$ and $t =$

$(x_t, y_t, z_t)$ are the centers of $S$ and $T$. According to the St. Venant's Principle, we can construct an affine mapping $\phi$ of $V$ such that the displacement and force feedback in $V$ could be adjusted according to different probe regions, but outside of $V$ they remain unchanged. To construct such a mapping, let $\phi$ satisfy $\phi(b_1) = b_1, \phi(b_2) = b_2, \phi(s) = t$, then this generates the following relation:

$$
\begin{pmatrix} x_{b_1} & x_{b_2} & x_t \\ y_{b_1} & y_{b_2} & y_t \\ z_{b_1} & z_{b_2} & z_t \end{pmatrix} = \begin{pmatrix} a_{11} & a_{12} & a_{13} \\ a_{21} & a_{22} & a_{23} \\ a_{31} & a_{32} & a_{33} \end{pmatrix} \begin{pmatrix} x_{b_1} & x_{b_2} & x_s \\ y_{b_1} & y_{b_2} & y_s \\ z_{b_1} & z_{b_2} & z_s \end{pmatrix}
$$

$$
= \phi \begin{pmatrix} x_{b_1} & x_{b_2} & x_s \\ y_{b_1} & y_{b_2} & y_s \\ z_{b_1} & z_{b_2} & z_s \end{pmatrix} \tag{10}
$$

where $\phi$ could be solved through the inversion of the $3 \times 3$ matrix on the right hand side of (10). Now $\phi$ has established a relation between the two coordinate systems, i.e, if $p$ is a free node, its coordinates are mapped to $q'(x', y', z')$ under $\phi$. Since each polynomial is associated with a node, we need to find the $q$ closest to $q'$ to use the pre-computed coefficients of $q$ for $p$.

To avoid searching the entire index table for $q$, we establish a local table for each node. The size of the table depends on the distance between $S$ and $T$. If the distance is increased, $V$ will be expanded until $\partial V$ meets $P_B$ and then $b_1$ and $b_2$ could be chosen from $P_B$. But this is the worst case for $\phi$ which is designed based on St. Venant's principle for a small vicinity $V$. The effect of such a mapping (i.e., $b_1, b_2 \in P_B$) is shown in Figure 1.

## 3. Results and Discussion

In the last section we specified two simulation approaches: the enhanced pre-computed FE method (EPFE) for the linear elastic model and the polynomial interpolation with an affine mapping (PIAM) for non-linear elastic models. Both EPFE and PIAM were tested by probing a brain model generated from an MRI volume. Compared to the pre-computed FE model (PEF) in [4] which involves approximately $3m \times 3k$ multiplications for each operation during the simulation, the proposed EPFE method requires $3m \times (3k + 3k) + k^3$ multiplications, where $m$ and $k$ denote the number of free nodes and the nodes in the contacted area respectively, and where $k^3$ operations are required to invert the small sub-matrix. If $k \ll m$ (e.g. $k=3$, $m=1,000$), the time to convert the sub-matrix is small relative to the overall computation time. Generally the three pre-computed FE methods PFE, EPFE and PIAM could be at least 10 times faster than the localized conjugate gradient method (LCG) described in [11]. The four methods were implemented using a tetrahedron of 2886 free nodes, generated with ICEM. Results are shown below.

|             | LCG       | PFE   | EPFE   | PIAM  |
|-------------|-----------|-------|--------|-------|
| Frames/sec  | 3         | 200+  | 50–100 | 30–40 |
| Flexibility | Very good | Poor  | Good   | Good  |

Our PIAM method was then compared to a gold standard FE approach. Experimental results show that the mean error of the displacements in the contacted nodes in the

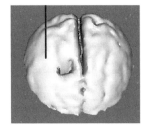 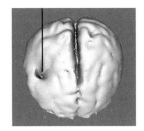 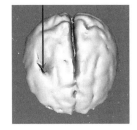

**Figure 1.** Results for a needle probing a site outside the pre-defined area using: (a) PFE (b) EPFE (c) PIAM.

preprocessing step and the nodes in the real-time simulation was reduced from 5.9 mm (using PFE) to 0.63 mm (PIAM). Although PFE computes deformations quickly, additional time is required to re-compute the linear system when the interaction occurs outside the pre-defined area. Otherwise, PFE may be inaccurate (Fig. ??a), reducing flexibility. EPFE is more flexible, and exhibits acceptable accuracy (Fig. 1b), even though more memory and computation time are required. PIAM addresses the same problems, but is applicable to non-linear elastic models.

## 4. Conclusions

In this paper we discussed the flexibility of pre-computed FE methods for linear and non-linear elastic models. In the linear case, we specified a direct link between the displacements of the contacted nodes and other free nodes. To realize real-time performance, the large global stiffness matrix must be inverted and saved at the preprocessing stage, as distinct from Cotin's work [4,5] where all the tensor must be computed in advance. It will double the computation time of [4] in real simulation situations, but it can provide the advantages of probing different regions and fixing more boundary nodes dynamically, which may give surgeons more flexibility in rehearsing their surgical plans. Efficiency may be further improved with parallel numerical approaches.

The polynomial approximation is appropriate for matching some hyper-elastic material models. Its time efficiency is similar to that in the precomputed tensor matrix model [4], but better than the tensor-mass model [5,12]. The affine mapping addressed earlier provides an approximate means of relocating the contacted nodes for non-linear models based on St. Venant's Principle. If the distance between $S$ and $T$ is small, the mapping $\phi$ can provide a proper displacement and haptic feedback for different perturbations within $V$, while the use of St. Venant's principle guarantees that points outside $V$ retain the same response as computed during the preprocessing stage. However if this distance is increased, the distribution of the displacements in $V$, especially in the contact area, will be reshaped due to the property of the affine mapping (see (c) in Figure 1).

## Acknowledgment

This work is funded by CIHR and ORDCF. The authors also thank Dr. Xinhua Yuan and Dr. Renata Smolíková-Wachowiak for valuable discussions.

# References

[1]  M.A. Audette, F. Ferrie, T.M. Peters, An Algorithmic Overview of Surface Registration Techniques for Medical Imaging, MED IMAGE ANAL, 5: 1-18, 1999.

[2]  J. Berkley, G. Turkiyyah, D. Berg, M. Ganter, S. Weghorst, Real-time finite element modeling for surgery simulation: an application to virtual suturing, IEEE T VIS COMPUT GR, 2004.

[3]  M. Bro-Nielsen, S. Cotin, Real-time volumetric deformable models for surgery simulation using finite element and condensation, Computer Graphics Forum, 15: 57-66, Eurographics'96, 1996.

[4]  S. Cotin, H. Delingette and N. Ayache, Real-time elastic deformations of soft tissues for surgery simulation, IEEE T VIS COMPUT GR, 5: 62-73, 1999.

[5]  S. Cotin, H. Delingette and N. Ayache, A Hybrid Elastic Model allowing Real-Time Cutting, Deformations and Force-Feedback for Surgery Training and Simulation. VISUAL COMPUT, 16: 437-452, 2000.

[6]  J. G. Eisley, Mechanics of elastic structures, Prentice-Hall, 1989.

[7]  K.V. Hansen, L. Brix, C.F. Pedersen, J.P. Haase, O.V. Larsen, Modelling of interaction between a spatula and a human brain, MED IMAGE ANAL, 8: 23-33, 2003.

[8]  W.E.Lorensen, H.E.Cline, Marching Cubes: A High Resolution 3D Surface Construction Algorithm, ACM Comp Graph. 21: 163-169, 1987.

[9]  P. Meseure and C. Chaillou, Deformable Body Simulation with Adaptative Subdivision and Cuttings, 361-370, In Proceedings of the WSCG'97.

[10]  Nastar and A. Ayache, Frequency-Based Nonrigid Motion Analysis: Application to Four Dimensional Medical Images, IEEE T PATTERN ANAL, 18: 1067-1079, 1996.

[11]  H.W. Nienhuys and A.F. van der Stappen, "Combining finite element deformation with cutting for surgery simulation", 19: 143-152, *Eurographics*, 2000.

[12]  Picinbono, H. Delingette, and N. Ayache, Non-linear and anisotropic elastic soft tissue models for medical simulation, In ICRA2001: IEEE International Conference Robotics and Automation, Seoul Korea, 2001.

*Medicine Meets Virtual Reality 13*
*James D. Westwood et al. (Eds.)*
*IOS Press, 2005*

# Cardiac MR Image Segmentation and Left Ventricle Surface Reconstruction Based on Level Set Method

Zeming ZHOU [a,1], Jianjie YOU [a], Pheng Ann HENG [b] and Deshen XIA [a]

[a] *Department of Computer, NUST, Nanjing, Jiangsu, China, 210094*
[b] *Department of Computer Science and Engineering, CUHK, Hong Kong*

**Abstract.** A two-stage segmentation algorithm is presented to solve the problems of inhomogeneity, weak edges and artifacts exhibited in the magnetic resonance imaging (MRI) images. First, the K-mean clustering algorithm is applied to classify the objects. Then, a speed function based on the clustering results is defined in order to search the rough boundary. Secondly, a speed function of the gradient intensity is constructed to locate the boundary accurately. Due to the lack of deformation information of the boundaries between MR slices, a deformable model is used to reconstruct the shape of the LV: a dynamic equation governing the surface deformation is given; from the slice data, external forces are constructed and elastic forces are provided with mean curvatures of the deformation surface. The level set method is applied to solve the dynamic equation for the LV shape. Experimental results demonstrate the effectiveness of the algorithm listed in the paper.

## 1. Introduction

MRI has been widely used in the diagnosis of the brain disease, and cardiac vessel, etc. However, some phenomena such as inhomogeneity, weak edges and artifacts are often found in the MRI images. This imposes difficulties on the segmentation algorithm based on the image gradient. To solve these problems, [1–3] propose to combine gradient and region information in order to obtain better segmentation results.

The algorithm used in our paper is as follows: the K-mean clustering algorithm and level set method are applied to segment the MRI images. After boundaries of cardiac muscle are achieved, the surface of the left ventricle can be reconstructed with a deformable model.

Section 2 proposes the segmentation and surface reconstruction algorithm of the left ventricle. Section 3 shows the experiment results. The final section is the conclusion.

---

[1]The work described in this paper is supported by a grant from the Research Grants Council of the Hong Kong Special Administrative Region,Chian (Project No. CUHK4180/01E).

## 2. MR image segmentation and surface reconstruction of the left ventricle

K-mean clustering is a statistical region-based image segmentation method. It is suitable for biomedical image segmentation [4] since the number of clusters is known according to the prior anatomy knowledge. For cardiac MRI images, we can assume an existence of three populations: the blood (bright); the muscles (gray); the air-filled lungs (dark gray). From the histogram of the cardiac MRI image, the gray values corresponding to the maximum points are chosen as the initial clustering centers. After the K-mean clustering is applied, we perform a morphological processing for the classified images to smooth edges and to erode the inhomogeneous regions inside the left ventricle. Let the pixel $I_i$ in the ROI belong to class $C_i$, its speed function is defined as $F = F_r V_0 + \varepsilon K$;

$$F_r = \begin{cases} 1, & \text{if } I_i \in C_i \\ -1, & \text{else} \end{cases}$$

In the first stage, we define the evolving equation as:

$$\phi_t = (-F_r V_0 + \varepsilon K)\|\nabla\phi\| \tag{1}$$

To solve equation (1), we can achieve a rough border of the endocardium by the curve evolving according to the clustering result.

In order to attract the curve which lies in the rough border to the true boundary, we construct a gradient vector flow (GVF) [5]: $V_G = (u(x, y), v(x, y))$. Compared with the traditional gradient force, it has a larger capture range of boundary and can overcome problems caused by weak edges effectively. The evolving equation of the second stage is:

$$\phi_t = -V_G \bullet \vec{N} \, \|\nabla\phi\| \tag{2}$$

where $\vec{N}$ is the normal vector of the evolving curve. Take the rough border of ROI as the initial zero-level curve and solve the level set equation (2) for the true boundary.

After the boundaries of the left ventricle in all slices are segmented, its surface can be reconstructed with the deformable model. Let $r(u, v, t)$ be the deforming surface, and its kinetic equation can be written as:

$$\frac{\partial\phi}{\partial t} + (V - \varepsilon K)\|\nabla\phi\| = 0 \tag{3}$$

where $\phi(r, t) = 0$, $V$ is the projection of exterior force along the unit normal vector, $K$ is the mean curvature of the surface. It can be used with the narrow band level set method [6].

We apply the seed filling algorithm to tag the points that lie inside or outside the boundaries. Beginning from the top image slice, search the boundary point in the next slice that is nearest to the above boundary point. Then we perform a linear interpolation between the two points in order to get the boundary points of the left ventricle along the image slices. We define the external force acting on the deforming surface at point P as follows:

$$V = \begin{cases} V_1; & P \in \Omega \\ V_1 - V_2; & P \in \partial\Omega \\ -V_2; & P \notin \overline{\Omega} \end{cases}$$

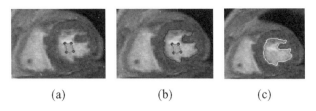

(a)                        (b)                        (c)

**Figure 1.** MR image segmentation with weak edges and local gradient maximum region (a) initial contour. (b) rough segmentation result. (c) more accurate segmentation result.

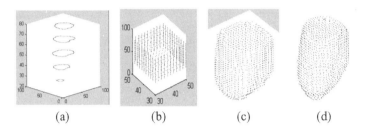

(a)               (b)               (c)               (d)

**Figure 2.** The surface reconstruction of the left ventricle. (a) the boundaries of the left ventricle in 5 slices. (b) initial deforming surface. (c) 20 steps. (d) 40 steps.

where $\Omega$ is the region made up of inner points and $\partial \Omega$ is the boundary of $\Omega$, $\bar{\Omega}$ is the union set of $\Omega$ and $\partial \Omega$.

## 3. Experimental results and analysis

First, we take Fig. 1 as an example. After the K-mean clustering algorithm is applied to classify objects in the images, the morphological operation is used to smooth the classified image. We define the speed function according to equation (1), (2); let $V_0 = 1$; $\varepsilon = 0.2$; $h = 1$; $\Delta t = 0.1$; the initial zero level curve, the rough boundary, and the segmentation result are shown in Fig. 1(a), Fig. 1(b) and Fig. 1(c).

Next we reconstruct the inner surface of the left ventricle based on the slices in the short axis direction. We have five slices and the distance between slices is thirteen pixels (Fig. 2 (a)). Set $V_1 = 1$; $V_2 = 1$; $\varepsilon = 0.2$, $h = 2$; $t = 0.1$. As we can see from Fig. 2, the surface is continuously deforming in the process of iteration. The initial cubic surface is shown in Fig. 2 (b); it deforms under the pressure of the external force and elastic force. Fig. 2 (c) is the result after 20 iterative steps, and Fig. 2 (d) is the final reconstruction result.

## 4. Conclusion

In this paper, we propose an algorithm to segment MRI images and reconstruct the surface of the left ventricle. Further research could include incorporating the shape constraint to the level set framework for better segmentation of cardiac MRI images and taking boundary points in images along the long axis direction as the constraint conditions for reconstruction of the surface.

# References

[1]  J. Deng, H. T. Tsui. A fast level set method for segmentation of low contrast noisy biomedical images. Pattern Recognition Letters. 2002,23: 161~169.
[2]  J. S. Suri, Leaking prevention in fast level sets using fuzzy models: An application in MR brain in Proc. Int. Conf. Inform. Technol. Biomedicine, Nov.2000: 220~226.
[3]  N. Paragios and R. Detiche. Coupled geodesic active regions for image segmentation: A level set approach. In Proceeding of 6th Eur. Conf. on Computer Vision,Dublin,2000:224~240.
[4]  M. Jolly, Combining edge, region, and shape information to segment the left ventricle in cardiac MR images. Medical Image Computeing and Computer-Asisted Intervention, Utrecht, The Netherlands: Springer-Verlag, 2001. 482-490.
[5]  C. Xu, J. L. Prince. Snakes, shapes and gradient vector flow. IEEE Trans on Imaging Processing. 1998,7(3):359~369.
[6]  D. Adalsteinsson, J. A. Sethian, A fast level set method for propagating interfaces. Journal of Computational Physics,1995,118(2):269~277.

*Medicine Meets Virtual Reality 13*
*James D. Westwood et al. (Eds.)*
*IOS Press, 2005*

633

# Author Index